T0380995

Essentials of Pediatric Anesthesiology

Essentials of Pediatric Anesthesiology

Edited by

Alan David Kaye, M.D., Ph.D.
Chairman and Director of Pain Services, Department of Anesthesiology, and Professor of Pharmacology, Louisiana State University School of Medicine, New Orleans, Louisiana, USA

Charles James Fox, M.D.
Professor and Chair, Department of Anesthesiology, Louisiana State University School of Medicine, Shreveport, Louisiana, USA

James H. Diaz, M.D., M.P.H., Dr.P.H., D.A.B.A., F.A.A.P.
Professor of Anesthesiology, Professor of Public Health and Preventive Medicine, and Director of Environmental and Occupational Health Sciences, Louisiana State University Health Sciences Center, New Orleans, Louisiana, USA

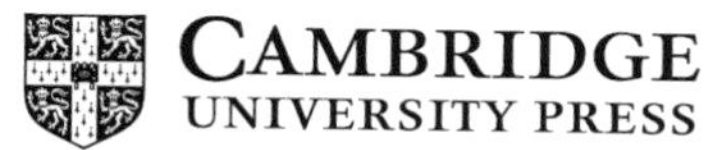

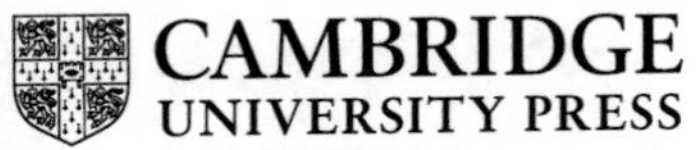

Shaftesbury Road, Cambridge CB2 8EA, United Kingdom

One Liberty Plaza, 20th Floor, New York, NY 10006, USA

477 Williamstown Road, Port Melbourne, VIC 3207, Australia

314–321, 3rd Floor, Plot 3, Splendor Forum, Jasola District Centre, New Delhi – 110025, India

103 Penang Road, #05–06/07, Visioncrest Commercial, Singapore 238467

Cambridge University Press is part of Cambridge University Press & Assessment, a department of the University of Cambridge.

We share the University's mission to contribute to society through the pursuit of education, learning and research at the highest international levels of excellence.

www.cambridge.org
Information on this title: www.cambridge.org/9781107698680

© Cambridge University Press & Assessment 2015

This publication is in copyright. Subject to statutory exception and to the provisions of relevant collective licensing agreements, no reproduction of any part may take place without the written permission of Cambridge University Press & Assessment.

First published 2015

A catalogue record for this publication is available from the British Library

Library of Congress Cataloging-in-Publication data
Essentials of pediatric anesthesiology / edited by Alan David Kaye, Charles James Fox, James H. Diaz.
p. ; cm.
Includes bibliographical references and index.
ISBN 978-1-107-69868-0 (Paperback)
I. Kaye, Alan David, editor. II. Fox, Charles J., III (Charles James), 1961– editor. III. Diaz, James H., editor. [DNLM: 1. Anesthesia. 2. Child. 3. Infant. WO 440]
RD139
617.906083–dc23 2014006200

ISBN 978-1-107-69868-0 Paperback

Additional resources for this publication at www.cambridge.org/9781107698680

Cambridge University Press & Assessment has no responsibility for the persistence or accuracy of URLs for external or third-party internet websites referred to in this publication and does not guarantee that any content on such websites is, or will remain, accurate or appropriate.

Every effort has been made in preparing this book to provide accurate and up-to-date information which is in accord with accepted standards and practice at the time of publication. Although case histories are drawn from actual cases, every effort has been made to disguise the identities of the individuals involved. Nevertheless, the authors, editors and publishers can make no warranties that the information contained herein is totally free from error, not least because clinical standards are constantly changing through research and regulation. The authors, editors and publishers therefore disclaim all liability for direct or consequential damages resulting from the use of material contained in this book. Readers are strongly advised to pay careful attention to information provided by the manufacturer of any drugs or equipment that they plan to use.

To my wife Dr. Kim Kaye and my children, Aaron and Rachel Kaye, for all their love and kindness.

To my mother Florence Feldman and my father Joel Kaye, the former Joseph Krakower, for providing me with thousands of enlightening lessons in life and for helping to shape me into the man I am today.

To my step parents the late Gideon Feldman and Andrea Bennett-Kaye, who helped raise me, providing love, support, and wisdom over the last 30-plus years.

To my brother Dr. Adam Kaye and my sister Sheree Kaye Garcia for always loving and supporting me.

To my lifelong friends, Barry Lustig, Brian Finerman, Jamie Johnson, Walter Eichinger, the late Steve Corty, Joe Walsh, Troy Cotter, and Torsten Andresen, I am grateful for each of you and the many lessons you taught me in life, especially when things did not go my way and when my future was uncertain.

Alan David Kaye, M.D., Ph.D.

To my parents, Charles James (Jimmy) Fox Jr. and Sandra Marie Blanchard Fox, for their hard work and dedication to our family; you have created a foundation on which generations will build.

Charles James Fox, M.D.

To Robert H. (Rob) Friesen, M.D., of the Denver Children's Hospital: mentor, colleague, friend; epitome of the clinician-researcher.

James H. Diaz, M.D., M.P.H., Dr.P.H., F.A.C.M.T.

Contents

Contributors

Naila A. Ahmad, M.D.
Assistant Professor, Congenital Cardiac Anesthesia Co-ordinator, Department of Anesthesiology and Critical Care Medicine, Saint Louis University School of Medicine, MO, USA

Dua M. Anderson, M.D., M.S.
Assistant Clinical Professor, Department of Anesthesiology and Pain Medicine, University of California Davis Medical Center, Sacramento, CA, USA

Jennifer Aunspaugh, M.D.
Assistant Professor of Anesthesiology, Arkansas Children's Hospital, Little Rock, AR, USA

Sabrina T. Bent, M.D., M.S.
Clinical Associate Professor of Anesthesiology and Pediatrics, Department of Anesthesiology, Tulane University School of Medicine, New Orleans, LA, USA

Adam Broussard, M.D.
Resident, Louisiana State University Health Sciences Center, New Orleans, LA, USA

Staci Cameron, M.D.
Assistant Professor, Division of Pediatric Anesthesia, University of Texas, Health Science Center Houston, TX, USA

Rahul Dasgupta, M.D.
Assistant Professor of Anesthesiology, Pediatric Cardiac Anesthesia Team, Arkansas Children's Hospital, University of Arkansas for Medical Sciences, Little Rock, AR, USA

Ravinder Devgun, D.O.
University at Buffalo Pediatric Anesthesiology Fellow, Buffalo, NY, USA.

Ofer N. Eytan, M.D.
Desert Eye Specialists Ltd., Peoria, AZ, USA

Sean H. Flack, M.B.Ch.B., F.C.A.
Associate Professor, Anesthesiology and Pain Medicine, University of Washington and Seattle Children's Hospital, Seattle, WA

Terry G. Fletcher, M.D., Ph.D.
Co-Director, Burn Anesthesia, Arkansas Children's Hospital Burn Center, Assistant Professor of Anesthesiology, UAMS COM Division of Pediatric Anesthesiology and Pain Medicine Little Rock, AR, USA

Charles James Fox, M.D.
Department of Anesthesiology, Louisiana State University Health Sciences Center, Shreveport, LA, USA

Mary Elise Fox, B.S.
Louisiana State University Health Sciences Center, New Orleans, LA, USA

Scott Friedman, M.D.
Department of Anesthesiology, Tulane University School of Medicine, New Orleans, LA, USA

Louise K. Furukawa, M.D., F.A.A.P.
Clinical Associate Professor, Stanford University School of Medicine, Menlo Park, CA, USA

Sonja Gennuso, M.D.
Associate Professor, Department of Anesthesiology, Louisiana State University Health Sciences Center and Clinical Attending Staff, Childrens Hospital, New Orleans, LA, USA

Stanley M. Hall, M.D., Ph.D.
Clinical Chief Anesthesiologist, Children's Hospital New Orleans; Clinical Professor of Nursing, Louisiana State University Health Sciences Center, New Orleans, LA, USA

Hani Hanna, M.D.
Assistant Professor of Anesthesiology, Arkansas Children's Hospital, University of Arkansas for Medical Sciences, Little Rock, AR, USA

Jacob Hummel, M.D.
Department of Anesthesiology, Tulane University School of Medicine, New Orleans, LA, USA

James E. Hunt, M.D.
Co-Director, Burn Anesthesia, Arkansas Children's Hospital Burn Center; Assistant Professor of Anesthesiology, UAMS COM Division of Pediatric Anesthesiology and Pain Medicine, Little Rock, AR, USA

Ranu Jain, M.D.
Assistant Professor, Division of Pediatric Anesthesia, University of Texas, Health Science Center Houston, TX, USA

Joe R. Jansen, M.D.
Assistant Professor of Anesthesiology, UAMS COM Division of Pediatric Anesthesiology and Pain Medicine, Arkansas Children's Hospital Burn Center, Little Rock, AR, USA

Deepa Kattail, M.D.
Assistant Professor, Anesthesiology and Critical Care Medicine, Division of Pediatric Anesthesiology, Johns Hopkins University, Baltimore, MD, USA

Alan David Kaye, M.D., Ph.D.
Professor and Chairman, Department of Anesthesiology, Louisiana State University Health Sciences Center; Professor, Departments of Anesthesiology and Pharmacology, Tulane School of Medicine, New Orleans, LA, USA

David J. Krodel, M.D.
Instructor in Anesthesiology, Northwestern University Feinberg School of Medicine Anesthesiologist, Ann & Robert H. Lurie Children's Hospital of Chicago, Chicago, IL, USA

Gregory J. Latham, M.D.
Department of Anesthesiology and Pain Medicine, Seattle Children's Hospital, University of Washington School of Medicine, Seattle, WA, USA

Sungeun Lee, M.D.
Assistant Clinical Professor, University of California, Davis, Sacramento, CA, USA

Michael G. Levitzky, Ph.D.
Professor of Physiology and Anesthesiology, Louisiana State University Health Sciences Center, New Orleans, LA, USA

Alexander Y. Lin, M.D.
Assistant Professor, Section Chief, Pediatric Plastic Surgery, Division of Plastic Surgery, Department of Surgery, Saint Louis University School of Medicine, MO, USA

Carl Lo, M.D.
Pediatric Anesthesiology Clinical Fellow, Johns Hopkins University, Baltimore, MD, USA

Hoa N. Luu, M.D.
Assistant Professor of Anesthesiology, Louisiana State University Health Sciences Center, Shreveport, LA, USA

Camila Lyon, M.D.
Pediatric Anesthesiology Clinical Fellow, Johns Hopkins University, Baltimore, MD, USA

Kelly A. Machovec, M.D., M.P.H.
Assistant Professor of Anesthesiology, Duke University School of Medicine, Durham, NC, USA

Lizabeth D. Martin, M.D.
Acting Assistant Professor, Anesthesiology and Pain Medicine University of Washington and Seattle Children's Hospital, Seattle, WA, USA

Maria Matuszczak, M.D.
Professor, Division Chief of Pediatric Anesthesia, University of Texas, Health Science Center Houston, TX, USA

Patrick S. McCarty, M.D.
Clinical Assistant Professor of Anesthesiology and Pediatrics, Department of Anesthesiology, Tulane University School of Medicine, New Orleans, LA, USA

Brenda C. McClain, M.D.
Medical Director, Section of Pediatric Anesthesia, Department of Anesthesiology and Critical Care Medicine, Saint Louis University School of Medicine, Missouri, MO, USA

J. Grant McFadyen, M.B.Ch.B., F.R.C.A.
Clinical Assistant Professor, Anesthesiology and Pain Medicine, Stanford University School of Medicine, Stanford, CA, USA

Helen Nazareth, M.D., Ph.D.
University at Buffalo Pediatric Anesthesiology Fellow

Dolores B. Njoku, M.D.
Associate Professor, ACCM, Pediatrics and Pathology, Director, The Fellowship in Pediatric Anesthesiolog, Lead Investigator, Drug-Induced, Immune-mediated Liver Injury, Johns Hopkins University, Baltimore, MD, USA

Christina M. Pabelick, M.D.
Departments of Anesthesiology, Physiology, and Biomedical Engineering, Mayo Clinic, Rochester, MN, USA

Shannon M. Peters, M.D.
Valley Anesthesiology and Pain Consultants, Phoenix, AZ, USA

Amit Prabhakar, M.D.
Department of Anesthesiology, LSU School of Medicine, New Orleans, LA, USA

Michael Richards, B.M., F.R.C.A.
Senior Resident, Department of Anesthesiology and Pain Medicine, Seattle Children's Hospital, University of Washington School of Medicine, Seattle, WA, USA

Kasia Rubin, M.D.
University Hospitals Case Medical Center, Cleveland, OH, USA

Joel A. Saltzman, M.D.
Medical Director, Anesthesiology, Le Bonheur Children's Hospital, Memphis, TN, USA

Lisgelia Santana, M.D.
Director of Pediatric Pain Management, Pediatric Anesthesiologist, Nemours Children's Hospital, Orlando, FL, USA

Gabriel Sarah, M.D.
Fellow, Pediatric Anesthesiology, University of Miami Miller School of Medicine, Miami, FL, USA

Katherine Stammen, M.D.
Louisiana State University Health Sciences Center, Shreveport, LA, USA

John Stork, M.D.
University Hospitals Case Medical Center, Cleveland, OH, USA

Kim M. Strupp, M.D.
Assistant Professor of Anesthesiology, Children's Hospital Colorado, University of Colorado, Aurora, CO, USA

Lalitha V. Sundararaman, M.D.
Assistant Professor of Clinical Anesthesia, Brigham and Women's Hospital, Harvard Medical School, Boston, MA, USA

Rosalie F. Tassone, M.D., M.P.H.
Associate Professor of Clinical Anesthesiology, University of Illinois at Chicago, Chicago, IL, USA

Douglas R. Thompson, M.D.
Department of Anesthesiology and Pain Medicine, Seattle Children's Hospital, University of Washington School of Medicine, Seattle, WA, USA

Nicole C. P. Thompson, M.D.
Assistant Professor, Department of Anesthesiology, University of Illinois College of Medicine, Chicago, IL, USA

Paul A. Tripi, M.D., F.A.A.P.
Associate Professor of Anesthesiology and Pediatrics, Chief, Division of Pediatric Anesthesiology, Rainbow Babies and Children's Hospital, University Hospitals Case Medical Center, OH, USA

Jacqueline L. Tutiven, M.D.
Assistant Professor of Clinical Anesthesiology, Director, Pediatric Anesthesia Fellowship Program,University of Miami Miller School of Medicine, Miami, FL, USA

Navyugjit Virk, M.D.
University at Buffalo Obstetric Anesthesiology Fellow, Buffalo, NY, USA

Stacey Watt, M.D.
Associate Professor, Pediatric Anesthesiology Fellowship Program Director, University at Buffalo Department of Anesthesiology, Buffalo, NY, USA

B. Craig Weldon, M.D.
Professor of Anesthesiology and Child Health, Chief, Division of Pediatric Anesthesia, University of Missouri School of Medicine, Columbia, MO, USA

Maria Zestus, M.D.
Department of Anesthesiology, Wayne State University School of Medicine, Detroit, MI, USA

Preface

My first experiences with pediatric anesthesia were as a four-year-old inpatient undergoing a tonsillectomy. I recall the following events very clearly – a premedication shot, likely morphine and atropine or scopolamine; the smell of ether; postoperative vomiting; and going home from the hospital the next day with a sore throat. Although intramuscular premedication injections and ether anesthesia have now been replaced by gentler selections for premediation and nonflammable halogenated agents for general anesthesia, nausea and vomiting still remain unwelcomed postoperative events for pediatric patients and anesthesiologists.

Years later, I joined the staff of that same hospital as a pediatric anesthesiologist and intensivist in a modern, new facility for multispecialty group practice. I had frequent access to my medical records over the years including the original anesthesia record for my tonsillectomy, which included the names of the anesthesiologist and surgeon, the anesthetic agents administered, and a few heart rate measurements. The anesthetic was conducted under mask ether without an endotracheal tube, precordial stethoscope, or an intravenous line for fluid therapy. No blood pressures and no temperatures were recorded. The equipment for transcutaneous oxygen saturation and end tidal carbon dioxide measurements had not been invented yet.

When I served as a pediatric anesthesiology fellow, the Jackson Rees modification of the Mapleson F circuit was used for endotracheal halothane in oxygen and nitrous oxide anesthesia during spontaneous assisted ventilation and the Bain modification of the Mapleson D circuit was used for controlled mechanical ventilation. Fentanyl had recently been introduced as an intravenous anesthetic adjunct, and pediatric surgeons infiltrated surgical wounds prior to closing with local anesthetics. There was only one textbook of pediatric anesthesia, Smith's *Anesthesia for Infants and Children*, which was updated in subsequent editions to include the anesthetic management of new procedures in cardiac surgery and neonatal surgery.[1] I had to supplement my pediatric anesthesia library with classic British texts, now out of print, including *Paediatric Anaesthesia* by Drs. G. Jackson Rees and Cecil T. Gray, and *Neonatal Anaesthesia and Perioperative Care* by Drs. David Hatch and Edward Sumner.[2,3] Later, I was invited to serve a summer fellowship with Drs. Hatch and Sumner at the Hospital for Sick Children on Great Ormond Street in London, where I learned how to incorporate regional blocks into general anesthetics, especially caudal injections, and to conduct cyclopropane inductions in the sickest neonates with congenital heart disease.

Although the modern operating room has eliminated the use of flammable anesthetics, such as ether and cyclopropane, caudal and lumbar epidural-administered local anesthetics and opioids are in increasingly frequent use today and provide excellent postoperative pain relief in children. Today, pediatric anesthesia techniques, anesthesia breathing systems, and cardiopulmonary function monitors have improved dramatically and continue to evolve rapidly. Endotracheal or laryngeal mask-administered anesthesia, the use of multiple intravenous and local anesthetic agents to control hemodynamics and provide perioperative analgesia, and the continuous monitoring of oxygen saturation, end tidal carbon dioxide, inspired anesthetic fraction, and body temperature are now regarded as national standards for the safe anesthesia care of infants and children. Newly installed electronic anesthetic records can capture all of the patient's physiologic measurements, and the anesthesiologist simply indicates the agents used and tubes inserted with a keystroke, completely eliminating the old paper anesthetic record. Pediatric anesthesiology is now its own multispecialty practice that includes fetal and neonatal anesthesia, anesthesia for complex congenital heart and craniofacial defects, pediatric organ transplant anesthesia, and many other specialized indications and techniques.

Although the United States (US) may have lagged behind the British and Canadians in earlier advancements in pediatric anesthesia equipment and techniques, US-trained pediatric anesthesiologists are at the forefront of the very latest advances today. *Essentials of Pediatric Anesthesiology* will allow anesthesiologists to prepare rapidly for the most complex cases, such as *in utero* fetal surgery, abdominal organ transplants, or separation of conjoined twins. Concise chapters are illustrated with diagrams and images and feature clear tables to organize information for quick recall. Single-answer pretest and post-test questions accompany each chapter to identify pre-existing knowledge and confirm newly acquired knowledge respectively.

With more approved anesthesiology residency programs and pediatric anesthesiology fellowship programs and a new American Board of Anesthesiology (ABA)-administered subspecialty board certification examination in pediatric anesthesiology, a new multi-authored textbook in pediatric anesthesiology is needed now. *Essentials of Pediatric Anesthesiology* is that text. *Essentials of Pediatric Anesthesiology* will effectively supplement the current multivolume treatises in the field and appeal to a broad audience of residents, fellows, attending anesthesiologists, pediatric intensivists, and other practitioners caring for pediatric patients in the perioperative period, especially those seeking rapid reviews before taking oral board and subspecialty board certification examinations. *Essentials of Pediatric Anesthesiology* will definitely be a valuable addition to any perioperative physician's library.

James H. Diaz, M.D., M.P.H., Dr.P.H., D.A.B.A., F.A.A.P.

Professor of Anesthesiology and Public Health
Louisiana State University
Schools of Medicine and Public Health
New Orleans, Louisiana

References

1. RM Smith. *Anesthesia for Infants and Children*. St. Louis, Missouri: Mosby; 1959.
2. G Jackson Rees, T Cecil Gray. *Paediatric Anaesthesia*. London: William Clowes (Beccles) Limited; 1981.
3. DJ Hatch, E Sumner. *Neonatal Anaesthesia and Perioperative Care*. London: Edward Arnold Publishers Limited; 1981.

Chapter 1

Anatomy

Maria Zestos

Introduction

The anatomical differences between the infant and the adult are numerous and can greatly affect the care of the infant and, most notably, the neonate. This chapter presents an overview of anatomical differences between the neonate and the adult, including general development, with a focus on the airway, body habitus, thermoregulation, and vascular cannulation.

General development

Airway

Respiratory development begins by the fourth week of gestation with a primitive pharynx, larynx, trachea, and bronchial bud. The trachea and the esophagus develop from the foregut, and then separate during division of the endoderm. If this separation fails, a tracheoesophageal fistula (TEF) lesion will result. With successive branching of the airways, the respiratory tree is formed. By 24 weeks gestation, respiratory bronchioles and primitive alveoli are present and surfactant begins to be produced. Adequate air exchange requires surfactants to maintain alveolar expansion and adequate lung exchange.[1] Even though surfactants can be administered after delivery, adequate air exchange for survival limits the viability of premature infants delivered before 23 weeks gestation. The alveoli continue to increase in number and size until 8 years of age, after which alveoli increase only in size.

Many morphological differences exist between the neonatal airway and the adult airway. In neonates, the epiglottis and tongue are relatively large. Other anatomical differences in the pediatric airway include large head, short neck, narrow nares, redundant soft tissues, and a high glottis. All these features can make mask ventilation and direct laryngoscopy a challenge.

Neonates are obligate nasal breathers, with about 22% of term infants being unable to breathe if the nares are occluded. Most infants gain the ability to compensate for nares occlusion with oral breathing by 5 months of age. The relatively large tongue of the neonate can result in upper airway obstruction, as can be seen in certain syndromes such as Beckwith–Wiedemann and Down syndrome. These anatomical differences along with the high oxygen consumption can make hypoxia more common and also more severe.

The anatomy of the airway changes with age. The glottis functions as an occlusive valve to protect the lower airway from the alimentary tract. The glottis is at the level of C3 in babies, moving caudad to the level of C4–5 in adults. The shape of the larynx also changes with age. Infants have a cricoid cartilage that is narrower than that of an adult. This creates a vocal cord aperture that is funnel shaped. As the child grows, the diameter of the cricoid cartilage also increases resulting in a cylindrical shape of the larynx by the age of 8 years. At the level of the cricoid, the cartilage forms a complete ring to prevent compression. The larynx at the subglottis is the narrowest portion of the respiratory system for all ages.

Delayed development in the neuromuscular tone of the supraglottic muscles can result in laryngomalacia with inward collapse of supraglottic structures, namely, the aryepiglottic folds or the anterior collapse of the arytenoid cartilages. As the neuromuscular tone improves during the first two years of life, symptoms also improve and often disappear completely.[2]

Body habitus

The degree of difference and variation between neonates and adults is striking. When compared to an adult, a newborn infant is 1/21 adult size in weight, 1/9 adult size in body surface area, and 1/3 adult size

Essentials of Pediatric Anesthesiology, ed. Alan David Kaye, Charles James Fox and James H. Diaz. Published by Cambridge University Press. © Cambridge University Press 2015.

in length. It is thus essential to choose carefully the variable used to compare patients of different sizes.[3] For medication administration, the actual body weight is most commonly used. Drug dosing can also be based on ideal body weight or lean body mass. Most obese patients have increased total body weight as well as lean body mass. For these patients, ideal body weight has been shown to be the best measurement for dose calculation, but this is not often used in clinical practice. Calculations for fluids and doses of medications can be based on body surface area (BSA), which requires both a height and a weight measurement. The BSA can be estimated by Mosteller's calculation:[4]

$$\text{BSA (m}^2) = [\text{ht (cm)} \times \text{wt (kg)}/3600]^{1/2}$$

Body fluid compartment composition also varies with age, with an abrupt fall in total body water (TBW) and extracellular fluid levels (ECF) over the first year of life, reaching adult levels by 2 years of age.[5]

Water volume and blood composition

Total body water (TBW) varies inversely with age. While the newborn has 85% TBW, this percentage steadily decreases to the adult level of 65% TBW by 3 years of age. Males also have a higher TBW compared to females. The body's water can be divided into intracellular fluid (ICF), which contains 67% of the water distribution and extracellular fluid (ECF), which contains 33% of the water distribution. Diffusion across the cell membrane results in fluid exchange between the ECF and the ICF. Fluid will move from an area of low osmolality to an area of high osmolality. The body regulates ECF volume by varying renal sodium excretion and controls renal osmolality by varying water intake and excretion.

Normal fluid management in the perioperative period includes administration of maintenance, preoperative deficit and replacement of ongoing losses. Maintenance requirements consist of replacing insensible losses through the skin and lungs, and urinary volume replacement.[6] Fluid requirements in infants are greater than adults because of greater surface-to-weight ratio and higher metabolic rate as well as reduced renal concentrating ability. In the newborn, day 1 maintenance fluids are decreased because of immature renal function that slowly improves during the first few days of life. For day 1 of life, $D_{10}W$ without added salt is administered at a rate of 80 ml/kg/day. By day 2 of life, sodium excretion from the kidney has begun and urine output improves, resulting in a change of maintenance fluids to include sodium replacement (2–3 mEq/dl NaCl). This is usually given in the form of $D_{10}W$ with 0.2 NS at a rate of 100 ml/kg/day. By day three of life, potassium replacement (1–2 mEq/dl KCl) is begun and total fluids are increased at a rate of 120 ml/kg/day. Outside of the neonatal period, the most commonly used formula for calculating hourly maintenance fluid perioperatively consists of the following calculation:[7]

"4–2–1 rule" for hourly maintenance fluid rate:
4 ml/kg/hr for the first 1–10 kg body weight plus
2 ml/kg/hr for each kg from 11–20 kg plus
1 ml/kg/hr for every kg $>$ 20 kg

Maintenance fluids routinely provide dextrose, usually as 5% dextrose, and sodium supplementation as 0.2–0.45 NS. However, in the operating room routine dextrose administration is no longer advised in healthy children. Moreover, isotonic fluids have been shown to be significantly safer than hypotonic fluids for protection against postoperative hyponatremia in children.[8] Thus perioperative maintenance fluids are usually replaced with a balanced salt solution such as Ringer's lactate or 0.9% normal saline solution, except in patients at risk for hypoglycemia, such as neonates, children receiving hyperalimentation, and children with endocrinopathies.

Fluid deficits must also be replaced, and may be significant in the presence of prolonged fasting, fever, vomiting, or diarrhea. Preoperative fasting should be minimized to avoid significant dehydration or hypoglycemia in infants. Specific instructions should be given for infants to be encouraged to ingest clear fluids up until two hours before elective surgery.

Third-space losses from surgical trauma, burns or infection result in isotonic fluid transfer from the ECF to the interstitial compartment with resultant plasma volume depletion. These losses can be as high as 10 ml/kg/hr for major intra-abdominal surgery and even 50 ml/kg/hr for a premature infant undergoing surgery for necrotizing enterocolitis. These losses can be replaced with Ringer's lactate solution. Administration of fluid should be titrated to the clinical response, with maintenance of appropriate hemodynamic variables and a minimum urine output of 0.5–1 ml/kg/hr.

In addition to fluid replacement, blood loss needs to be closely monitored with prompt replacement as needed. Blood loss is initially replaced with a crystalloid such as lactated Ringer's as 3 ml per 1 ml

Table 1.1: Estimated blood volume

	Premature	Newborn	1 year	3 years	9 years	Adult
EBV (ml/kg)	100	90	80	75	70	65

blood lost to an acceptable minimal hematocrit, after which packed red cells should be administered. Factors that determine the maximum allowable blood loss (MABL) include the patient's estimated blood volume (EBV), body weight and starting hematocrit (HCT). Estimated blood volume decreases with age (see Table 1.1). The MABL can be calculated with the following formula:

$$MABL = EBV \times [HCT_{start} - HCT_{low}]/HCT_{start}$$

Thermoregulation

Under normal conditions, body temperature is one of the most accurately maintained physiologic parameters. The outer skin serves as a shell with the muscle compartment acting as a buffer. Thermoregulatory mechanisms including vasoconstriction can spare body heat and decrease heat loss up to 50%. In adults, shivering is a main component of this process. In infants and neonates, brown fat provides nonshivering thermogenesis. Brown fat can represent 2–6% of neonatal body weight and is found in the scapulae, axillae, mediastinum, adrenal glands, and the kidneys. Nonshivering thermogenesis from brown fat is the main thermoregulatory response to cold stress in the neonate and can double metabolic heat production during cold exposures.[9] This ability persists up to two years of age.

General anesthesia disrupts thermoregulation by producing vasodilation by two mechanisms. It reduces the vasoconstriction threshold below core temperature, inhibiting centrally mediated thermoregulatory constriction, and also causes direct peripheral vasodilation.[10] This results in internal redistribution of body heat as the core temperature decreases with a proportional increase in peripheral tissue temperature. The body heat content remains constant. During the first few hours of anesthesia, redistribution contributes 65% of the total decrease in core temperature.[11]

In addition to redistribution of body heat during anesthesia, total body heat is lost through four mechanisms: radiation, conduction, convection, and evaporation. Heat transfer is minimal if the temperature of the body surface and the environment are similar but increase proportionally as the temperature difference increases.[9] **Radiation** is the transfer of heat from one surface to another without direct contact and results in 39% of the heat loss in a neonate. Radiation does not depend at all on the temperature of the intervening air. Radiant heat loss can be reduced by warming the room and by covering the patient. Because of the greater surface area to body mass ratio, infants have a greater radiative heat loss than adults. It is thus essential to increase the temperature of the operating room to help stabilize the temperature of small infants and especially neonates.[12] **Conduction** is the direct transfer of heat from the contact of one object to a second object, and accounts for about 3% of neonatal heat loss. Conductive losses can be avoided by warming the IV fluids and the table and by insulating the patient. Infants have less subcutaneous fat and a greater surface area to body ratio resulting in larger conductive heat losses than adults. **Evaporation** is the transfer of heat by vaporization of water and represents 24% of the neonatal heat loss. Evaporative losses include sensible losses such as sweating and insensible losses through the skin or surgical wound. Insensible loss from the skin in the adult is minimal but is significant in infants, particularly in the premature, who have less epidermal keratin, resulting in larger evaporative losses. Evaporative losses can be reduced by keeping the skin dry and by warming and humidifying gases in the breathing circuit. There is also substantial evaporative loss from within surgical incisions. **Convection** is the transfer of heat from an object to air or liquid and accounts for 34% of heat loss in the neonate. Convection removes heat to the environment, and is responsible for the wind-chill effect. Convection can be reduced by insulating barriers such as a plastic drape that prevent movement of air along the skin.

Anatomy for procedures

Airway management

Management of the pediatric airway begins with the adequate opening of the airway and effective bag-mask ventilation. The ability to maintain airway patency and ventilation can prevent an unexpected airway problem from becoming an airway emergency.

The neonatal airway can be particularly difficult with a relatively large tongue and redundant tissues. Maintaining a degree of mouth opening while placing a tight mask seal can compensate for the large tongue and redundant tissues and make bag-mask ventilation successful. For those who have not mastered the neonatal airway, insertion of an oral airway can achieve the same effect, if the patient is adequately anesthetized to tolerate insertion of an oral airway. Once a tight mask fit is achieved with a patent airway, the application of constant positive airway pressure (CPAP) can assist in achieving adequate ventilation.

Many airway tools exist to facilitate airway management in children. Many supraglottic airway devices exist but the most widely used is the laryngeal mask airway (LMA). Anatomical differences in the infant larynx can affect airway instrumentation with a supraglottic device. The shape of the infant larynx makes the LMA more difficult to position in infants less than 10 kg, resulting in more leaks and partial obstruction by the epiglottis, especially during positive-pressure ventilation. This occurs because the smaller LMA is a scaled-down version of the adult LMA, in which the anatomical differences of the larynx are not accounted for, making positioning more difficult.[13] Performing a jaw thrust during insertion of the LMA in an infant can minimize this complication. Although leak pressures in an LMA are rarely measured in clinical practice, maintaining the leak pressure at 40 cmH_2O can minimize leaks around the cuff as well as the incidence of sore throat.

The small size of infants and children also makes regional anesthesia of the airway more difficult. Most laryngeal nerve block techniques normally performed in adults are not commonly used in children. One exception is the subcutaneous lateral approach which allows bilateral subcutaneous administration of local anesthetic just lateral to the hyoid bone.[14]

Intubation can be challenging in the infant, whose large occiput and large tongue can hinder the alignment of the oral, pharyngeal and tracheal axes during direct laryngoscopy (DL). Placement of a shoulder roll can assist in aligning these axes. The infant epiglottis is narrow and angled away from the axis of the trachea, making a straight blade preferable for tracheal intubation in an infant or neonate. Despite these anatomic challenges, direct laryngoscopy is successful in the majority of infants and children. When laryngoscopy is difficult, the use of muscle relaxant to facilitate intubation in infants and children in conjunction with sevoflurane anesthetic is associated with fewer adverse respiratory events and should be considered while investigating the use of other advanced airway devices.[15]

The videolaryngoscope (VL) can provide improved view of the glottis specifically when the oral, pharyngeal and tracheal axes are not well aligned. In this misalignment, the epiglottis partially obstructs the glottic view or, in the worst case scenario, even the epiglottis is unable to be visualized under DL. In these patients, the VL has been shown to be a successful rescue technique for unsuccessful DL. Moreover, utilizing a VL blade smaller than that based on weight can further improve the visualization. Thus, changing to a smaller VL blade can clinically improve successful intubation in the infant or child with a difficult airway.[16]

Difficult airway: Although data is limited for the incidence of the difficult pediatric airway, it has been calculated to be anywhere from 0.58% up to 3%, which is significantly less than the 9–13% often reported in adults.[17] Both younger age and ASA III/IV status is associated with difficult laryngoscopy. Many studies have found a significantly higher risk of difficult intubation in infants under one year of age with a rate as high as 5%. Similar to adults, being overweight alone is not a predictor for difficult airway but, unlike adults, being underweight in children is associated with a difficult airway. The Mallampati score is less useful in the uncooperative pediatric patient or infant. However, in the cooperative pediatric patient, the Mallampati score can be a helpful tool to predict difficult laryngoscopy.[18] Despite many available videolaryngoscopic devices, fiberoptic intubation remains the gold standard for securing the difficult airway for both the adult and pediatric airway.

Should a surgical airway be needed in an emergency, needle cricothyroidotomy may be more difficult in the infant because of less room between the chin and the cricothyroid membrane. Caution must be given to correct placement as the target is small and the trachea is compressible making passage through the back wall of the trachea and into the esophagus a calculated risk in this procedure.[19]

Vascular cannulation

Successful cannulation of central veins requires a thorough understanding of the anatomy of relevant structures. Central access in infants can be technically more difficult due to the small vein size, and the variable anatomy. As with many pediatric procedures, once the vessel is identified, the actual cannulation can be hindered by difficulty threading the guidewire into the vessel and by kinking or dislodging of small-caliber guidewires when threading the catheter over the guidewire.

The decision to place a central venous line should be given serious thought before placing the line as the complications can be devastating. Due to the smaller caliber of the vessels in infants and children, thrombus formation and vessel occlusion are increased risks. Many other complications exist depending on the site chosen for central access and will be discussed with the individual sites. Despite the risk, central venous access is often required in infants and children for central venous pressure monitoring, administration of vaso-active medications, and hyperalimentation. The most commonly used sites for central venous cannulation in infants and children include the umbilical vein, the subclavian vein, the internal jugular vein, the femoral vein, and percutaneous intravenous access (PICC). Preferred sites depend upon the age of the patient, the type of surgery and practitioner preference. In neonates, undergoing cardiac surgery, central access is represented by all sites, including internal jugular/subclavian (38.8%), femoral (27.2%) and umbilical/central (32.9%). For infants out of the neonatal period undergoing cardiac surgery, internal jugular/subclavian is the site of choice with 70.5% of infants having access from these sites.[20]

Real-time ultrasound guidance has been definitively shown to be beneficial in adults, but pediatric data is less clear-cut. The use of real-time ultrasound in adults has been shown to decrease risks of cannulation failure, arterial puncture, hematoma, and hemothorax.[21] Although pediatric studies exist, data to evaluate outcomes in pediatric patients remain limited. Current evidence in the pediatric literature supports ultrasound use especially with inexperienced operators. For inexperienced operators,[22] ultrasound guidance versus landmark techniques can improve successful cannulation and decrease the number of needle passes needed to cannulate the vessel. In the pediatric intensive care setting, ultrasound guidance has been shown to decrease the time needed for residents to cannulate a vessel but does not offer such a benefit for experienced providers.[23]

Umbilical vein: The umbilical cord contains two umbilical arteries and one umbilical vein. The umbilical vein can be used in a neonate up to one week of age, after which atresia of the vessel makes cannulation unlikely. Use of this vessel has its limitations because of significant complications including necrotizing enterocolitis, thrombus in the vena cava or thrombus in the portal vein. Signs of umbilical vein thrombus formation include renal dysfunction and systemic hypertension. Umbilical vein cannulation can be life-saving, especially in the resuscitation of a newborn in distress at the time of delivery. Skilled practitioners can place such an umbilical line within minutes, providing much needed vascular access.[24]

Femoral vein: Femoral vein cannulation may be preferred in some patients when hemothorax, pneumothorax or local hematoma is of concern or when access is required without interfering with the airway. However, femoral venous access has been reported to have a higher incidence of thrombosis and infections as long-term complications. Femoral head necrosis is another risk, especially in the premature infant, and is avoided if possible in the premature infant. The femoral vein lies midway between the anterior superior iliac spine and the symphysis pubis and can be accessed just below the inguinal ligament at the inguinal crease. The femoral vein is medial to the femoral artery. Appropriate positioning can improve both cross-sectional area of the femoral vein and minimize overlap with the artery. This includes reverse Trendelenburg, external rotation of the hip and 60° abduction of the leg.[25] Although two-dimensional ultrasound is not required for femoral vein cannulation, ultrasound has been shown to improve the overall success rate, decrease the incidence of arterial puncture, decrease the incidence of hematoma, and decrease the number of needle passes for successful cannulation. The use of ultrasound guidance by trainees for femoral cannulation decreases the time of insertion, markedly improves first attempt success, and lowers the median number of passes for success.[22]

Upper body central cannulation: Upper body central lines in the internal jugular veins or the subclavian veins can be placed in neonates, infants, and small children. Upper body central lines provide reliable vascular access and accurate central venous pressure monitoring with a decreased risk of infection when compared to lower body central lines.[26] However, these vessels are sometimes avoided in small children with single-ventricle cardiac physiology due to a potential risk of stenosis or thrombosis of the

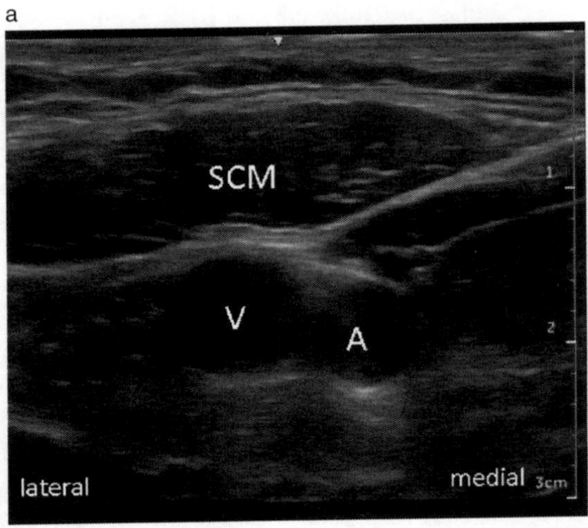

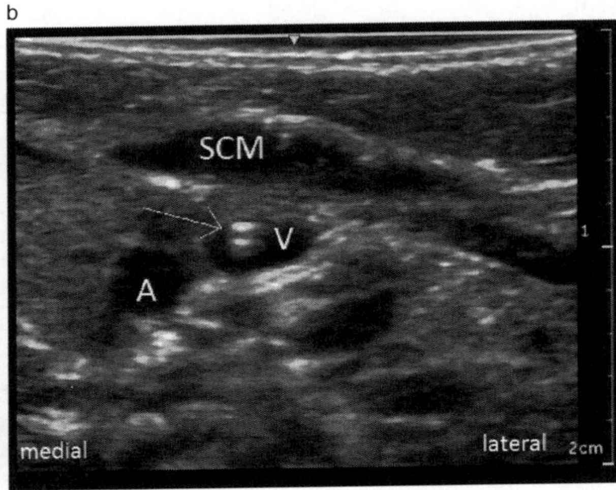

Figure 1.1 Ultrasound pictures of the internal jugular vessels. **Figure 1.1a.** shows the left neck vessels in a 3-year-old. **Figure 1.1b.** shows the right neck vessels in a newborn. A = carotid artery, V = internal jugular vein, SCM = sternocleidomastoid muscle. The arrow is pointing to the central line within the IJ lumen after cannulation. IJ = internal jugular.

superior vena cava. Stenosis or thrombosis of vessels in the upper body can result in "superior vena cava syndrome," a post-thrombotic syndrome with marked elevated pressures in the head and neck, facial swelling, and headaches. However, studies have shown minimal risk of clinically significant catheter-associated vessel thrombosis or stenosis in patients with single-ventricle physiology, especially when the right internal jugular access is used.[20]

Subclavian vein: The subclavian vein can be accessed via an infraclavicular approach using the landmarks of the lower border of the clavicle just lateral to the intersection of the clavicle with the first rib. This is also the lowest part of the "bend" of the clavicle. Complications such as pneumothorax and arterial puncture can be avoided with a flat angle of approach so the needle stays adjacent to the clavicle to avoid unwanted structures.

Internal jugular vein: The internal jugular anatomy has easily identified landmarks both anatomically and via ultrasound. Cannulation success rate can be improved with optimal positioning. This includes Trendelenburg position with the table tilted down 15° and passive leg elevation of 50° to increase the cross-sectional area of the IJ vessel.[27] The head should be turned only 45° from midline, as extreme turning of the head will cause more overlap of the internal jugular (IJ) and carotid, making carotid puncture more likely. Ultrasound is recommended for improved cannulation success. The straighter course of the right internal jugular vein towards the heart makes this the preferred site of access with less difficulty passing the guidewire and catheter into the heart and a lower thrombotic risk to the patient from catheter placement. Figure 1.1 depicts the anatomical view of the left and right neck anatomy. Figure 1.1a shows the ultrasound view of the left neck in a 3-year-old child. Note the depth of the vessels at 2 cm and the well-developed sternocleidomastoid muscle. Figure 1.1b shows the right neck in a newborn. Note the vessels are shallower at a depth of 1 cm with a less developed sternocleidomastoid muscle. The cross-sectional areas of the vessels in the neonate are smaller than those seen in the older child.

References

1. P.J. Davis, F.P. Cladis, E.K. Motoyama. *Smith's Anesthesia for Infants and Children*, 8th Edition. Philadelphia PA, Elsevier Mosby, 2011, p. 14.
2. B. Bissonnette and B. Dalens. *Pediatric Anesthesia: Principles and Practice*. New York NY, McGraw-Hill, 2002, p. 1215.
3. P.J. Davis, F.P. Cladis, E.K. Motoyama. *Smith's Anesthesia for Infants and Children*, 8th Edition, Philadelphia PA, Elsevier Mosby, 2011, p. 7.
4. R.D. Mosteller. Simplified calculation of body-surface area. *N Engl J Med* 1987; **317**: 1078.

5. H.I. Hochman, M.A. Grodin, R.K. Crone. Dehydration, diabetic ketoacidosis, and shock in the pediatric patient. *Pediatr Clin North Am* 1979; **26**: 803.
6. J.D. Crawford, M.E. Terry, G.M. Rourke. Simplification of drug dosage calculation by application of the surface area principle. *Pediatrics* 1950; **5**: 783–90.
7. A.G. Bailey, P.P. McNaull, E. Jooste, J.B. Tuchman. Perioperative crystalloid and colloid fluid management in children: where are we and how did we get here? *Anesth Analg* 2010; **110**: 375–90.
8. K. Choong, S. Arora, J. Cheng, *et al.* Hypotonic versus isotonic maintenance fluids after surgery for children: a randomized controlled trial. *Pediatrics* 2011; **128**: 857–66.
9. A. Sarti, D. Recanati, S. Furlan. Thermal regulation and intraoperative hypothermia. *Minerva Anestesiol* 2005; **71**: 379–83.
10. D. Sessler. Perioperative heat balance. *Anesthesiology* 2000; **92**: 578–96.
11. D. Galante. Intraoperative hypothermia. Relation between general and regional anesthesia, upper- and lower-body warming: what strategies in pediatric anesthesia? *Pediatr Anesth* 2007; **17**: 821–3.
12. B. Tander, S. Baris, D. Karakaya, *et al.* Risk factors influencing inadvertent hypothermia in infants and neonates during anesthesia. *Pediatr Anesth* 2005; **15**: 574–9.
13. C. Park, J.H. Bahk, W.S. Ahn, S.H. Do, K.H. Lee. The laryngeal mask airway in infants and children. *Canadian J Anaesth* 2001; **48**: 413–17.
14. B. Bissonnette and B. Dalens. *Pediatric Anesthesia: Principles and Practice*. New York, McGraw-Hill, 2002, p. 571.
15. R.A. Sunder, D.T. Haile, P.T. Farella, A. Sharma. Pediatric airway management: current practices and future directions. *Review Article Ped Anesth* 2012; **22**: 1008–15.
16. J.H. Lee, Y.H. Park, H.J. Byon, *et al.* A comparative trial of the glidescope® videolaryngoscope to direct laryngoscope in children with difficult direct laryngoscopy and an evaluation of the effect of blade size. *Anesth Analg* 2013; **117**: 176–81.
17. S. Heinrich, T. Birkholz, H. Ihmsen, *et al.* Incidence and predictors of difficult laryngoscopy in 11, 219 pediatric anesthesia procedures. *Pediatr Anesth* 2012; **22**: 729–36.
18. C. Sims, B. von Ungern-Sternber. The normal and the challenging pediatric airway. *Pediatr Anesth* 2012; **22**: 521–6.
19. J. Stacey, A.M. Heard, G. Chapman, *et al.* The 'Can't Intubate Can't Oxygenate' scenario in pediatric anesthesia: a comparison of different devices for needle cricothyroidotomy. *Pediatr Anesth* 2012; **22**: 1155–8.
20. J.W. Miller, D.N. Vu, P.J. Chai, *et al.* Upper body central venous catheters in pediatric cardiac surgery. *Pediatr Anesth* 2013; **23**: 980–8.
21. S. Wu, Q. Ling, L. Cao, *et al.* Real-time two-dimensional ultrasound guidance for central venous cannulation. A meta-analysis. *Anesthesiology* 2013; **118**: 361–75.
22. M.T. Aouad, G.E. Kanazi, F.W. Abdallah, *et al.* Femoral vein cannulation performed by residents: a comparison between ultrasound-guided and landmark technique in infants and children undergoing cardiac surgery. *Anesth Analg* 2012; **111**: 724–8.
23. C.R. Grebenik, A. Boyce, M.E. Sinclair, *et al.* NICE guidelines for central venous catheterization in children: is the evidence base sufficient? *Br J Anaesth* 2004; **92**: 827–30.
24. G. Ancora, S. Soffritti, G. Faldella. Diffuse and severe ischemic injury of the extremities: a complication of umbilical vein catheterization. *Am J Perinatol* 2006; **23**: 341–4.
25. A.A. Eldabaa, A.S. Elgebaly, A.A. Abd Elhafz, A.S. Bassun. Comparison of ultrasound-guided versus anatomical landmark-guided cannulation of the femoral vein at the optimum position in infants. *Annals of Pediatric Surgery* 2012, **8**: 65–8.
26. S.T. Verghese, W.A. McGill, R.I. Patel, *et al.* Ultrasound-guided central venous catheter placement decreases complications and decreases placement attempts compared with landmark techniques in the patient in the pediatric intensive care unit. *Crit Care Med* 2009; **37**: 1090–6.
27. W.H. Kim, J. H. Lee, S.M. Lee, *et al.* The effect of passive leg elevation and/or Trendelenburg position on the cross-sectional area of the internal jugular vein in infants and young children undergoing surgery for congenital heart disease. *Anesth Analg* 2013; **116**: 178–84.

Chapter 2

Anesthesia equipment

Hoa N. Luu

In this chapter, we will review anesthesia equipment as it relates to respiration. The one major focus would be on the breathing circuits that connect the anesthesia machine to the patient. Another focus is ventilation devices and ventilation techniques used.

The anesthesia machine is a huge subject that we will briefly discuss in this chapter. You should be aware that there is no dedicated anesthesia machine for the pediatric patient but we use the normal adult anesthesia machine. Thus, when providing anesthesia to the pediatric patient it is important for us to know the limitations of the anesthesia machine.

When connecting the patient to the anesthesia machine, we are all familiar with the standard semi-closed circle absorber system used in adults. With this breathing system, the use of two unidirectional valves allows for the anesthetic gases to flow in one direction and prevent rebreathing of carbon dioxide with the carbon dioxide absorber. This circle system allows for rebreathing of the anesthetic gas mixture, thus, cutting the cost by minimizing waste of anesthetic gases and conserving heat and moisture. The limitations of this system are that it is more bulky in size and there is increased resistance in the circuit if the patient is breathing spontaneously. In the pediatric patient, there are more options. While these options are rarely used today, except at some children's hospital operating rooms, it is important for us to learn about because they are continued to be used for transporting pediatric patients in the hospital.

Before we discuss the Mapleson systems, we will first talk about what practical options we have when a pediatric patient comes to the operating room. While some argue that the standard adult circuit can still be used, most hospitals do have the modified pediatric circuit. This modified pediatric circuit would consist of a shorter, stiffer, and smaller-diameter tubing and smaller rebreathing bag. The advantage of having this modified circuit would be having a decreased compression volume that means less compliance of the circuit. In addition, smaller CO_2 canisters can be used to minimize resistance to breathing.

Now we will learn about the Mapleson circuits that are semiclosed rebreathing systems. There are six different types of Mapleson circuits (A to F) that we are familiar with (Figure 2.1). Each circuit is different from the others by the location of its components. The five components are fresh gas inflow, expiratory valve, corrugated tubing, reservoir bag, and an adaptor for a face mask or endotracheal tube.

Depending on the locations of the components and mode of ventilation, it affects the amount of rebreathing that occurs. For simplicity, I like to divide the Mapleson circuits into three groups so it will help you remember the location of the components in each circuit. We will discuss the Mapleson systems as three groups as well because it will help us memorize which circuits are better for spontaneous or controlled ventilation.

The Mapleson A circuit has the expiratory valve close to the patient with the corrugated tubing separating away the fresh gas inflow and reservoir bag at the end. The Mapleson A circuit is the most efficient circuit for spontaneous ventilation because there is no rebreathing when the fresh gas flow is more than 80% of the minute ventilation. However, it is the least efficient circuit for controlled ventilation so it would require a much larger fresh gas flow to prevent rebreathing. We do not use the Mapleson A circuit today in the operating room because of the proximal location of the valve to the patient. It is potentially hazardous because the weight of the valve could inadvertently extubate an endotracheal tube.

Both Mapleson B and C circuits have the expiratory valve close to the patient with the fresh gas inflow

Essentials of Pediatric Anesthesiology, ed. Alan David Kaye, Charles James Fox and James H. Diaz. Published by Cambridge University Press. © Cambridge University Press 2015.

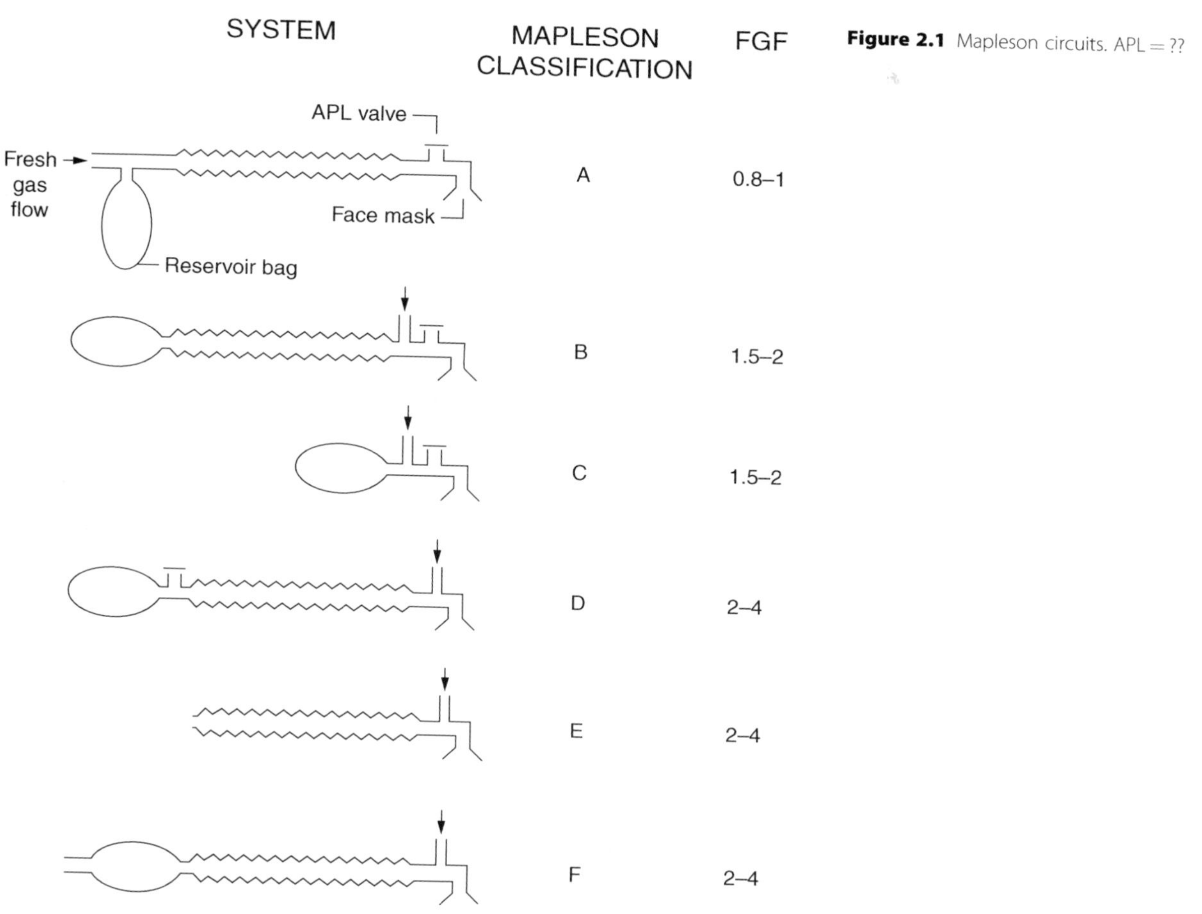

Figure 2.1 Mapleson circuits. APL = ??

nearby as well. The difference is that there is a corrugated tube separating the reservoir bag in Mapleson B while there is no corrugated tube in Mapleson C. Both of these circuits are seldom used today because of the proximity of the expiratory valve to the patient and high fresh gas flow required to prevent rebreathing.

The Mapleson D, E, and F circuits have the fresh gas inflow close to the patient. In the Mapleson D circuit, the expiratory valve is between the corrugated tube and reservoir bag. While the Mapleson D does require a little more fresh gas flow to prevent rebreathing than Mapleson A during spontaneous ventilation, it is the most efficient circuit during controlled ventilation. Bearing in mind both modes of ventilation, Mapleson D requires the lowest fresh gas flow rate; thus, explains it is the most commonly used Mapleson circuit. Mapleson E is the basically the Ayre T-piece while the Mapleson F is a modified Ayre T-piece with reservoir bag and tubing. They are grouped together also because they have similar rebreathing characteristics.

To help determine which circuits are better for spontaneous or controlled ventilation, there is a mnemonic that is easy to remember. For spontaneous ventilation, it's "**A**ll **D**ogs **C**an **B**ite." (A > DEF > CB) Thus, there is the least rebreathing in Mapleson A. For controlled ventilation, it's "**D**og **B**ites **C**an **A**che." (DEF > BC > A) Thus, there is the least rebreathing in Mapleson D, E, and F. To remember which phrase goes with which mode of ventilation, I just modify the first one to "**A**ll **D**ogs **C**an **B**ite **S**pontanously."

Now we will discuss ventilation devices. The focus will be devices we particularly use once the airway is secured. The discussion of airway management will be

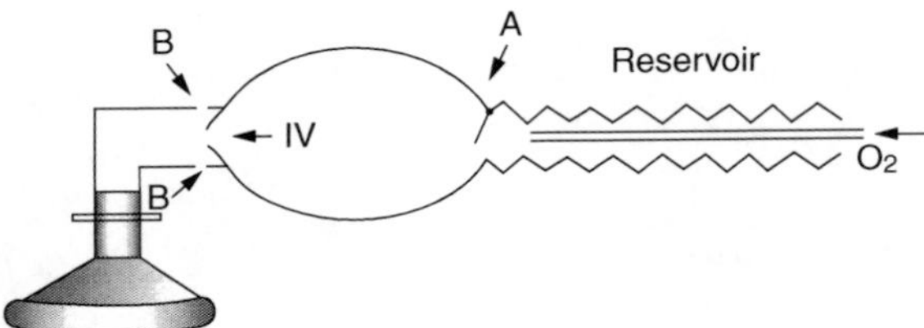

Figure 2.2 Self-inflating bag.

discussed later in the book. In that section, you will learn about the devices and techniques for both mask ventilation and endotracheal intubation.

As you can see, we have already talked about the most important ventilation device which is our anesthesia machine and the different circuits to connect it to the patient. But what happens when there is a machine failure or malfunction? The answer brings us to the last device we will discuss: the self-inflating bag (Figure 2.2).

The self-inflating bag can provide positive-pressure ventilation to ventilate the patient's lungs with room air or air enriched with oxygen if an oxygen supply is available. The Mapleson circuit would require compressed gas, thus, you would not be able to ventilate the patient with the circuit alone. You do not need to worry about rebreathing with the self-inflating bag because there is an one-way valve (B) near the patient which opens at expiration and closes at inspiration. When you squeeze the bag, the air within it would flow to the adaptor that connects to the face mask or endotracheal tube since the valve (A) would be closed. When the self-inflating bag re-expands, the valve (A) would open allowing the gas in the reservoir tubing to fill the bag. This gas can just be room air or be oxygen-enriched air if it is connected to an oxygen source. Thus, it is very important to have a self-inflating bag and alternate oxygen source prior to the start of every anesthesia case.

I hope you have a better understanding of the anesthesia equipment regarding breathing circuits now so you can address the limitations when caring for the pediatric patient.

Further reading

1. Y.C. Lin. Paediatric anaesthetic breathing systems. *Pediatr Anaesth* 1996; **6**: 1–5.
2. T. Smith. *Fundamentals of Anaesthesia*. Cambridge, Cambridge University Press, 2009.
3. J. Cote. *A Practice of Anesthesia for Infants and Children*. Philadelphia PA, Elsevier, 2009.
4. P.J. Davis. *Smith's Anesthesia for Infants and Children*. Philadelphia PA, Elsevier, 2011.
5. R.D. Miller. *Miller's Anesthesia*. Philadelphia PA, Elsevier, 2009.
6. T.Y. Euliano. *Essential Anesthesia*. Cambridge, Cambridge University Press, 2004.

Chapter 3

Methods for monitoring

Patrick S. McCarty and Sabrina T. Bent

Brain

Electroencephalogram

Electroencephalogram (EEG) is a signal that reflects the electrical activity of neurons in the cerebral cortex (1). Intraoperative EEG monitoring is most commonly performed in daily practice as a monitor of awareness or, more accurately, the depth of anesthesia or depth of hypnosis. The EEG is used also in congenital heart surgery to monitor brain activity during cardiopulmonary bypass and deep hypothermic circulatory arrest. Use of EEG in congenital heart surgery is usually part of a multimodal neuromonitoring protocol in most institutions. However, no studies have clearly shown a correlation between intraoperative EEG findings and neurologic outcomes (2). The effect of anesthetics on EEGs above the age of one year is comparable to that seen in adults. However, the concentration of the anesthetic agent required to produce a given effect may be correlated with age (1). The EEG in the awake state varies along with cerebral maturation and neuronal myelination from birth to adolescence. The newborn EEG has a predominance of slow oscillations. In the first year of life there is a rapidly progressive increase in the dominant frequency along with a decrease in amplitude of oscillations of the EEG. These changes continue with increasing age, but at a more gradual pace (1).

The pharmacodynamics of anesthetics on the EEG in infants is not well understood and therefore EEG monitors may not be indicative of depth of anesthesia in this age group (1).

Several EEG monitors are used in clinical practice including:

1. *Bispectral Index* (BIS), a proprietary algorithm (Aspect Medical Systems, Natick, MA) that converts a single channel of frontal electroencephalograph into an index of hypnotic level (BIS). The BIS values are scaled from 0 to 100, with specific ranges reported to reflect a low probability of consciousness under general anesthesia.
2. *Entropy* (GE Healthcare Technologies, Waukesha, WI) describes the irregularity, complexity, or unpredictability characteristics of a signal. Two entropy values are reported, state entropy (SE) and response entropy (RE). The SE is an index ranging from 0 to 91 (awake), computed over the frequency range from 0.8 to 32 Hz, reflecting the cortical state of the patient. The RE is an index ranging from 0 to 100 (awake), computed over a frequency range from 0.8 to 47 Hz (3).
3. *Narcotrend* (MonitorTechnik, Bad Branstedt, Germany) is derived from a system developed for the visual classification of the electroencephalographic patterns associated with various stages of sleep. Processed EEG results are calculated and given as a number, a Narcotrend index (NI) ranging from 0 (very deep hypnosis) to 100 (awake) (3) (4).
4. *Patient State Ana*lyzer. The Patient State Index (PSI; Physiometrix, North Billerica, MA) is derived from a four-channel EEG. The PSI has a range of 0–100, with decreasing values indicating decreasing levels of consciousness or increasing levels of sedation (3).
5. *SNAP Index*. The SNAPII (Everest Biomedical Instruments, Chesterfield, MO) calculates a "SNAP index" from a single channel of electroencephalograph. The index calculation is based on a spectral analysis of electroencephalographic activity in the 0 to 18 Hz and 80 to 420 Hz frequency ranges and a burst suppression algorithm.

Essentials of Pediatric Anesthesiology, ed. Alan David Kaye, Charles James Fox and James H. Diaz. Published by Cambridge University Press. © Cambridge University Press 2015.

6. *Cerebral State Monitor/Cerebral State Index.* The Cerebral State Monitor (Danmeter A/S, Odense, Denmark) is a handheld device that analyzes a single channel EEG and presents a Cerebral State "Index" scaled from 0 to 100. In addition, it also provides electroencephalographic suppression percentage and a measure of electromyographic activity (75–85 Hz) (3).

The American Society of Anesthesiologists task force on intraoperative awareness suggests that multiple modalities be used to monitor depth of anesthesia including clinical techniques (i.e., checking for purposeful movement), use of conventional monitors (i.e., electrocardiogram, blood pressure, heart rate, end-tidal anesthetic analyzer and capnography), and brain function monitors on a case-by-case basis, but not as a routine monitor. This consensus is based on the fact that a given monitor and its associated numerical value may not correlate with a specific depth of anesthesia. Additionally, the measured values do not have uniform sensitivity across different anesthetic drugs or types of patients (3).

Near-infrared spectroscopy

Near-infrared spectroscopy (NIRS) is based on the Beer–Lambert law which states that the concentration of a substance is proportional to the absorption of light and thickness of the substance. Clinically the most widely used NIRS monitor is the INVOS™ (Covidien, Mansfield, Massachusetts) which utilizes near-infrared light at two wavelengths, 730 nm and 810 nm, which are absorbed by hemoglobin. The light travels from the sensor's light-emitting diode to either a proximal or distal detector permitting separate data processing of the surface tissues (skin and skull) from the deep tissues (brain) (5). The NIRS samples the nonpulsatile optical component which is highly correlated with capillary–venous hemoglobin oxygen saturation, rSO_2 (6). Adult data has shown that a cerebral rSO_2 of 50 or a 20% decline from baseline may be associated with increase morbidity (6). The NIRS monitor noninvasively measures continuous regional tissue oxygenation. It has been used in a variety of clinical settings including pediatric congenital and adult heart surgery, vascular surgery, orthopedic surgery, and critical care.

Current evidence of NIRS monitoring in human studies over the past decade is consistent with class IIB recommendations according to the American Heart Association and the American College of Cardiology Task Force on Practice Guidelines (6).

Transcranial Doppler ultrasound

Transcranial Doppler ultrasound (TCD) was first introduced in 1982 (7). The use of TCD monitoring provides real-time cerebral blood flow velocity and detection of cerebral emboli. It is most commonly used in pediatric congenital heart surgery. The probe for the TCD is usually placed on the temporal bone near the temporal artery where it measures the velocity in the proximal segment of the middle cerebral artery, which provides approximately 70% of the blood flow to the ipsilateral cerebral hemisphere (2) (8). Many centers utilize TCD as part of a multimodal monitoring approach to guide treatment during cardiopulmonary bypass as a strategy to prevent neurologic injury (2) (9).

Limitations to use of TCD include that it is operator-dependent, it can be difficult to reproduce, especially at low blood flow, and up to 25 percent of patients cannot be assessed through the temporal window (8) (10). Additionally, there is an absence of a signal during low flow and during deep hypothermic circulatory arrest (8).

Jugular venous bulb saturation

Jugular venous bulb saturation, $S_{jv}O_2$, is used to measure the global cerebral oxygenation. The $S_{jv}O_2$ is a global measure of cerebral oxygen supply and demand and has a normal range between 60–75%. Values of $S_{jv}O_2$ less than 50% are indicative of cerebral ischemia. Focal areas of pathology and ischemia may not be detected by $S_{jv}O_2$ (11). Proper placement of an oximetric catheter for continuous sampling or a standard catheter for intermittent sampling can be technically challenging. Intraoperatively, it can be inserted by the surgeon in cardiac cases where the heart is exposed. However, NIRS, another surrogate of cerebral oxygenation, is noninvasive and has nearly replaced $S_{jv}O_2$ as a standard monitor (10).

Brain tissue oxygenation

Recently, small oxygen electrodes have been used to measure brain tissue oxygenation, $P_{bt}O_2$. These electrodes are relatively atraumatic and are frequently placed in the penumbra region (area surrounding an ischemic tissue) (10) (11). The electrodes are usually placed through a burr hole by surgeons. The Licox™

(Integra Lifesciences) and Neurovent™ (Neurovent Research Inc.) multiparameter probes have been investigated for clinical use. Normal ranges for $P_{bt}O_2$ are 25–30 mm of Hg in patients with normal intracranial and cerebral perfusion pressures. When the $P_{bt}O_2$ is less than ~20 mmHg, intervention is usually indicated (10). These interventions may involve increasing cerebral oxygenation through increased hemoglobin, vasodilation, and increased F_iO_2 or decreasing cerebral oxygen demand with sedation, treatment of fevers, and seizures (10).

Current use is mainly in the critical care setting in patients with traumatic brain injury. Although data is limited, initial studies have not clearly shown improved outcomes with monitoring $P_{bt}O_2$ and interventions (10) (11).

Spinal cord

Somatosensory evoked potentials

Somatosensory evoked potentials, SSEPs, are a noninvasive measure of function in pathways between the primary somatosensory cortex and peripheral nerves. The SSEPs are performed on the median and ulnar nerves in the upper limbs and the tibial and peroneal nerves in the lower limbs (12). Needles are placed in the scalp following the international 10–20 system, and recording sites include the brain stem, dorsal column nuclei, thalamus, and the primary sensory cortex on the postcentral gyrus (2). Usually an electrical stimulus with a duration of 100 μsec, intensity of 5–30 volts and a constant current between 5–30 mA is used to elicit a response (12). Preincision baseline values are obtained. The standard alarm criteria include either a 10% increase in latency or a 50% decrease in amplitude from the baseline preincision values (2) (12).

When abnormalities occur intraoperatively, interventions are made often by both the surgeon and the anesthesiologist. As in scoliosis repair, rod placement may be altered or blood pressure increased in an effort to improve SSEPs.

The SSEPs, when used as the sole mode of neuromonitoring, have a wide range of reported sensitivity (0–92%) and specificity of 95– 100%) for new postoperative motor deficits (13). Although SSEPs have excellent specificity, they have relatively low sensitivity for motor deficits. The SSEPs averaging of evoked responses leads to significant delays in signal changes; it may lag up to 16 minutes behind motor evoked potentials. Additionally they may remain unchanged with anterior spinal artery injury (13).

All sedatives, including barbiturates, benzodiazepines, propofol, opioids, and volatile anesthetics affect latency and amplitude of evoked potentials in a dose-concentration dependent manner. Ketamine causes an increase in amplitude and latency. Neuromuscular blocking agents do not affect SSEPs at normal clinical doses. All antiepileptics slow central conduction velocity and proportion to serum drug levels (12).

The SSEPs are commonly monitored in orthopedic, neurosurgery, and in some centers, congenital heart surgery (2) (12).

Motor evoked potentials

Motor evoked potentials, MEPs, are noninvasive transcranial electrical stimulations applied to the motor cortex utilizing a train of 3–7 stimuli, with recordings of muscle motor evoked responses (compound muscle action potentials) from the limbs (14).

The MEPs are primarily monitored to ensure the integrity of the motor cortex, corticospinal tract, nerve root, and peripheral nerves. The MEPs are most commonly used in conjunction with SSEPs.

Usually corkscrew or needle electrodes are placed in the scalp according to the international 10–20 system. Use of these electrodes is relatively contraindicated in infants with open fontanels and in children with shunt systems to avoid injury due to misplacement of the corkscrew or needle (14). Frequently only six electrodes are placed (15). The nerve roots and corresponding muscles that are commonly used for MEPs are: C8–T1 (thenar muscle); C5–C6 (biceps or brachioradialis); S1–S2 (abductor halluces); L4–L5 (tibialis anterior); S1–S2 (gastrocnemius); L2–L4 (vastus lateralis); L2–L4 (rectus femoris) (14). The range of voltages used to elicit MEPs is patient dependent, but varies from 300 to 1000 V (16).

In spinal surgery, MEPs are considered abnormal if there is an absence of response, the all-or-nothing criterion. However, during brain surgery, a $>$ 75–80% drop of MEP amplitude from baseline values after stimulation should be avoided as these may correlate with long-lasting motor deficits (14) (15). The MEPs have nearly 100% sensitivity for motor deficits (13).

Complications from MEPs are relatively rare. However, tongue lacerations are the most commonly reported complication. It is imperative that the anesthesiologist position and secure the bite block(s) carefully to prevent the teeth from coming in contact with the tongue; that is, the tongue should be placed behind the teeth (16). Patient movement during stimulation is potentially a risk to injury if the surgeon is not notified in advance of the stimulation.

Anesthesia for MEPs usually consists of a total intravenous anesthetic without the use of neuromuscular blockade, with exception to that used for induction. Even partial neuromuscular blockade confounds the interpretation of MEPs especially with respect to amplitude changes and thereby introduces a poorly controlled source of variability. This in turn reduces the reliability of MEPs as early indicators of evolving spinal cord or spinal nerve root injury, and inappropriately calls into question the overall value of the test. Depth of anesthesia also plays an important role in minimizing or eliminating patient movement following MEPs. The anesthesiologist must be vigilant to ensure an adequate anesthetic plane without having the patient so deep that it will preclude triggering of MEPs with optimal amplitudes (16)

Because of the immaturity of the pediatric central nervous system compared with the adult central nervous system, anesthetic drugs in general have more potent and longer lasting effects during the surgical procedure. Particularly with halogenated anesthetic agents, cortical potential amplitudes can be significantly attenuated with smaller percent doses compared with adults. Both amplitude and latency are affected in a dose-dependent fashion with inhalational anesthetics, and this is particularly true in those under the age of 3 years (14).

Electromyographic potentials

Electromyographic potentials, EMG, can be either spontaneous, SEMG or evoked, EEMG. The difference in the two is dependent on whether the recording is continuous spontaneous muscle activity, SEMGs, or elicited from direct nerve stimulation of the nerve causing muscle contraction, EEMGs.

Spontaneous electromyographs

Spontaneous electromyographic potentials, SEMGs, are recordings of the spontaneous electrical activity of muscle cells, otherwise known as muscle action potentials, MAPs (17). The SEMGs are highly sensitive for nerve root injury, but also have a high rate of false positives. Additionally, SEMGs are extremely sensitive to temperature changes (cold irrigation or electrocautery) (13).

Evoked electromyographs

Evoked electromyographic potentials, EEMGs, recordings are produced when the nerve innervating a muscle is stimulated with a voltage and current that is somewhat supraphysiologic (of the order of 0.5 mA), for the purpose of spatial identification of nerves to preserve them from injury, usually during operations (17). Advantages of EEMGs are: they are highly sensitivity for medial pedicle breach in spine surgery, useful in minimally invasive surgery where anatomical landmarks may be challenging to visualize, and they are relatively easy to perform and interpret. Disadvantages of EEMGs include: optimal alarm criteria are not firmly established, they may provide false-positive alarms if multiple passes have been made through the pedicle or if the operative field is bloody in spine surgery (13).

In an effort to monitor the recurrent laryngeal nerve and the vagus nerves which innervate the vocalis muscle, a specially designed endotracheal tube with embedded wire surface electrodes (e.g., NIM™ tube, Xomed, Jacksonville, FL, USA) has been used for the dedicated task of monitoring spontaneous and evoked potentials of the vocalis muscle. This is commonly utilized in neck surgeries involving the thyroid, parathyroid, neck dissections, carotid endarterectomy, and other surgeries in the anterior cervical region. Abnormalities of the NIM tube EMG signals is defined as a of loss of signal being either a change from initial satisfactory EMG; no signal or quantitatively low EMG response (i.e., ≤ 100 mV) with stimulation using a stimulus of 1 to 2 mA, and with dry surgical field conditions; or no laryngeal twitch or observed glottic twitch visualized (17).

The facial nerve is also commonly monitored utilizing EMGs during tympanic, mastoid, and parotid surgeries. The EMG monitoring during operations involving the base of the skull or neck dissections include: the ansa cervicalis (omohyoid muscle, sternohyoid muscle, sternothyroid muscle, thyrohyoid muscle, geniohyoid muscle) or ansa hypoglossi nerves, the phrenic nerve, C3–5, (diaphragm) and the lower cranial nerves, CN (VII–XII). The cranial nerves and corresponding muscles monitored with EMG include those nerves emerging from the middle cranial fossa: CN III (rectus medialis and rectus inferior), CN IV (obliquus superior), CN V (digastricus and masseter), CN VI (rectus lateralis); and nerves emerging from the posterior cranial fossa: CN VII (frontalis, orbicularis oris, mentalis, and orbicularis oculi), CN IX (stylopharyngeus), CN X (vocalis), CN XI (trapezius and sternocleidomastoideus), CN XII (hypoglossus and genioglossus) (17).

Other surgical procedures where EMG monitoring is utilized includes: scoliosis repairs with posterior spinal fusions, tethered cord releases where the anal sphincter muscle is monitored, selective dorsal rhizotomy is performed for the treatment of spasticity (i.e., in cerebral palsy) where tibialis anterior, medial gastrocnemius, vastus lateralis, and gluteus maximus muscles are often monitored (14).

In posterior spinal fusions, the nerve roots and corresponding muscles that are commonly recorded for EMGs include: C5–C6 (biceps, brachioradialis, deltoid); C7–C8 (triceps); C8–T1 (thenar ms. group, primarily abductor pollicus brevis and hypothenar ms. group); T6–T12 (intercostal, abdominal, paraspinal); L1–L2 (iliopsoas); L2–L4 (quadriceps, vastus lateralis or medialis); L4–L5 (tibialis anterior); S1–S2 (abductor hallucis, gastrocnemius) (14).

Anesthesia for EMG monitoring usually consists of a total intravenous anesthetic, often consisting of continuous infusions of propofol and an opioid, where neuromuscular blockade is avoided except for use during intubation.

The wake-up test

The wake-up test, formerly the Stagnera wake-up test, named after one of the original implementers, is currently infrequently used but still remains a valuable tool as a supplement to other intraoperative monitoring tests such as SSEPs and MEPs.

This intraoperative test involves the gradual lightening of the anesthetic until the patient can voluntarily move their extremities to command. Symmetry of movement is gauged by an unscrubbed person. The test is usually 100% accurate in detecting gross motor changes. Sensory and fine motor deficits are not tested (18).

Disadvantages of the wake-up test include the following: one time measure of function as opposed to continuous, risk of air embolism, risk of self-extubation, recall for event, self-induced contamination, positional changes resulting in neural compression, and lack of nerve root injury information (18).

As in most multimodal intraoperative neurophysiologic monitoring, the anesthetic is usually a total intravenous anesthetic without neuromuscular blockade. The anesthetic choices should lend itself to easy reversibility or lightening within approximately 15 to 20 minutes of notification by the surgeon. Immediately following the test the patient is reanesthetized to allow adequate depth of anesthesia to avoid awareness, provide good surgical conditions, and continued quality neurophysiologic testing.

Neuromuscular function

Neuromuscular blockade, NMB, is most commonly monitored by a peripheral nerve stimulator. The most common nerve–muscle unit used for neuromuscular monitoring is the ulnar nerve–adductor pollicis muscle. Another common site for monitoring is the facial nerve and either the orbicularis oculi or corrugator supercilii muscles. It is recommended that the two electrocardiogram electrodes be placed no greater than 6 cm apart (19).

It is appropriate to use the facial nerve–corrugator supercilii muscle for monitoring optimal intubation conditions or paralysis of the diaphragm and the abdominal wall muscles following NMBs whereas the ulnar nerve–adductor pollicis unit is the better choice if information about pharyngeal muscle recovery is desired. The recommended electrical stimulus is 15–20% above the level of maximum muscular response, referred to as the supramaximal stimulus (SMS). The stimulation patterns that are most often used in the clinical setting are the single twitch stimulation, the train-of-four stimulation (TOF), tetanic stimulation, post-tetanic count stimulation (PTC), and the double-burst stimulation (DBS) (19).

The single twitch is an SMS to the nerve with a frequency between 0.1–1.0 Hz. The single twitch has limited value. It does not provide reliable information either about the neuromuscular recovery or onset of block (19).

The TOF stimulation allows more reliable tactile assessment of a NMB. The TOF consists of four twitches at 2 Hz. A stimulation-free period of at least 10 seconds should be allowed between repetitive TOF stimulations to avoid fade during measurement. The loss of the responses and corresponding residual neuromuscular blockade is: 4th (75–80%), 3rd (85%), 2nd (90%) and 1st (98–100%). The TOF ratio is defined as the amplitude of the 4th response divided by the amplitude of the 1st response of the TOF. Tactile estimation is accurate in detecting fade during TOF stimulation only if the TOF ratio is <0.4. Clinically, a TOF ratio of 0.7 and >0.9

corresponds to adequate diaphragmatic and pharyngeal muscle recovery, respectively (19).

Tetanic stimulation is a high frequency (50–200 Hz) stimulation pattern usually applied for 5 seconds. Visual fading of this pattern has relatively low sensitivity (70%) and specificity (50%). However, in light of this, a visual absence of fading after a 100 Hz, 5-second tetanic stimulation may be comparable to a TOF ratio of 0.85 (19).

Post-tetanic count, PTC, allows a visual or tactile evaluation of a deep nondepolarizing NMB that does not respond to TOF stimulation. The PTC stimulation consists of a 50 Hz tetanic stimulation applied for 5 seconds followed by a single 1 Hz SMS after a pause of 3 seconds. The resulting count should be zero for a very deep NMB. If 5–7 counts are obtained, the return of the TOF is imminent (19).

Double-burst stimulation, DBS, consists of two bursts of stimuli at 50 Hz with an interval of 750 ms usually combined as a series of three and two impulses, referred to as a DBS 3, 2. Fading of the second impulse series compared to the first correlates with an incomplete NMB comparable to a TOF ratio < 0.6. The DBS method is more sensitive for tactile evaluation of the fade than using TOF stimulation (19).

The three most commonly used pieces of equipment for the monitoring of NMB are: acceleromyography (AMG), mechanomyography (MMG), and electromyography. *Acceleromyography* is inexpensive and easy to utilize. With AMG, a stimulating electrode is placed on the target nerve and a piezoelectric element is placed over the muscle innervated by the nerve. The isotonic acceleration of the stimulated muscle is measured. The basis for AMG is Newton's second law, force = mass x acceleration. Since muscle mass is constant, the force of the muscle can be calculated from the measured acceleration of the muscle. The movement of the muscle generates a voltage in the piezoelectric element that correlates with the acceleration of the muscle. Intraoperatively, AMG measurements can be influenced by movement artifacts and unstable twitch responses. Therefore, fixation of fingers and forearm is recommended when using the thumb as the target muscle. The AMG overestimates neuromuscular recovery when compared to mechanomyography (19).

Mechanomyography measures the isometric contraction of a muscle following nerve stimulation. A force transducer converts the force of contraction of the muscle to an electric signal. A preload of 200–300 g must be applied for stabilization of the signal and the limb must be immobilized. Using MMG is time consuming and requires large equipment. It is not utilized clinically, but is considered the "gold standard" for investigation of new neuromuscular blockers (19).

Electromyography is the oldest technique for measuring NMB. It is based on the fact that the force of muscular contraction is proportional to the compound action potential of the muscle; the device records the electrical activity of the stimulated muscle. The amplitude of the signal is a sum of the compound action potential. There is good correlation with MMG. However, electromyography is used primarily in research (19).

Cardiac rhythm

Electrocardiogram

The electrocardiogram, ECG, is a recording of cardiac electrical activity of the heart that causes the cardiac myocytes to contract. Intraoperatively, either a three-lead or five-lead ECG is utilized. The three-lead ECG allows for basic cardiac rate and rhythm determination, it does not provide good evaluation of ST segments. The three-lead ECG is normally acceptable for patients without any cardiac history undergoing minor procedures where the risk for ischemia and hemodynamic instability is unlikely.

The American Society of Anesthesiologists (ASA) considers ECG to be part of standard monitors for anesthesia and requires that every patient receiving anesthesia shall have the electrocardiogram continuously displayed from the beginning of anesthesia until preparing to leave the anesthetizing location (20).

There are some characteristics of ECG that are specific or unique to pediatric patients that are important to be familiar with. The normal pediatric ECG changes throughout childhood. These changes that occur in the ECG reflect the anatomical dominance of the right ventricle during neonatal life. At birth, the right ventricle is thick as a result of high pulmonary artery pressure in utero. With the expected fall in pulmonary artery pressure during infancy, right ventricular wall stress and thickness decrease until right ventricular pressure approximates that of the adult, typically by 6 months of age (21).

The normal mean heart rate for newborn infants 1 to 6 months of age ranges from 125 to 145 beats/min (bpm) with the normal resting heart rate of 80 bpm in adults typically not achieved until mid-adolescence. These changes can be accounted for by the gradual increase in vagal tone that accompanies aging (21).

Bradyarrhythmias are uncommon causes of ECG abnormalities in children without congenital heart disease. But in general a heart rate less than 100 beats per minute (bpm) in children younger than 3 years old, less than 60 bpm in children 3 to 9 years old, less than 50 bpm in children 9 to 16 years old, and less than 40 in older children and adolescents should entertain the diagnosis of sinus bradycardia (22).

The rate for tachycardia rhythms are age dependent but general guidelines exist; heart rates greater than 160 bpm in infants and greater than 140 bpm in children suggest sinus tachycardia. Supraventricular tachycardia, SVT, is one of the most common arrhythmias encountered in pediatric patients. However, atrial flutter and atrial fibrillation are quite rare in pediatric patients (22).

Incomplete right bundle branch blocks, RBBB, are commonly seen in pediatric ECGs.

Ventricular arrhythmias are uncommon in children and usually arise in the setting of severe electrolyte disarray, ingestion, or rare inherited disorders of cardiac conduction.

Premature ventricular contractions (PVCs) are a frequent finding in children and may be cause for concern in rare cases. Premature ventricular contractions of uniform morphology are less concerning than those of multiple forms. The most common syndrome associated with pre-excitation in children and adults is the Wolff–Parkinson–White (WPW) syndrome. In patients with WPW, the most commonly encountered arrhythmia is a paroxysmal re-entry SVT. Congenital long QT syndrome is a cause of pediatric sudden death and has been associated with sudden death during sleep, exercise, and perhaps a small subset of infants dying of sudden infant death syndrome (22).

A special group of pediatric patients are susceptible to arrhythmias, those with congenital heart disease. Approximately 1% of newborns are affected by congenital heart disease (CHD), and although many lesions of CHD have trivial hemodynamic and clinical implications, some clinically significant lesions are asymptomatic in the immediate newborn period. However, the ECG is an insensitive and nonspecific screening method in the diagnosis of CHD, unless an arrhythmia is present. Patients who have undergone repair for CHD are at increased lifetime risk of arrhythmias, symptomatic and asymptomatic (23).

Precordial and esophageal stethoscopes

Precordial (PCS) and/or esophageal stethoscopes (ES) have been used in anesthesia for more than 100 years. The first description of the use of the stethoscope during anesthesia appears to be that by Kirk at the Glasgow Western Infirmary in 1896. He began by using an ordinary binaural stethoscope with a Ford's type bell, but soon substituted a Phonendoscope, commonly referred to as the flat-sided diaphragm part of the modern stethoscope. The first use of the esophageal stethoscope during anesthesia was described by Code Smith from the Hospital for Sick Children in Toronto in 1954 (24).

The PCS or ES can be used to auscultate the evolution of an S_3 cardiac gallop rhythm, cardiac arrhythmias and murmurs, accumulation of airway secretions, air embolism, wheezing, circuit or ventilator disconnect, and detection of a right mainstem intubation. These stethoscopes are inexpensive and may provide earlier indications of potential problems prior to more advanced and expensive monitors (25) (26).

Complications from use of PCS and ES are rare, but include: hypoxemia, vocal cord paralysis, esophageal or pharyngeal traumatic injury, and small bowel obstruction (25).

Pulse oximetry

Pulse oximetry and the plethysmography that is displayed on most monitors can be used as a surrogate monitor of both heart rate and rhythm. A heart rate is usually measured and displayed. This visual information, combined with the auditory signal that is available on most devices, can alert the anesthesiologist to changes in rate and rhythm. Although the exact nature of the arrhythmia cannot be determined, general information regarding classification (i.e., bradycardia, tachycardias, ectopic beats, perfusion, and regularity) can be ascertained.

Vascular pressures

Arterial

The most common method of measuring arterial pressure is with the use of the noninvasive automated oscillometric blood pressure monitor. The ASA standard for basic anesthetic monitoring states that:

1. Every patient receiving anesthesia shall have arterial blood pressure and heart rate determined and evaluated at least every five minutes (20).
2. And every patient receiving general anesthesia shall have, in addition to the above, circulatory function continually evaluated by at least one of the following: palpation of a pulse, auscultation of heart sounds, monitoring of a tracing of intra-arterial pressure, ultrasound peripheral pulse monitoring, or pulse plethysmography or oximetry (20).

Oscillometric blood pressure

The automated oscillometric blood pressure method involves placing a pneumatic cuff which is then inflated around the arm to a pressure greater than systolic; oscillations are recorded from the cuff, reflecting pulsation upstream in the occluded artery. When the cuff is deflated, the oscillations suddenly increase when the cuff pressure approaches the intra-arterial systolic pressure. On further deflation, the oscillations steadily increase in amplitude to a maximum and then begin to decrease. The point at which there is an abrupt decrease in the large oscillations is considered to coincide with diastolic pressure. The cuff pressure at the point of maximal amplitude corresponds to the mean intra-arterial pressure (27). Noninvasive blood pressure monitoring with a digital automated oscillometric "traditional" blood pressure cuff monitors, are known to produce inaccurate readings. Only 60 to 86% of the measured values were within 5 mmHg of the observed value when multiple devices were tested (28). In neonates, the oscillometric technique has been shown to be an accurate trend monitor for heart rate and blood pressure for stable neonates with greater bias at lower blood pressures (29).

Arterial pressure transducers

Arterial pressure can be measured by cannulation of a variety of arteries, usually a function of the surgical site, patient imposed limitations, and technical success. The arteries most commonly utilized include: radial, femoral, umbilical (neonates), dorsalis pedis, posterior tibial, brachial, ulnar, and axillary. Intra-arterial blood pressure (ABP) monitoring is considered the gold standard for arterial pressure. Using ABP monitoring is based on the principle of transmitting pressure changes from a column of compressible fluid (in an ideally incompressible tube) to a mechanical transducer. The mechanical transducer is basically a displaceable diaphragm, which converts physical fluid displacement into a proportional electrical signal, which is processed and displayed (29). The ABP also has inherent errors, such as overdampening, underdampening, and require zeroing at the appropriate level.

The ABP catheterization can be accomplished by percutaneous, Seldinger technique, and cut-down. Studies have shown that the minor complications, such as pain, bleeding, transient loss of pulse occurs in approximately 10% of cases. Major complications such as distal ischemia and loss of limb occur in approximately 1–2% cases. Complication rates may be increased with the Seldinger technique, use of the brachial artery, and in children less than 10 years of age (29).

Flotrac™

Flotrac™ (Edwards Lifesciences, Irvine, USA) is a special transducer that connects to an arterial line and provides additional information beyond arterial systolic/diastolic pressure. The Flotrac™ uses a clinically validated algorithm to provide continuous cardiac output (CCO), stroke volume (SV), and stroke volume variation (SVV) in real time (30). This system is approved for use in patients with a body weight $\geq$ 40 kg. Advantages of this system include that it does not require external calibration, is easy to use, and does not require recalibration. Disadvantages include that it depends on a regular rhythm; it has decreased accuracy in the setting of altered vascular tone, and limited accuracy during hemodynamic instability (31) (32).

PiCCO®

The PiCCO® (Pulsion, Munich, Germany) system combines arterial waveform analysis (AWA) with the thermodilution technique to determine real-time CO, SVV, pulse pressure variation (PPV), global end-diastolic volume (GEDV), and extravascular lung water (EVLW), a marker of pulmonary edema. Advantages include that it is very robust during hemodynamic instability with frequent recalibration, it requires a central arterial line and central venous lines, and it requires frequent recalibration. Pediatric use is limited (32).

LiDCO™

The LiDCO™ (LiDCO, Cambridge, UK) system combines AWA with lithium indicator dilution for continuous SV and SVV monitoring. Continuous CO is also provided. Advantages include that it is very robust during hemodynamic instability with frequent recalibration and is easy to use via peripheral or central artery. Disadvantages include that it requires frequent recalibration; it requires intravenous injection of lithium and may have interference with the use of some neuromuscular blockers (32). Pediatric use is limited.

ccNexfin®

A newer technology, ccNexfin® (Nexfin CO-Trek, Edwards Lifesciences, Irvine, USA) uses a noninvasive finger cuff to measure beat-to-beat arterial blood pressure, CO, heart rate, SV, systemic vascular resistance, SVV, and PPV. This device uses a pulse contour method determined from a three-element Windkessel model in which the nonlinear effect of mean pressure and the influence of the patient's age, height, weight, and sex on aortic mechanical properties are incorporated (33). The ccNexfin® is currently approved for adults, but future studies may lead to pediatric use, especially in older children.

Central venous pressure

Central venous pressure (CVP) is usually measured with an invasive catheter in one of the central veins. The internal jugular vein is the most commonly used vein, but other veins include: subclavian, external jugular, femoral, and umbilical (neonates). Both CVP and arterial pressure transducers function similarly. Complications from CVP insertion include infection, hematoma formation, vessel dissection, thrombosis, pneumothorax, hemothorax, and hemopericardium. The CVP is often inappropriately used to assess volume status. Cardiac output is dependent on left ventricular end-diastolic volume, which is poorly estimated by CVP (29). The central venous wave form can provide information regarding cardiac rhythm and valvular regurgitation through changes in the atrial and ventricular components in the tracing. Many central venous catheters have the ability to measure central venous oxygen saturation, $S_{cv}O_2$, which has gained popularity in the pediatric population.

PediaSat™

PediaSat™ (Edwards Lifesciences, Irvine, California) is an oximetry catheter that provides both continuous CVP and $S_{cv}O_2$. Venous oxygen saturation is measured through reflection spectrophotometry. Light is emitted from an LED through one of the two fiber-optic channels into the venous blood; some of this light is reflected back and received by another fiber-optic channel, which is read by a photodetector. The amount of light that is absorbed by the venous blood (or reflected back) is determined by the amount of oxygen that is saturated or bound to hemoglobin. Keeping $S_{cv}O_2$ values above 70% has been proven to lead to better patient outcomes (34).

$S_{cv}O_2$ is a surrogate for mixed venous oxygenation, S_vO_2 and can provide information regarding global oxygen demand and supply. Several studies have demonstrated the use of $S_{cv}O_2$ in goal-directed therapy in both adult and pediatric studies treating sepsis and congenital heart disease. It is important to recognize the limitations of $S_{cv}O_2$. Values may vary depending on the sampling site. Additionally, as a marker of global oxygen delivery, it may be normal, or even high, in the face of regional perfusion abnormalities or impaired oxygen uptake and thus be falsely reassuring. Conversely, an abnormally low value is extremely specific for low cardiac output states and in the absence of significant anemia or hypoxia can be used as a therapeutic target (35).

Two things are important to note when monitoring this value. First, the relationship between $S_{cv}O_2$ and CO is nonlinear. Second, it is assumed that oxygen consumption and arterial oxygen content are stable (35).

Pulmonary artery catheter

The pulmonary artery catheter (PAC) was first introduced in 1970. The PAC can be inserted via the internal jugular, subclavian, femoral, and antecubital veins. However, the most limiting factor in pediatric patients is the catheter size, as the smallest PAC available is 5 Fr diameter (which includes cardiac output). Intraoperative use of PACs is limited and rarely performed in children. The directly measured physiological data available from the PAC include the pressures in the right atrium, right ventricle, pulmonary artery (PA), and PA occlusion pressure; mixed venous oxygenation; cardiac output (CO); and temperature. Additional calculated information, including stroke volume, systemic vascular resistance, pulmonary vascular resistance, oxygen transport, oxygen consumption, and oxygen extraction ratio can also be obtained (36).

Complications of PAC placement include problems with vessel cannulation, insertion, and maintenance. Vessel cannulation problems may include: arterial puncture, pneumothorax, hemothorax, hydrothorax, air embolism, thoracic injury, and bronchial injury. Insertion problems include: arrhythmias, cardiac conduction disturbances, catheter looping and knotting, pulmonary artery perforation, and valve damage. Maintenance problems include pulmonary infarction, venous thrombosis, infections, aseptic endocarditis, thrombocytopenia, and balloon rupture. Additional complications can include pulmonary hypertensive crisis and cardiac arrest (36).

There are a variety of methods which can be utilized to measure cardiac output, as described previously. Transpulmonary thermodilution CO is considered the gold standard in children. Clinical uses of PACs in pediatric patients include determination of fluid responsiveness, pulmonary hypertension, shock, and acute lung injury. The effect of fluid therapy can be determined by measuring CO before and after a fluid bolus. When CO (or, more precisely, SV) increases by > 10% to 15%, the patient is considered fluid responsive (37).

Recommendations for the use of right heart or PA catheterization in the assessment of pediatric pulmonary hypertension are as follows: 1. hemodynamic catheterization is recommended to confirm the diagnosis and establish severity (class I, level of evidence C); and 2. right heart catheterization with vasodilator testing is recommended to guide initial determination of therapy (class I, level of evidence B). The standard diagnostic criteria for pulmonary hypertension include the presence of mean pulmonary artery pressure > 25 mmHg with pulmonary artery occlusion pressure < 15 mmHg and pulmonary vascular resistance > 3 Wood units/m^2 (36).

Recommendations for the use of PAC in the assessment and management of shock are that the PA catheter can be used in those patients who remain in shock despite therapies directed to clinical signs of perfusion, mean arterial pressure–central venous pressure, central venous oxygen saturation, and echocardiographic analyses (class IIa, level of evidence C). Goal-directed therapy in shock includes interventions to maintain mixed venous oxygen saturation > 70%, cardiac index > 3.3 l/min/m^2, and a normal perfusion pressure for age (mean arterial pressure–central venous pressure) with the ultimate goal of restoration of normal perfusion (36).

Recommendations for the use of a PAC in the management of patients with ARDS or pulmonary edema are: 1. the PAC may be useful in selected pediatric patients with ARDS (class IIb, level of evidence C); and 2. the PAC may be useful in the diagnosis and management of uncertain causes of pulmonary edema (class IIb, level of evidence C). Strategies for managing ARDS include not only the manipulation of mechanical ventilation, but also nonventilatory modalities such as fluid restriction and selective use of pulmonary vasodilators. The PAC can be invaluable in assessing these therapies (36).

Oxygenation

Monitoring of oxygenation, ventilation, and gas concentration are three of the most important intraoperative tools anesthesiologists use to safely deliver general anesthesia (38). Monitoring oxygenation in pediatric anesthesia is even more important due to the increased oxygen consumption as compared to adults. The small functional residual capacity also can lead to increased hypoxemia when infants and children are rendered apneic, making oxygenation even more important. Inadequate ventilation is one of the most frequent things noted in the American Society of Anesthesiologists closed claims database (39). Reviews of closed claims, specifically in children, note respiratory complications as the most common event (39). Standard equipment should always be used in determining the adequacy of respiration, including but not limited to a stethoscope to auscultate breath sounds.

Pulse oximetry

Oxygenation is measured by pulse oximetry. Two wavelengths of light are used to differentiate between oxyhemoglobin and deoxyhemoglobin. Pulsations are noted in a probe that differentiates between two wavelengths of 660 nm and 930 nm (38). The probe has a built in algorithm that allows it to measure the oxyhemoglobin. Oxygenated blood absorbs a different wavelength than deoxygenated blood. This absorption is related to the percentage of saturation according to the Beer–Lambert law (38). The probe differentiates between systole and diastole, secondary to more blood flow during systole. Saturations in the range of 80% to 100% are considered accurate, with saturations less than 80% becoming increasingly less accurate.

Pulse oximetry can detect hypoxemia early in pediatric patients. It can be a warning to the quickness in which hypoxemia develops (40). The use of pulse oximetry has been shown to decrease the incidence of hypoxia and increase recognition of adverse events in dealing with oxygenation. Cote, *et al.* displayed the merit of the monitoring making this a standard monitor used during pediatric anesthesia (40). Pulse oximetry is a continuous monitor, but it does not reflect arterial saturation in real time. The measurement lags behind, with the monitor displaying an average for several of the last saturations. Pulse oximeters should be used as an early warning, not quantitative devices (38).

Pulse oximeters have a variety of limitations both in technical nature and clinical situations (38). Motion of an extremity is a major limitation and can be large in the pediatric population, especially upon induction of anesthesia. This problem can cause the sensor to interpret the motion as saturation or display nothing. Manufacturers have included different equations and safeguards to try and decrease the number of inaccurate readings and reduce false alarms (38). Other problems include being sensitive to operating room lighting. The probe can be sensitive to peripheral circulation and body temperature. Hemoglobin modalities other than normal adult or fetal hemoglobin can affect the pulse oximeter (40).

Cutaneous oxygenation monitors can also be used. Their use in pediatric anesthesia is especially helpful due to the thin layers of skin in neonates and infants, thus increasing the accuracy of the device (41). The patient's skin is warmed and a probe can detect the underlying oxygen concentration, which can be used to correlate with arterial oxygen concentration (42). Problems arise with thicker skin and occasional burns from the heating of the probe. This monitor is also highly variable and if possible should not be the only device used to determine oxygenation (40) (42).

Near infrared spectroscopy

Oxygenation can also be approximated using near infrared spectroscopy (NIRS). This monitoring provides information noninvasively about oxygenation in different parts of the body from cerebral to peripheral oxygenation (43). NIRS relies on similar aspects of the absorption of light in response to differing degrees of oxygenation or hypoxia. Light that is returned to the skin from the probe is analyzed and displayed through different algorithms (38). The use of NIRS does not rely on pulsatile flow and can be used in certain states such as cardiopulmonary bypass and circulatory arrest. The data from this monitor must be interpreted in the context of a clinical situation. The NIRS can be an accurate monitor of cerebral oxygenation (43). Significant decreases in reported number of NIRS approximating cerebral oxygenation has been shown to correlate with an actual decrease in cerebral oxygen concentration. In pediatric patients cerebral oximetry measured with NIRS revealed an improved neurologic score in patients undergoing treatment for hypoplastic left heart syndrome (44).

Ventilation

Ventilation is the discharge of carbon dioxide. It is the complicated exchange of carbon dioxide and oxygen in the lungs so the oxygen can be delivered to the tissues and carbon dioxide can be expelled (38). Ventilation is measured by capnometry and capnography. Capnometry measures the carbon dioxide at any point and time in the breathing circuit. This information is shown on a monitor in graphic display. Infrared light absorption is the measurement tool, and is accomplished by sampling gas. The gas can be sampled in mainstream or sidestream (45).

Mainstream sampling utilizes a sensor placed directly into the breathing circuit. The measurement is instant and does not require transport of gas to an analyzer. In pediatric anesthesia this type of sampling can prove to be dangerous in that the sensor is large and needs to be attached close to the y-piece adapter for accurate sampling (38). The sensor is heavy and could cause the dislodgment of smaller endotracheal tubes specifically in pediatric anesthesia. Dead space can also be added by a mainstream analyzer (46). Sidestream analyzers sample from the circuit and transport it to a machine some distance away. The tubing is usually long and thin. The added weight to the circuit with sidestream is negligible, but the problem arises in the sample tubing which can become occluded, kinked, or otherwise dislodged (38).

Capnography

Capnography differs from capnometry in the display of a graphic feature. Capnography is the graphic display of the measurement – capnometry, of exhaled carbon dioxide (47). This provides information on respiratory rate, breathing pattern, and can give information on degree of neuromuscular blockade. Capnography is the standard for confirming tracheal intubation (38). The method is not infallible with positive detection of carbon dioxide occurring with esophageal intubation from previously instilled gas into the stomach during mask ventilation. Capnography can be an early detection for many cardiovascular and metabolic disturbances. Carbon dioxide detection can be falsely negative with endotracheal intubation (40) within states with very low cardiac output including hypotension and cardiac arrest, high fresh gas flows, or any instance in which pulmonary blood flow is inefficient for gas exchange (38).

The normal end-tidal carbon dioxide begins with a rapid upstroke indicating the beginning of exhalation. The next part is a long plateau where tracheal dead space continues to generate carbon dioxide. The plateau carries a small upslope that continues until a peak is reached which equates to the end-tidal carbon dioxide measurement. The last part of the waveform is a rapid return to baseline that signifies inspiration. Many different pathologies and etiologies can be ascertained by the shape, slope, and overall location of the carbon dioxide waveform on the graph. For example, if the final down stroke does not reach zero then rebreathing can be occurring from increased dead space, pulmonary embolus, or a faulty expiratory valve (38).

Pediatric patients have differences in capnography from adult patients (48). In smaller infants there is not a plateau phase in the waveform. This is due to an increased respiratory rate, a large leak around the endotracheal tube, or a high sampling rate. In pediatrics it is sometimes difficult to use the end-tidal carbon dioxide waveform to accurately and reliably make decisions about ventilation secondary to the aforementioned reasons (46). Pediatric patients can have increases in the capnography waveform that can represent hypoventilation, but the increase can also occur from increased production of carbon dioxide, such as occurs with malignant hypothermia. A low number can indicate an increase in dead space ventilation or a problem in the sampling. Specific to pediatric congenital heart surgery, congenital heart diseases can also display inaccurate end-tidal measurements (38). Right to left intracardiac shunting causes blood to bypass the pulmonary artery and the lung, reducing the amount of blood participating in gas exchange.

Patient end-tidal carbon dioxide measurements approximate arterial carbon dioxide measurements (46). There are many issues and circumstances in which this approximation is not accurate. Accurate measurements rely on flow rate and volume of exhaled gas, the flow rate of the gas being aspirated to measure, fresh gas flow rate, location of sampling mechanism, and the type of breathing circuit (38). In smaller neonates and infants, these variables are even more important secondary to the very small exhaled tidal volumes.

Gas concentration

Other respiratory and anesthetic gases are measured to provide information regarding the patient and the concurrent physiology. The measurement is accomplished with a gas chromatograph, which works by accelerating particles in the presence of a magnet and the radius with which the particle is moved correlates with size (38). Algorithms analyzing size and movement can then display the concentration of differing gases such as volatile agents or nitrogen. The newer machines can analyze multiple gases at once. Volatile anesthetics can be a cardiac depressant and can have profound effects especially when used in very high concentrations, and the determination of levels at the conclusion of cases can be a valuable tool in emergence from anesthesia (49) (38). Finally, nitrogen can provide information on adequate preoxygenation, and can be helpful in the diagnosis of a venous air embolism (38).

Temperature

The American Society of Anesthesiologists has published guidelines for the intraoperative monitoring of pediatric patients under anesthesia (50). The body has a very effective regulatory system for temperature, including blood flow to areas of skin, changes in minute ventilation, sweat production, and metabolism; but this system can also be easily overwhelmed (51). Core and peripheral temperature are monitored in different and numerous ways. Core temperature includes the temperature of well-perfused organs, while peripheral temperature is primarily a part of the peripheral system and the musculoskeletal system (52). Hypothermia has often been accepted as an unfortunate but acceptable response to anesthesia and a surgical procedure.

Temperature regulation occurs primarily in the hypothalamus with an acceptable range of 36.8–37.2 degrees Celsius (51). Heat-sensitive areas are located in the preoptic area of the hypothalamus (52). The body uses peripheral sensors and efferent input to blood vessels, sweat glands, muscles, brown fat, and respiratory centers. Efferent output to receptors is both behavioral and autonomic (38) (51). Infants are more inclined to increased heat loss compared to adults, with the most important reason for this difference being the increased body surface area to weight ratio. Infants also have decreased shivering and need to generate heat through the metabolism of brown fat in order to liberate ATP and heat. This mechanism is active at birth and continues until two years of age (53).

Heat loss

Heat loss in the operating room occurs in four different mechanisms including radiation, convection, evaporation, and conduction. Radiant heat loss includes loss of heat from the body to the surroundings. The difference in temperature between the body and objects in the environment affect the rate of loss of body heat (54). Radiant heat loss is the single largest factor in heat loss in infants and children, and can be decreased by increasing the operating room temperature. Covering the patient also decreases radiant heat loss. Heat loss by convection deals with movement of air in contact with the body and the liberation of heat. The temperature gradient between the air and the body directly affects the amount of heat lost (55).

Evaporative loss accounts for at least one quarter of total heat loss (53). Evaporation heat loss occurs through the skin and the lungs. Infants are especially vulnerable due to the thin skin and have greater loss secondary to increased minute ventilation per kilogram of body weight as compared to adults. Increased heat loss can occur if the patient comes into contact with wet drapes or if the patient is wet (56). Conductive heat loss occurs between two surfaces that are in direct contact, including intravenous fluids and irrigation solutions. Conductive heat loss accounts for less than 3% of heat loss (56). The patient's skin should be kept away from cold metallic surfaces and fluids and irrigation should be warmed. Heat lost during the first hour of anesthesia is due to redistribution from the central compartment to the periphery (55).

Measures should be taken to keep the patient normothermic. Core temperature will drop 0.5–1 degree Celsius per hour (38). Morbidity associated with hypothermia includes delayed wound healing, impaired immune function, increased infection, and decreased coagulation. Other issues with hypothermia include a decrease in minimum alveolar concentration, cardiac depression, arrhythmias, and hypotension. Oxygen consumption increases with increasing hypothermia with infants and children while under general anesthesia. This can be a larger problem in the pediatric population because cardiac output in children is limited with an upper threshold (55).

Ideal temperature monitoring should accurately reflect core temperature in a safe manner (55). Monitoring in the perioperative setting is accomplished with thermocouples and thermistors. A thermocouple consists of two different metals that are aligned in a way that a current exists between the metals. The magnitude, of the difference in current, correlates with the temperature. A thermistor is type of thermometer consisting of a resistor made with a piece of metal. The resistance change when exposed to an object of a certain temperature is analyzed and the information is displayed (56). Infrared thermometers are generally used in the postanesthesia care unit, but these cannot give a continuous measurement (38). Temperature varies widely when measured in different parts of the body and differing compartments. The central temperature is thought to be the blood directly reaching the hypothalamus through the carotid arteries (53). Pulmonary artery catheters, esophageal, tympanic, and nasopharyngeal probes all measure the temperature of blood. Bladder and rectal temperature can also be used for central temperature. These can be used to approximate the temperature of the blood in the carotid arteries and therefore central temperature. Peripheral temperature can be measured with skin and oral probes (55).

Peripheral temperature measurement

Peripheral temperature is thought to be lower than core temperature and changes more quickly than core temperature. Peripheral temperature measurements do not accurately reflect core temperature, rather a regional temperature (57). This type of monitoring has minimal morbidity and is the most convenient. The measurements can vary widely between locations. Regional temperature is affected by regional blood flow. Sites of peripheral temperature measurement include skin, oral, and sometimes rectal (38). Skin temperature measurements are frequently made on forehead and in axilla. Skin temperature can be influenced by skin perfusion, equipment problems, and improper placement of the probe (57). Use of forced air warming can also influence skin temperature making the readings erroneous. The axillary temperature is the most often employed skin temperature (56). It has been reported to be as accurate as any other noninvasive method at measuring central temperature. The probe must be placed directly over the axillary artery for an accurate measurement, and misplacement is the largest problem. Oral probes are positioned in the oropharynx. These probes can be influenced by a number of things including oral secretions, entrapped air, and other devices, namely endotracheal tubes. Oral measurement is generally felt to be inaccurate and is not routinely used (38). Rectal temperature can mark peripheral temperature. Problems include stool, which can act as an insulator and the change lagging behind actual core temperature measurements (57).

Core temperature measurement

Core temperature can be approximated noninvasively with tympanic membrane, nasopharyngeal, and esophageal probes (38). Tympanic membrane temperature can be used to provide an easy and accurate approximation of central core temperature. The first thermometers designed for use in the ear carried significant risk. The more recent tympanic membrane temperature measurement devices use infrared technology making risk to the ear minimal. However, this measurement can be adversely influenced by air entrapment into the ear canal (57). Immediately post-cardiopulmonary bypass, the tympanic membrane does not correlate with the core temperature. Nasopharyngeal probes should be located in the posterior nasopharynx to reflect accurately the core temperature. Problems with this measurement include bleeding from the nasopharynx during insertion and cooling with ventilator gases when used with an uncuffed endotracheal tube, a mask or a laryngeal masked airway (55) (56). Esophageal temperature probes are becoming increasingly popular in the pediatric population. These probes are easily inserted and can be used as an esophageal stethoscope. The tip must be placed in the distal third of the esophagus for an accurate reading (58). Invasive core monitoring includes bladder and pulmonary artery catheter measurement. Bladder catheter temperature monitoring can be as accurate as pulmonary artery monitoring (56). Inaccuracy occurs with decreased urine output. The gold standard for core temperature monitoring is pulmonary artery temperature. Secondary to the invasive nature, this monitoring should be done only in critically ill infants and children who also need advanced monitoring (55). The site of measurement of body temperature should be driven by the surgical procedure as well as the associated comorbidities of the infant or child. More invasive and complicated surgical procedures will require invasive monitoring of perhaps more than one site; however, short procedures without much change in hemodynamics can usually be performed with axillary or skin temperature measurement (56).

References

1. Constant I, Sabourdin N. The EEG signal: a window on the cortical brain activity. *Pediatr Anesthes*. 2012; **22**: 539–52.
2. Clark JB, Barnes ML, Undar A, Myers JL. Multimodality neuromonitoring for pediatric cardiac surgery: our approach and a critical appraisal of the available evidence. *World J Pediatr Congenit Heart Surg*. 2012; **3**(I): 87–95.
3. The American Society of Anesthesiologists Task Force on Intraoperative Awareness. Practice advisory for intraoperative awareness and brain function monitoring. *Anesthesiology*. 2006; **104**: 847–64.
4. Münte S, Klockars J, van Gils M, *et al.* The Narcotrend index indicates age-related changes during propofol induction in children. *Anesth Analg*. 2009; **109**(1): 53–9.
5. Covidien. [Online]; 2010 [cited 2013 August 20. Available from: http://www.covidien.com/imageServer.aspx/doc229415.3.2.1_Adult%20Brochure.pdf?contentID=27528&contenttype=application/pdf.
6. Ghanayem S, Wernovsky G, Hoffman GM. Near-infrared spectroscopy as a hemodynamic monitor in critical illness. *Pediatr Crit Care Med*. 2011; **12**(Suppl): S27–32.

7. Smith M. Perioperative uses of transcranial perfusion monitoring. *Anesthesiology Clin.* 2007; **25**: 557–77.
8. Guarracino F. Cerebral monitoring during cardiovascular surgery. *Curr Opin Anaesthesiol.* 2008; **21**: 50–4.
9. Nelson DP, Andropoulos DB, Fraser Jr. CD. Perioperative neuroprotective strategies. *Semin Thorac Cardiovasc Surg Pediatr Card Surg Ann.* 2008; **11**: 49–56.
10. Grocott HP, Davie S, Fedorow C. Monitoring of brain function in anesthesia and intensive care. *Curr Opin Anaesthesiol.* 2010; **23**: 759–64.
11. Umamaheswara Rao GS, Durga P. Changing trends in monitoring brain ischemia: from intracranial pressures to cerebral oximetry. *Curr Op Anesthes.* 2011; **24**: 487–94.
12. Freye E. Cerebral monitoring in the operating room and the intensive care unit – an introduction for the clinician and a guide for the novice wanting to open a window to the brain. *J Clin Monit Comput.* 2005; **19**: 77–168.
13. Lall RR, Lall RR, Hauptman JS, *et al.* Intraoperative neurophysiological monitoring in spine surgery: indications, efficacy, and role of the preoperative checklist. *Neurosurg Focus.* 2012; **33**(5): 1–10.
14. Galloway G, Zamel K. Neurophysiologic intraoperative monitoring in pediatrics. *Pediatr Neurol.* 2011; **44**: 161–70.
15. Sala F, Manganotti P, Grossauer S, *et al.* Intraoperative neurophysiology of the motor system in children: a tailored approach. *Childs Nerv Syst.* 2010; **26**: 473–90.
16. Schwartz DM, Sestokas AK, Dormans JP, *et al.* Transcranial electric motor evoked potential monitoring during spine surgery: is it safe? *Spine.* 2011; **36**: 1046–9.
17. Dillon FX. Electromyographic (EMG) neuromonitoring in otolaryngology-head and neck surgery. *Anesthesiology Clin.* 2010; **28**: 423–42.
18. Malhotra NR, Shaffrey CI. Intraoperative electrophysiological monitoring in spine surgery. *Spine.* 2010; **35**(25): 2167–79.
19. Fuchs-Buder T, Schreiber JU, Meistelman C. Monitoring neuromuscular block: an update. *Anaesthesia.* 2009; **64**(Suppl. 1): 82–9.
20. ASA House of Delegates. American Society of Anesthesiologists. [Online]; 2010 [cited 2013 August 25. Available from: http://www.asahq.org/For-Members/Standards-Guidelines-and-Statements.aspx.
21. O'Connor M, McDaniel N, Brady WJ. The pediatric electrocardiogram Part I: Age-related interpretation. *Am J Emerg Med.* 2008; **26**: 506–12.
22. O'Connor M, McDaniel N, Brady WJ. The pediatric electrocardiogram Part II: Dysrhythmias. *Am J Emerg Med.* 2008; **26**: 348–58.
23. O'Connor M, McDaniel N, Brady WJ. The pediatric electrocardiogram Part III: Congenital heart disease and other cardiac syndromes. *Am J Emerg Med.* 2008; **26**: 497–503.
24. Westhorpe RN BC. Precordial and oesophageal stethoscopes. *Anaesth Intensive Care.* 2008;**36**(4):479.
25. Prielipp RC, Kelly S, Roy RC. Use of esophageal or precordial stethoscopes by anesthesia providers: are we listening to our patients? *J Clin Anesth.* 1995; **7**: 367–72.
26. Watson A, Visram A. Survey of the use of oesophageal and precordial stethoscopes in current paediatric anaesthetic practice. *Pediatr Anesth.* 2001; **11**: 437–42.
27. van Montfrans GA. Oscillometric blood pressure measurement: progress and problems. *Blood Pressure Monitoring.* 2001; **6**: 287–90.
28. Wan Y, Heneghan C, Stevens R, *et al.* Determining which automatic digital blood pressure device performs adequately: a systematic review. *J Hum Hypertens.* 2010; **24**: 431–8.
29. Sivarajan VB, Bohn D. Monitoring of standard hemodynamic parameters: Heart rate, systemic blood pressure, atrial pressure, pulse oximetry, and end-tidal CO2. *Pediatr Crit Care Med.* 2011; **12**(4 (Suppl.)): S2–11.
30. Edwards Lifesciences. [Online]; 2013 [cited 2013 August 30. Available from: http://www.edwards.com/products/mininvasive/Pages/flotracfaqs.aspx.
31. Hashim B, Lerner AB. The flotract system: measurement of stroke volume and the assessment of dynamic fluid loading. *Int Anesthesiol Clin.* 2010; **48**(1): 45–56.
32. Montenij LJ, de Waal EEC, Buhre WF. Arterial waveform analysis in anesthesia and critical care. *Curr Opin Anaesthesiol.* 2011; **24**: 651–6.
33. Bogert LWJ, Wesseling O, Schraa, EJ. *et al.* Pulse contour cardiac output derived from non-invasive arterial pressure in cardiovascular disease. *Anaesthesia.* 2010; **65**: 1119–25.
34. Frazier J. Edwards Lifesciences. [Online]; 2009 [cited 2013 August 31. Available from: http://ht.edwards.com/scin/edwards/sitecollectionimages/edwards/products/presep/ar04011pediasatwhpaper.pdf.
35. Spenceley N, MacLaren G, Kissoon N, Macrae DJ. Monitoring in pediatric cardiac critical care: A worldwide perspective. *Pediatr Crit Care Med.* 2011; **12**(Suppl.): S76–80.

36. Perkin RM, Anas N. Pulmonary artery catheters. *Pediatr Crit Care Med.* 2011; **12**(Suppl.): S12–20.
37. Lemson J, Nusmeier A, van der Hoeven JG. Advanced hemodynamic monitoring in critically ill children. *Pediatrics* 2011; **128** (3):560–71.
38. Litman RS, Cohen DE, Sclabassi RJ. *Anesthesia for Infants and Children*, 7th edn. Motoyama EK Davis PJ, eds. Philadelphia PA: Mosby Inc., 2006.
39. Morray JP, Geiduschek JM Caplan RA, *et al.* A comparison of pediatric and adult anesthesia closed malpractice claims. *Anesthesiology.* 1993; **78**(3): 461–7.
40. Cote CJ, Rolf N, Liu LMP, *et al.* A single-blind study of combined pulse oximetry and capnography in children. *Anesthesiology.* 1991; **74**(6): 980–7.
41. Monaco F, Nickerson B, Mcquity J. Continuous transcutaneous oxygen and carbon dioxide monitoring in the pediatric ICU. *Critical Care Medicine.* 1982; **10**(11): 765–6.
42. Cote CJ. Oxygenatinon and pediatric anesthesia. *Anesthesiology.* 1993 June; **6**(3): 532–6.
43. Tortorielo TA, Strayer SA Mott AR, *et al.* A noninvasive estimation of mixed venous oxygen saturation using near-infrared spectroscopy by cerebral oximetry in pediatric cardiac surgery patients. *Pediatr Anesth.* 2005; **15**(6): 495–503.
44. Hoffman GM, Stuth EA, Jaquiss RD, *et al.* Changes in cerebral and somatic oxygenation during stage 1 palliation of hypoplastic left heart syndrome using continuous regional cerebral perfusion. *J Thorac Cardiovasc Surg.* 2004; **127**(1): 223–33.
45. Stock M. Noninvasive carbon dioxide monitoring. *Crit Care Clin.* 1988; **4**(3): 511–26.
46. Wiedemann H, McCarthy K. Noninvasive monitoring of oxygen and carbon dioxide. *Clin Chest Med.* 1989; **10**(2): 239–54.
47. McQuillen KK, Steele DW. Capnography during sedation/analgesia in the pediatric emergency department. *Pediatric Emergency Care.* 2000; **16**(6): 401–4.
48. Krauss M B, Hess DR. Capnography for procedural sedation and analgesia in the Emergency Department. *Annals Emerg Med.* 2007; **50**(2): 172–81.
49. Roth DM, Swaney JS, Dalton ND, Gilpin EA, Ross Jr. J. Impact of anesthesia on cardiac function during echocardiography in mice. *Am J Physiol – Heart Circ Physiol* 2002 June; **282**(H2134–2140).
50. American Academy of Pediatrics. Guidelines for the pediatric perioperative anesthesia environment. *Pediatrics.* 1999; **103**(2): 512–15.
51. Morimoto T IT. Thermoregulation and body fluid osmolality. *JBasic Clin Physiol Pharmacol.* 1998; **9**(1): 51–72.
52. Bissonnette, B, Sessler, DI, Laflamme. Intraoperative temperature monitoring sites in infants and children and the effect of inspired gas warming on esophageal temperature. *Anesthes Analg.* 1989; **69**: 192–6.
53. Martin KA. Can there be a standard for temperature measurement in the pediatric intensive care unit? *AACN Adv Crit Care.* 2004; **15**(2): 254–6.
54. Sessler,DI. Temperature monitoring and perioperative thermoregulation. *Anesthesiology.* 2008; **2**(109): 318–38.
55. Pate MFD. *Critical Care Nursing of Infants and Children.* Second Edition ed. Curley MAQ, Moloney-Harmon PA, editors. Philadelphia PA: WB Saunders Company, 2001.
56. Barash PG, Cullen BF, Steolting RK, *et al. Clinical Anesthesia.* Sixth Edition., Philadelphia PA: Lippincott Williams and Wilkins, 2009.
57. Bailey JRP. Axillary and tympanic membrane temperature recording in the preterm neonate: A comparative study. *J Adv Nurs.* 2001; **34**: 465–74.
58. Holtzclaw B. Monitoring body temperature. *AACN Clinical Issues.* 1993; **4**: 44–55.

Anesthetic pharmacology: Physiologic states, pathophysiologic states, and adverse effects

Camila Lyon and Dolores B. Njoku

Pharmacokinetics and pharmacodynamics

Blood–brain barrier[1–3]

The blood–brain barrier (BBB) regulates the entry of proteins, electrolytes, vitamins, minerals, fatty acids, peptides, and medicines into the CNS. The regulation mechanisms mature with age and can be altered by disease. The primary function of the blood brain barrier is threefold: 1. inhibition of intercellular passage of molecules by tight junctions between endothelial cells; 2. inhibition of intracellular passage because of inherent low pinocytic activity; and 3. specific transport systems within endothelial cells that actively transport nutrients into the brain while toxins are actively transported out. Adult BBB permeability is reached by two months of age. Physical and enzymatic barrier functions within tight junctions exist to maintain brain homeostasis in children. Thus, drug metabolizing proteins actively metabolize lipophilic drugs such as fentanyl and/or promote drug efflux. However, barbiturates and morphine penetrate the blood–brain barrier in neonates and are in essence "trapped" when compared to adults.

Drug absorption[4,5]

Oral medications are a commonly used form in children. Neonates have a higher gastric pH, slower gastric and intestinal motility, slower intestinal drug transport, and limited bacterial flora. Therefore neonates, infants, and small children may have a slower onset of action of per oral (PO) medications. Intramuscular drugs have a higher bioavailability in neonates and infants due to increased muscle capillaries in this vessel-rich group. Immature livers can lead to higher bioavailability in rectally administered medications that undergo first-pass metabolism. Rectal drugs may also be expelled more quickly. Thinner skin, large surface area, and increased perfusion increase the bioavailability of transdermal medications.

Drug distribution[6,7]

Drug distribution is affected by total body water, fat, and protein. Neonates and infants have a larger body water percentage than children and adults. This results in larger volume of distribution for hydrophilic drugs and lower intravascular drug concentration. With time. extracellular water decreases while intracellular water increases to reach adult levels. Lipophilic drugs are less affected by distribution outside of the brain even though body fat has a sharp increase at 3–6 months of age. Total body protein is relatively lower in children. Hence, decreased albumin and alpha-1-acid glycoprotein concentrations in neonates may result in increased free drug concentrations.

Neuromuscular system[8,9]

Neuromuscular transmission pathways include the spinal cord, motor neurons, and endplates between nerves and muscle fibers. Acetylcholine nicotinic receptors involved in the transmission of impulses are clustered at these endplates. Adult receptors are predominant at birth, with few fetal (also called extra-junctional receptors) that can proliferate in cases of nerve damage. These endplate receptors are the main site of action of neuromuscular blocking drugs, with some activity in presynaptic receptors as well.

At birth, the neuromuscular system is not completely developed and continues to mature throughout childhood. Motor nerve conduction velocities increase throughout gestation with slow synaptic transmission and acetylcholine release rates at birth. Myotubules continue the process of connecting to

Essentials of Pediatric Anesthesiology, ed. Alan David Kaye, Charles James Fox and James H. Diaz. Published by Cambridge University Press. © Cambridge University Press 2015.

muscle fibers, acetylcholine receptors mature in function and distribution, slow twitch fibers increase in the diaphragm and intercostal muscles in the first 6 months of life. All of these changes make infants less than 2 months old have a greater degree of block for a specific plasma concentration which fade at higher rates of stimulation and lower TOF ratios. Neonates and infants are more sensitive to neuromuscular blockade than children and adults, with premature neonates showing the highest sensitivity.

There are two types of drugs that can stop neuromuscular transmission: depolarizing and nondepolarizing neuromuscular blockers. Nondepolarizing blockers competitively bind to the α subunit of postsynaptic acetylcholine receptors preventing action potentials. High frequency stimulation and TOF fade is characteristic. Since these drugs are competitive antagonists, they can be antagonized by high levels of acetylcholine provided by acetylcholinesterase inhibitors such as neostigmine and edrophonium, as well as low-dose succinylcholine. Of the depolarizing medicines, only succinylcholine is available in the USA. The drug depolarizes endplate and extrajunctional receptors and remains in the receptor causing desensitization and preventing the action potential. Because it is an agonist of the receptor, muscle firing or fasciculations are seen when it first binds, followed by relaxation. Twitch height decrease is observed but minimal TOF and tetanic fade. When an infusion, a second dose, or very high doses of succinylcholine is given, TOF and tetanic fade is apparent and this is called phase II or nondepolarizing block, which can be antagonized by neostigmine.

The ED_{95} is the dose of neuromuscular blocker that produces 95% adductor pollicis blockade. For most nondepolarizers, this dose is higher in children than in infants and adults, with the exception of atracurium. The onset of action tends to be faster in children. Duration of action is measured as the time to return to 25% of baseline (T_{25}); at this time four twitches using TOF stimulation are present. If further relaxation is needed, 0.25–0.3 times the intubation dose should be given as maintenance. Reversal agents should be given at T_{25} for full recovery.

Biotransformation and excretion

Drug metabolism occurs in the liver, kidneys, intestines, lungs, blood, and other tissues. The majority of drug metabolism is performed by the liver (80%), and this is true of sedatives, opioids, and neuromuscular blockers. Hence biotransformation will be affected by enzymatic activity as well as blood flow to the liver. Phase I reactions (oxidation, reduction, hydrolysis) modify drug structure to make the drug more water soluble. The bulk of these reactions use cytochrome P450. Phase II reactions (glucoronidation, sulphation, glutathione conjugation) add a molecule to the drug to make it more water soluble. Before the first month of life there is very low phase I metabolism, and drugs such as midazolam will have a long clearance time.

Phase I metabolism approximates adult levels at 1 year of age. The timing of reaching adult levels for phase II metabolism depends on the enzyme system. Sulfotransferases are mature at birth and have increased activities when compared to adult levels. However, glucuronidation reaches adult levels by 6 – 18 months and N-acetyl transferase 2 reaches adult levels by 1–3 years of age. As examples, morphine clearance is conjugated by phase II enzymes that reach adult levels by as early as 2 – 3 months but certainly by 6 months for most infants. Acetaminophen undergoes both phase I and phase II metabolism, and clearance is markedly higher at 1 year of age compared to neonates. Esterase activity is similar to adults, and drugs such as remifentanil and esmolol will have similar clearance.

In infants, kidney metabolism is predominant for water-soluble drugs, as hepatic metabolism is immature. When renal excretion plays a large role in metabolism, clearance rates resemble renal function (GFR). The GFR is 10% of adult levels at term and reaches adult levels by one year. Clearance is also affected by coexisting disease and drug interactions.

Pharmacogenetics

Genetic variation is a growing field in medicine and may explain why patients react differently to medications. Polymorphism of enzymes that activate or metabolize medications can affect a drug's maximum effect as well as clearance. Cytochrome P450 CYP2D6 metabolizes around 25% of current drugs including opioids; 74 allelic variants of this cytochrome have been reported.[12] Patients can be poor or ultrafast metabolizers of codeine, which affects levels of plasma morphine in their system.[13] Gene polymorphisms have been found to affect postoperative response to pain after morphine.[14] Future research will likely elucidate more information on what population perceives more pain as well as medication tailoring.

Nonopioid analgesics

Nonopioid analgesics are commonly used adjuncts to opioid analgesia. In this group, nonsteroidal anti-inflammatory agents (NSAIDs) work by attenuating increased prostaglandin levels triggered by noxious stimuli. Ketorolac, a commonly used NSAID, can be given orally, intravenously, and intranasally. The IV route is commonly used with a dose of 0.5 mg/kg. Single-dose pharmacokinetics is similar in adults and children.[16] In addition to analgesia, antiemetic properties as well as the ability to decrease bladder spasm has been attributed to ketorolac. Because it is an NSAID, there are concerns about kidney damage. Two studies found no changes in renal function post cardiac surgery with the use of ketorolac; one of the studies noted no increased need of transfusions.[17, 18] One study in infants 6–18 months old showed no increased surgical drain output, changes in renal or hepatic function tests, and one study in infants 2–6 months old showed no adverse effects[20,21] Another concern is the possibility of decreased bone healing. In a study of posterior spinal fusions, children receiving ketorolac had the same incidence of pseudo-orthosis as the children who did not receive it.[19] Ketorolac does induce platelet dysfunction secondary to reversible inhibition of cyclo-oxygenase. Platelet dysfunction recovers once the NSAID is excreted.

Although almost never utilized in children because of past associations with Reye's syndrome, aspirin is also a member of the NSAID group. Aspirin also increases bleeding time from platelet dysfunction caused by irreversible cyclo-oxygenase inhibition. Thus, for resolution of platelet dysfunction following ketorolac, the drug must be excreted and disassociated from cyclooxygenase; however, for resolution of platelet dysfunction following aspirin, additional platelets have to be formed.

Acetaminophen is another nonopioid analgesic. Acetaminophen has antipyretic and analgesic effects, likely due to inhibition of prostaglandins. Oral and IV forms are available at doses of 10–15 mg/kg for a maximum of 60 mg/kg/day for infants and children. Total daily dose should not exceed 4 grams. Rectal doses may be higher, up to 30–40 mg/kg. Overdose may cause liver damage. Infants appear to generate less of a hepatotoxic compound through metabolism and therefore may have a wider margin of safety. However, clearance is decreased in neonates, and acetaminophen in premature infants may have an even longer half-life.

Opioid analgesics

In general, opioid analgesics are more potent in neonates and infants than in adults. There are age-dependent differences in pharmacokinetics and pharmacodynamics. Lipophilic drugs readily cross the BBB in neonates and infants.

Fentanyl is a short-acting opioid given in an IV (1–10 mcg/kg), patch, intranasal (1–2 mcg/kg), and transmucosal formulations. The fentanyl buccal tablet is reserved for adults because of the high doses needed. High doses may cause bradycardia and chest wall rigidity. Preterm neonates have decreased fentanyl clearance, but term neonates have clearances similar to adults. A slow wean from continuous infusions is a must because of the rapid development of "tolerance" in this format.

Sufentanil (1–3 mcg/kg) has a shorter elimination half-life, less respiratory depression, and longer analgesia duration than fentanyl. Neonates have longer half-lives than older children. Alfentanil is another short-acting analog of fentanyl with one-third the duration of action. It is metabolized by CYP3A5 and therefore has high individual variability. Patients with liver and kidney disease have decreased protein binding which may increase alfentanil's free fraction. Newborns have longer elimination half-lives, but older infants have normal clearances. Patients with kidney disease show an increased volume of distribution and those with liver disease show an increased half-life. Respiratory depression and muscle rigidity can happen with sufentanil and alfentanil. Heart rate, MAP, and SVR may decrease with alfentanil and it does not block the neuroendocrine stress response as well as fentanyl and sufentanil. Fentanyl, sufentanil, and alfentanil cause a significant but transient increase in ICP, decrease in MAP, and CPP.[25]

Remifentanil is an ultra-short-acting opioid metabolized by blood and tissue esterases. It has an extremely short half-life of 10 minutes. The half-life does not change with age and it is unaffected by cardiopulmonary bypass. Remifentanil may cause tolerance and hyperalgesia demonstrated by increased opioid requirements after surgery. These effects have been associated with remifentanil doses greater than 0.4 mcg/kg/min.[26]

Morphine is a long-acting opioid drug with a half-life of 2–3 hours that is available in oral (0.3 mg/kg) and parenteral (0.1–02 mg/kg) forms. It is metabolized by the liver (and possibly the intestines and kidneys) and excreted in the kidneys. The metabolites have analgesic and respiratory activity and high plasma concentrations of these metabolites can be seen in chronic kidney disease. There is large individual variability, but morphine clearance is slower in preterm, younger, and critically ill neonates possibly caused by accumulation of morphine 3 glucuronide.[23] By one year of age, clearance is almost at adult levels. Intranasal morphine has been used in adults.[24] Meperidine is available in oral and parenteral forms. The active metabolite normeperidine can cause tremors and seizures in patients with decreased kidney function. It has opioid and local anesthetic properties. It is commonly used for postoperative shivering.

Methadone is a long-acting opioid with a half-life of 24–36 hours. It is available in IV (0.1–0.2 mg/kg with 0.05 mg/kg supplemental dose every 4–12 hours) and PO (0.2–0.4 mg/kg) forms. It is effectively used in the perioperative period, with studies suggesting longer analgesia, fewer postoperative opioid doses, and lower cumulative postoperative opioid use. The onset of action is fast at 4–8 minutes. Methadone may prolong the QT interval, an effect that may be enhanced by hypokalemia.

Oxycodone (0.1 mg/kg) and hydrocodone (0.05–0.1 mg/kg) are oral opioids often used to transition from IV opioids to oral. Oxycodone has high individual variability, has a peak concentration in 25 minutes, and a clearance that increases with age reaching adult levels by 2–6 months.[28] Patients with hepatic or renal impairment have longer half-lives. Hydrocodone is a semisynthetic derivative of codeine.[29] Codeine is also a commonly used oral opioid (1 mg/kg), also available in rectal and intramuscular forms. Peak effect is seen in 30 minutes. Codeine is metabolized to morphine in order to have an effect and this is accomplished by CYP2D6. However, genetic variability of this enzyme – some patients are poor metabolizers and some extensive metabolizers – affects efficacy in the population. Because of the variability in metabolism triggered by wide variations in CYP2D6, and the potential for dangerous levels of morphine in some patients, many anesthesiologists are favoring other drugs instead of codeine.

Sedative and anxiolytic agents

Sedatives and anxiolytics can be utilized as adjuncts for opioids as well as inhaled halogenated gas. In some cases these agents are utilized for total intravenous anesthesia. In general, increased total body water results in a large volume of distribution for these agents. Termination of drug effect is determined by redistribution. In the neonate duration of action may be affected by changes in the blood brain barrier.

Benzodiazepines can be used for anterograde amnesia, sedation, reducing anxiety, and as an adjunct during induction and in balanced anesthesia. Diazepam is the traditionally used benzodiazepine. At doses of 0.2–0.3 mg/kg, diazepam sedates with less cardiac depression than barbiturates. The drug's metabolism slows with younger ages and it can cause pain on injection.

Midazolam has minimal venous irritation and pain, amnesia, short duration, and a short mild respiratory depression time. It decreases blood pressure and increases heart rate. It can be safely administered to children with cyanotic congenital heart disease. It is given at doses of 0.15 mg/kg IV with a half- life of 70 minutes. Peak times for IM, rectal, and oral administration are 15, 30, and 53 minutes. Commonly used oral midazolam doses are 0.5 mg/kg; however, 0.2–0.3 mg/kg has been suggested as adequate.[32] Midazolam can be given rectally at doses of 0.3mg/kg and intranasally at doses of 0.2–0.3 mg/kg. Teens absorb the drug half as fast as children and have a slower half-time after IV administration. Full-term neonates clear the drug 1.6 times faster than preterm neonates. Side effects include paradoxical agitation, dysphoria, loss of balance, blurred vision, and hiccups. Metabolism of midazolam is inhibited by drugs or agents that reduce cytochrome oxidase: grapefruit juice, erythromycin, calcium channel blockers, and protease inhibitors. Benzodiazepines can be reversed by flumazenil.

Etomidate is a short-acting sedative with an onset of 5–15 seconds and duration of 3–5 minutes. The drug has minimal effects on cardiovascular function and blood pressure and therefore may be helpful in compromised patients. Side effects include myoclonus, pain on injection, and adrenal suppression. Even a single dose can impair adrenal function and increase mortality in critically ill children.[33] Etomidate can also cause epileptiform activity in known seizure disorder patients. The induction dose is 0.3–0.4 mg/kg.

Propofol is a rapidly distributed and metabolized drug that can be used in infusions without significant buildup. The context-sensitive half- life of a propofol infusion is 10–20 minutes. Blood pressure decreases and cardiac output mildly decreases. Despite these hemodynamic changes, propofol does not appear to change shunt fractions in congenital heart disease.[34] Propofol decreases cerebral blood flow. It can cause pain on injection and spontaneous excitatory movements. It has some antiemetic effect. Propofol doses are 3 mg/kg for infants, 2.5 mg/kg for children, and 1–1.5 mg/kg for older children. Higher induction doses for infants and young children reflect the large volume of distribution in these age groups. There are concerns with using this drug for long-term ICU management (greater than 12 hours) because of the risk for propofol infusion syndrome. Propofol infusion syndrome includes arrhythmia, lipemic plasma, hepatomegaly, metabolic acidosis, myocardial failure, and rhabdomyolysis.

Ketamine is a phencyclidine derivative that provides sedation while maintaining muscle tension, laryngeal irritability, and the gag reflex. Respiration and blood pressures are maintained, although ketamine has direct negative inotropic effects that may be seen in catecholamine-depleted patients. In normal patients, tachycardia and hypertension are usually seen in addition to salivation, postoperative nausea and vomiting and hallucinations. Ketamine can cause increased EEG seizure activity, increased CSF pressures, and increased ocular pressures as well as nystagmus. Infants require higher dosing to decrease movement but have slower clearance than older children. These high doses may induce apnea. Dysphoria can be noted in older children. Oral ketamine is dosed at 3–6 mg/kg and IV 0.5–2 mg/kg.

Clonidine and dexmedetomidine are central α2 agonists. Clonidine can be used for premedication, as an adjunct, or to prolong analgesia in regional and central blocks. Clonidine can cause hypotension and bradycardia, often requiring atropine premedication. Epidural clonidine may increase apnea in infants. It can be given in doses of 1–2 mcg/kg. Dexmetomidine is more selective than clonidine for α2 receptors. It can be used as a sedative, anxiolytic, and analgesic without respiratory depression. Hypertension is usually seen when first injected, followed by hypotension. Bradycardia may also be an affect. Doses are 1 mcg/kg loading dose over 10 minutes followed by 0.2–0.7 mcg/kg/hr infusion for the IV route and 1–2 mcg/kg intranasally. The half-life is 2 hours. It can be used to treat postoperative delirium and shivering. Clearance increases with age.

Barbiturates were formerly the predominant sedative given but are now rarely used due to observed side effects, alternative medications available and drug shortages. Barbiturates cross the blood brain barrier more on neonates than adults, and neonates have a decreased ability to metabolize these drugs. Thiopental is a short-acting barbiturate that is useful as an antiepileptic and in the treatment of increased ICP. Doses are 3 mg/kg for neonates and 6 mg/kg for infants and older children. Methohexital is even shorter acting, and often used for electroconvulsive therapy as it lowers seizure thresholds. It can be given in doses of 1–2 mg/kg.

Antiemetics

Postoperative nausea and vomiting is a common cause of delayed discharge from PACU and unplanned admission of ambulatory patients. Risk factors include postpuberty females, nonsmokers, history of postoperative nausea and vomiting or motion sickness, increased length of surgery, use of volative anesthetics, nitrous oxide, neostigmine, and opioids. Other possible risk factors include history of migraine, perioperative anxiety, decreased IV fluids, and duration of anesthesia. Postoperative vomiting is infrequent in children less than 1 year of age and the use of antiemetics may be unwarranted[35]

If postoperative nausea and vomiting is predicted, available antiemetics include 5-hydroxytryptamine type 3 receptor antagonists (ondansetron, granisetron, dolasetron, tropisetron), steroids (dexamethasone), dopamine antagonists (metoclopramide, prochlorperazine perphenazine), and antihistamines (dimenhydrinate, promethazine). The 5-HT3 antagonists are superior to metaclopramide in the prevention of postoperative vomiting in children and therefore first choice. Dual therapy is more effective than monotherapy; patients at moderate to high risk should receive two or more interventions.[38] Other measures that may be beneficial include preoperative anxiolysis, aggressive hydration, propofol as the anesthetic agent, avoiding nitrous oxide, minimizing opioids through the use of adjuvant pain medications and regional anesthesia, slow titration of PO intake, and slow ambulation.[39]

Ondansetron is one of the most widely used 5-HT3 antagonists. Usual doses are 0.1–0.15 mg/kg every 6 hours with a max of 4 mg/dose. A second dose may be repeated if nausea persists in children > 2 years of age; the half-life is decreased in children younger than 2 years by 50% making repeated dosing unnecessary.[40] These medications are well tolerated;

however, common side effects include fever, headache, dizziness, and constipation. In 2011, the FDA issued a warning that ondansetron may prolong the QT interval. Ondansetron is the only drug in this class approved for children < 2 years of age, with dolasetron approved for children aged 2 and older. The dose for dolasetron is 0.35 mg/kg.

Dexamethasone is also utilized to reduce postoperative nausea and vomiting. Dexamethasone's dose is 0.15 mg/kg with a maximum dose of 8 mg. Dexamethasone may also improve pain control in tonsillectomy patients. There's evidence that the best available treatment is a combination of dexamethasone and a 5-HT3 antagonist.[41]

Other antiemetics are usually utilized as an adjunct to ondanestron and dexamethasone. In this category, the antihistamine diphenhydramine has an effect at a dose of 0.5 mg/kg up to 25 mg, and promethazine in a dose of 0.25–1 mg/kg up to 25 mg; both drugs may cause significant sedation. Metoclopramide has direct effects on the chemoreceptor trigger zone and it stimulates gastric emptying through the antagonism of dopamine. Doses are 0.15 mg/kg every 6 hours. Prochlorperazine is a dopamine antagonist effective at doses of 0.1–0.13 mg/kg every 8–12 hours and should not be used in patients with WBC < 1000.

Droperidol is another dopamine antagonist that has been used at doses of 0.01–0.015 mg/kg up to 1.25 mg. Recent concerns with extrapyramidal symptoms and cardiac effects have caused many pediatric anesthesiologists to refrain from using it in children. Perphenazine is only available as an oral formulation in the USA and is given at doses of 0.07 mg/kg. All of the dopamine antagonists may prolong the QT interval and therefore caution must be observed when multiple QT-prolonging drugs are given or in patients with risk factors for torsades de pointes.

Inhaled anesthetics

Inhaled anesthetics are the most commonly used anesthetic agents in children. The amount of anesthetic delivered is dependent upon three factors: inspired concentration, alveolar ventilation, and functional residual capacity. Differences in neonates and infants can increase rate of alveolar (FA) to inspired (FI) concentration in neonates. Even so alveolar ventilation, specifically ventilation to FRC ratio is the primary determinant of the rate of delivery when comparing neonates and adults: 5:1 in neonates compared to 1.5:1 in adults. Moreover, this is effect is more pronounced in more soluble anesthetics. Cardiac output is the primary determinant of rate of removal or uptake from the lungs. Hence, the rate of rise of FA/FI is inversely proportional to cardiac output. Neonates represent a special situation where this relationship may produce a directly proportional effect. In this situation, while neonates have higher cardiac output, preferential distribution to the vessel-rich group may increase anesthetic delivery. The currently used anesthetics for inhalation include sevoflurane, isoflurane desflurane, and nitrous oxide.

The MAC rises during the neonatal period, peaks in infancy, and declines for the rest of life. Sevoflurane is an exception, with MAC peaking in neonates. All halogenated inhalational anesthetics cause hypotension in a dose-dependent fashion and can cause tachycardia. Desflurane may have direct inhibition effects on the myocardium, with neonates being the most sensitive to this. The decrease in blood pressure is higher with younger patients.

All the agents depress ventilatory drive and the response to increased CO_2, although they cause rapid shallow breathing at low MAC. Isoflurane and sevoflurane are bronchodilators; desflurane can worsen respiratory dynamics in children with airway reactivity.[44] Desflurane can produce carbon monoxide when exposed to desiccated soda lime or baralyme. Sevoflurane can produce compound A, which has been found to cause kidney damage in rats. Although there is no evidence of human damage, some recommend keeping fresh gas flow at least at 2 l/min when using closed circuits with baralyme or soda lime and sevoflurane. All volatile agents decrease cerebral metabolic rates, cause direct cerebral vasodilation, and alter CO_2 responsiveness. They may trigger malignant hyperthermia in susceptible individuals.

Nitrous oxide can be used to speed the uptake of the volatile anesthetics. Side effects include expansion of air-filled cavities, including the middle ear, which may cause postop discomfort in children. This would also include the ocular globe, the cranium, GI, endotracheal tube cuff, and pneumothoraxes.

Local anesthetics

Local anesthetics act through sodium channel blockade which results in preventing action potentials in nerve cells. They may also have effects on G-protein receptors. All local anesthetics are weak bases.

Lipophilicity, degree of ionization, pH of the solution, and protein binding determine the potency and duration of action of local anesthetics.[47] The pH of the solution determines the ionization fraction and therefore activity of the drug. This property can be exploited by adding bicarbonate to increase the onset of the drug action.

Local anesthetics are used in central blocks through spinals, epidurals, and caudals, as well as peripheral nerve blocks. The speed of absorption and peak plasma concentration varies depending on the site. Therefore, although maximum bolus dosing is recommended by manufacturers for each local anesthetic, this will depend on the site of injection. The order of absorption from highest to lowest is intercostal, tracheal, caudal, epidural, brachial plexus, and subcutaneous. Epinephrine can be added to the solution to decrease absorption through vascular constriction. Epinephrine should not be used for penile blocks.

Local anesthetics are bound to proteins, especially alpha1-acid glycoprotein (AAG), with 65% of lidocaine and 95% of bupivacaine, and ropivacaine bound. Neonates and infants have lower levels of AAG, and free fraction of local anesthetic is increased. Infants 0–3 months have higher free ropivacaine than infants 3–12 months. The concentration of AAG increases with inflammation, which can be protective. This effect only lasts 48 hours, at which time some recommend terminating continuous infusions in infants under 6 months as total bupivacaine concentration in plasma tends to increase. Local anesthetics also bind to RBCs and polycythemia may be protective. Acidosis changes protein binding and increases risk of toxicity.

Two main groups of local anesthetics include amides and esters. Amide local anesthetics are metabolized by the liver. The clearance of bupivicaine is only one-third the adult clearance at 1 month and two-thirds at 6 months. Ropivicaine's clearance is not as low as expected and the drug may be used in younger patients, but clearance won't reach normal levels until age 5.[48] Lidocaine has a longer half life in children compared to adults. The lungs extract amide local anesthetics and infants with right-to-left cardiac shunts may be at higher risk of toxicity. The duration of action is shorter in neonates and infants possibly due to age-related pharmacodynamics and immaturity of the nervous system. With regards to ester local anesthetics, decreased neonatal plasma pseudocholinesterase may be a factor in utilizing these agents even though 2,3 chlorprocaine may be preferred for neonates since there is less ion trapping. Methmoglobin reductase is also immature in neonates and must be considered.

Doses of commonly used local anesthetic depend on the drug and the site of injection. For single shot caudal epidural 0.25% bupivacaine and 0.2% ropivacaine can be given at doses of 0.5–1.25 ml/kg depending on the level desired. Maximum bolus dose of bupivacaine is 3 mg/kg, lidocaine 5 mg/kg, and lidocaine with epinephrine 7 mg/kg. For bupivacaine infusions after single-bolus rates of 0.2–0.4 mg/kg/hr for infants and 0.2–0.75 mg/kg/hr for children have been utilized.

Local anesthetic toxicity presents initially with CNS signs – tinnitus, changes in taste, altered mental status, seizures – followed by cardiac toxicity, including arrhythmias, heart blocks, and asystole. Neonates may be more prone to myocardial toxicity due to higher heart rates. Hypoxia, acidosis, hypothermia, and electrolyte abnormalities all increase toxicity. Drugs that only have one enantiomer such as ropivacaine and L-bupivacaine have less cardiac toxicity. If toxicity is detected, intralipid can be used as a sink for local anesthetic at doses of 1.5 ml/kg of 20% lipid emulsion bolus followed by 0.25 ml/kg/min for at least 10 minutes after return of stability. The maximum dose is 10 ml/kg per 30 minutes. More information can be obtained at lipidrescue.org.

Neuromuscular blocking and reversal agents[49–51]

Neuromuscular blocking agents facilitate intubation, immobility during surgery, and ventilation in the operating room and ICU. They decrease metabolic demand, prevent shivering and nonsynchronous ventilation, and may decrease ICP. The average doses of these drugs in children is similar to adults, but the variability of dose requirements is greater. Infants have a larger volume of distribution, but a higher number of extrajunctional receptors in skeletal muscles and a greater degree of block for a specific plasma concentration. Neuromuscular blockage should be monitored as a guide to dosage. Volatile anesthetics, including nitrous oxide, augment neuromuscular blockage intensity. Blockade is also augmented by some antibiotics, hypothermia, acidosis, hypocalcemia, and hypermagnesemia.

Succinylcholine is the only depolarizing neuromuscular blocking agent currently available in the USA. It has the fastest onset of action of the neuromuscular blockers of 0.5–0.9 minutes and therefore it is the ideal drug for rapid sequence intubation. However, studies have shown that propofol and remifentanil can produce good intubating conditions compared to propofol and succinylcholine. Doses are 2 mg/kg IV in infants, 1 mg/kg in children, and 3–4 mg/kg IM in both age groups (onset 3–4 minutes). The duration of action is 5.2 minutes, making this drug safest for possible cannot-intubate-or-ventilate scenarios where muscle relaxation is needed. As IV succinylcholine causes bradycardia commonly in children and may lead to asystole, atropine or glycopyrrolate premedication is recommended. The IM route has a minimal effect on heart rate. It can cause life-threatening hyperkalemia in patients with myopathies, and thus should not be given routinely to children as they may be too young to have signs of these disorders. The only recommended use in children is in emergency control of airways. Hyperkalemia may also be seen in patients with burns or strokes. Succinylcholine can cause masseter spasms, myalgias, and may trigger malignant hyperthermia in susceptible individuals.

The remaining neuromuscular blockers are in the nondepolarizer group. These drugs are usually divided into intermediate-acting and short- and long-acting groups. Rocuronium is an intermediate-acting blocker. It is the alternative to succinylcholine for rapid sequence intubation with an onset of 1.3 minutes in children (+2 minutes in 1–5 year olds) and 0.6 minutes in infants at a dose of 0.6 mg/kg. The average recovery time is 26 minutes in children and 42 minutes in infants. It may cause tachycardia in children and pain on injection. Rocuronium can have prolonged and unpredictable recovery time in neonates and therefore some pediatric anesthesiologists do not use this drug in children younger than 6 months. Recovery times range from 45–100 minutes. Intramuscular rocuronium may not produce satisfactory intubating conditions. Vecuronium is another intermediate-acting agent with onset time of 1.3–1.5 minutes at doses of 0.1 mg/kg. It has a longer duration of action in neonates and infants (73 minutes) than children (35 minutes) and adults (53 minutes). Both of these drugs undergo metabolism in the liver and kidneys. Cisastracurium is an intermediate-acting agent that undergoes Hoffman elimination and therefore is the choice agent for patients with moderate–severe kidney and liver dysfunction. At doses of 0.15 mg/kg the onset is 1.2 minutes in infants, and 2.2 minutes in children. Duration is longer in infants (55 minutes) than in children (34 minutes). Pancuronium is the only drug in the long-acting group. This long-acting nondepolarizing blocker has vagolytic properties in children (minimal in infants), which may improve cardiac output. In the past years there have been several short-acting nondepolarizers that have been developed; however, when these agents were released on the market, it was soon discovered that they actually belonged in the intermediate-acting group. Gantacurium is the only ultra-short acting nondepolarizing blocker in development.

Neuromuscular blockade reversal is recommended when T_{25} is reached, that is, when 3–4 twitches are present of the TOF. At this point, 70–75% of receptors are blocked. Reversal can be accomplished with acetylcholinesterase inhibitors, increasing the concentration of acetylcholine at the neuromuscular junction. Neostigmine is the classically used drug for neuromuscular blockade reversal. The recommended dose of neostigmine is 50 mcg/kg, edrophonium 0.5–1 mg/kg and pyridostigmine 350 mcg/kg. Another drug, edrophonium is more rapid than neostigmine but less effect to reserve profound blocks. Glycopyrrolate should be administered with neostigmine and atropine with edrophonium to block muscarinic effects. Higher doses of neostigmine may cause nausea. Sugammadex is an agent that uncapsulates rocuronium reversing its blockade and turning it into a short-acting agent. It has not yet been approved in the USA.

Sympathetic and parasympathetic agents[52,53]

Hypotension can occur in the operating room in critically ill and even in healthy children during the administration of a seemingly routine anesthetic. It is imperative that the pediatric anesthesiologist recognizes hypotension in children and understands the available sympathetic agents that can reverse this process.

Sympathetic agents are usually classified by the mechanisms with which they produce their effects. Phenylephrine can be given at doses of 1–10 mcg/kg and up to 30 mcg/kg. It is a direct acting alpha1 receptor agonist and will increase systemic vascular resistance causing a baroreceptor reflex that decreases the heart rate. Ephedrine doses are 0.2–0.3 mg/kg and the drug will increase both systemic vascular resistance and heart rate through indirect alpha (α) and β effects, through the release of norepinephrine from sympathetic nerves. For severe hypotension, arrest or anaphylaxis, epinephrine is the drug of choice, at doses of 1–10 mcg/kg. It will increase SVR, heart rate, and has inotropic effects with direct α and β effects. It also has β2 affects that cause bronchodilation and will therefore be the drug of choice in anaphylactic shock. Intense vasoconstriction will result from epinephrine administration, which may compromise flow to nonvital organs such as kidneys and small intestine.

Some sympathetic agents are best administered by infusion. Dopamine has direct and indirect effects, and effects depend on dosing. Low-dose dopamine (< 2 mcg/kg/min) will cause vasodilation and increased renal blood flow, 2–5 mcg/kg/min begins to activate β and will increase chronotropy and inotropy as well as cause vasodilation. Infusions higher than 10 mcg/kg/min have intense α effects and vasoconstriction. Dobutamine can be infused at 2–20 mcg/kg/min and has direct β effects, increasing inotropy and decreasing SVR. Milrinone is a phosphodiesterase inhibitor that is often used in congenital heart disease surgery. This drug causes increased inotropy, dromotropy, and lusitropy, decreased pulmonary vascular resistance, and decreased afterload. High doses or long-term use may cause thrombocytopenia. Milrinone has a loading dose of 50 mcg/kg over 30 minutes as is infused at 0.5–1 mcg/kg/min. Vasopressin can also be used and will cause intense vasoconstriction through direct effects on V1 receptors at doses of 0.5 U/kg/dose or an infusion of 0.3–2 milliUnit/kg/min. Vasopressin may be particularly useful in cases were vasoplegia is suspected.

Parasympathetic agents are also utilized in the operative period. Atropine is a commonly used drug (0.01–0.02 mg/kg with a minimum of 0.15 mg) to increase the heart rate through reduced vagal tone. It is used to reliably prevent bradycardia from succinylcholine injection, increased parasympathetic tone from laryngoscopy or manipulation of the viscera, and the oculocardiac reflex during ophthalmologic surgery. Glycopyrrolate may also be used for similar reasons in older children.

Agents affecting coagulation

Newborn babies have low levels of vitamin K-dependent factors at birth. By 6 months of age these factors are at adult levels. Factors 2 and 7 are less than adult levels for most of childhood. Factor 9 reaches adult levels at 9 months. The vWF factors are increased at birth and return to normal values between 2–6 months. Overall, newborns have delayed thrombin formation and will often receive vitamin K supplementation.

In cases of refractory bleeding, fresh frozen plasma, cryoprecipitate, and procoagulants may be given. Also FFP and cryoprecipitate may be administered alone or in conjunction with packed red cells or other procoagulant agents. The DDAVP analog (0.3 mcg/kg) is an analog of vasopressin that induces the release of von Willebrand factor and factor VIII from endothelial storage granules. It can be used in von Willebrand disease and uremic platelet dysfunction. Factor VIII has a high concentration of vWF and can be used in vWF deficiencies. Recombinant factor VIIa binds to tissue factor and activated platelets, resulting in thrombin production. Doses of 90–120 mcg/kg every 2–3 hours can significantly help with hemostasis. It can be useful in a variety of conditions including hepatic dysfunction, platelet dysfunction, dilutional coagulopathy, DIC, and after bypass for rescue therapy.[59] Prothrombin complex concentrate includes factors 2, 9, 10 or 2, 7, 9, 10. Antifibrinolytic agents (aminocaproic acid and tranexamic acid) can be useful as adjuvants in the treatment of hemophilia and are used during surgeries that are high risk for profuse bleeding, including major spine surgery and re-do sternotomies.

Anticoagulants are often given to adult patients as well as some adolescent postoperative patients to prevent deep venous thrombosis. Anticoagulants are also utilized during cardiac or veno-venous bypass, and for patients at risk of clotting. Platelet aggregation inhibitors include COX-1 inhibitors (ASA), ADP platelet receptor P2Y12 antagonists (ticlopidine), and $\alpha_{II2}\beta_3$ activated platelet binding blockers. Vitamin K antagonists (warfarin) inhibit factors 2, 7, 9, 10, and protein C and S production in the liver. Heparin is an antithrombin agonist that inactivates thrombin and factor Xa. Direct factor Xa inhibitors include low molecular weight heparins and fondaparinux; LMWH is increasingly replacing heparin in the treatment of pediatric thrombotic disease.[55,56] Direct thrombin inhibitors include lepirudin, bivalirudin, and argatroban. Argatroban has been used in an infant with HIT for bypass.[57]

References

1. Davis P, Cladis F, Motoyama E. *Smith's Anesthesia for Infants and Children.* 2013; **7**: 197–209.
2. Lynn AM, McRorie TI, Slattery JT, *et al.* Age-dependent morphine partitioning between plasma and cerebrospinal fluid in monkeys. *Dev Pharmacol Ther.* 1991; **17**(3–4): 200–4.
3. Banks WA. Physiology and pathology of the blood–brain barrier: implications for microbial pathogenesis, drug delivery and neurodegenerative disorders. *J Neurovirol.* 1999; **5**(6): 538–55.
4. Davis P, Cladis F, Motoyama E. *Smith's Anesthesia for Infants and Children.* 2013; **7**: 183–4.
5. Tayman C, Rayyan M, Allegaert K. Neonatal pharmacology: extensive interindividual variability despite limited size. *J Pediatr Pharmacol Ther.* 2011; **16**(3): 170–84.
6. Davis P, Cladis F, Motoyama E. *Smith's Anesthesia for Infants and Children.* 2013; **7**: 184.
7. Tayman C, Rayyan M, Allegaert K. Neonatal pharmacology: extensive interindividual variability despite limited size. *J Pediatr Pharmacol Ther.* 2011; **16**(3): 170–84.
8. Davis P, Cladis F, Motoyama E. *Smith's Anesthesia for Infants and Children.* 2013; **7**: 239–57.
9. Barash P, Cullen B, Stoelting R, *et al. Clinical Anesthesia*, 6th edition. Philadelphia PA, Lippincott Williams & Wilkins, 2009.
10. Davis P, Cladis F, Motoyama E. *Smith's Anesthesia for Infants and Children.* 2013; **7**: 182–84.
11. Johnson TN, Thromson M. Intestinal metabolism and transport of drugs in children: the effects of age and disease. *J Pediatr Gastroenterol Nutr.* 2008; **47**(1): 3–10.
12. Zhou SF. Polymorphism of human cytochrome P450 2D6 and its clinical significance: Part I. *Clin Pharmacokinet.* 2009; **48**(11): 689–723.
13. Kirchheiner J, Schmidt H, Tzvetkov M, *et al.* Pharmacokinetics of codeine and its metabolite morphine in ultra-rapid metabolizers due to CYP2D6 duplication. *Pharmacogenomics J.* 2007; **7**(4): 257–65.
14. Chou WY, Yang LC, Lu H, *et al.* Association of mu-opioid receptor gene polymorphism (A118G) with variations in morphine consumption for analgesia after total knee arthroplasty. *Acta Anaesthesiol Scand.* 2006; **50**(7): 787–92.
15. Davis P, Cladis F, Motoyama E. *Smith's Anesthesia for Infants and Children.* 2013; **7**: 258–60.
16. Dsida RM, *et al.* Age-stratified pharmacokinetics of ketorolac tromethamine in pediatric surgical patients. *Anesth Analg.* 2002; **94**(2): 266–70.
17. Inoue M, *et al.* Safety and efficacy of ketorolac in children after cardiac surgery. *Intensive Care Med.* 2009; **35**(9): 1584–92.
18. Dawkins TN, *et al.* Safety of intravenous use of ketorolac in infants following cardiothoracic surgery. *Cardiol Young.* 2009; **19** (1): 105–8.
19. Sucato DJ, *et al.* Postoperative ketorolac does not predispose to pseudoarthrosis following posterior spinal fusion and instrumentation for adolescent idiopathic scoliosis. *Spine (Phila Pa 1976).* 20081; 33(10): 1119–24.
20. Lynn AM, *et al.* Postoperative ketorolac tromethamine use in infants aged 6–18 months: the effect on morphine usage, safety assessment, and stereo-specific pharmacokinetics. *Anesth Analg.* 2007; **104**(5): 1040–51.
21. Lynn AM, *et al.* Ketorolac tromethamine: stereo-specific pharmacokinetics and single-dose use in postoperative infants aged 2–6 months. *Paediatr Anaesth.* 2011; **21**(3): 325–34.
22. Davis P, Cladis F, Motoyama E. *Smith's Anesthesia for Infants and Children.* 2013; **7**: 208–23.
23. K. J. S. Anand, *et al.* Morphine pharmacokinetics and pharmacodynamics in preterm and term neonates: secondary results from the NEOPAIN trial. *Br J Anaesth.* 2008 November; **101** (5): 680–9.
24. Stoker DG, *et al.* Analgesic efficacy and safety of morphine-chitosan nasal solution in patients with moderate to severe pain following orthopedic surgery. *Pain Med.* 2008 Jan-Feb; **9**(1): 3–12.
25. Albanèse J, *et al.* Sufentanil, fentanyl, and alfentanil in head trauma patients: a study on cerebral hemodynamics. *Crit Care Med.* 1999 Feb; **27**(2): 407–11.
26. Zhao M, Joo DT. Enhancement of spinal N-methyl-D-aspartate receptor function by remifentanil action at delta-opioid receptors as a mechanism for acute opioid-induced hyperalgesia or tolerance. *Anesthesiology.* 2008 Aug; **109**(2): 308–17.
27. Kharasch ED. Intraoperative methadone: rediscovery, reappraisal, and reinvigoration? *Anesth Analg.* 2011 Jan; **112**(1): 13–16.
28. Pokela ML, *et al.* Marked variation in oxycodone pharmacokinetics in infants. *Paediatr Anaesth.* 2005; **15**: 560–5.
29. Marco CA, *et al.* Comparison of oxycodone and hydrocodone for the treatment of acute pain associated with fractures: a double-blind, randomized, controlled trial. *Acad Emerg Med.* 2005; **12**: 82.

30. Drendel AL, *et al.* A randomized clinical trial of ibuprofen versus acetaminophen with codeine for acute pediatric arm fracture pain. *Ann Emerg Med.* 2009 Oct; **54**(4): 553–60.

31. Davis P, Cladis F, Motoyama E. *Smith's Anesthesia for Infants and Children.* 2013; **7**: 197–208

32. Reed MD, *et al.* The single-dose pharmacokinetics of midazolam and its primary metabolite in pediatric patients after oral and intravenous administration. *J Clin Pharmacol.* 2001 Dec; **41**(12): 1359–69.

33. den Brinker M, *et al.* One single dose of etomidate negatively influences adrenocortical performance for at least 24h in children with meningococcal sepsis. *Intensive Care Med.* 2008 Jan; **34**(1): 163–8.

34. Gozal D, Rein AJ, Nir A, Gozal Y. Propofol does not modify the hemodynamic status of children with intracardiac shunts undergoing cardiac catheterization. *Pediatr Cardiol.* 2001 Nov-Dec; **22**(6): 488–90.

35. Cote C, Lerman J, Anderson B. *A Practice of Anesthesia for Infants and Children.* 2013; **6**: 146–7.

36. Lerman J. Surgical and patient factors involved in postoperative nausea and vomiting. *Br J Anaesth.* 1992; **69**(7 Suppl 1): 24S–32.

37. Mondick JT, *et al.* Population pharmacokinetics of intravenous ondansetron in oncology and surgical patients aged 1–48 months. *Eur J Clin Pharmacol.* 2010 Jan; **66**(1): 77–86.

38. Gan TJ, *et al.* Society for Ambulatory Anesthesia guidelines for the management of postoperative nausea and vomiting. *Anesth Analg.* 2007 Dec; **105**(6): 1615–28.

39. Cote C, Lerman J, Steward D. *Manual of Pediatric Anesthesia.* 2010: **7**: 218–19.

40. Davis P, Cladis F, Motoyama E. *Smith's Anesthesia for Infants and Children.* 2011; **13**: 378–9.

41. Gombar S, *et al.* Superior anti-emetic efficacy of granisetron–dexamethasone combination in children undergoing middle ear surgery. *Acta Anaesthesiol Scand.* 2007 May; **51**(5): 621–4.

42. Gan TJ. Risk factors for postoperative nausea and vomiting. *Anesth Analg.* 2006 Jun; **102**(6): 1884–98.

43. Davis P, Cladis F, Motoyama E. *Smith's Anesthesia for Infants and Children.* 2013; **7**: 223–35.

44. von Ungern-Sternberg BS, *et al.* Desflurane but not sevoflurane impairs airway and respiratory tissue mechanics in children with susceptible airways. *Anesthesiology.* 2008 Feb; **108**(2): 216–24.

45. Davis P, Cladis F, Motoyama E. *Smith's Anesthesia for Infants and Children.* 2013; **7**: 235–9.

46. Hollmann MW, Strümper D, Durieux ME. The poor man's epidural: systemic local anesthetics for improving postoperative outcomes. *Med Hypotheses.* 2004; **63**(3): 386–9.

47. Heavner JE. Local anesthetics. *Curr Opin Anaesthesiol.* 2007 Aug; **20**(4): 336–42.

48. Mazoit JX, Dalens BJ. Pharmacokinetics of local anaesthetics in infants and children. *Clin Pharmacokinet.* 2004; **43**(1): 17–32.

49. Davis P, Cladis F, Motoyama E. *Smith's Anesthesia for Infants and Children.* 2013; **7**: 240–57, **13**: 379.

50. Cote C, Lerman J, Steward D. *Manual of Pediatric Anesthesia.* 2010; **3**: 68.

51. Fotopoulou G, Theocharis S, Vasileiou I, Kouskouni E, Xanthos T. Management of the airway without the use of neuromuscular blocking agents: the use of remifentanil. *Fundam Clin Pharmacol.* 2012 Feb; **26**(1): 72–85.

52. Davis P, Cladis F, Motoyama E. *Smith's Anesthesia for Infants and Children.* 2013; **38**: 1250–23.

53. Barash P, *et al. Clinical Anesthesia.* 6th edition. 2009; **15**: 353

54. Davis P, Cladis F, Motoyama E. *Smith's Anesthesia for Infants and Children.* 2013; **36**: 1144–63.

55. Merkel N, Gunther G, Schobess R. Long-term treatment of thrombosis with enoxaparin in pediatric and adolescent patients. *Acta Haematol.* 2006; **115**(3–4): 230–6.

56. U Nowak-Göttl, *et al.* Pharmacokinetics, efficacy, and safety of LMWHs in venous thrombosis and stroke in neonates, infants and children. *Br J Pharmacol.* 2008 Mar; **153**(6): 1120–7.

57. Malherbe S, Tsui BC, Stobart K, Koller J. Argatroban as anticoagulant in cardiopulmonary bypass in an infant and attempted reversal with recombinant activated factor VII. *Anesthesiology.* 2004 Feb; **100**(2): 443–5.

58. Kaw D, Malhotra D. Platelet dysfunction and end-stage renal disease. *Semin Dial.* 2006 Jul–Aug; **19**(4): 317–22.

59. Guzzetta NA, Russell IA, Williams GD. Review of the off-label use of recombinant activated factor VII in pediatric cardiac surgery. *Anesth Analg.* 2012 Aug; **115**(2): 364–78.

60. Horlocker TT, Wedel DJ, Rowlingson JC, Enneking FK. Regional anesthesia in the patient receiving antithrombotic or thrombolytic therapy: American Society of Regional Anesthesia and Pain Medicine Evidence-based Guidelines *(Third Edition).* Reg Anesth Pain Med. 2010 Jan–Feb; 35(1): 102–5.

Chapter 5

Respiratory system

Adam J. Broussard, Stanley M. Hall, and Michael G. Levitzky

Respiratory system: anatomy and physiology

Prenatal and postnatal development

The respiratory system comprises the respiratory control centers in the brainstem; central and peripheral chemoreceptors; several nerves including the phrenic, intercostals, hypoglossal, and vagus; the bones, cartilage and muscles of the thorax; airways from nares to alveoli; and other lung tissues including bronchial and pulmonary vasculatures. These components develop and mature at differing rates. Although some of the components of the respiratory system are functional at birth, growth of the lungs continues until 8–10 years of age.

Brain maturation is incomplete at birth. The pontine and medullary structures involved in respiratory rhythm generation establish fetal breathing efforts prenatally. These efforts appear to be necessary for the growth and development of the respiratory system (especially the respiratory musculature) and to prepare for postnatal breathing. These in utero ventilatory efforts are affected by fetal hypoxia, hypercarbia, and acidosis. During severe distress, evacuation of meconium from the bowels in conjunction with gasping ventilatory efforts can cause meconium aspiration. Functioning of the peripheral and central chemoreceptors requires integration with maturing brain pathways and may be responsible for conditions such as sudden infant death syndrome (SIDS) and apnea of prematurity.

Respiratory system function depends primarily on both cardiac and pulmonary components. The heart starts to form 18–19 days after fertilization, with blood flow beginning in only the third week of development. The more-slowly developing lungs are derived from the laryngotracheal groove, an outpouching of the embryonic pharynx during the fourth week of gestation. This outpouching is called the respiratory diverticulum (Fig. 5.1A). During the end of the fourth week of gestation, the developing tracheobronchial tree splits into the two bronchial buds (Fig. 5.1B). The three stages of lung development based on histological appearance are designated as: the *pseudoglandular stage* (5 to 16 weeks), the *canalicular stage* (16 to 26 weeks) and the *alveolar stage* (26 weeks to birth).

Pseudoglandular Stage- The bronchial buds grow into the pleural cavities and become the two main-stem bronchi. During the fifth week post-conception, the right bronchopulmonary bud forms three secondary buds which become the three lobes of the right lung, while the left bronchopulmonary bud forms two secondary buds that become the two lobes of the left lung (Fig. 5.1C-E). Tertiary buds shown in Fig. 5.1F develop into the ten bronchopulmonary segments of the right lung and the eight bronchopulmonary segments of the left lung.

The nascent tracheobronchial tree begins development at this time, starting with the trachea and progressing peripherally. The endodermal lining of the laryngotracheal tube is surrounded with mesenchymal cells that give rise to the cartilage, smooth muscle and connective tissue of the larynx and trachea. The columnar epithelium and mucous glands lining the lumen of the tracheobronchial tree are derived from the endoderm. Tracheal cartilages begin to appear during the eighth post-conception week, cilia begin to develop on the tracheal lining by about the tenth week. Mucous glands first appear in the upper part of the tracheobronchial tree at about the twelfth week of development and are seen farther down the developing airway soon thereafter. Cartilage develops in the main-stem bronchi by the tenth week and in the segmental bronchi by about the twelfth week.

Essentials of Pediatric Anesthesiology, ed. Alan David Kaye, Charles James Fox and James H. Diaz. Published by Cambridge University Press. © Cambridge University Press 2015.

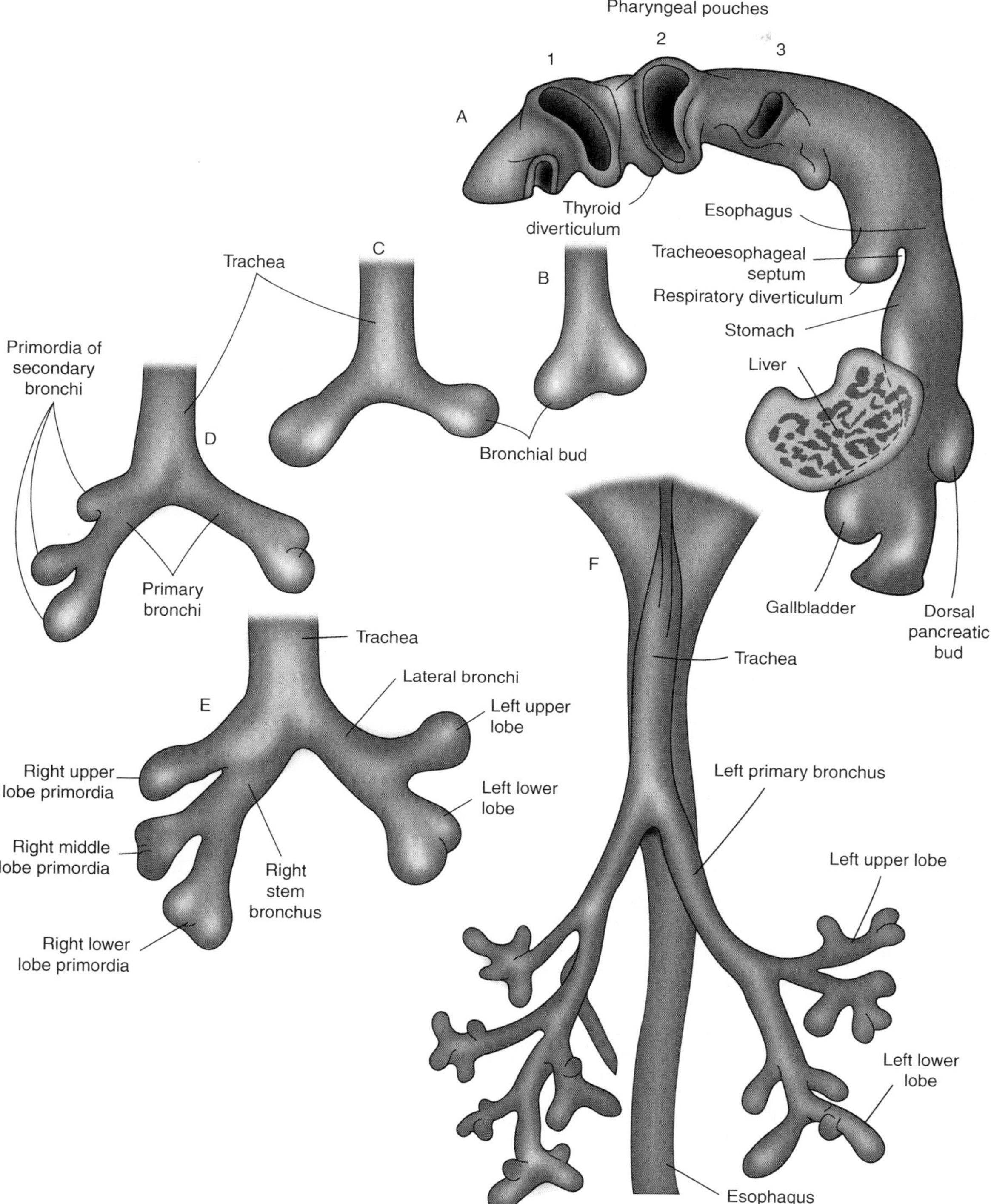

Figure 5.1 Illustration of ventral views of the development of the fetal tracheobronchial tree at about 4 weeks of development: **A**. Lateral view of pharynx. **B**. At 4 weeks. **C**. At about 32 days. **D**. At about 33 days. **E**. At the end of the fifth week. **F**. Early in the seventh week. (Reproduced with permission from Carlson BM. *Human Embryology and Developmental Biology*. St. Louis, MO; Mosby; 1994.)

Cilia develop on the epithelium of the main-stem bronchi in the twelfth week and in the segmental bronchi during the thirteenth week. The mucous glands that appear in the bronchi during the thirteenth week begin to produce mucous about a week later.

Pulmonary arteries develop from the sixth aortic arch artery during the fifth and sixth weeks following conception. Growth of the pulmonary arteries parallels the growth of the two main-stem bronchi. At about the fourth week after conception, the pulmonary veins begin to develop from the wall of the left atrium. The bronchial arteries sprout from the dorsal aorta during the seventh and eighth weeks, forming many anastomoses with the pulmonary circulation (which will contribute to anatomic shunting).

The lower portions of the tracheobronchial tree, including the functional alveolar-capillary gas exchange units, develop during the second and third stages of fetal lung development; the canalicular stage and then the alveolar stage.

Canalicular stage (16 to 26 weeks) – Until about the fifteenth to sixteenth week of fetal development, the lungs resemble glands because they consist of small branching future airways lined with large numbers of mucous glands (and hence the term pseudoglandular stage). During the subsequent canalicular stage, the lumens of the developing airways enlarge and the terminal bronchioles give rise to the respiratory bronchioles. Respiratory bronchioles divide into alveolar ducts and the terminal air sacs, which later become the alveolar sacs. Some references (Langston 1984) state that respiratory bronchioles do not form until after birth but this distinction may be due to the difficulty defining the end of the bronchial circulation and the beginning of the pulmonary circulation. Also, alveolarization of the future respiratory bronchioles is scarce until after birth. The epithelium lining the lumen begins to differentiate into two populations: one becoming flattened squamous alveolar type 1 cells and the other becoming cuboidal secretory alveolar type 2 cells (responsible for surfactant production and secretion.) Pulmonary capillaries and lymphatics also begin to form during this period.

Alveolar stage (26 weeks to birth) – the pulmonary capillary network proliferates around the developing alveoli during this final stage of lung development. In adulthood, the ratio of pulmonary capillaries to alveoli is 1000:1. Surfactant production normally begins after about the seventh month of gestation although this aspect of lung maturation can be greatly accelerated by administering glucocorticoids to the mother (achieving nearly normal newborn lung function as early as the 24th gestational week.) Prolonged intra-uterine stress can also speed up fetal lung maturation. Additionally, aerosolized exogenous surfactant (mentioned later in this chapter) can ease transition of the premature newborn's lungs to their gas exchange function and reduce the likelihood of development of infant respiratory distress syndrome (IRDS). At term, almost all of the 23 generations of airways have developed, although only one tenth of the adult number of alveolar ducts and one fifteenth of the final adult number of alveoli have formed. Most alveolar formation occurs during the first 12 to 18 months of postnatal life. At that time, alveolar development is essentially complete although growth and development of the lungs and surrounding thorax continues through the first decade of life.

Lung volumes

Newborns were believed to have a smaller FRC per kg body weight when compared to adults until methods for accurate microspirometric measurement of newborn lung volumes and capacities were developed and revealed that spontaneously breathing neonates have an FRC that is fairly equivalent to adult FRC per kg body weight. In an adult, the FRC is that lung volume at which the outward recoil of the chest wall is equal to the inward recoil of the lungs. Although the lungs have high compliance in the newborn, the compliance of the chest wall is much higher than in an adult. The outward recoil of the neonate's chest wall is much less than the inward recoil of the lungs, which tends to diminish the FRC. Neonates elevate their FRC by glottis closure and also by postinspiratory stimulation of the inspiratory muscles during expiration. These measures have a "braking" effect on exhalation which is otherwise passive and depends on elastic recoil. This effect has been called the "active FRC of the newborn." However, under general anesthesia (especially with muscle relaxation), the very compliant infant cartilaginous rib cage, the poorly developed chest wall muscle mass and high compliance of newborn lungs combine to promote lung collapse and atelectasis formation. High lung compliance in the newborn is partially due to the fact that lung elastic fibers do not develop until the postnatal period. Similarly, geriatric lungs also have high compliance due to brittle and nonfunctional

Table 5.1. Causes of rapid arterial desaturation following onset of infant apnea

1. Increased Metabolic Rate: Oxygen consumption rate is about twice of adults per body weight or surface area: Infants: 6–7 ml O_2 consumed/kg/min. Adults: 3–3.5 ml O_2 consumed/kg/min.
2. FRC in spontaneously breathing infants is comparable to adult FRC = 30 ml/kg. Under general anesthesia, infant FRC decreases, reducing oxygen reserves during apnea.
3. Closing capacity is increased at extremes of age (pediatric and geriatric individuals). Closing capacity consists of poorly ventilated alveoli distal to collapsed airways.
4. Patent foramen ovale (PFO) is more common in infants and can result in cyanotic shunting when PVR is high. PFO declines progressively with age.
5. Artifact: Venous pulsations can lead to a falsely low estimation of arterial oxygen saturation. Causes of significant venous pulsations include severe tricuspid regurgitation, use of intra-aortic balloon pump, and high airway pressures such as during a Valsalva maneuver.

elastic fibers. These are the main reasons why closing volume is increased at the extremes of age.

Combining these factors with the approximately double rate of oxygen consumption/ body weight or surface area (when compared to adults) explains the very rapid rate of arterial desaturation that occurs following the onset of infant apnea (Table 5.1).

Respiratory mechanics

At birth, the neonate must generate intrapleural pressures estimated to be from -30 to -70 cm H_2O in order to inflate the lungs and begin breathing. During the later stages of gestation, the fetus begins to make ventilatory efforts in utero. These movements are believed to be necessary to stimulate ventilatory muscle development and to help expel some of the fluid produced by the lungs. This fluid expands the airways, stimulating lung growth and development while contributing about one third of the total amniotic fluid volume.

Much fetal lung fluid is expressed from the airways by the compressive forces of passing through the birth canal during vaginal delivery. This task is assumed by the neonatologist by thorough suctioning of the airway following C-section. Residual fluid leaves the lungs via the pulmonary capillaries and lymphatics during the first few days of life. This improves the compliance of the lungs and decreases the work of breathing for the easily fatigued newborn. Delivery from the aqueous amniotic environment at birth and the subsequent water loss from all body tissues explain the loss in weight usually seen in the days following birth.

Control of breathing

Rhythmic breathing at birth is initiated and maintained by several factors such as clamping the umbilical cord and the increasing arterial oxygen tensions from breathing air. Prenatal hypoxia can evoke gasping ventilatory efforts in utero associated with meconium aspiration as discussed previously. These gasping efforts are independent of the rhythmic breathing efforts. The mechanisms responsible for control of breathing gradually evolve in the newborn and are not mature until at least 42 to 44 weeks post conception, especially the response to hypoxia. Hypoxia depresses or abolishes rhythmic breathing both in utero and in the newborn. Clamping of the umbilical cord reinforces rhythmic breathing. The breathing pattern is relatively unaffected by the $PaCO_2$ in the newborn. Newborns respond to hypercapnia by increasing ventilation but less so than do older infants. The slope of the CO_2 response curve increases with age. In adults, the CO_2 response curve shifts to the left in the presence of hypoxemia while in the newborn, it shifts to the right. Additionally, $PaCO_2$ in the newborn normally is lower than that found in older children and adults.

During the first 2 to 3 weeks of life, both term and premature infants in a warm environment respond to hypoxemia with a transient increase in ventilation followed by sustained ventilatory depression. In a cold environment, the initial period of transient hyperpnea is abolished. By about three weeks after birth, hypoxemia induces sustained hyperpnea in term infants as it does in adults and older children. This response is delayed in prematurely born infants. In all ages, hypoxic ventilatory drive can be abolished by as little as 0.1 MAC of inhaled anesthetic.

Periodic breathing, in which rhythmic breathing is interrupted with repetitive short apneic episodes lasting 5 to 10 seconds, occurs normally in healthy neonates and young infants. The incidence of periodic breathing is much higher in preterm than in full-term neonates. However, central apnea of infancy lasts for 15 seconds or longer or else is associated with bradycardia and/ or arterial desaturation. Central apnea is strongly associated with the degree of prematurity and lower birth weights (less than 2 kg.) It is believed to be associated with immature respiratory control mechanisms. Development and maturation of central and peripheral chemoreceptors as well as overall maturation (and myelination) of the newborn brain may be responsible for this poor ventilatory control.

Due to the risk of life-threatening postoperative apneic episodes in infants who had been born prematurely, it has been recommended that even term infants younger than 44–46 weeks post-conception should be admitted for overnight observation after general anesthesia and surgery. This topic remains controversial among pediatric anesthesiologists with the most conservative mandate not allowing outpatient surgery for infants who had been born prematurely (born at < 37 weeks post conception) until 60 weeks post-conception (Cote). A sliding scale has also been proposed that postpones outpatient surgery for a variable time depending on extent of prematurity:

Degree of Prematurity	Post-conception age at which outpatient surgery allowed
< 37 weeks	50–52 weeks
< 35 weeks	54 weeks
< 32 weeks	56 weeks

These guidelines are tempered by various issues such as the frequency of apneic episodes and the interval since the last episode. Anemia, hypothermia, coexisting diseases, and the need for large doses of postoperative narcotics increase the risk of postoperative apnea. Outpatient surgery occasionally is allowed early for an ex-premature infant if the parents already possess and are experienced with a home apnea monitor. Regional anesthesia (such as a spinal for inguinal hernia) may reduce the risk of postoperative apnea.

Cardiopulmonary transition

Starting with the first breath, as the lungs expand with air, pulmonary artery pressure and vascular resistance (PVR) fall dramatically while pulmonary blood flow markedly increases (Fig. 5.2).

These changes are due to the release of the effects of hypoxic pulmonary vasoconstriction (HPV) present in the uninflated lungs in utero. The first breath raises alveolar PO_2 and pH while lowering the PCO_2 and reducing the number of uninflated (atelectatic) alveoli, all of which affect HPV. In addition, the tethering effect of alveolar inflation likewise uncoils and straightens the pulmonary capillaries that line the walls of every alveolus reducing PVR (about 1000 capillaries for each alveolus). At the same time, systemic vascular resistance (SVR) increases due to loss of the low vascular resistance placenta, which was in parallel circulation with the other organs of the body. These hemodynamic changes occurring at the time of birth (increased systemic vascular resistance and pressure coupled with decreased pulmonary vascular resistance and pressure) change the pressure gradient across the atria and act to close the foramen ovale, which usually functions as a right-to-left one-way valve.

Anatomic closure of the foramen ovale is progressive with age but up to 20% of 80-year-olds can have a patent foramen ovale. With newborn lung disease such as infant respiratory distress, meconium aspiration or congenital diaphragmatic hernia, alveolar hypoxia and atelectasis maintain a high level of HPV, and the foramen ovale remains open, shunting blood flow right-to-left. The cyanotic newborn is then said to have persistent fetal circulation.

The dramatic increase in blood flowing into the pulmonary vasculature at normal birth exposes prostaglandins in the blood to pulmonary metabolic mechanisms (discussed later) which almost completely remove the vasodilating prostaglandins E and F. The reduction in these prostaglandins is usually adequate enough to result in closure of the ductus arteriosus but, if necessary, NSAID administration to the newborn (indomethacin in the USA, ibuprofen in Europe) can further reduce prostaglandin levels and frequently results in closure. Unfortunately, NSAIDs do increase risk of intracerebral bleeding. With certain cyanotic congenital heart diseases such as pulmonary or tricuspid atresia, pulmonary blood flow is dependent on patency of the ductus arteriosus so prostaglandin F2alpha infusion is administered to maintain ductal flow.

Ventilation

Spontaneous infant alveolar ventilation (100–150 ml/kg/min) is about twice that of an adult (60 ml/kg/min). Dead space (2–2.5 ml/kg) and tidal volume

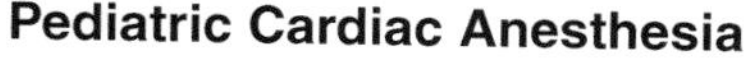

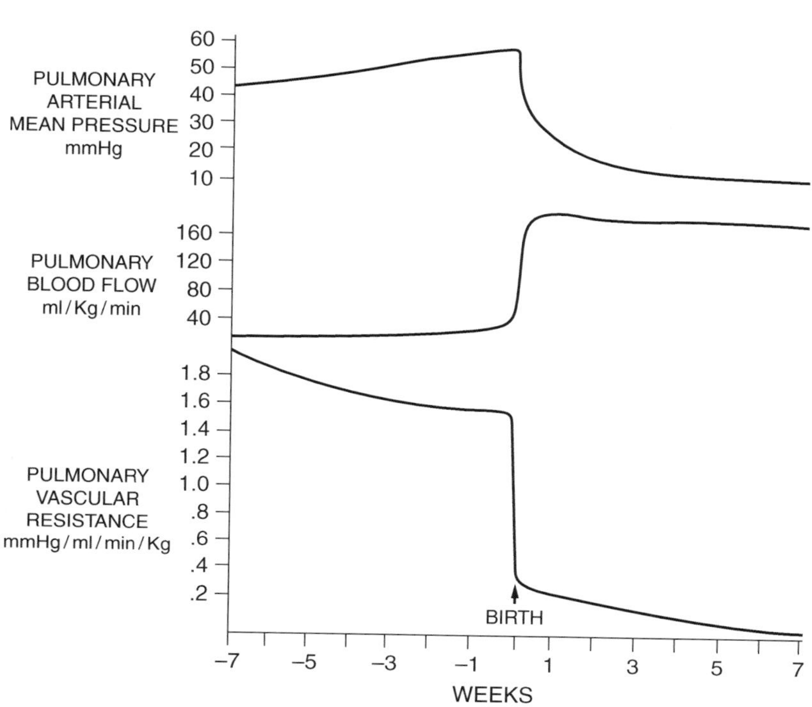

Figure 5.2 Pulmonary artery pressure and vascular resistance.

(7 ml/kg) are comparable for infants and adults on a per kilogram basis. Mechanical lung protection ventilation (ventilator tidal volume of 6–7 ml/kg) has been shown to be beneficial in adult ICU patients and is undergoing trials during adult surgery. This technique using low tidal volumes may be beneficial for pediatric patients but may require occasional sigh breathing to reverse the tendency toward atelectasis. Tidal volume is normally set at 10–12 ml/kg with an I/E ratio of 1:2. The addition of 3–5 cm H_2O PEEP will also reduce the development of atelectasis but can produce undesirable (for the surgeons) lung distention during intrathoracic procedures. Ventilator frequency should be set at 20 to 30 breaths/min for infants, 14 to 20 breaths per min for children, and 19 to 14 breaths per min for adolescents. Infants need these high ventilator rates because of their high oxygen demand and their normal spontaneous ventilatory rate is 30–50 breaths per min.

Capnography is an intraoperative monitoring standard for pediatric and adult surgery. End-tidal PCO_2 normally underestimates arterial PCO_2 by 2–3 torr but this gradient can widen unpredictably in conditions associated with increased alveolar dead space (such as high airway pressure or low pulmonary perfusion.) Capnography also is an unreliable predictor of arterial PCO_2 in pediatric patients with cyanotic heart disease (see Table 5.2).

Ventilation/perfusion matching

In utero, the lungs are not ventilated with air and the circulation mainly bypasses the pulmonary vasculature via the right- to- left shunts of the foramen ovale and ductus arteriosus. At the time of birth, the expansion of the lungs, coupled with increased pulmonary blood flow, produce the abrupt transition to extrauterine gas exchange. Ventilation is fairly well matched with perfusion in the newborn although the large amount of lung water lowers lung compliance and increases work of breathing.

Additionally, the rapid decrease in FRC associated with general anesthesia causes V/Q mismatch. When shunting and arterial desaturation occurs during inhalational induction of a pediatric patient, it is proper to increase the FiO_2 to 100%. However, the addition of 100% O_2 to poorly ventilated (but well-perfused) alveoli can rapidly lead to absorption

Table 5.2 Effects of cyanotic heart disease on end-tidal/arterial PCO_2 gradient (ΔPCO_2)

End-tidal PCO_2 underestimates arterial PCO2
ΔPCO_2 of cyanotic patients was significantly greater than for acyanotic patients
ΔPCO_2 is not stable intraoperatively in the cyanotic patients
ΔPCO_2 increases by 2–3 torr for each 10% decrease in SpO_2

atelectasis and persistent shunting. Re-expansion of the alveoli with sigh breaths (40–60 cmH_2O airway pressure) can reduce shunting and improve compliance.

Oxygen transport

In the newborn, blood affinity for oxygen is very high (O_2–Hb dissociation curve is shifted to the left) because 2,3-DPG levels are low and fetal hemoglobin (HbF) interacts poorly with 2,3-DPG. Thus in the newborn the P_{50} is only 18 to 19 mmHg (adult $P_{50} = 27$ mmHg). Therefore the PO_2 in neonatal tissues is low but this is compensated by the normally high hemoglobin levels of the newborn. Total hemoglobin and HbF levels fall rapidly after birth reaching their lowest levels by 2 to 3 months of age (so-called physiologic anemia of infancy). This anemic period is usually sooner, longer-lasting, and with a lower hematocrit in infants born prematurely. The P_{50} levels then rise (as HbA production increases) reaching their peak at about 10 months of age ($P_{50} = 30$ mmHg).

Lung cellular physiology

At the level of the alveolar–capillary interface, three types of cells play differing roles in either gas exchange, lung defense, or the production of a variety of local and humoral substances. Flattened squamous alveolar type I cells cover about 80% of the air-facing surface. They are fairly limited metabolically and when damaged, alveolar type II cells multiply and transform to replace them. These multipotent type II cells produce varied metabolic and enzymatic activities in addition to surfactant production. Alveolar macrophages (alveolar type III cells) perform important immunologic and phagocytic lung defense, respond to infection, and contribute to the inflammatory response.

Surfactant and surface tension

Fetal pulmonary surfactant production begins between weeks 24–28 and adequate levels for normal lung function are reached naturally by about the 35th week. Surfactant (composed of six lipids and four proteins, mainly dipalmitoylphosphotidylcholine) reduces surface tension, the work of breathing and the tendency to develop atelectasis. Surfactant preferentially lowers surface tension in the small alveoli (which are the ones most susceptible to collapse) and helps stabilize them. Surface tension is present at air–liquid interfaces and contributes to the elastic forces that tend to reduce alveolar size, leading to atelectasis. Surfactant also reduces the movement of fluid from the pulmonary capillaries into the alveolar air-containing spaces. By these mechanisms, surfactant increases lung compliance, reducing ventilatory work for the newborn. Certain proteins (SP-A and SP-D) in surfactant function as opsins for macrophages, coating bacteria and viruses, enhancing immune function.

When premature delivery is likely, the administration of corticosteroids to the mother accelerates maturation of the fetal lungs and endogenous surfactant production. Prolonged intrauterine stress can also enhance fetal lung maturation. Additionally, liquid synthetic or animal-derived surfactant can be administered to premature newborns via endotracheal tube and can greatly improve their lung function and chance of survival.

At birth, lung ventilation results primarily from diaphragmatic contractions due to later development of the intercostal muscles. The diaphragm consists of two muscle types: type 1 are slow twitch, sustained contraction fibers with low fatigability, while type 2 give fast contractions but fatigue easily. The mature diaphragm (after 2 years old) has about 55% type 1 fibers while newborns have only about 25% type 1 and premature newborns as little as 10%. Thus newborns, especially premature newborns, risk diaphragmatic fatigue when work of breathing is increased.

Metabolism

The lungs convert or remove multiple substances contained in the pulmonary blood and also produce, store, and release substances used locally in the lung or elsewhere in the body. While pulmonary surfactant is most notable, lung cells produce several other substances. Mast cells release bradykinin, prostaglandins,

Table 5.3 Uptake of conversion by the lungs of chemical substances in mixed venous blood

Substance in mixed venous blood	Result of a single pass through the lung
Prostaglandins E_1, E_2, $F_{2\alpha}$	Almost completely removed
Prostaglandins A_1, A_2, I_2	Not affected
Leukotrienes	Almost completely removed
Serotonin	85–95% removed
Acetylcholine	Inactivated by cholinesterases in blood
Histamine	Not affected
Epinephrine	Not affected
Norepinephrine	Approximately 30% removed
Isoproterenol	Not affected
Dopamine	Not affected
Bradykinin	Approximately 80% inactivated
Angiotensin I	Approximately 70% converted to angiotensin II
Angiotensin II	Not affected
Vasopressin	Not affected
Oxytocin	Not affected
Gastrin	Not affected
ATP, adenosine monophosphate	40–90% removed
Endothelin 1	Approximately 50% removed

Reproduced with permission from Levitzky MG. *Pulmonary Physiology*, 8th edition. McGraw-Hill, 2013.

leukotrienes, serotonin, lysosomal enzymes, platelet-activating factor, neutrophil and eosinophil chemotactic factors, and histamine (Table 5.3). Substances produced in the lung and released into the airways include mucus and other tracheobronchial secretions, surface enzymes, proteins, and immunologically active substances such as opsins. These substances are produced by submucosal gland cells, goblet cells, Clara cells, and macrophages.

The pulmonary vascular endothelium almost completely removes prostaglandins E_1, E_2, F_{2a} (this promotes closure of the ductus arteriosus in the newborn) and leukotrienes in a single pass. Endothelin 1 is almost 50% removed; while 80–90% of bradykinin is inactivated in a single pass. Norepinephrine is 30% removed while 70% of angiotensin I is converted to angiotensin II in a single pass. Prostaglandins A1, A2, prostacyclin, epinephrine, and dopamine are unaffected. Thus, some substances can be removed from the blood entering the lungs then added back to the blood by different cells.

Overall pediatric metabolism tends to be faster than adult metabolism. Adults consume 3–3.5 ml O_2/kg/min while neonatal oxygen consumption is about twice that (7–9.5 ml O_2/kg/min). This is one of the factors that lead to a very rapid decline in oxyhemoglobin saturation when a pediatric patient becomes apneic.

Respiratory system: pathophysiology and anesthesia concerns

Airway obstruction in pediatric anesthesia

Upper airway

Pediatric airway anatomy causes children to be at greater risk of airway obstruction when compared to adults. Infants and toddlers are much more susceptible to severe airway obstruction of both upper and lower airways due to their having much smaller absolute airway diameters than those in adults. Thus, even relatively mild airway edema, inflammation or secretions can lead to much greater increases in airways resistance (compared to in adults). Poiseuille's equation states that airways' resistance is inversely proportional to their radius to the fourth power.

Children have large heads, small necks and small mandibles in relation to their large tongues. In addition, children are more likely to attempt to ingest foreign bodies that can become lodged in the airway. Foreign body obstruction can occur at any level of the airway. Symptoms can range from cough to complete airway obstruction.

Clinical care: If the child is stable, radiographic evidence can be obtained prior to attempted removal. If there are any signs of respiratory distress, proceeding directly to the operating room for retrieval should not be delayed. Inhalational induction while maintaining spontaneous ventilation should occur prior to retrieval. Positive pressure or assisted ventilations may force the object further down the airway or risk aspiration. Airway edema may be present following retrieval.

Airway masses: Neoplastic or other types of masses can occur at any level of the tracheobronchial tree. Spontaneous ventilation should be maintained anytime there is a known mass. Muscle relaxation can cause airway collapse because the airway stenting from spontaneous ventilation is lost. This is especially important for mediastinal masses that may compress the airway distal to the endotracheal tube and compromise ventilation. Mediastinal masses can also cause compression of the superior vena cava (SVC syndrome), pulmonary arteries, or the heart. Anterior mediastinal masses (AMM) are especially associated with adverse perioperative events. Posterior mediastinal masses are usually of neurogenic origin and do not cause such high anesthetic risks. These issues should be investigated at the preoperative visit.

Clinical care: A patient with dyspnea that worsens upon lying in the supine position can experience complete airway collapse following induction of deep sedation or general anesthesia. Positive-pressure ventilation and even endotracheal intubation may be unsuccessful. In this dire situation, consider using a very small diameter endotracheal tube and attempt to pass it beyond the obstruction into the main-stem bronchus. Ideally, this situation should be avoided by maintaining spontaneous ventilation.

Imaging (CXR and CT) should be acquired to assess for airway compromise and difficulty of intubation. An ECHO can be obtained to access the degree of cardiac and pulmonary artery compression. For diagnostic biopsy procedures, local with minimal sedation (with ketamine and/or dexmedetomidine) should be attempted. Once diagnosis is established, a plan to shrink the tumor with radiation or chemotherapy should be made prior to procedures requiring general anesthesia. If general anesthesia is absolutely required prior to this time, an ENT surgeon with rigid bronchoscopy skills and also femoral–femoral bypass can be on standby during the procedure but is unlikely to be established in time for an emergency situation. Antisialagogues may be given if a fiberoptic intubation is planned. Patients should be awakened fully prior to extubation. Due to the relatively small airway size, pediatric patients are at a greater risk for airway complications compared to adults. Even an asymptomatic patient with AMM is at risk for airway complications. If the patient cannot tolerate the supine position, consider if the procedure can be done in the lateral or prone position (with spontaneous ventilation). Also, in the presence of SVC syndrome, remember to establish IV access in the lower extremity to assure delivery of injected medications in a timely manner.

As seen in Figure 5.3(c), an intrathoracic airway compressing lesion (such as an AMM) obstructs exhalation due to dynamic compression of the airways. These lesions are usually very vascular and become engorged as intrathoracic pressure rises, which further increases airway compression. As air trapping increases and the chest distends, further inflation becomes impossible. Figure 5.3(b) shows the effects of an obstruction from an extrathoracic lesion (such as laryngomalacia or stenosis), where obstruction worsens during inspiration.

Numerous congenital abnormalities and syndromes further increase the likelihood of pediatric airway obstruction. Cleft palate, isolated or as part of a syndrome, further amplifies the risk of obstruction. Mandibular hypoplasia is a key component of several syndromes with varying degrees of potential airway obstruction. These syndromes include: Pierre Robin Syndrome, Treacher Collins Syndrome, Goldenhar syndrome, and Nager syndrome.

Clinical care: Preoperative evaluation is essential in determining the risk and degree of airway obstruction for the individual child. Special attention should be given to airway exam, cardiovascular status, and the symptoms of chronic hypoxemia and pulmonary hypertension. Antisialagogues may be given preoperatively, but respiratory depressants should be avoided. Spontaneous ventilation should be maintained throughout induction and intubation and the patient should be fully awake prior to extubation.

Acute epiglottitis (AE): this is a life-threatening upper airway infection that requires emergent recognition and treatment. Haemophilus influenzae type B is the predominant cause but its incidence has decreased since vaccination has begun. An AE typically occurs in children 2–7 years old and presents as rapidly evolving febrile illness with inspiratory stridor. Emergent intubation in the operating room should occur in the presence of a practitioner able to establish a surgical airway if necessary.

Obstructive sleep apnea (OSA): secondary to adenotonsilar hypertrophy, OSA is common in children with large tonsils, Down syndrome, craniofacial anomalies, prematurity, and obesity. They often present for tonsillectomy and adenoidectomy. Endotracheal intubation is preferred for all cases. As with other chronic obstructive processes, careful attention

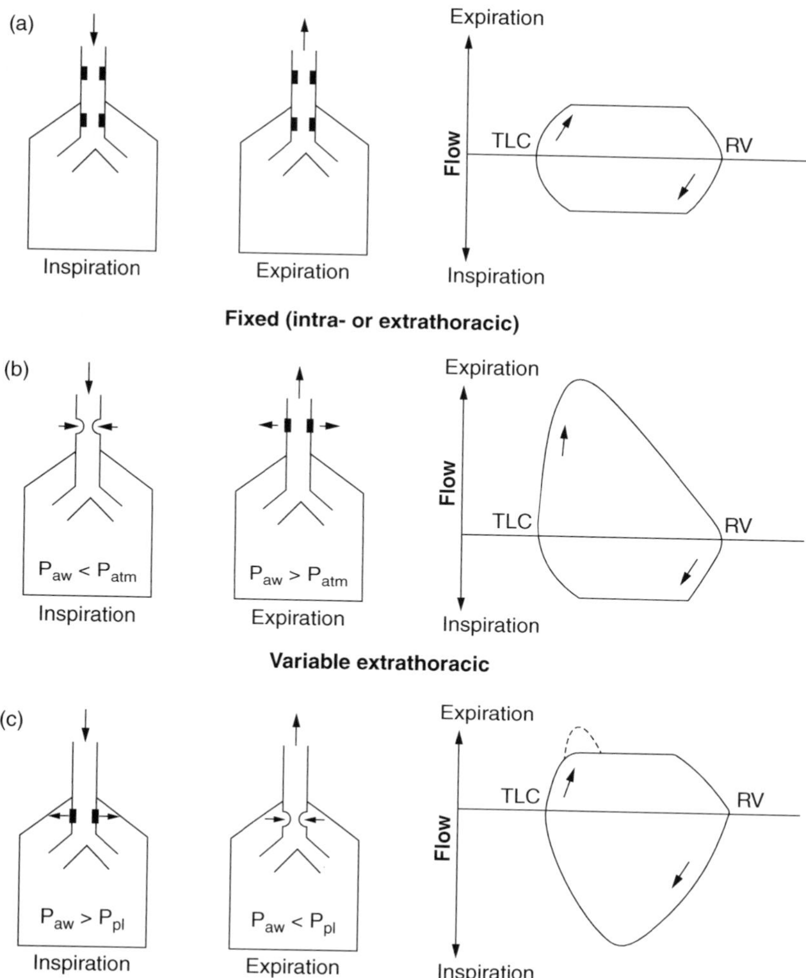

Figure 5.3 Inspiratory and expiratory flow–volume curves representing the patterns in: **(a):** Fixed intra- or extrathoracic obstruction. **(b):** Variable extrathoracic obstruction. **(c):** Variable intrathoracic obstruction. P_{atm} = atmospheric pressure; P_{aw} = airway pressure; P_{pl} = intrapleural pressure; RV = residual volume; TLC = total lung capacity. (Reproduced with permission from Burrows B, Knudson RJ, Quan SF, Kettel LJ. *Respiratory Disorders: A Pathophysiologic Approach*. 2nd edn. Chicago, IL: Year Book Medical Publishers; 1983.)

should be given to cardiovascular status and effects of chronic hypoxemia. These patients should be extubated awake and monitored closely postoperatively for obstruction.

Laryngomalacia: this is an upper airway obstruction that results from the collapse of soft cartilage of the upper larynx during inspiration. This results in an inspiratory stridor during infancy that usually resolves over time.

Tracheobronchial conditions

Croup (laryngotracheobronchitis) is typically caused by a viral infection causing airway obstruction at the level of the cricoid rings. Barking-like inspiratory stridor occurs because of mucosal swelling. Croup usually affects children between 6 months and 6 years of age. Croup rarely requires emergent intubation unlike epiglottitis. Treatment for mild to moderate croup includes steroids, humidified oxygen, and racemic epinephrine. In the event that intubation is required, it should be performed in the operating room with surgeons present as noted in the discussion of epiglottitis.

Subglottic stenosis can be a result of prolonged intubation or tracheostomy or congenital conditions (congenital heart disease, Down syndrome, and tracheoesophageal fistula). Subglottic stenosis from prolonged intubation or tracheostomy is more likely to be clinically significant in young children due to their airway anatomy. Even minimal airway edema can cause near complete airway obstruction. Postintubation edema risk is higher following prolonged intubation, and with traumatic intubation, children under 4 years of age, tight-fitting endotracheal tubes, a history of infectious or postintubation croup, neck or airway surgery, or Down syndrome. Postintubation stenosis typically presents with stridor (inspiratory if above the vocal cords or expiratory if below the vocal cords), cough, hoarseness, retractions, hypoxia, or mental status changes. Presentation is usually within one hour of extubation. Symptoms peak around 4 hours and resolve within 24 hours. The severity of symptoms dictates the treatment.

Clinical care: Observation or aerosolized racemic epinephrine hourly until symptoms resolve may be used for mild to moderate symptoms. More severe symptoms may require surgical airway placement or heliox (a commercially available mixture of helium and oxygen. This low-density gas mixture is easier for the asthmatic patient to breathe than room air.) Congenital stenosis usually requires a tracheostomy and surgical repair. Following surgery, the patient should remain sedated to allow for healing.

Parenchymal disorders

The common lower airway disorders seen in children include bronchopulmonary dysplasia, cystic fibrosis, bronchial asthma, reactive airway disease associated with gastroesophageal reflux, and congenital heart disease with left-to-right shunting and pulmonary hypertension.

Bronchopulmonary dysplasia (BPD) is a parenchymal and small airways disorder affecting former prematurely born children who required mechanical ventilation. Diagnosis is made if the child requires oxygen therapy beyond 36 weeks gestational age. The BPD presents with airway hyper-reactivity and elevated airways resistance, impaired pulmonary compliance, hypoxia, hypercarbia, ventilation-to-perfusion mismatch, and possible right heart failure.

Clinical care: Treatment entails maintaining adequate oxygenation ($PaO_2 > 55$ mmHg and $SaO_2 > 94\%$). Airway management requires careful attention to rapid desaturation, possible subglottic stenosis, and airway hyper-reactivity. A surgical level of anesthesia should be established prior to airway instrumentation due to hyper-reactivity. Increased FiO_2 and peak airway pressure may be needed to maintain adequate ventilation and oxygenation; however, both should be at the lowest possible level to achieve this goal. In addition, fluid management and fluid status must be monitored to avoid pulmonary edema, especially in infants with known cor pulmonale.

Asthma is the most common cause of wheezing in the pediatric population. Asthma is a recurrent and reversible airway obstruction resulting from chronic inflammation, smooth muscle hypertrophy, mucus hypersecretion, and airway hyper-reactivity. Patients with allergies and atopy have a strong association with asthma.

Clinical care: Treatment includes various bronchodilators and inhaled or systemic steroids, depending on the severity and frequency of attacks. During attacks, airway obstruction can lead to air trapping and hyperinflation. This leads to decreased compliance, increased work of breathing, V/Q mismatch, atelectasis, and dead space ventilation. These characteristics result in hypoxemia. Initially, the increased work of breathing and tachypnea result in hypocarbia, but increased obstruction and fatigue cause additional hypoxia and hypercarbia. Wheezing may no longer be heard as obstruction progresses and the child fatigues. Intubation and inhaled anesthetics may be necessary for refractory asthma. When an asthmatic child presents for surgery, a careful history and physical examination must be performed. Special attention should be paid to inciting factors, recent upper respiratory tract infection (URI), frequency and severity of attacks, medication regime, and cardiopulmonary exam. Make sure that the patient receives his or her daily maintenance medications. Preoperative anxiolytics can help prevent acute attacks. Intravenous steroids should be given if the patient is on chronic oral steroid therapy. Induction can be performed with sevoflurane or IV propofol or ketamine. Although ketamine is a bronchodilator, increased secretions may put the patient at increased risk for bronchospasms. Avoidance of or minimal airway manipulation is preferred. Histamine releasing agents should be avoided. If wheezing occurs intraoperatively, mechanical causes must be first ruled out. Once ruled out, anesthesia should be deepened, albuterol may be given, lidocaine administered, and inspiratory: expiratory ratio decreased (↓I:E) to allow complete expiration and prevent air trapping. Permissive hypercarbia is allowed to limit peak inspiratory pressure. Deep extubation may be preferred for patients with easily intubated airways to limit the risk of bronchospasm.

Cystic fibrosis morbidity and mortality is most often pulmonary in nature. Pulmonary complications result from abnormally thick mucus. This causes chronic sinusitis and respiratory infections and inflammation due to impaired mucociliary transport. Mucus pooling can cause airway obstruction and provide a substrate for infection. As patients age, pulmonary scarring and inflammation increase until bronchiectasis and moderate emphysema, ventilation/perfusion mismatching, and hypoxemia occur and lung transplant is required.

Clinical care: Cystic fibrosis patients typically present for nasal polyp removal and long-term IV access for therapy. Pulmonary exam and assessment is important preoperatively. Elective cases should be scheduled for later in the day because secretions are worse in the morning. Aggressive chest physiotherapy should occur prior to surgery. Patients should be allowed clear liquids until 2 hours prior to surgery to decrease the thickness of secretions. Any bronchodilators or other respiratory medications should be taken on the operative day. An IV induction should be used due to possible airway irritation from inhaled agents and the more prolonged induction. Use humidified gas and frequent airway suctioning to clear secretions. Euvolemia should be maintained to avoid mucus plugging or excessive secretions. Regional/local anesthesia and minimal respiratory depressant drugs should be used. The patient should be extubated awake following the procedure and chest physiotherapy should be performed in the post-anesthesia care unit (PACU).

Restrictive diseases in pediatric anesthesia

Pediatric **restrictive disorders** occur primarily from limitations of chest wall movement due to disorders such as scoliosis, chest wall deformities, pleural effusions, obesity, or abdominal distention. Intrapulmonary lesions such as bullae, cysts, and alveolar filling defects can also cause restrictive patterns. In restrictive diseases, all lung volumes and compliance are reduced, but expiratory rate is maintained. Acute restrictive disorders, such as pleural effusions or abdominal distention, should be treated and the patient optimized prior to elective procedures. Chronic restrictive disorders or emergent surgery for patients with acute issues require low tidal volumes and higher rates to decrease the risk of hemodynamic compromise and barotrauma.

Diaphragmatic hernia is the herniation of abdominal contents into the thoracic cavity through a defect in the diaphragm. The most common manifestation is a left-sided lesion via the foramen of Bochdalek. Right-sided lesions do occur via the foramen of Morgagni but are less serious. Herniation of the abdominal contents compresses the developing lungs in utero and results in pulmonary hypoplasia. This presents as respiratory distress soon after birth. Neonates present with tachypnea, scaphoid abdomen, absent breath sounds, or presence of bowel sounds on the affected side.

Clinical care: It is important to not bag/mask ventilate as this can further distend the abdomen and worsen the thoracic compression. The child should be intubated immediately. Chest X-ray confirms the diagnosis by showing bowel in the chest cavity that is displacing the heart and mediastinum. Persistent fetal circulation with right to left shunting further worsens the hypoxemia. In response, pulmonary vascular resistance is further increased. Surgical correction is delayed until the patient has been medically optimized. Following intubation, the infant is placed on low pressure mechanical ventilation and pulmonary vasodilators. High peak airway pressures may result in a contralateral tension pneumothorax. Sedation, paralysis, surfactant, high-frequency ventilation, or even cardiopulmonary bypass (extracorporeal membrane oxygenation) may be needed to stabilize the patient. Once stabilized, the infant can proceed to surgery. The patient will likely present to the operating room already intubated. Right-sided radial arterial line and pulse ox should be placed to monitor preductal oxygenation. Intraoperative management should be focused on minimizing pulmonary hypertension exacerbation. In addition, low-volume tidal volumes should be delivered to prevent contralateral tension pneumothorax. Patients typically return to the ICU intubated following the procedure.

Muscular dystrophy patients can present with a restrictive breathing pattern. Muscular weakness can lead to kyphoscoliosis thus restricting lung expansion. In addition, inspiratory muscle weakness causes chronic hypoventilation. Expiratory muscle weakness diminishes the ability to cough leading to the increase of infection and aspiration.

Clinical care: Respiratory depressants should be avoided or used sparingly. Succinylcholine should be avoided to prevent hyperkalemia and cardiac arrest. Nondepolarizing blockers may have prolonged action. As with other restrictive diseases, these patients should be awakened completely prior to extubation. These patients may require postoperative ventilation because of the extended action of the neuromuscular blockade.

One-lung ventilation: Many thoracic procedures require or are aided by one lung-ventilation (OLV.)

Clinical care: In young children, OLV must be carefully planned preoperatively. The smallest double lumen tube is 26F, which has the outer diameter of a 6.5 single lumen tube. This would be acceptable for a 7–8 year old child. For younger children, other methods of OLV must be chosen. The simplest technique is to intentionally insert a normal endotracheal tube into the appropriate mainstem bronchus. A tube one size smaller than would normally be used should be chosen. Positioning should be confirmed with fiberoptic bronchoscopy (FOB.) If the left bronchus is intended to be intubated, it may require FOB guidance. The downside of this technique is the inability to suction the operative lung, possible contamination of the nonoperative lung, and difficulty obtaining a seal. In addition, the right upper lobe may not be ventilated. Hypoxemia may require withdrawing the tube to ventilate both lungs and repositioning once the patient is stable.

Univent tubes are single lumen tubes that contain a blocker that is advanced from the tube and inflated in the bronchus. Positioning is once again confirmed with FOB. Univent tubes have an internal lumen in the blocker which allows for suctioning of the operative lung. Since the blocker is attached to the tube, the positioning is less likely to be disturbed.

Alternatively, a pulmonary artery balloon catheter, Foley catheter, or Fogarty balloon catheter may be used as a bronchial blocker. The bronchus should be intubated with a single lumen tube. A guide wire is then placed through the lumen of the tube and the tube is removed. The chosen balloon catheter is advanced over the guide wire. Once placed, the single lumen tube is then replaced. It is possible for the balloon catheter to be displaced and completely occlude the trachea.

Video-assisted thoracoscopic surgery (VATS)

Infants have a higher oxygen demand which leads to rapid desaturation. When placed in lateral decubitus position, the dependent lung receives greater perfusion, while the upper lung receives greater ventilation. This causes V/Q mismatch. Single-lung ventilation tends to improve the V/Q mismatch through hypoxic pulmonary vasoconstriction. Medications that inhibit HPV should be avoided to ensure improved ventilation and perfusion match. Careful attention should be given to desaturations and possible displacement of any bronchial blockers. High FiO_2 may be needed to maintain oxygen saturation. Thoracic epidural may be helpful for postoperative pain.

Further reading

1. Fishman AP. Non-respiratory function of the lung. *Chest* 1977; **72**: 84.
2. Merrill JD, Ballard RA. Pulmonary surfactant for neonatal respiratory disorders. *Curr Opin Pediatr* 2003; **15**: 149.
3. Wright JR. Host defense functions of pulmonary surfactant. *Biol Neonate* 2004; **85**(4): 326–32.
4. Engle WA. Surfactant- replacement therapy for respiratory distress in the preterm and term neonate. *Pediatrics* 2007; **120**: 272.
5. Langston C, Kida K, Reed M, *et al.* Human lung growth in late gestation and in the neonate. *Am Rev Respir Dis* 1984; **129**:607.
6. Cheung SL, Lerman J. Mediastinal masses and anesthesia in children. *Anesth Clin North Am* 1998; **16**: 893–910.
7. Cote CJ, Zaslavsky A, Domes JJ, *et al.* Postoperative apnea in former preterm infants after inguinal herniorraphy. *Anesthesiology* 1995; **82**: 809–21.
8. Kurup V. Respiratory diseases. In Hines RL, Marschall KE, editors. *Stoeling's Anesthesia and Co-existing Diseases*, 5th edn. Philadelphia, PA: Churchill Livingstone; 2008.
9. Lee C, Luginbuehl I, Bissonnette B, Mason LJ. Pediatric diseases. In Hines RL, Marschall KE, editors. *Stoeling's Anesthesia and Co-existing Diseases*, 5th ed. Philadelphia, PA: Churchill Livingstone; 2008.
10. Lerman J, Cote CJ, Stewart DJ. *Manual of Pediatric Anesthesia*, 6th edn. Philadelphia, PA: Churchill Livingstone; 2010.
11. Firth PG, Haver KE. Essentials of pulmonology. In Cote CJ, Lerman J, Todres ID, editors. *A Practice of Anesthesia for Infants and Children*, 4th edn. Philadelphia, PA: Saunders Elsevier; 2009.

12. Wheeler M, Cote CJ, Todres ID. The pediatric airway. In Cote CJ, Lerman J, Todres ID, editors. *A Practice of Anesthesia for Infants and Children*, 4th edn. Philadelphia, PA: Saunders Elsevier; 2009.
13. Hammer GB. Anesthesia for thoracic surgery. In Cote CJ, Lerman J, Todres ID, editors. *A Practice of Anesthesia for Infants and Children*, 4th edn. Philadelphia, PA: Saunders Elsevier; 2009.
14. Crean P, Hicks E. Essentials of neurology and neuromuscular disease. In Cote CJ, Lerman J, Todres ID, editors. *A Practice of Anesthesia for Infants and Children*, 4th edn. Philadelphia, PA: Saunders Elsevier; 2009.
15. Fletcher RL. The relationship between the arterial to end-tidal PCO_2 difference and hemoglobin saturation in patients with congenital heart disease. *Anesthesiology*. 1991; **72**: 210–16.
16. Stricker L, Berkowitz D. Pectus excavatum repair. In Litman RS, editor. *Pediatric Anesthesia Practice*, 2nd edn. New York: Cambridge University Press; 2007.
17. Stricker P. Anterior mediastinal mass. In Litman RS, editor. *Pediatric Anesthesia Practice*, 2nd edn. New York: Cambridge University Press; 2007.
18. Bhananker SM. Asthma. In Litman RS, editor. *Pediatric Anesthesia Practice*, 2nd edn. New York: Cambridge University Press; 2007.
19. Litman, RS. Obstructive sleep apnea. In Litman RS, editor. *Pediatric Anesthesia Practice*, 2nd edn. New York: Cambridge University Press; 2007.
20. Litman, RS. Video-assisted thoracoscopic surgery. In Litman RS, editor. *Pediatric Anesthesia Practice*, 2nd edn. New York: Cambridge University Press; 2007.
21. Litman, RS. Mediastinoscopy. In Litman RS, editor. *Pediatric Anesthesia Practice*, 2nd edn. New York: Cambridge University Press; 2007.
22. Mazurek, M. Congenital diaphramatic hernia repair. In Litman RS, editor. *Pediatric Anesthesia Practice*, 2nd edn. New York: Cambridge University Press; 2007.
23. Cote CJ, Lerman J, and Stewart DJ. General and thoracoabdominal surgery In Lerman J, Cote CJ, Stewart DJ, editors. *Manual of Pediatric Anesthesia*, 6th edn. Philadelphia, PA: Churchill Livingstone; 2010, pp. 336–97.

Chapter 6

Cardiovascular system

Douglas R. Thompson, Gregory J. Latham, and Michael Richards

Anatomy and physiology

Prenatal and postnatal development

Embryologic formation of the cardiovascular system

The heart is the first functional organ of the embryo and forms between the second and eighth weeks of life. On day 15, the mesoderm differentiates from the ectoderm and gives rise to the straight heart tube, which will form the atria, ventricles, bulbus cordis, and truncus arteriosis. The primitive heart tube begins to beat by day 23 and gives rise to embryonic circulation by day 30. Various factors, including differential growth rates, constrictions at sites of future structures, genetic factors, cell differentiation, and influence from the surrounding pericardium and neural crest cells chaperone ongoing formation of the heart over the next several weeks.[1–3]

Over the next 4–6 weeks, the structure of the heart matures almost completely into that seen at the end of gestation. Cardiac looping on day 21 causes the primitive heart tube to fold on to itself, migrating the eventual cardiac chambers and great vessels into their relative positions. Subsequent development includes septation and heart chamber formation, formation of heart valves, formation of the pulmonary vascular system, formation of the conduction and coronary artery system, and septation and formation of the outflow tracts and great arteries. Abnormal cardiac development that leads to congenital heart disease likely occurs through a complex relationship of genetic and environmental factors in utero. Further discussion of embryology is beyond the scope of this chapter, but excellent reviews are available for the interested reader.[1–3]

Postnatal cardiovascular development

Although myocardial mechanics are qualitatively similar from embryonic stages through childhood, several pertinent differences exist that impact overall cardiac function.[4] Compared with the adult, the immature neonatal myocardium cannot generate the same contractile force. The neonatal myocardium is comprised of less contractile elements and more connective tissue than adults, and the myofibrils are less organized. Neonatal myocardium relies more on extracellular calcium for contractility, compared to immediate release and uptake by the sarcoplasmic reticulum in adults, which may explain the exaggerated sensitivity in infants to hypocalcemia from rapid transfusion of blood products. Additional reasons for less contractile force exist in the neonatal period, including contractile protein immaturity, inefficient energy storage and utilization, and immature cellular regulation of the action potential compared to the adult.[5]

Traditionally, it has been believed the neonatal cardiac output is primarily heart rate dependent; however, this view has been challenged. Neonatal hearts do respond to alterations in preload and afterload, but the effect is not as great as in adults. Poor ventricular compliance and likely a very narrow Frank–Starling curve predisposes the neonatal heart to have less of an ability to alter cardiac output based on stroke volume, preload, and afterload, thus having a greater reliance on heart rate for cardiac output. Overall, because of the high metabolic demands of the heart and other developing tissues, the neonatal heart operates at near-maximal capacity at most times.[5]

The neonatal and even fetal heart does respond to sympathetic stimulation. The sympathetic nervous innervation of the heart, however, is immature at birth, and parasympathetic innervation dominates, leading to potentially exaggerated vagal responses to a number of stimuli. The sympathetic nervous system becomes mature by late infancy.[5, 6]

Essentials of Pediatric Anesthesiology, ed. Alan David Kaye, Charles James Fox and James H. Diaz. Published by Cambridge University Press. © Cambridge University Press 2015.

Fetal, transitional, and adult circulation

Fetal circulation

Fetal growth occurs in a relatively hypoxic environment. The PO_2 of umbilical vein blood entering the fetus is approximately 30 mmHg and is approximately 16 mmHg when returning to the placenta via the umbilical arteries. Several mechanisms, most notably fetal shunts, are in place to best utilize the limited O_2 available to the developing tissues. The three fetal shunts are the ductus venosus, foramen ovale, and ductus arteriosus.[4, 7, 8]

The ductus venosus aids in directing the oxygenated blood from the placenta directly to the heart. This bypass of the portal venous system maintains the high oxygenation and velocity of placental blood into the inferior vena cava (IVC) and heart. The remainder of IVC flow is from the fetal lower body and the hepatic vein and is both deoxygenated and low velocity.[4, 7, 8]

As IVC flow enters the right atrium (RA), the eustachian valve preferentially streams most of the high-velocity, oxygenated umbilical venous blood from the ductus venosus toward the foramen ovale and into the left atrium (LA) and left ventricle (LV). Conversely, the low-velocity, desaturated blood from the lower body and hepatic vein enters the right atrium and mixes with deoxygenated blood return from the superior vena cava (SVC). Most of this deoxygenated venous return preferentially streams across the tricuspid valve and into the right ventricle (RV). Thus, the RV contains lower saturated blood, and the LV contains higher saturated blood.[4, 7, 8]

The LV ejection sends the relatively oxygenated blood to the ascending aorta and aortic arch vessels, providing blood with an SaO_2 of 60–65% to the highly metabolic heart and brain. The RV ejection sends the deoxygenated blood into the pulmonary artery. The high pulmonary vascular resistance (PVR) directs 90% of the RV output across the third fetal shunt, the ductus arteriosus, and into the descending aorta. Two-thirds of the descending aorta blood, with an SaO_2 of 50–55%, returns to the placenta, and the rest perfuses the abdominal organs and lower body.[4, 7, 8]

Fetal oxygen delivery (DO_2) in this relatively hypoxic state is augmented by four factors: (1) relatively high cardiac output, (2) high hemoglobin concentrations, (3) greater oxygen affinity of hemoglobin F for enhanced O_2 binding at the placenta, and (4) increased 2,3-diphosphoglycerate in fetal tissues for enhanced O_2 release to the tissues.[6]

Transitional circulation

At birth, several acute changes occur that profoundly impact the circulation, leading to a state called the transitional circulation. In the transitional state, the pulmonary arterial pressures are still high (although much lower than in utero), and flow reverses in the ductus arteriosus from right-to-left in utero to left-to-right. Maturation to the adult circulation occurs over a few weeks. However, reversal to or persistence of the fetal circulation is possible during this period, especially with various congenital heart lesions or isolated increases in PVR (see below).

Clamping of the umbilical vessels at birth removes the large, low-resistance vascular bed of the placenta, causing an acute elevation of SVR and LV afterload. At the same time, lung expansion and the start of postnatal ventilation elicits a dramatic decrease in PVR and is associated with an eight- to ten-fold increase in pulmonary blood flow and subsequent LA filling. The combined increase in pulmonary venous return and increased LV afterload results in a sudden increase in LA pressure. As LA pressure exceeds that of the RA minutes after birth, the flap-like foramen ovale functionally closes, signaling closure of the first fetal shunt. Complete anatomic closure, however, occurs more slowly or not at all. An anatomically patent foramen ovale can be found in over 50% of infants 2–6 months of age and in 25% of adults, most of which have little clinical significance.[6, 9–11]

Within hours after birth, the rise in SVR and fall in PVR leads to a reversal of flow to left-to-right across the ductus arteriosus. The elevation in PO_2 and decrease of circulating prostaglandins after birth leads to constriction of the ductus arteriosus tissue. Functional closure of the duct occurs in over half of newborns by day 2 and in 98% by day 4; within 2–3 weeks, ductal fibrosis occurs, resulting in the ductal remnant called the ligamentum arteriosum.[6, 10] Premature babies may require significantly longer time for ductal closure or may require surgical closure in cases of pulmonary overcirculation and systemic steal.

When the umbilical cord is clamped, flow through the ductus venosus stops, and portal venous flow dramatically decreases. Functional closure of the ductus venosus occurs in 1–2 weeks, and ongoing fibrosis results in the ligamentum venosum within months.[6]

Persistent fetal circulation

Persistence of or reversal to the fetal circulation, that is right-to-left flow across the foramen ovale and/or ductus arteriosus, can occur in two newborn scenarios: (1) various forms of cyanotic congenital heart disease that maintain patency of the fetal shunts, and (2) persistent pulmonary hypertension of the newborn (PPHN). The numerous complex congenital heart lesions that cause persistence of ductal flow or intracardiac mixing at the atrial level are beyond the scope of this chapter and not further reviewed.

Persistent pulmonary hypertension of the newborn occurs when PVR fails to decrease at birth, and symptoms are present immediately at birth or shortly thereafter. The most common cause of PPHN is parenchymal lung disease, including meconium aspiration and respiratory distress syndrome. Other causes include sepsis, alveolar-capillary dysplasia, surfactant dysfunction, and severe lung hypoplasia (e.g., congenital diaphragmatic hernia).[11, 12]

Continued elevation of PVR after birth limits pulmonary venous return to the LA, thus maintaining right-to-left shunt across the atrial septum and failure of foramen ovale closure. Furthermore, the elevated PVR promotes right-to-left shunt across the ductus arteriosus. Hypoxemia ensues from poor ventilation at the alveolar level and from the right-to-left shunts at the ductus arteriosus and foramen ovale. A vicious cycle occurs whereby the hypoxia further potentiates the elevated PVR and patency of the ductus arteriosus.[11, 12] Mild forms may just require supplemental oxygen by nasal cannula to lessen PVR, but severe forms may require inotropic support or extracorporeal membrane oxygenation (ECMO).[11]

Anesthetic management of the newborn with PPHN requires meticulous management to ensure adequate oxygenation and preservation of myocardial function and systemic perfusion. The newborn pulmonary vasculature strongly reacts with vasoconstriction to several stimuli, most notably hypoxia. Additional stimuli include acidosis, elevation of leukotrienes and thromboxane, catecholamine release (including crying and light anesthesia), atelectasis, and excessive PEEP.[6, 11] While oxygen therapy causes potent vasodilation and improved PO_2, hyperoxia can be harmful to the newborn, and maximal dilation occurs at relatively low O_2 levels. Thus, oxygen should be titrated to the lowest acceptable levels, with a PaO_2 of 60–90 mmHg as the goal. Normocapnia is ideal; hypercapnia induces pulmonary vasoconstriction, and excessive alkalinization through hyperventilation may be harmful.[11] Inhaled nitric oxide (NO) is a potent selective pulmonary vasodilator and may be required perioperatively in the newborn. Lastly, adequate systemic perfusion must be ensured, which may require inotropic support in newborns that are severely ill.[6, 11]

Newborn resuscitation

In the fetus, the saturation of blood is approximately 65% in the LA and is 55% in the descending aorta. Immediately after birth, right-to-left shunting across the ductus arteriosus slows and then reverses over a few hours. Normal arterial PO_2 increases from 50 mmHg 10 minutes after birth, to 62 at 1 hour after birth, and to 75–83 over the next several hours or day.[10, 13] The normal arterial saturation 5 minutes after birth is 90%, which gradually increases over the next day. Therefore, resuscitation of the hypoxic newborn to SaO_2 and PO_2 values greater than these normal values is not only unnecessary but is probably harmful.[14]

Based upon the potential harm of hyperoxia in newborns, the following are a subset of recommendations from the 2010 International Consensus on Cardiopulmonary Resuscitation and Emergency Cardiovascular Care Science With Treatment Recommendations – Neonatal Resuscitation:[15]

- Oximetry should be used for evaluation of oxygenation because assessment of color is unreliable.
- For babies born at term it is best to begin resuscitation with air rather than 100% oxygen.
- Administration of supplementary oxygen should be regulated by blending oxygen and air, and the concentration delivered should be guided by oximetry.

Thus, resuscitation with room air or cautious escalation of fractional inspired O_2 should target normal postnatal saturations. In the newborn, goal saturations of 88–92% are commonly regarded as the best balance between the risks or hypoxia with lower goal saturations and hyperoxia with higher saturations.[14]

Effects on the cardiovascular system of commonly used anesthetic medications

This section will focus on understanding the effects of commonly used anesthetic medications on the cardiovascular system. Most studies that have examined these effects have several confounding variables, and frequently the medication being studied is used in combination with other anesthetic agents. Many pediatric studies examine the hemodynamic effects of drugs in patients with underlying congenital cardiac disease, raising the question of whether results in such patients can be extrapolated to a normal physiological state. Finally some studies look at drug effects in isolated cardiac muscle preparations, which although a useful model may not reflect the in vivo effects (such as ketamine as will be discussed below).

To help make this discussion more relevant, consider the following case scenario:

A 21-month-old female requires anesthesia for a cardiac catheterization procedure. Her past medical history is significant for coarctation of the aorta, mild mitral stenosis, and moderate aortic stenosis. On day 4 of life she underwent a repair of her coarctation, but no intervention on her mitral or aortic valve was performed. She had an excellent surgical result from her coarctation repair but was lost to follow-up. She presented to an outside institution in poorly compensated heart failure thought due to her unrepaired aortic stenosis and was transferred to your institution for an aortic valvuloplasty. She has been started on an inotrope to improve her cardiac function. Her most recent cardiac echo shows no residual coarctation, mild mitral stenosis, and moderate aortic stenosis in the context of severely depressed left ventricular function, raising the likelihood that the degree of aortic stenosis is being underestimated. Right ventricular function and the remainder of the echo is normal.

Question: What anesthetic agents would you choose to anesthetize this patient for her catheterization? Bear in mind the hemodynamic goals for a patient with aortic stenosis include maintenance of preload and afterload, avoidance of bradycardia and tachycardia, and avoidance of hypotension; tachycardia and hypotension adversely affect the balance between myocardial oxygen supply and demand.

Propofol

Propofol has found ubiquitous use in the operative arena, especially with the recent withdrawal of thiopental from the market. Propofol allows for both a rapid induction of anesthesia as well as emergence. Regarding its hemodynamic effects, in a study of healthy Chinese children without congenital heart disease (CHD), propofol used for induction of anesthesia (2.5 mg/kg) resulted in a 28–31% reduction in mean arterial pressure (MAP).[16] In a later study on ASA I and II pediatric patients undergoing elective surgery, hemodynamic measurements after induction with propofol revealed that although there was no significant change in heart rate (HR), there was a reduction in MAP of 15% at induction, increasing to 25% at 5 minutes after induction. In this study, systemic vascular resistance (SVR) decreased by 14% and 27% respectively at induction and 5 minutes, and when echocardiography was used to assess contractility, a significant decrease compared to awake values was noted.[17] Although such hemodynamic perturbations are well tolerated in healthy children, caution would be advised in those with impaired contractility or when maintenance of SVR is important. These considerations may make propofol a less desirable agent in the care of our catheterization patient.

Thiopental

Although no longer available in the USA, thiopental is still widely used in other areas of the world. The cardiovascular depressant effects of thiopental are generally considered to be less profound than those caused by propofol and are primarily due to venodilation (reducing venous return) as well as direct myocardial depression. In their study, Wodey *et al.*[17] found that thiopental did not lead to a significant reduction in systolic blood pressure (SBP), MAP or SVR, although there was a significant reduction in shortening fraction. Thiopental has also been safely used in neonates without dramatic changes in either HR or blood pressure;[18] therefore, where available thiopental is an attractive choice for use during our catheterization procedure.

Ketamine

Ketamine is thought to act as an NMDA receptor antagonist to produce a dissociative anesthetic state. In many regards, ketamine is almost a complete anesthetic agent in and of itself, providing amnesia, unconsciousness, and analgesia. Ketamine is widely considered one of the least hemodynamically depressant anesthetic agents, and many studies seem to support this.[19–21] Ketamine also causes little if any change in pulmonary artery pressure (PAP) or pulmonary vascular resistance (PVR).[20] The purported hemodynamic stability of ketamine is thought to be due to CNS mediated sympathomimetic excitation and inhibition of neuronal uptake of catecholamines,[22] often leading to an increase in HR, MAP, and SVR.[23] Thus ketamine would seem an attractive choice for our cath procedure; however, there are studies which might cause us to pause.

When examined in isolated cardiac muscle cells, ketamine has been shown to have negative inotropic effects as a result of reduced movement of calcium across the sacroplasmic reticulum.[24] In a series of 12 critically ill adult patients, Waxman *et al.*[25] showed half the patients suffered a decrease in cardiac contractility and a decrease in SVR following intravenous ketamine induction. These authors hypothesize that given the critically ill nature of these patients, "adrenocortical and catechol stores had been depleted prior to ketamine administration... setting the stage for possible adverse effects." This was also implicated in a child with end-stage cardiomyopathy who developed pulseless electrical activity following induction with ketamine.[26] Furthermore, Christ *et al.* showed that patients receiving long-term infusions of β agonist exhibited adverse hemodynamic consequences after ketamine infusion with a reduction in cardiac output (CO) of 21%.[27] This may be due to a downregulation of adrenergic receptors causing a weaker response to any endogenously released catecholamines.

Etomidate

Etomidate is a rapidly acting induction agent that exerts its effects via the GABA receptor to induce unconsciousness. Etomidate is purported to have minimal cardiovascular effects, even in children with little hemodynamic reserve. It allowed for an uneventful anesthetic induction in a patient that arrested 10 days earlier during induction of anesthesia with ketamine (see above).[26] Dhawan *et al.* studied the effects of a single dose of etomidate at 0.3 mg/kg in a series of 30 patients with congenital cardiac shunts undergoing cardiac catheterization procedures. There were no significant changes in HR, SBP, MAP, or systemic blood flow.[28] This study agrees with a later study by Sarkar *et al.*, which demonstrated no change in aortic pressure and no significant changes in PAP after etomidate bolus.[29] In addition to use as an induction agent, use of etomidate for maintenance of anesthesia has also been described in children.[30]

Despite these favorable effects on hemodynamics, etomidate is not routinely utilized for the induction of anesthesia in children given the undesirable effects of the drug, including pain on injection, myoclonic movements, nausea and vomiting, and perhaps most importantly adrenal suppression leading to a decrease in cortisol levels. The significance of etomidate-induced adrenal suppression continues to be debated in the literature. In a meta-analysis of 21 studies, Albert *et al.* compared etomidate versus nonetomidate anesthesia in critically ill patients and found a significantly increased rate of adrenal insufficiency AND mortality in patients who received etomidate.[31] More recently, a retrospective review of septic patients that received etomidate for intubation reported no association between single-dose etomidate and mortality or adverse clinical outcomes.[32] It is difficult to generalize these results to pediatrics, but clearly prudence is advised.

Midazolam

Midazolam may be used as the sole anesthesia induction agent; however, induction is slow compared to thiopental, and even high-dose midazolam unreliably induces anesthesia.[33] Midazolam has been used as a sole anesthetic for procedures, typically during procedures that are quick and not very painful.[34] More often, midazolam is used as a premedication or in combination with other anesthetic/analgesic agents. When given as a bolus, Shekerdemian *et al.* demonstrated that midazolam caused a significant decrease in arterial blood pressure (BP) as well as a 24% reduction in CO.[35] These parameters tended to return to baseline within an hour, but this study was done in children with a normal CO. It is also important to note that severe hypotension is possible when midazolam is given as a bolus in neonates also receiving fentanyl.[36] Similarly midazolam–fentanyl infusions during surgery for repair of CHD have been associated with significantly decreased HR, BP, and CO; however, cardiac contractility is preserved.[37]

Hemodynamic effects aside, midazolam by itself or in combination with fentanyl is certainly a viable option for the anesthetic management of our cath procedure, yet it could be challenging to conduct the anesthetic in a manner conducive to extubation at the conclusion of the procedure, which would be desirable.

Dexmedetomidine

Dexmedetomidine is an α-2 specific adrenergic agonist, producing analgesia, anxiolysis, and sedation via spinal cord and centrally mediated actions. It has found use as an adjunct during general anesthesia and as a sedative for procedures. In a small case series of four infants requiring direct laryngoscopy and bronchoscopy, general anesthesia was adequately induced and maintained with dexmedetomidine as a sole agent; one patient did require the addition of propofol however.[38]

An advantage of dexmedetomidine over other commonly used sedatives/anesthetics is its minimal effect on ventilation.[39] In the pediatric population, dexmedetomidine has been associated with a decrease in HR[40] and an accompanying decrease in BP; the hypotension associated with use in pediatric patients was within 20% of baseline measurements in one study,[41] and *hypertension* with the use of dexmedetomidine in children undergoing electrophysiologic studies has been described in another study.[42] The effects of dexmedetomidine on HR and MAP are thought to be secondary to sympathetic output from the central nervous system.

Opioids

There have been many studies of the hemodynamic effects of opioids in neonates and infants. Here we will concentrate primarily on synthetic opioids:

Fentanyl use has been well studied in children and remains one of the most commonly used opioids during general anesthesia in neonates, infants, and children. Fentanyl (in combination with pancuronium) has also been described as the sole anesthetic in patients undergoing repair of CHD and was found to provide hemodynamic stability at doses of 50–75 mcg/kg.[43] In a study by Duncan *et al.*, investigators found that as part of a balanced anesthetic, fentanyl at doses of 25 to 50 mcg/kg blunted the hemodynamic and stress response in the precardiopulmonary bypass period.[44] It is known though that opioids used as a sole anesthetic may not reliably provide amnesia, and as mentioned above, caution is warranted when using fentanyl and midazolam in combination given the possibility of profound hypotension.

Similarly, sufentanil use in children undergoing cardiac surgery has been studied, and, similar to fentanyl, sufentanil has been shown be maintain hemodynamic stability. In their study on infants undergoing repair of complex CHD, Hickey *et al.* found that after premedication with morphine and atropine, sufentanil in doses of 5 to 10 mcg/kg (in combination with pancuronium) provided excellent hemodynamic stability, even in the face of sternotomy.[45]

Remifentanil is an ultra-short acting synthetic opioid that can exert a powerful opioid effect with relative cardiovascular stability. In a study comparing remifentanil versus fentanyl in infants undergoing cardiac surgery, remifentanil was noted to provide good hemodynamic stability; however, significant increases in HR and MAP did occur.[46] Other studies suggest that it may have a negative chronotropic effect,[47] and the common use of remifentanil during controlled hypotension may suggest a hypotensive effect.

Nitrous oxide (NO_2)

Incapable of producing a full MAC of anesthesia, NO_2 is used primarily as an adjunct during maintenance of anesthesia. Given the lack of pungent odor, it is also commonly used in the anesthetic induction of pediatric patients as well. While its use has been reported to increase PVR in adults, no such evidence exists in children, even in those with elevated baseline PVR.[48] In contrast to the minimal impact on PVR, at least two studies in pediatrics have demonstrated a small but significant decrease in HR and CI with the use of NO_2; however, in the study by Murray *et al*, ejection fraction and stroke volume were unchanged.[48, 49]

Volatile anesthetics

The impact of volatile anesthetics on SVR in pediatric patients generally shows that all the inhalational agents will decrease BP; the degree to which that occurs depends on the particular agent used. The reduction in BP is most profound with halothane (no longer available in the USA).[50] In a study of sevoflurane in children one year of age or older, there was a 0–11% reduction in SBP at 1 MAC,[51] and in a separate study of desflurane in children one year or older, the decrease in SBP was between 22 and 28%.[52] In both these studies neonates and infants were shown to be more sensitive to volatile anesthetic-induced hemodynamic depression,[51] which may be due to maturational differences in the sarcoplasmic reticulum, muscle contractile elements, and calcium homeostasis.[53]

Most studies also show that volatile anesthetics lead to a decrease in cardiac contractility to varying degrees. This depression is most profound with halothane and less so with isoflurane, sevoflurane, and desflurane. The mechanism by which this occurs is thought to be related to decreasing intracellular Ca^{2+} flux via actions on the sarcoplasmic reticulum, Ca^{2+} channels, and ion pumps.[54]

Effects on the cardiovascular system of commonly used vasoactive medications

Using the example patient with aortic stenosis for a cardiac catheterization procedure, we will examine the effect of some *common* vasoactive medications.

Epinephrine

Epinephrine is an endogenous catecholamine that acts on both α and β adrenergic receptors. The physiologic response to epinephrine depends on the dose administered as well as the preponderance of adrenergic receptor subtype present in the organ or tissue bed in question. At lower doses (less than 0.05 mcg/kg/min),[55] SBP increases primarily as a result of β-adrenergic stimulation, leading to increased in inotropy and chronotropy. Increasing the dose of epinephrine leads to an increase in α mediated actions and an increase in SVR and PVR. Given the effect on HR and the concomitant effect on myocardial oxygen demand, epinephrine may not be the ideal choice for an inotrope for managing our patient's heart failure.

Norepinephrine

Similar to epinephrine, norepinephrine acts on both α and β adrenergic receptors. In clinical use, norepinephrine is used for its potent effect on α_1 receptors, leading to an increase in SVR as well as systolic and diastolic BP. The CO may decrease due to increases in afterload, and the HR may exhibit a reflex slowing secondary to the effects of the baro-receptor reflex. Norepinephrine is listed as a first-line agent in the international guidelines for management of severe sepsis and septic shock.[56] Extravasation of norepinephrine may lead to tissue necrosis; thus administration via a central line is advised. Given the primary action on α_1 receptors, norepinephrine has little role in the management of heart failure.

Dopamine

Dopamine is a catecholamine with varying affinity for dopamine (DA) receptors as well as β and α adrenergic receptors. At lower doses (infusion rates of 0.5 to 2 mcg/kg/min) activation of DA_1 and DA_2 receptors occurs, leading to vasodilation in the renal, mesenteric, and coronary vascular beds. At such doses, a decreased diastolic pressure and slight increase in HR may be seen.[57] At intermediate doses of 2 to 10 mcg/kg/min, activation of β adrenergic receptors occurs with an increase in chronotropy and inotropy; concomitant systemic vasodilation and venoconstriction yields a net effect of an increase in CO with minimal changes on BP. Infusion rates of 10 mcg/kg/min or greater lead to greater α receptor activation, resulting in higher vascular resistances and BP. At low doses dopamine may be of use in cardiogenic shock, but the increase in chronotropy may limit its use in our hypothetical patient.

Dobutamine

Dobutamine is a synthetic analog of dopamine. Unlike dopamine, dobutamine activates primarily β_1 receptors with a smaller effect on α_1 and β_2 adrenergic receptors. As such, dobutamine results in increased inotropy and chronotropy, with a resultant increase in CO. Reductions in SVR may occur given the β_2 effects of dobutamine, particularly at higher infusion rates. Left ventricular filling pressures are decreased as a result of the vasodilation in pulmonary vasculature,[58] making dobutamine useful in the treatment of right-sided heart failure. Dobutamine may also be of benefit to our catheterization patient, as long as dramatic increases in myocardial oxygen demand as a result of increases in HR and contractility are avoided.

Milrinone

A phosphodiesterase III enzyme inhibitor, milrinone increases cyclic AMP with a resultant increase in intracellular calcium stores, leading to an increase in inotropism, decreased SVR (reduced afterload), and diastolic relaxation. The sum of these effects is to increase CO and oxygen delivery without the deleterious effect of increased myocardial oxygen demand. Taking advantage of these properties, milrinone has found use in treating chronic heart failure, pulmonary hypertension, and diastolic dysfunction associated with cardiac surgery.[59] With its beneficial effects on inotropism (without increasing myocardial oxygen demand), milrinone may be of great benefit to our catheterization patient in heart failure.

Isoproterenol

Isoproterenol is a nonselective β adrenergic agonist with little effect on α receptors. As such it leads to vasodilation with a decrease in both PVR and SVR (β_2 actions) and to an increase in chronotropy and inotropy. These effects will increase myocardial oxygen demand and, in the compromised heart, may induce ischemia; as such it is usually not considered a first-line agent in the treatment of chronic heart failure or myocardial dysfunction (as in the case of our hypothetical patient). Clinically, isoproterenol finds use in electrophysiologic studies, where it is used to increase the heart rate, or in the management of complete heart block, as may occur following cardiac surgery.

Phenylephrine

Phenylephrine is considered a pure α agonist and is commonly used to treat low BP or SVR as may occur after induction of anesthesia. It causes venoconstriction, leading to an increase in cardiac preload as well as afterload. The CO may remain unchanged given the reflex slowing in heart rate that may result from the baroreceptor reflex. The rapidity of its onset and short duration of action make it one of the most commonly used medications to raise SVR. In pediatric anesthesiology, it may find use treating tetralogy "spells" where right ventricular outflow obstruction and a relatively low SVR leads to an increase in right-to-left shunting and cyanosis. Phenylephrine may be useful in our patient to increase BP after induction of anesthesia but plays little role in the treatment of her heart failure.

Ephedrine

Both a direct and indirect α and β receptor agonist, ephedrine is a common vasoactive medication found in the operating room. The primary mode of action is via indirect actions leading to the release of norepinephrine from postsynaptic nerve terminals. Tachyphylaxis through depletion of norepinephrine stores may limit the utility of this drug.[60] The α agonism of ephedrine leads to both venoconstriction and vasoconstriction; with the concomitant β receptor effect of increased ionotropy and chronotropy, the net effect of ephedrine administration is an increase in CO and BP.

Vasopressin

Vasopressin is a synthetic preparation of antidiuretic hormone, which is secreted by the posterior pituitary in response to decreasing filling pressures. Vasopressin works via effects on the V1 and V2 receptors, causing vasoconstriction and antidiuretic effects respectively. Traditionally used as adjunct therapy in gastrointestinal bleeding, its list of indications in adults has expanded to include pressure support in septic shock, cardiac arrest from ventricular fibrillation/ventricular tachycardia, and pulseless electrical activity/asystole. Although there are few studies examining the use of vasopressin in pediatrics, a recent multicenter randomized trial failed to show that low-dose vasopressin was beneficial in the treatment of vasodilatory shock in children.[61] It may be of benefit to those infants undergoing cardiac surgery with a deficiency of arginine vasopressin,[62] but given that it is a vasoconstrictor, it may be detrimental in a patient with low CO.

Sodium nitroprusside

Sodium nitroprusside (SNP) acts directly on vascular smooth muscle, leading to dilation of both arterial and venous beds by releasing nitric oxide. Due to the short half-life, SNP facilitates tight control of BP and systemic vascular resistance. In those patients with poor ventricular function and a compensatory increase in SVR, SNP may be of benefit by decreasing afterload and thus facilitating increased stroke volume and CO. A key side effect of SNP to consider is cyanide toxicity, which results from metabolism of SNP to produce cyanide as a byproduct; the development of an unexplained metabolic acidosis, tachyphylaxis, and increased mixed venous oxygen content are all harbingers of developing cyanide toxicity.[63] Toxicity is more likely to occur at higher doses (10 mcg/kg/min) and with administration lasting more than several hours. If cyanide toxicity is suspected, treatment consists of inhaled amyl nitrate and administration of sodium nitrite followed by sodium thiosulfate. Cyanide poisoning kits are commercially available.

Summary

The anesthetic management of complex CHD necessitates a good working knowledge of developmental anatomy, physiology, pathophysiology, and pharmacology. With these tools the anesthesiologist can make well-informed and appropriate decisions during the management of complex cases, allowing for the patient to be supported in the best manner possible.

References

1. R. Abdulla, G. A. Blew, M. J. Holterman. Cardiovascular embryology. *Pediatr Cardiol* 2004 Jun; **25**(3): 191–200.

2. A. C. Gittenberger-de Groot, M. M. Bartelings, M. C. Deruiter, *et al.* Basics of cardiac development for the understanding of congenital heart malformations. *Pediatr Res* 2005 Mar; **57**(2): 169–76.

3. M. E. Mitchell, T. L. Sander, D. B. Klinkner, *et al.* The molecular basis of congenital heart disease. *Semin Thorac Cardiovasc Surg* 2007; **19**(3): 228–37.

4. D. F. Teitel, S. C. Cassidy, J. R. Fineman. Circulation physiology. In Moss A. J., Allen H. D., eds. *Moss and Adams' Heart Disease in Infants, Children, and Adolescents: Including the Fetus and Young Adult*: Wolters Kluwer Health/ Lippincott Williams & Wilkins; 2008.

5. V. C. Baum, B. W. Palmisano. The immature heart and anesthesia. *Anesthesiology* 1997 Dec; **87**(6): 1529–48.

6. A. Y. Schure, J. A. Dinardo. Cardiac physiology and pharmacology. In Coté C. J., Lerman J., Anderson B. J., eds. *Coté and Lerman's a Practice of Anesthesia for Infants and Children*. 5th edn. Philadelphia, PA: Elsevier; 2013.

7. A. M. Rudolph. Congenital cardiovascular malformations and the fetal circulation. *Arch Dis Child Fetal Neonatal Ed* 2010 Apr 01; **95**(2): F132–6.

8. T. Kiserud. Physiology of the fetal circulation. *Semin Fetal Neonatal Med* 2005 Dec; **10**(6): 493–503.

9. D. Connuck, J. P. Sun, D. M. Super, *et al.* Incidence of patent ductus arteriosus and patent foramen ovale in normal infants. *Am J Cardiol* 2002 Feb 15; **89**(2): 244–7.

10. M. D. Freed. Fetal and transitional circulation. In Keane J. F., Lock J. E., Fyler D. C., eds. *Nadas' pediatric cardiology*. 2nd edn. Philadelphia, PA: Saunders; 2006.

11. G. G. Konduri, U. O. Kim. Advances in the diagnosis and management of persistent pulmonary hypertension of the newborn. *Pediatr Clin North Am* 2009 Jul; **56**(3): 579–600.

12. J. E. B. Cabral, J. Belik. Persistent pulmonary hypertension of the newborn: recent advances in pathophysiology and treatment. *J Pediatr (Rio J)* 2013 Jun; **89**(3): 226–42.

13. N. H. Hillman, S. G. Kallapur, A. H. Jobe. Physiology of transition from intrauterine to extrauterine life. *Clin Perinatol* 2012 Dec; **39**(4): 769–83.

14. J. P. Goldsmith, J. Kattwinkel. The role of oxygen in the delivery room. *Clin Perinatol* 2012 Dec; **39** (4): 803–15.

15. J. M. Perlman, J. Wyllie, J. Kattwinkel, *et al.* Part 11: Neonatal resuscitation: 2010 International Consensus on Cardiopulmonary Resuscitation and Emergency Cardiovascular Care Science With Treatment Recommendations. *Circulation* 2010 Oct 19; **122**(16 Suppl 2): S516–38.

16. C. S. Aun, R. Y. Sung, M. E. O'Meara, *et al.* Cardiovascular effects of i.v. induction in children: comparison between propofol and thiopentone. *Br J Anaesth* 1993 Jun; **70**(6): 647–53.

17. E. Wodey, L. Chonow, X. Beneux, *et al.* Haemodynamic effects of propofol vs. thiopental in infants: an echocardiographic study. *Br J Anaesth* 1999 Apr; **82**(4): 516–20.

18. A. Bhutada, R. Sahni, S. Rastogi, *et al.* Randomised controlled trial of thiopental for intubation in neonates. *Arch Dis Child Fetal Neonatal Ed* 2000 Jan; **82**(1): F34–7.

19. V. Stanley, J. Hunt, K. W. Willis, *et al.* Cardiovascular and respiratory function with CI-581. *Anesth Analg* 1968 Nov–Dec; **47** (6): 760–8.

20. J. P. Morray, A. M. Lynn, S. J. Stamm, *et al.* Hemodynamic effects of ketamine in children with congenital heart disease. *Anesth Analg* 1984 Oct; **63**(10): 895–9.

21. M. Tugrul, E. Camci, K. Pembeci, *et al.* Ketamine infusion versus isoflurane for the maintenance of anesthesia in the prebypass period in children with tetralogy of Fallot. *J Cardiothorac Vasc Anesth* 2000 Oct; **14**(5): 557–61.

22. P. Chang, K. E. Chan, A. Ganendran. Cardiovascular effects of 2-(O-chlorophenyl)-2-methylaminocyclohexanone (CI-581) in rats. *Br J Anaesth* 1969 May; **41**(5): 391–5.

23. W. Berman, Jr., R. R. Fripp, M. Rubler, *et al.* Hemodynamic effects of ketamine in children undergoing cardiac catheterization. *Pediatr Cardiol* 1990 Apr; **11**(2): 72–6.

24. B. F. Rusy, J. K. Amuzu, H. A. Bosscher, *et al.* Negative inotropic effect of ketamine in rabbit ventricular muscle. *Anesth Analg* 1990 Sep; **71**(3): 275–8.

25. K. Waxman, W. C. Shoemaker, M. Lippmann. Cardiovascular effects of anesthetic induction with ketamine. *Anesth Analg* 1980 May; **59**(5): 355–8.

26. W. S. Schechter, C. Kim, M. Martinez, *et al.* Anaesthetic induction in a child with end-stage cardiomyopathy. *Can J Anaesth* 1995 May; **42**(5 Pt 1): 404–8.

27. G. Christ, G. Mundigler, C. Merhaut, *et al.* Adverse cardiovascular effects of ketamine infusion in patients with catecholamine-dependent heart failure. *Anaesth Intensive Care* 1997 Jun; **25**(3): 255–9.

28. N. Dhawan, S. Chauhan, S. S. Kothari, *et al.* Hemodynamic responses to etomidate in pediatric patients with congenital cardiac shunt lesions. *J Cardiothorac Vasc Anesth* 2010 Oct; **24**(5): 802–7.

29. M. Sarkar, P. C. Laussen, D. Zurakowski, *et al.* Hemodynamic responses to etomidate on induction of anesthesia in pediatric patients. *Anesth Analg* 2005 Sep; **101**(3): 645–50.

30. B. Kay. Total intravenous anesthesia with etomidate. I. A trial in children. *Acta Anaesthesiol Belg* 1977; **28**(2): 107–13.

31. S. G. Albert, S. Ariyan, A. Rather. The effect of etomidate on adrenal function in critical illness: a systematic review. *Intensive Care Med* 2011 Jun; **37**(6): 901–10.

32. L. C. McPhee, O. Badawi, G. L. Fraser, *et al.* Single-dose etomidate is not associated with increased mortality in ICU patients with sepsis: analysis of a large electronic ICU database. *Crit Care Med* 2013 Mar; **41**(3): 774–83.

33. M. Salonen, J. Kanto, E. Iisalo, *et al.* Midazolam as an induction agent in children: a pharmacokinetic and clinical study. *Anesth Analg* 1987 Jul; **66**(7): 625–8.

34. R. Singh, N. Kumar, H. Vajifdar. Midazolam as a sole sedative for computed tomography imaging in pediatric patients. *Paediatr Anaesth* 2009 Sep; **19**(9): 899–904.

35. L. Shekerdemian, A. Bush, A. Redington. Cardiovascular effects of intravenous midazolam after open heart surgery. *Arch Dis Child* 1997 Jan; **76**(1): 57–61.

36. P. Burtin, P. Daoud, E. Jacqz-Aigrain, *et al.* Hypotension with midazolam and fentanyl in the newborn. *Lancet* 1991 Jun 22; **337** (8756): 1545–6.

37. S. M. Rivenes, M. B. Lewin, S. A. Stayer, *et al.* Cardiovascular effects of sevoflurane, isoflurane, halothane, and fentanyl-midazolam in children with congenital heart disease: an echocardiographic study of myocardial contractility and hemodynamics. *Anesthesiology* 2001 Feb; **94**(2): 223–9.

38. M. Shukry, K. Kennedy. Dexmedetomidine as a total intravenous anesthetic in infants. *Paediatr Anaesth* 2007 Jun; **17**(6): 581–3.

39. J. P. Belleville, D. S. Ward, B. C. Bloor, *et al.* Effects of intravenous dexmedetomidine in humans. I. Sedation, ventilation, and metabolic rate. *Anesthesiology* 1992 Dec; **77**(6): 1125–33.

40. C. Chrysostomou, S. Di Filippo, A. M. Manrique, *et al.* Use of dexmedetomidine in children after cardiac and thoracic surgery. *Pediatr Crit Care Med* 2006 Mar; **7** (2): 126–31.

41. K. P. Mason, D. Zurakowski, S. E. Zgleszewski, *et al.* High-dose dexmedetomidine as the sole sedative for pediatric MRI. *Paediatr Anaesth* 2008 May; **18**(5): 403–11.

42. G. B. Hammer, D. R. Drover, H. Cao, *et al.* The effects of dexmedetomidine on cardiac electrophysiology in children. *Anesth Analg* 2008 Jan; **106**(1): 79–83.

43. D. D. Hansen, P. R. Hickey. Anesthesia for hypoplastic left heart syndrome: use of high-dose fentanyl in 30 neonates. *Anesth Analg* 1986 Feb; **65**(2): 127–32.

44. H. P. Duncan, A. Cloote, P. M. Weir, *et al.* Reducing stress responses in the pre-bypass phase of open heart surgery in infants and young children: a comparison of different fentanyl doses. *Br J Anaesth* 2000 May; **84**(5): 556–64.

45. P. R. Hickey, D. D. Hansen. Fentanyl- and sufentanil-oxygen-pancuronium anesthesia for cardiac surgery in infants. *Anesth Analg* 1984 Feb; **63**(2): 117–24.

46. E. A. Akpek, C. Erkaya, A. Donmez, *et al.* Remifentanil use in children undergoing congenital heart surgery for left-to-right shunt lesions. *J Cardiothorac Vasc Anesth* 2005 Feb; **19**(1): 60–6.

47. C. Chanavaz, O. Tirel, E. Wodey, *et al.* Haemodynamic effects of remifentanil in children with and without intravenous atropine. An echocardiographic study. *Br J Anaesth* 2005 Jan; **94**(1): 74–9.

48. P. R. Hickey, D. D. Hansen, M. Strafford, *et al.* Pulmonary and systemic hemodynamic effects of nitrous oxide in infants with normal and elevated pulmonary vascular resistance. *Anesthesiology* 1986 Oct; **65**(4): 374–8.

49. D. J. Murray, R. B. Forbes, D. L. Dull, *et al.* Hemodynamic responses to nitrous oxide during inhalation anesthesia in pediatric patients. *J Clin Anesth* 1991 Jan–Feb; **3**(1): 14–19.

50. R. S. Holzman, M. E. van der Velde, S. J. Kaus, *et al.* Sevoflurane depresses myocardial contractility less than halothane during induction of anesthesia in children. *Anesthesiology* 1996 Dec; **85**(6): 1260–7.

51. J. Lerman, N. Sikich, S. Kleinman, *et al.* The pharmacology of sevoflurane in infants and children. *Anesthesiology* 1994 Apr; **80**(4): 814–24.

52. R. H. Taylor, J. Lerman. Minimum alveolar concentration of desflurane and hemodynamic responses in neonates, infants, and children. *Anesthesiology* 1991 Dec; **75**(6): 975–9.

53. Y. S. Prakash, I. Seckin, L. W. Hunter, *et al.* Mechanisms underlying greater sensitivity of neonatal cardiac muscle to volatile anesthetics. *Anesthesiology* 2002 Apr; **96**(4): 893–906.

54. V. C. Baum, B. W. Palmisano. The immature heart and anesthesia. *Anesthesiology* 1997 Dec; **87**(6): 1529–48.

55. M. J. Allwood, A. F. Cobbold, J. Ginsburg. Peripheral vascular effects of noradrenaline, isopropylnoradrenaline and dopamine. *Br Med Bull* 1963 May; **19**: 132–6.

56. R. P. Dellinger, M. M. Levy, A. Rhodes, *et al.* Surviving sepsis campaign: international guidelines for management of severe sepsis and septic shock: 2012. *Crit Care Med* 2013 Feb; **41**(2): 580–637.

57. J. O. Johnson, L. Grecu, N. W. Lawson. Autonomic nervous system. In Barash P. G., editor. *Clinical Anesthesia*. 6th edn. Philadelphia, PA: Wolters Kluwer/Lippincott Williams & Wilkins; 2009; p. 353.

58. K. Harada, M. Tamura, T. Ito, *et al.* Effects of low-dose dobutamine on left ventricular diastolic filling in children. *Pediatr Cardiol* 1996 Jul–Aug; **17**(4): 220–5.

59. T. M. Hoffman, G. Wernovsky, A. M. Atz, *et al.* Efficacy and safety of milrinone in preventing low cardiac output syndrome in infants and children after corrective surgery for congenital heart disease. *Circulation* 2003 Feb 25; **107**(7): 996–1002.

60. J. Moss, D. Glick. The autonomic nervous system In: Miller R. D., editor. *Miller's Anesthesia.* 6th edn. New York: Elsevier/Churchill Livingstone; 2005; p. 650.

61. K. Choong, D. Bohn, D. D. Fraser, *et al.* Vasopressin in pediatric vasodilatory shock: a multicenter randomized controlled trial. *Am J Respir Crit Care Med* 2009 Oct 1; **180**(7): 632–9.

62. C. W. Mastropietro, N. F. Rossi, J. A. Clark, *et al.* Relative deficiency of arginine vasopressin in children after cardiopulmonary bypass. *Crit Care Med* 2010 Oct; **38**(10): 2052–8.

63. A. C. Shukla, J. M. Steven, F. X. McGowan. Cardiac physiology and pharmacology. In Cote C. J., Lerman J., Todres I. D., eds. *A Practice of Anesthesia for Infants and Children.* 4th edn. Philadelphia, PA: Saunders; 2008; p. 381.

Chapter 7

Cardiovascular system

David J. Krodel

Introduction

Special considerations are needed when providing perioperative care for children who have congenital or acquired heart disease. This is true for the cardiac operating room, but increasingly these children are undergoing noncardiac procedures in various stages of palliation both at and outside of specialized centers. It is likely with the successes of modern congenital cardiac surgery that this population will continue to increase in coming years. Understanding of congenital cardiac physiology and anatomy (including post-palliation) will be paramount for the pediatric anesthesiologist and for the general anesthesiologist taking care of adults with congenital heart disease.

General considerations

Cardiovascular effects on anesthetic uptake and delivery

Induction is a particularly critical time in any anesthetic, but particularly so for the child or adult with congenital heart disease (CHD). Understanding how the pharmacology of inhaled anesthetics is affected by underlying CHD is mainly dictated by the presence or absence of intracardiac shunts. Shunting of blood affects the relative pulmonary to systemic blood flow (Qp/Qs), which is 1 under normal conditions. A right to left intracardiac shunt, which decreases Qp/Qs, will slow the uptake of inhaled anesthetic, prolonging induction times due to decreased pulmonary blood flow relative to systemic. A large left to right shunt, which increases Qp/Qs, speeds the uptake of inhaled anesthetic due to the increase of pulmonary blood flow assuming that the cardiac output is relatively normal; however, smaller left to right shunts have a negligible effect on uptake. It is also important to consider that shunting may be dynamic and that decreased SVR may decrease Qp/Qs and even reverse some left to right shunts. The overall effect of this would be to prolong induction. The effect of shunting on uptake increases as solubility decreases, therefore nitrous oxide and desflurane will be more affected than the relatively soluble isoflurane.

Conversely intravenous anesthetics have a quickened onset of action in the presence of a right to left shunt as the pulmonary circulation is bypassed and anesthetic is more quickly available to the brain. Therefore in cases where a rapid induction is desirable in the presence of a right to left shunt (e.g., pulmonary hypertension in the presence of an ASD) an intravenous induction may be preferable to an inhalational induction. Intravenous anesthetics are minimally affected by the presence of a left to right shunt. However it should be noted that in the presence of low cardiac output, the perceived potency of intravenous anesthetics may be higher and the duration of action prolonged, due to both slower uptake into nonvessel rich tissues and to lower clearance rates.

Anesthetic effects on the cardiovascular system

All anesthetic agents have profound effects on the autonomic nervous system, and many may depress cardiac function. These effects are magnified in children with CHD and especially in those with depressed cardiac function, hypovolemia or both. Propofol causes reductions in blood pressure due both to decreases in systemic vascular resistance (SVR) and to cardiac output. This is most frequently seen with bolus administration at the induction of anesthesia and must be used carefully in the presence of CHD.

Essentials of Pediatric Anesthesiology, ed. Alan David Kaye, Charles James Fox and James H. Diaz. Published by Cambridge University Press. © Cambridge University Press 2015.

Similarly the inhaled anesthetics all cause decreases in SVR and direct myocardial depression. They also cause increased susceptibility to arrhythmias, which may further compromise cardiac output. Distinctions in cardiovascular effects between the inhaled potent anesthetics (i.e., isoflurane, sevoflurane, desflurane) currently in use are relatively minor as compared to halothane. Desflurane is notable, however, for sometimes causing sympathetic stimulation at high concentrations leading to tachycardia and hypertension. This effect is unfortunately less reliable than that of ketamine, which may be chosen for this property.

Nitrous oxide has less cardiovascular depressant effects than the potent agents, but has additive decreases in SVR and myocardial depression in combination with other inhaled anesthetics or opioids. Unlike in the adult population there is no evidence of nitrous oxide increasing PVR in children and it is thought to be safe even in the presence of pulmonary hypertension and right heart failure. Concern for enlarging microbubbles means that nitrous oxide should be avoided for cases with potential right to left shunts.

The other intravenous anesthetics are better at preserving hemodynamics. Etomidate causes little change in hemodynamics, even in the presence of hypovolemia. Ketamine reliably causes endogenous release of catecholamines causing increases in heart rate, blood pressure, and cardiac output. It causes direct myocardial depression, which is clinically significant only when catecholamine stores have been depleted, such as severe cardiomyopathy. Midazolam has little effect on hemodynamics. Opioids have relatively few hemodynamic effects. Fentanyl while maintaining SVR and PVR, causes bradycardia, which can decrease cardiac output significantly in some children. Morphine may cause a decrease in SVR. Histamine release by morphine, which is more likely with rapid administration, can produce profound decreases in SVR transiently. Remifentanil may cause bradycardia and related systemic hypotension. Dexmedetomidine is known to cause bradycardia and potentially systemic hypotension, but, in children, tachycardia is also seen and therefore its cardiovascular effects in this population can be unpredictable.

Vasoactive medications

Dobutamine is a primarily beta-1-agonist that functions as a positive inotrope and chronotrope while providing systemic vasodilation.

Dopamine is an agonist at dopamine receptors, but also at catecholamine receptors at higher concentrations. At low infusion rates (i.e., < 5 mcg/kg/min) it may cause vasodilation preferably in the renal vasculature. At higher rates (i.e., 5–10 mcg/kg/min) is a positive inotrope and chronotrope via its action at beta-adrenergic receptors. At the highest rates (> 10 mcg/kg/min) it increases SVR through action at alpha-adrenergic receptors in the vasculature. It also increases susceptibility to tachyarrhythmias.

Epinephrine is a potent adrenergic agonist both at beta- and alpha- type receptors. It produces increases in contractility, heart rate, and systemic vascular resistance.

Isoproterenol is a non-selective beta-agonist used mainly as a positive chronotrope although it also has positive inotropic effects and dilates systemic blood vessels.

Milrinone is a phosphodiesterase-type-3(PDE-3) inhibitor that functions as a positive inotrope and provides systemic vasodilation by inhibiting the breakdown of cAMP by PDE in cardiac myocytes.

Nicardipine is a dihydropyridine-type calcium channel blocker (CCB), causing decreases in systemic vascular resistance. Its myocardial depressant effects are minimal, which makes it distinct from other CCBs; however, like all CCBs should be used with caution in the setting of cardiomyopathy.

Nitrogylcerin is a vasodilator that acts primarily on veins, but also has vasodilatory properties on the coronary arteries. It is a nitrate and its mechanism of action like all nitrates is through its conversion to nitric oxide.

Nitroprusside is a potent nitrate vasodilator that acts both on arterioles and veins. Prolonged infusions may cause cyanide toxicity.

Norepinephrine is a potent adrenergic agonist that preferentially acts at alpha-adrenergic receptors, but also increases myocardial contractility via beta-adrenergic stimulation. It is a poor chronotrope and causes less tachycardia than epinephrine and dopamine, and has less potential for arrhythmias.

Phenylephrine is primarily alpha-adrenergic, increasing SVR, which may cause a reflex bradycardia, and does not have inotropic properties.

Vasopressin increases systemic vascular resistance via its activity at vasopressin receptors in the vasculature. It has no effect on myocardium. It is useful in the catecholamine-depleted patient as well as in patients that have refractory hypotension due to angiotensin converting enzyme inhibitors (ACEi) and angiotensin receptor blockers (ARB).

Disease states

Congenital cardiac disease may be classified in a number of ways, most often divided into cyanotic and acyanotic categories.

Cyanotic lesions

Tetralogy of Fallot (TOF) is the most common cyanotic heart condition consisting of VSD, overriding aorta, pulmonary infundibular stenosis, and right ventricular hypertrophy. The physiology is dominated by the ratio of pulmonary to systemic blood flow. A "tetralogy spell" or "tet spell" occurs when the right ventricular outflow tract is obstructed, resulting in decreased pulmonary blood flow and cyanosis. This may be compensated for by increasing systemic vascular resistance. In patients with mild right ventricular outflow tract (RVOT) obstruction cyanosis may be minimal or absent giving rise to the term "pink tet." At the other extreme pulmonary atresia or pulmonic stenosis can complicate repair. Double-outlet right ventricle is another variant of TOF in which the aorta overrides the ventricular septum by more than 50%. Usually the patient undergoes repair in a single stage during the first year of life. Neonates with severe cyanosis may require percutaneous pulmonary valvuloplasty if the stenosis is valvar, or early surgical intervention. Perioperatively patients with TOF require adequate SVR to prevent severe cyanosis, sufficient intravascular volume for adequate right ventricular filling, and avoidance of medications that may depress RV function.

Hypoplastic left heart syndrome (HLHS) continues to be one of the most challenging anomalies in modern congenital heart surgery. These patients are born cyanotic with ductal dependence for systemic perfusion and require staged palliative surgery within a few days of birth. The first operation is usually the Norwood operation. For a description of this operation see palliative procedures below. The Norwood procedure establishes systemic circulation from the right ventricle and is accompanied by a modified Blalock–Taussig shunt (mBTS) (see below) to provide pulmonary circulation although sometimes a Sano shunt is performed instead. The second stage is a bidirectional Glenn shunt, which is usually performed around 3–6 months of age and finally a Fontan procedure usually around age 2. Mortality is high with stage 1 mortality potentially as high as 25%, but discharge home is fraught with risk as interstage (the period after initial hospital discharge, but prior to stage 2) mortality remains high (> 10%). Mortality after stage 2 is lower, but not insignificant.

Ebstein anomaly is an anomaly of the tricuspid valve in which the septal and posterior leaflets are displaced towards the apex. A small RV chamber results, and often there is an accompanying ASD which allows right to left shunting and cyanosis. While some patients are symptomatic as neonates, others may not have problems until later in life. Arrhythmias are prevalent, especially SVT. Medical management is common, but surgical repair of the valve may be needed in some cases. Occasionally, the Glenn procedure is performed in an effort to reduce right ventricular volume overload and tricuspid regurgitation.

Tricuspid atresia is a congenital absence of the tricuspid valve, which leads to hypoplasia of the right ventricle. These patients must be palliated by a single ventricle pathway. Alprostadil may be administered at birth to maintain a patent ductus arteriosus. Surgical intervention includes an mBTS at a few days of age, a bidirectional Glenn at 3–6 months, and Fontan at around 2 years. In contrast to HLHS, patients with a left-sided single ventricle have less long-term ventricular dysfunction and heart failure.

Double-inlet left ventricle (DILV) is the third most common indication for a single ventricle palliation that is similar to that of tricuspid atresia. In DILV, both atria open into a large left ventricle and a hypoplastic right ventricle receives little or no blood flow. The right ventricle may be completely absent. These children may have other anomalies such as pulmonary stenosis or atresia, d-TGA, and coarctation of the aorta.

Transposition of the great arteries (TGA, d-TGA) is a severe anomaly that creates two parallel circulations and is incompatible with life unless a communication exists in the form of an ASD, VSD, or a patent ductus arteriosus. If no such communication exists one needs to be performed emergently such as an atrial septostomy. A patent ductus may be maintained with alprostadil in the first few days of life. Typically a Jatene arterial switch is performed, in which the pulmonary artery and the aorta are divided from their left ventricular and right ventricular outflow tracts, respectively, and reanastomosed in the correct orientation. Buttons around the coronary ossa are created such that the coronary arteries are reimplanted into the aorta to preserve adequate coronary blood flow. The Mustard or Senning atrial switch operations are also performed for this indication, but recently the Jatene arterial switch has become the more common approach. While atrial switch restores serial circulation, the right ventricle remains the systemic ventricle, leading to heart failure after several decades of life.

Truncus arteriosus causes cyanosis due to complete mixing at the level of the great arteries. In this anomaly a single vessel originates from both the right and left ventricular outflow tracts, and subsequently branches into the systemic and pulmonary circulations. To repair, the pulmonary artery is divided from the main truncus and anastomosed to the right ventricle via a valved conduit. The outflow tract VSD is closed. The conduit will need to be replaced to allow for growth several times during childhood.

Total anomalous pulmonary venous return (TAPVR). Anomalous pulmonary venous return is the result of one or more of the pulmonary veins not returning to the left atrium. When none of the pulmonary veins return to the left atrium it is termed TAPVR otherwise it is termed partial anomalous pulmonary venous return (PAPVR). In TAPVR, it is essential that an atrial communication is present to provide systemic blood flow and an atrial septostomy can be performed if necessary. In half the cases the pulmonary veins will drain into the SVC or the brachiocephalic vein (supracardiac). Less commonly (~20%) the veins return directly to the right atrium or the coronary sinus (intracardiac). The remainder (~20%) returns to the portal or hepatic veins (infracardiac). About 10% of the time a mixed picture occurs. Oxygenated and deoxygenated blood mix at the level of the atria or above and a right to left shunt provides mixed blood to the systemic circulation. When obstruction to pulmonary venous blood flow occurs, severe cyanosis mandates emergency surgery at birth. Without obstruction the procedure can be performed in the first few weeks to months of life. Correction involves locating the major pulmonary veins and implanting them into the left atrium, ligation of the minor veins, and closure of the ASD. This can be performed as a staged procedure, but some centers have shown improved long-term outcomes with a longer single-stage procedure.

Acyanotic lesions

Atrial septal defect (ASD). An ASD is a defect in the atrial septum that may occur in isolation or combination with other defects. Usually it presents as a low velocity left to right shunt which causes few symptoms. Over time increased right-sided flow can lead to right atrial enlargement and arrhythmias. Pulmonary hypertension and right ventricular failure may also develop later in life, which stresses the importance of repair either with a transcatheter device or surgically. The patient is also at risk for strokes from paradoxical embolism from the venous to the arterial circulation. There are four major types of ASD including septum secundum and septum primum, which represent failures in the development in those septae. Often septum secundum defects can be closed by transcatheter devices whereas primum defects more commonly require surgical intervention. Patent foramen ovale (PFO), which is a failure of the fusion of the two septae after birth, is present in about 25% of the adult population and intervention is only warranted if symptoms occur. With normal atrial pressures the PFO is physiologically closed and therefore anatomic closure is not completely necessary in the asymptomatic patient although paradoxical embolism precautions should be taken in patients known to have a PFO. Sinus venosus ASD represents an abnormal insertion of the sinus venosus such that there is a communication between atria. This usually requires surgical intervention.

Ventricular septal defect (VSD). A VSD is a defect in the ventricular septum. This is usually characterized by a left to right shunt and leads to right- and left-sided volume overload over time. Small defects present at birth may be observed as they are largely asymptomatic and may close over the first few years of life. Surgical repair is necessitated in cases with heart failure refractory to medical therapy, associated pulmonary hypertension, associated pulmonic stenosis, and associated aortic regurgitation. Perimembranous defects are most common, but muscular, subaortic, and inlet defects also occur. Failure to recognize and treat a VSD long term places the patient at risk for volume overload, pulmonary overcirculation, pulmonary hypertension, and Eisenmenger syndrome, although this complication is rarely seen today due to early recognition and closure. A small subset of patients may undergo transcatheter device closure.

Patent ductus arteriosus (PDA). Patent ductus arteriosus may be asymptomatic or cause heart failure due to a left to right shunt. There is a high incidence of this defect in preterm neonates. Closure may be accomplished by NSAIDs such as ibuprofen or indomethacin, but often the muscular, large ductus of preterm infants will require surgical closure via a left posterior thoracotomy. Risks of this procedure are low, but ligation of the descending aorta or pulmonary artery has been described. Smaller defects may be hemodynamically insignificant or not appreciated until the patient is older. Older patients may be candidates for percutaneous closure via a device. Some young patients 1 - or 2-years-old may present with heart failure and failure to thrive, but often these patients are asymptomatic and presence of the PDA is suggested by a continuous murmur on auscultation and confirmed by echocardiogram. These patients require closure to prevent pulmonary overcirculation and subsequent pulmonary hypertension, which may become irreversible leading to right heart failure.

Endocardial cushion defect. Also known as atrioventricular (AV) canal (partial or complete), these defects are most commonly associated with patients with Down syndrome (although VSD is the most common heart anomaly in Down syndrome, not AV canal). Complete AV canal refers to a defect in the atrial septum primum, AV valves, and an inflow tract ventricular septal defect. Partial AV canal typically refers to a defect only involving the atria and the AV valve, but no communication in the ventricles. Rastelli described three types of CAVC (A, B and C) based on the morphology of the common AV valve in relation to the septum. Repair is always surgical and consists of closure of the ASD, VSD, and valvuloplasty of the common AV valve to create a left and right AV valve. Often a pericardial or synthetic patch is used in the repair. These patients are at high risk for arrhythmias involving the AV node postoperatively and temporary pacing wires are commonly used. The CAVC occurring in the presence of morphologically normal right and left ventricles is referred to as "balanced." Unbalanced AV canal occurs when there is hypoplasia of either the right or, more commonly, the left ventricle making closure of the defect hemodynamically difficult or impossible. In these cases, if biventricular repair is not possible, the infant may go down a single-ventricle palliation pathway starting with a Norwood procedure.

Coarctation of the aorta. Coarctation of the aorta is characterized by a narrowing in the aortic arch, typically at the area of the insertion site of the ductus arteriosus. This is usually immediately distal to the origin of the left subclavian artery. Infants may present with heart failure and metabolic acidosis due to poor perfusion of the viscera and lower extremities. Four extremity blood pressures should be taken and pulse oximetry should be monitored on the right hand and on the left hand or a lower extremity. Frequently these infants need alprostadil to maintain an open ductus arteriosus. Repair is often performed by resection and reanastomosis, but a synthetic graft may be required. Patients with sufficient collateral circulation may not be identified at birth as they will not be in extremis nor will they have lower extremity cyanosis. They may be identified at a later time as their collateral circulation may become insufficient as they grow and they may only have symptoms of insufficiency with exertion. Frequently lower extremity pulses will be absent or very difficult to palpate in these patients, even if flow is sufficient.

Aortic stenosis. In the adult, aortic stenosis is a disease that causes pressure overload of the left ventricle leading to hypertrophy and ultimately failure. Additionally systemic and coronary perfusion may be compromised as high aortic valve gradients may lead to systemic hypoperfusion. The coronary circulation is particularly at risk both because diastolic pressures may be reduced and left ventricular perfusion pressure requirement may be increased due to a hypertrophic left ventricle. Therefore drops in systemic blood pressure are very poorly tolerated and restoration of spontaneous circulation (ROSC) is difficult after cardiac arrest. Induction of anesthesia is a particularly precarious time for patients with severe or critical aortic stenosis.

Bicuspid aortic valve is the most common valvular anomaly and usually leads to valve sclerosis and stenosis in the elderly, but stenosis may occur earlier and is not uncommon in the fifth or sixth decade. Aortic valve replacement is the treatment of choice with the option of a mechanical valve (requiring anticoagulation) or bioprosthetic valve (requiring earlier replacement).

Congenital aortic stenosis is very different in its physiology to the adult disease. An important difference is that due to low flow through the fetal left ventricular outflow tract, the left ventricle is often hypoplastic. These patients are often ductal dependent and furthermore may require an emergent atrial septostomy to facilitate outflow of oxygenated blood from the lungs, assuming that a native ASD or VSD does not exist. If the left ventricle is sufficiently developed a balloon aortic valvuloplasty may be attempted to avoid open valve repair. Open repair in infancy will usually consist of the Ross procedure which utilizes the patient's pulmonary valve as an aortic autograft and replace the pulmonary valve with a cadaveric allograft. Patients with hypoplastic left hearts will undergo the Norwood procedure

Idiopathic hypertrophic subaortic stenosis (IHSS). Please refer to the section on cardiomyopathy.

Williams syndrome. Patients with Williams syndrome often have supravalvular aortic stenosis. In addition to supravalvular stenosis, coronary artery stenosis may occur as well as pulmonic stenosis or pulmonary artery hypoplasia. In light of these abnormalities as well as reports of cardiac arrest under anesthesia, a comprehensive cardiac work-up prior to anesthesia is recommended. Cardiac catheterization may be necessary to delineate coronary abnormalities, but anesthesia and coronary catheterization is not without risk in this population as well. There have also been case reports of possible malignant hyperthermia in these patients, but no clear connection has been determined between the two.

Mitral stenosis. Mitral stenosis is characterized by left atrial hypertension and pulmonary venous congestion. Left ventricular function is dependent on adequate preload and sufficient filling time and slow heart rates are preferred. Mitral valvuloplasty is preferred if possible since valve replacement requires anticoagulation, and repeat replacement is likely in a young patient.

Congenital. When isolated this is most often approached by valvuloplasty.

Rheumatic. Mitral stenosis is the most common complication of rheumatic heart disease. When stenosis becomes severe, repair of the valve is preferred to replacement.

Congenitally corrected transposition of the great arteries (cc-TGA, l-TGA) is a condition in which the orientation of the right and left ventricles has been switched during development. The right ventricle provides systemic output and receives oxygenated blood from the lungs. This lesion is compatible with life and may be asymptomatic. As these patients age they may suffer from heart failure due to long term use of the right ventricle as the systemic ventricle. To prevent this long-term complication, a so-called double-switch operation can be performed. The double-switch procedure consists of both a Jatene arterial switch and a Mustard or Senning atrial switch performed at the same time.

Palliative procedures

Blalock–Taussig shunt (BTS). Also known as the Blalock–Thomas–Taussig shunt, the BTS is a palliative procedure performed as an alternative to maintained ductus arteriosus blood flow. Originally developed for palliation of failing, cyanotic tetralogy of Fallot, it is now rarely used for that indication unless pulmonary atresia occurs. It was described originally as division of the left subclavian artery with anastomosis to the left pulmonary artery. In the modern era a synthetic graft is used to anastomose the right subclavian artery to the right pulmonary artery, which is often termed a modified BTS (mBTS). It is most commonly used in neonates with a single ventricle (in conjunction with a Norwood procedure for those with HLHS) or those with severely diminished pulmonary blood flow.

Sano shunt. This is a shunt between the right ventricle and the pulmonary artery with a synthetic graft. This may be performed in conjunction with a Norwood operation in place of an mBTS.

Norwood procedure. The Norwood procedure consists of division of the main pulmonary artery from its branches and anastomosis to the ascending aorta. It is performed in conjunction with a mBTS or Sano shunt as a first-stage palliation of HLHS.

Glenn shunt (classic or bidirectional). A Glenn shunt is an anastomosis between the superior vena cava, which is divided from the right atrium, and the right pulmonary artery. It is performed to restore venous blood supply to the pulmonary circulation after an mBTS or Norwood procedure. Classically the pulmonary artery was divided to accomplish the anastomosis but now division of the artery is not typically performed and this is usually termed a "bidirectional Glenn."

Fontan procedure (atriopulmonary or cavopulmonary anastomosis). The final operation of a single ventricle pathway, this operation creates a conduit from the IVC to the pulmonary artery/Glenn shunt, thereby redirecting all venous blood flow directly to the pulmonary circulation. For success, pulmonary pressures must be near normal. While high pulmonary pressures after a Glenn shunt will lead to cyanosis, after a Fontan heart failure will occur. For that reason sometimes a fenestration will be created in the Fontan conduit to allow outflow of blood into the right atrium if Fontan pressures become elevated. This is thought to prevent fulminant heart failure due to pulmonary hypertension, but with improvements in surgical technique and medical care for these patients, the fenestration is now often omitted from the operation in selected patients. The connection between the IVC and the PA/Glenn shunt may be intra- or extracardiac. Intracardiac or atriopulmonary Fontan procedures were performed commonly in the past, but now extracardiac or cavopulmonary conduits are more common. It is not uncommon for adult survivors with intracardiac Fontan shunts to undergo conversion to the extracardiac shunt to improve hemodynamics and decrease arrhythmias. An ablation procedure may accompany the conversion for this reason. Long-term success of patients who receive a Fontan procedure is a remarkable 80% survival rate without transplant at 15–20 years at one large center. These patients are at risk for thromboembolism, heart failure, and sudden death as major causes of mortality. Other long-term complications include plastic bronchitis, which is rare, but has a high mortality, and protein-losing enteropathy, which occurs in about 10% of cases. These patients may require a pacemaker or automatic implantable cardioverter defibrillator (AICD) in the future as well as other procedures that may require them to come to the noncardiac operating room. Knowledge of their palliated anatomy and familiarity with these types of patients is key to ensuring safe perioperative patient care in this population.

Pulmonary artery (PA) band procedure. A band is placed on the PA to reduce pulmonary blood flow to prevent overcirculation and increase systemic output prior to definitive repair.

Atrial septostomy. A communication is made between the atria. This may be performed by a transcatheter technique or by open surgery.

Atrial switch procedure. The Mustard and Senning procedures utilize baffles to redirect blood flow from the right atrium to the left ventricle and from the left atrium to the right ventricle. In the past this was commonly performed as a repair of transposition of the great arteries (d-TGA), but now the Jatene arterial switch is more commonly performed.

Central shunts. These are direct shunts between the aorta and main (or main branch) pulmonary arteries. These are rarely utilized due to the difficulty of controlling flow through the shunt.

Potts shunt (aka. Potts–Smith–Gibon). This is a connection between the descending aorta and the left pulmonary artery. Originally an alternative to the BTS, the Potts shunt is sometimes performed now in children with pulmonary hypertension and right ventricular failure and has also been described by a transcatheter technique.

Waterston–Cooley shunt. This is a side-to-side anastomosis between the ascending aorta and the right pulmonary artery.

Schumacher–Mandelbaum shunt. A shunt between the ascending aorta and either the right or left pulmonary artery or the main pulmonary artery

Redo–Ecker shunt. A synthetic prosthesis anastomosed end-to-side between the aorta and the main pulmonary artery, just distal to the origins of these vessels within the pericardium

Pulmonary hypertension

Pulmonary artery hypertension (PAH) is defined as an increased pulmonary arterial pressure above normal. For adults, a mean pulmonary artery pressure > 25 mmHg is defined as abnormal. Association of a pulmonary artery occlusion pressure (PAOP) < 15 mmHg further subclassifies it as precapillary, versus PAOP > 15 mmHg which is postcapillary. No specific definition is used for children or infants. In the normal infant, pulmonary artery pressures fall dramatically at birth with clamping of the umbilical cord and taking the first breath. Pressures may remain elevated as compared to normal adult values for the first few months of life as the pulmonary vasculature and alveoli continue to develop. The Dana Point classification of pulmonary hypertension (2008) creates categories based on etiology: pulmonary arterial hypertension, pulmonary hypertension owing to left heart disease, pulmonary hypertension owing to lung disease and/or hypoxia, chronic thromboembolic pulmonary hypertension, and miscellaneous. Especially relevant to the pediatric population is pulmonary hypertension associated with congenital heart disease and persistent pulmonary hypertension of the newborn, which are subcategories of pulmonary arterial hypertension. Certainly pulmonary hypertension due to left heart disease can also be seen in the pediatric population, and less commonly due to other etiologies (e.g., interstitial lung disease, sleep-disordered breathing, Gaucher syndrome, and other metabolic disorders).

Pulmonary hypertension is a major consideration in the perioperative care of children with congenital heart disease. Patients with pulmonary hypertension are at risk for right heart failure as well as for intraoperative complications with a 1–5% mortality rate for patients with severe pulmonary hypertension. Induction is a particularly precarious time for patients with pulmonary hypertension as physiologic changes may exacerbate their heart disease. Reduced preload may result in right heart failure. Increases in pulmonary hypertension due to hypoxia or hypercarbia may lead to right heart failure, exacerbation of right to left shunting, or reversal of left to right shunting leading to further hypoxia and hypercarbia. Decreases in SVR may have similar effects on shunts, therefore the patient with severe pulmonary hypertension and/or right heart failure merits careful consideration of induction agents and conditions to maintain cardiovascular hemodynamics. Premedication is warranted in this population to ensure a smooth induction. Many congenital heart defects have pulmonary hypertension as a result of increased pulmonary blood flow and indeed repair is indicated to prevent irreversible changes in pulmonary vasculature in the first two decades of life. Treated prior to adulthood, many of these children will have normalization of pulmonary pressures early in the postoperative period. Conventional medical therapy for PAH is directed at reducing the symptoms of right heart failure and preventing pulmonary embolism typically using diuretics, digoxin, and anticoagulants, but this has never been systematically studied. Targeted medical therapies include phosphodiesterase-type-5 (PDE-5) inhibitors (e.g., sildenafil) and endothelin receptor antagonists (e.g., bosentan, ambrisentan). Prostacyclin (PGI2) analogs (e.g., epoprostenol, treprostinil, ilioprost) have been used with benefit in patients with World Health Organization (WHO) Functional Class II–IV, but have the disadvantage of having a short half-life necessitating continuous intravenous or subcutaneous infusion. Ilioprost and treprostinil also have inhaled forms that require frequent dosing. Patients whose pulmonary arterial pressures are responsive (decrease) to inhaled nitric oxide, epoprostenol, or adenosine may benefit from calcium channel blockers (e.g., diltiazem, nifedipine), but these should be avoided in severe heart failure as they can exert a negative inotropic effect. In the operating room and intensive care unit, inhaled nitric oxide (iNO) is often used for children with pulmonary hypertension and is the gold standard therapy for patients in extremis.

Infectious diseases

Infectious diseases involving the heart fall mainly into three categories: bacterial, viral, and inflammatory postinfectious syndromes.

Infectious endocarditis (IE) remains a concern for all patients with congenital heart disease. The perioperative recommendations for IE prophylaxis are an ongoing responsibility for anesthesiologists and their cardiology colleagues. The recommendation of the American Heart Association (AHA) and American College of Cardiology (ACC) for congenital heart disease were updated in 2008. Prophylaxis is no longer recommended for these patients, but it was deemed reasonable for dental procedures that involved manipulation of gingival tissue or the periapical region of teeth or perforation of the oral mucosa for the following high risk patients: patients with prosthetic cardiac valves or prosthetic material used for cardiac valve repair, patients with previous infective endocarditis, patients with unrepaired cyanotic CHD including palliative shunts and conduits, completely repaired congenital heart defect repaired with prosthetic material or device during the first 6 months following the procedure, repaired CHD with residual defects at the site or adjacent to the site of a prosthetic patch or prosthetic device, cardiac transplant recipients with valve regurgitation due to a structurally abnormal valve. Prophylaxis for IE is reasonable to consider for women delivering vaginally at the time of membrane rupture if they have prosthetic cardiac valves or prosthetic material used for cardiac valve repair or they have unrepaired or palliated cyanotic CHD, including palliative shunts and conduits. Prophylaxis is not recommended for patients undergoing nondental procedures in the absence of active infection, except in the case of procedures involving incision of the respiratory tract mucosa (e.g., tonsillectomy, adenoidectomy). In addition to considering

AHA/ACC guidelines, consultation with the patient's cardiologist and/or cardiac surgeon may help to stratify the patient's risk and necessity of IE prophylaxis for a given procedure. Prophylaxis with amoxicillin is recommended for dental procedures requiring prophylaxis unless unable to take oral medication in which case ampicillin, cefazolin, or ceftriaxone may be substituted. Patients with allergies to penicillins may receive cephalexin, cefazolin, ceftriaxone, clindamycin, azithromycin, or clarithromycin for prophylaxis. Cephalosporins should be avoided in patients with a history of anaphylaxis, angioedema, or urticaria with penicillins. Bacterial IE maybe either acute or subacute and if treatment with intravenous antibiotics is unsuccessful may require valve replacement surgery. Patients with congenital heart disease with IE are at high risk and should consult with a cardiac surgeon soon after diagnosis of IE due to the possibility of rapid deterioration.

Myocarditis is most commonly caused by viral infection and is a major cause of acquired cardiomyopathy in children. Causative vectors are usually common respiratory viruses (e.g., parvovirus B19), but nonviral etiologies include Lyme disease (*Borrelia burgdorferi*) and Chagas disease (*Trypanosoma cruzi*). Treatment is typically supportive unless a specific nonviral etiology is found. Myocarditis is a major indication for heart transplantation in children.

Pericarditis. Viral infection may also be responsible for pericarditis where again treatment is mainly supportive, although anti-inflammatory drugs (i.e., NSAIDs, aspirin, colchicine) may be used. The most common cause of pericarditis worldwide is infectious pericarditis due to tuberculosis and antibiotic therapy is the primary treatment. Associated pericardial effusion may cause tamponade physiology and require pericardial drainage either by percutaneous or surgical methods. Constrictive pericarditis may also cause symptoms of heart failure and require surgical pericardectomy.

Rheumatic fever. Many immunologic diseases may cause heart sequelae, but rheumatic fever is most relevant to the pediatric population since most primary occurrences are in the first two decades of life. Rheumatic fever may manifest with rheumatic heart disease, and is the primary cause of acquired heart disease in children worldwide. It is relatively uncommon in the USA since most occurrences of group A streptococcal pharyngitis are treated with antibiotics, which reduces the subsequent incidence of rheumatic fever. In the USA, it may be seen in immigrants and populations with reduced access to pediatric care. Acute rheumatic heart disease may present as myocarditis, endocarditis, or pericarditis, but frequently new onset mitral valve insufficiency and heart failure are the significant findings. The aortic valve, and then the tricuspid may also be affected, but rarely if ever is the pulmonic valve involved. Aspirin is a mainstay of therapy reducing all symptoms except chorea, but the association of aspirin and Reyes syndrome in children and young adults is a major caution to this approach and corticosteroids may also be used. Antibiotics are also administered to eradicate potential residual streptococcal infection. Patients, especially if untreated, may go on to have chronic rheumatic heart disease, which leads to valve fibrosis, stenosis, and insufficiency (mitral > aortic > tricuspid). Patients with a history of rheumatic fever with or without heart disease should receive benzathine penicillin G intramuscularly every three or four weeks to prevent reinfection and recurrence, and should be followed for the development of chronic rheumatic heart disease.

Cardiomyopathies

Hypertrophic cardiomyopathy is characterized by a thickening of the ventricular myocardium. It may exist with or without ventricular outflow track obstruction. Many children with this condition are largely asymptomatic, but can present with syncope, palpitations, or chest pain. Examination may reveal a systolic ejection murmur that decreases with increased afterload. Echocardiography reveals ventricular hypertrophy without dilation. Genetic causes are usually a result of defects in the sarcomere. Medical management typically consists of negative inotropes like beta blockers or calcium channel blockers as opposed to positive inotropes. Some children may require pacemaker-defibrillators to treat potentially fatal arrhythmias. Some patients will benefit from surgical myotomy to reduce left ventricular outflow tract obstruction.

Dilated cardiomyopathy is characterized by enlargement of the ventricular cavity associated with ventricular wall thinning and impaired systolic function. There are many causes, including genetic, metabolic, toxic, degenerative, and infectious. Specific etiologies may inform severity, progression, and prognosis. Acute failure may require treatment with positive inotropes, but once stabilized, afterload reduction through beta blockers or angiotensin converting enzyme (ACE) inhibitors should be commenced. Dilated cardiomyopathy is the leading indication for heart transplantation in children.

Restrictive cardiomyopathy is relatively uncommon and it has a poor prognosis. It may be due to a variety of infiltrative processes (e.g., amyloidosis, hemochromatosis, sarcoidosis). Diastolic dysfunction is due to poor ventricular relaxation and leads to poor ventricular filling. This may lead to enlarged atria, pulmonary and systemic congestion, and venous pulmonary hypertension. These children are at high risk for venous blood clots. They are dependent on high central venous pressures to maintain preload, and therefore aggressive diuresis is contraindicated. Inotropic agents may not be helpful, as systolic function is not decreased. These children may be candidates for transplantation given the poor prognosis and lack of other beneficial therapies.

Ischemic cardiomyopathy is relatively rare in children, and is usually a consequence of congenitally abnormal coronary anatomy or Kawasaki disease. Kawasaki disease is more common in Asian populations and has also been termed mucocutaneous lymph node syndrome. It most often affects children under the age of 5. It is characterized by high fevers poorly responsive to acetaminophen and ibuprofen. Other signs and symptoms include "strawberry" tongue, conjunctivitis, palmar, and plantar erythema with dorsal edema, desquamation of the fingers, at least one large cervical lymph node, and a maculopapular trunkal rash, although not all cases will have all the classic symptoms. Treatment is with intravenous IgG (IVIG) and high-dose aspirin. The most severe complications are coronary artery aneurysms, which are at risk of rupture and can lead to permanent coronary stenosis even if rupture does not occur. These children may present for angioplasty, coronary stenting, and coronary artery bypass grafting.

Pericardial disease

Pericardial disease, most often pericarditis, is characterized by chest pain and pericardial effusion. Effusion may or may not lead to tamponade physiology. Pericarditis may have infectious, immunologic etiologies or be idiopathic. Pericarditis can be treated by anti-inflammatory medications usually NSAIDs and also colchicine. Antibiotics are indicated for bacterial causes of pericarditis such as tuberculosis. Some medications can cause pericarditis, therefore these should be identified and stopped. Symptomatic effusions can be treated with percutaneous pericardiocentesis and persistent effusion can be treated surgically by the creation of a pericardial window.

Less commonly pericardial disease can be chronic (greater than 6 months) and this may lead to constrictive pericarditis. Constrictive pericarditis has similar physiology to restrictive cardiomyopathy and differentiating the two may be difficult. Definitive treatment is pericardial stripping, but the procedure is high risk due to pericardial adhesions to myocardium and coronary vessels.

Intracardiac masses

Intracardiac masses in children, as in adults, are most commonly benign. Unlike adults the most common histology is rhabdomyomas and then fibromas, not myxomas. The majority of patients with rhabdomyomas also have tuberous sclerosis. Rhabdomyomas tend to be multiple in number and can range in size. While some of these tumors may have effects on cardiac hemodynamics or cause arrhythmias due to size or position, many do not and they are rarely excised, as they tend to regress with age. In general, symptoms of benign intracardiac tumors are directly related to the location of the tumor and its effects on hemodynamics (i.e., outflow tract or valvular obstruction) and arrhythmogenicity, not its histology. Excision is only indicated in cases of hemodynamic compromise or severe arrhythmia generation. Tuberous sclerosis is associated with rhabdomyomas in infants, but these regress over time and a minority of adults with the condition have them. The other common pediatric tumor, fibroma, is typically large, singular and identified mostly in infancy and more commonly resection is indicated at the time of diagnosis.

Malignant neoplasms are less common. Angiosarcomas represent the most common primary malignancy of the heart in children. Metastases of angiosarcomas, which are extremely common, travel to distant sites via the bloodstream and are widely dispersed leading to the impression of systemic disease. Rhabdomyosarcomas and fibrosarcomas are also seen in children.

Arrhythmic lesions

Children may present to both the operating room and the catheterization laboratory with a variety of arrhythmias. Transient lesions may be caused by drugs, toxins, infections, or immunologic diseases and can be triggered or exacerbated by common anesthetic agents. Permanent lesions are more often congenital in nature and frequently due to re-entrant tracts, although many of these are largely asymptomatic or at least well tolerated, and may be treated by ablation electively. Less commonly emergent life-threatening arrhythmias require attempted ablation or placement of pacemakers and/or AICDs in the operating room. Special attention should be paid to the patient with the combination of anatomical congenital heart disease (both uncorrected and palliated) or cardiomyopathy and arrhythmias since these patients may not tolerate tachy- nor brady arrhythmias that the otherwise healthy child would find largely benign. Here are described several arrhythmias that have an increased incidence or particular relevance to the pediatric population.

Supraventricular tachycardias

Atrioventricular (AV) re-entrant tachycardia is one of the more common pediatric arrhythmias. When an antegrade accessory pathway is apparent during normal sinus rhythm, this is termed Wolff–Parkinson–White (WPW) syndrome. While WPW is well tolerated in the majority of patients, a rapidly conducting antegrade pathway may allow atrial fibrillation to induce ventricular fibrillation. Tachycardia in this syndrome may either be orthodromic (conducted anterograde across the AV node) leading to a typical narrow complex tachycardia, or antidromic (conducted anterograde across the accessory pathway and retrograde across the AV node), leading to wide complex tachycardia with the potential for degeneration, especially if atrial fibrillation occurs. Patients with WPW are often treated with beta blockade. Digoxin and calcium channel blockers may be avoided due to risk of increasing conduction via the accessory pathway. Patients without pre-excitation (nonWPW re-entrant tachycardia) may be treated with propranolol, but digoxin and calcium channel blockers are also used in these patients. Acutely, vagal maneuvers such as Valsalva or ice to the face may terminate the tachycardia. If these fail adenosine is typically used in stable patients, but beta-blockers, phenylephrine, edrophonium, and type I antiarrhythmic agents have been successfully used as well. Unstable patients should undergo synchronized cardioversion. Definitive treatment for this syndrome is catheter ablation of the accessory pathway(s) and is often performed under general anesthesia.

AV nodal re-entrant tachycardia is similar to AV re-entrant tachycardia in symptoms and treatment. In this syndrome the AV node provides both the antegrade and retrograde pathways. It is more frequently seen in adolescents and more frequently associated with syncope.

Junctional ectopic tachycardia (JET) is an arrhythmia of childhood that is not typically seen in adults. This is especially relevant to anesthesiologists since is it frequently seen in the postoperative period after cardiac surgery. Management characterized by decreasing adrenergic infusion rates if possible and aggressively treating fever. It usually resolves a few days after surgery. Nonpostsurgical JET is especially difficult to control and is treated with antiarrhythmics and ablation.

Other arrhythmic lesions

AV nodal block may be seen in children congenitally and also be acquired after surgery or myocardial infection. Congenital complete heart block is seen in infants born to mothers with systemic lupus erythematosus (SLE) or Sjögren syndrome, but also in the absence of maternal autoimmune disease. As in adults, children with high-grade heart block will usually require a pacemaker and occasionally an AICD. Small children will often require epicardial leads due to both the difficulty of placing transvenous leads and the fact that they would outgrow their transvenous leads leading to potential vascular complication.

Ventricular tachycardia (VT) is less common than SVT in pediatric patients and its treatment is similar to adult algorithms. Unlike adults, overdrive pacing is sometimes successful, but carries the risk of inducing fibrillation.

Long QT syndrome (LQTS) is a genetic abnormality of repolarization and associated with syncope or sudden death. These patients usually have a QTc greater than 450 ms, although this may only become apparent in high-catecholamine states. Not all patients with a prolonged QT have this syndrome and many pharmacologic agents have the potential to prolong the QT interval. These agents should be avoided in long QT syndrome. The usual therapy for long QT syndrome is beta-blockade to blunt the heart rate response to exercise. This may necessitate the use of a pacemaker to treat beta-blocker induced bradycardia, and an AICD may be indicated for patients with continued syncope or a history of cardiac arrest.

Heart transplantation

Heart transplantation is indicated in patients with heart failure who have a low life expectancy with other treatments. In infants congenital heart disease is the most common indication, but it is cardiomyopathy for older children. One-third of transplantations are in infants, one-third in toddlers through school-age children, and one-third in adolescents. A detailed assessment of potential recipients is undertaken to identify factors that may potentially exclude patients. Hemodynamic measurements via catheterization are also considered with emphasis on pulmonary vascular resistance (PVR). Elevated PVR (> 5 Wood U/m^2) or transpulmonary gradient greater than 15 mmHg is associated with increased mortality due to donor right heart failure, although experienced centers may choose to transplant children with PVR up to 12 Wood U/m^2, especially if reversibility with nitric oxide can be demonstrated. Central nervous system, renal, or hepatic dysfunction may exclude patients from consideration, as can some infections, malignancies, and chromosomal abnormalities. Donor matching is based on size and ABO typing as well as blood antibody screening and cross-matching. Pretransplant exposure to blood products causes increased sensitization to HLA antigens, and therefore transfusion should be avoided in potential candidates if possible. Since ischemic times less than 6 hours are preferred to improve graft function, donors must be relatively nearby. Orthotopic heart transplant from a brain-dead donor is by far the most common and most successful surgical approach although others are still performed (e.g., heterotopic, domino, cardiac death donor). While the original technique popularized by Lower and Shumway utilized right and left atrial cuffs, many centers are performing IVC and SVC anastomoses directly (i.e., bicaval approach) with smaller (sometimes two) left atrial cuffs containing the native pulmonary veins. This technique while technically more challenging may lead to fewer atrial arrhythmias. Anesthetic considerations during transplant in the prebypass period must take into consideration the patient's underlying cardiac disease, systemic disease, presence of pulmonary hypertension, and surgical history (e.g., sternotomy, heart surgery for congenital lesions, ventricular assist devices). The post-bypass period may be affected greatly by the ischemic time as well as by pulmonary hypertension that could lead to graft right heart failure. Use of inhaled nitric oxide is common in patients with elevated pulmonary pressures prior to transplant. Overall survival is approximately 80% at one year and among one-year survivors it is greater than 50% at twenty years. Long-term immunosuppression is required in recipients, which predisposes them to infection and malignancy. Medications to prevent rejection include corticosteroids, calcineurin inhibitors, azathioprine, mycophenolate mofetil, and tacrolimus. Rejection is an ongoing concern and close follow-up including myocardial biopsies and left heart catheterization is routine. Graft vasculopathy also contributes significantly to long-term mortality. Transplant patients may also develop renal insufficiency due to cardiopulmonary bypass, low cardiac output, and chronic calcineurin inhibitor use. Hypertension and hyperlipidemia are also relatively common. Despite improvements in graft survival many children are living long enough to require retransplant after both early and late graft failure. Over 4% of pediatric recipients are retransplants and additionally many pediatric recipients will require retransplant as adults.

Acknowledgments

The author would like to thank Drs. C. Hardy and H.J. Przybylo for their helpful comments and guidance in preparing this chapter.

Further reading

Alphonso N, Baghai M, Sundar P, *et al.* Intermediate-term outcome following the Fontan operation: a survival, functional and risk-factor analysis. *Eur J Cardiothorac Surg* 2005; **28**: 529–535.

Bacha EA, Daves S, Hardin J, *et al.* Single-ventricle palliation for high-risk neonates: the emergence of an alternative hybrid stage I strategy.

J Thoracic Cardiovasc Surg 2006; **131**: 163–171.

Baum VC. Pediatric cardiac surgery: an historical appreciation. *Paediatr Anaesth* 2006; **16**: 1213–1225.

Baum VC, Barton DM, Gutgesell HP. Influence of congenital heart disease on mortality after noncardiac surgery in hospitalized children. *Pediatrics* 2000; **105**: 332–335.

Bragg K, Fedel GM, DiProsperis A. Cardiac arrest under anesthesia in a pediatric patient with Williams syndrome: a case report. *AANA J* 2005; **73**: 287–293.

Butera G, Lucente M, Rosti L, *et al.* A comparison between the early and mid-term results of surgical as opposed to percutaneous closure of defects in the oval fossa in children aged less than 6 years. *Cardiol Young* 2007; **17**: 35–41.

Canter CE, Shaddy RE, Bernstein D, *et al.* Indications for Heart Transplantation in Pediatric Heart Disease. A Scientific Statement From the American Heart Association Council on Cardiovascular Disease in the Young; the Councils on Clinical Cardiology, Cardiovascular Nursing, and Cardiovascular Surgery and Anesthesia; and the Quality of Care and Outcomes Research Interdisciplinary Working Group. *Circulation* 2007; **115**: 658–676.

Cardenas L, Panzer J, Boshoff D, *et al.* Transcatheter closure of secundum atrial defect in small children. *Catheter Cardiovasc Interv* 2007; **69**: 447–452.

Cote CJ, Lerman J, Todres ID. *A Practice of Anesthesia for Infants and Children*, 4th Edition. 2009. Philadelphia, PA: Saunders–Elsevier.

Gelatt M, Hamilton RM, McCrindle BW, *et al.* Risk factors for atrial tachyarrhythmias after the Fontan operation. *J Am Coll Cardiol* 1994; **24**: 1735–1741.

Gillum RF. Epidemiology of congenital heart disease in the USA. *Am Heart J* 1994; **127**: 919–927.

Hagen PT, Scholz DG, Edwards WD. Incidence and size of patent foramen ovale during the first 10 decades of life: an autopsy study of 965 normal hearts. *Mayo Clin Proc* 1984; **59**: 17–20.

Holzman RS, van der Velde ME, Kaus SJ, *et al.* Sevoflurane depresses myocardial contractility less than halothane during induction of anesthesia in children. *Anesthesiology* 1996; **85**: 1260–1267.

Hörer J, Schreiber C, Cleuziou J, *et al.* Improvement in long-term survival after hospital discharge but not in freedom from reoperation after the change from atrial to arterial switch for transposition of the great arteries. *J Thorac Cardiovasc Surg* 2009; **137**: 347–354.

Horowitz PE, Akhtar S, Wulff JA, *et al.* Coronary artery disease and anesthesia-related death in children with Williams syndrome. *J Cardiothorac Vasc Anesth* 2002; **16**: 739–741.

Hraška V, Mattes A, Haun C, *et al.* Functional outcome of anatomic correction of corrected transposition of the great arteries. *Eur J Cardiothorac Surg* 2011; **40**: 1227–1234.

Hu P, Zhou JX, Liu J. Blood solubilities of volatile anesthetics in cardiac patients. *J Cardiothorac Vasc Anesth* 2001; **15**: 560–562.

Jacobs JP, Giroud JM, Quintessenza JA, *et al.* The modern approach to patent ductus arteriosus treatment: complementary roles of video-assisted thoracoscopic surgery and interventional cardiology coil occlusion. *Ann Thorac Surg* 2003; **76**: 1421–1427.

Joffs C, Sade RM. Congenital Heart Surgery Nomenclature and Database Project: palliation, correction or repair? *Ann Thorac Surg* 2000; **69**: S369–S372.

Kawakami H, Ichinose F. Inhaled nitric oxide in pediatric cardiac surgery. *Int Anesthesiol Clin* 2004; **42**: 93–100.

Kugler JD, Danford DA, Deal BJ, *et al.* Radiofrequency catheter ablation for tachyarrhythmias in children and adolescents. The Pediatric Electrophysiology Society. *N Engl J Med* 1994; **330**: 1481–1487.

Lammers AE, Adatia I, Cerro MJ, *et al.* Functional classification of pulmonary hypertension in children: Report from the PVRI pediatric taskforce, Panama 2011. *Pulm Circ* 2011; **1**: 280–285.

Laussen PC, Hansen DD, Perry SB, *et al.* Transcatheter closure of ventricular septal defects: hemodynamic instability and anesthetic management. *Anesth Analg* 1995; **80**: 1076–1082.

Lee C, Mason LJ. Pediatric cardiac emergencies. *Anesthesiol Clin North America* 2001; **19**: 287–308.

Lim HG, Kim WH, Lee JR, Kim YJ. Long-term results of the arterial switch operation for ventriculo-arterial discordance. *Eur J Cardiothorac Surg* 2013; **43**: 325–334.

Marianeschi SM, McElhinney DB, Reddy VM, *et al.* Alternative approach to the repair of Ebstein's malformation: intracardiac repair with ventricular unloading. *Ann Thorac Surg* 1998; **66**: 1546–1550.

Marijon E, Mirabel M, Celermajer DS, Jouven X. Rheumatic heart disease. *Lancet* 2012; **379**: 953–964.

Martin GR, Beekman RH 3rd, Mikula EB, *et al.* Implementing recommended screening for critical congenital heart disease. *Pediatrics* 2013; **132**: e185–192.

Masura J, Gavora P, Podnar T. Long-term outcome of transcatheter secundum-type atrial septal defect closure using Amplatzer septal occluders. *J Am Coll Cardiol* 2005; **45**: 505–507.

Masura J, Tittel P, Gavora P, Podnar T. Long-term outcome of transcatheter patent ductus arteriosus closure using Amplatzer duct occluders. *Am Heart J* 2006; **151**: e7–e10.

Mavroudis C, Backer CL, Deal BJ, *et al.* Evolving anatomic and electrophysiologic considerations associated with Fontan conversion. *Semin Thorac Cardiovasc Surg Pediatr Card Surg Annu* 2007; 136–145.

Medley J, Russo P, Tobias JD. Perioperative care of the patient with Williams syndrome. *Paediatr Anaesth* 2005; **15**: 243–247.

Nishimura RA, Carabello BA, Faxon DP, *et al.* ACC/AHA 2008 guideline update on valvular heart disease: focused update on infective endocarditis: a report of the American College of Cardiology/ American Heart Association Task Force on Practice Guidelines. *J Am Coll Cardiol* 2008; **52**: 676–685.

Nollert G, Fischlein T, Bouterwek S, *et al.* Long-term survival in patients with repair of tetralogy of Fallot: 36-year follow-up of 490 survivors of the first year after surgical repair. *J Am Coll Cardiol* 1997; **30**: 1374–1383.

Ohye RG, Devaney EJ, Hirsch JC, Bove EL. The modified Blalock–Taussig shunt versus the right ventricle-to-pulmonary artery conduit for the Norwood procedure. *Pediatr Cardiol* 2007; **28**: 122–125.

Ono M, Boethig D, Goerler H, *et al.* Clinical outcome of patients 20 years after Fontan operation – effect of fenestration on late morbidity. *Eur J Cardiothorac Surg* 2006; **30**: 923–929.

Raja SG, Pollock JC. Current outcomes of Ross operation for pediatric and adolescent patients. *J Heart Valve Dis* 2007; **16**: 27–36.

Rémond MG, Wheaton GR, Walsh WF, Prior DL, Maguire GP. Acute rheumatic fever and rheumatic heart disease – priorities in prevention, diagnosis and management. A report of the CSANZ Indigenous Cardiovascular Health Conference, Alice Springs 2011. *Heart Lung Circ* 2012; **21**: 632–638.

Rosenthal DN, Hammer GB. Cardiomyopathy and heart failure in children: anesthetic implications. *Paediatr Anaesth* 2011; **21**: 577–584.

Rowley AH, Shulman ST. Kawasaki syndrome. *Pediatr Clin North Am* 1999; **46**: 313–329.

Russell HM, Johnson SL, Wurlitzer KC, Backer CL. Outcomes of surgical therapy for infective endocarditis in a pediatric population: a 21-year review. *Ann Thorac Surg* 2013; **96**: 171–174.

Scheurer MA, Hill EG, Vasuki N, *et al.* Survival after bidirectional cavopulmonary anastomosis: analysis of preoperative risk factors. *J Thorac Cardiovasc Surg* 2007; **134**: 82–89.

Schure AY, Kussman BD. Pediatric heart transplantation: demographics, outcomes, and anesthetic implications. *Paediatr Anaesth* 2011; **21**: 594–603.

Simonneau G, Robbins IM, Beghetti M, *et al.* Updated clinical classification of pulmonary hypertension. *J Am Coll Cardiol* 2009; **54**: S43–S54.

Simsic JM, Bradley SM, Stroud MR, Atz AM. Risk factors for interstage death after the Norwood procedure. *Pediatr Cardiol* 2005; **26**: 400–403.

Stasik CN, Gelehrter S, Goldberg CS, *et al.* Current outcomes and risk factors for the Norwood procedure. *J Thorac Cardiovasc Surg* 2006; **131**: 412–417.

Stoelting RK, Longnecker DE. The effect of right-to-left shunt on the rate of increase of arterial anesthetic concentration. *Anesthesiology* 1972; **36**: 352–356.

Tanner GE, Angers DG, Barash PG, *et al.* Effect of left-to-right, mixed left-to-right, and right-to-left shunts on inhalational anesthetic induction in children: a computer model. *Anesth Analg* 1985; **64**: 101–107.

Task Force for Diagnosis and Treatment of Pulmonary Hypertension of the European Society of Cardiology (ESC); European Respiratory Society (ERS); International Society of Heart and Lung Transplantation (ISHLT), Galiè N, Hoeper MM, Humbert M, *et al.* Guidelines for the diagnosis and treatment of pulmonary hypertension. *Eur Respir J* 2009; **34**: 1219–1263.

Turina MI, Siebenmann R, von Segesser L, *et al.* Late functional deterioration after atrial correction for transposition of the great arteries. *Circulation* 1989; **80**: 1162–1167.

Tutar E, Ekici F, Atalay S, Nacar N. The prevalence of bicuspid aortic valve in newborns by echocardiographic screening. *Am Heart J* 2005; **150**: 513–515.

Warnes CA, Williams RG, Bashore TM, *et al.* ACC/AHA 2008 guidelines for the management of adults with congenital heart disease: a report of the American College of Cardiology/American Heart Association Task Force on Practice Guidelines (Writing Committee to Develop Guidelines for the Management of Adults with Congenital Heart Disease). *Circulation* 2008; **118**: e714–e833.

Williams GD, Hammer GB. Cardiomyopathy in childhood. *Curr Opin Anaesthesiol* 2011; **24**: 289–300.

Wilson NJ, Clarkson PM, Barratt-Boyes BG, *et al.* Long-term outcome after the Mustard repair for simple transposition of the great arteries: 28-year follow-up. *J Am Coll Cardiol* 1998; **32**: 758–765.

Wilson W, Taubert KA, Gewitz M, *et al.* Prevention of infective endocarditis. Guidelines from the American Heart Association. A Guideline from the American Heart Association Rheumatic Fever, Endocarditis, and Kawasaki Disease Committee, Council on Cardiovascular Disease in the Young, and the Council on Clinical

Cardiology, Council on Cardiovascular Surgery and Anesthesia, and the Quality of Care and Outcomes Research Interdisciplinary Working Group. *J Am Dent Assoc* 2007; **138**: 739–760.

Wu ET, Wang JK, Lee WL, *et al.* Balloon valvuloplasty as an initial palliation in the treatment of newborns and young infants with severely symptomatic tetralogy of Fallot. *Cardiology* 2006; **105**: 52–56.

Congenital heart disease: Arrhythmias, cardiopulmonary bypass, and "grown-ups"

Katherine Stammen, Sonja Gennuso, Mary Elise Fox, Charles James Fox, and Alan David Kaye

Congenital heart disease (CHD) outcomes have experienced significant improvement in the last two decades. Today over 85% of patients born with CHD survive to adulthood. Tremendous enhancement in equipment, technique, and knowledge are responsible for this progress. For every CHD lesion there now exists a surgical or interventional procedure responsible for cure, repair, or palliation.

The residual effects or sequelae associated with these defects are commonly dealt with by cardiologists or surgeons. One of the more frequent issues dealt with by pediatric cardiologists is arrhythmias. Pediatric cardiologists now possess the knowledge and devices to diagnose and treat most of the arrhythmias associated with specific CHD lesions. Many patients today present to the operating room with devices in place. Surgical ability has expanded due to improvements with cardiopulmonary bypass. Low-volume circuits equipped to provide ultrafiltration have expanded capabilities and improved outcome. This chapter will expand on issues related to treatment of arrhythmias, implanted arrhythmia devices, cardiopulmonary bypass, and adults with congenital heart disease.

Cardiac rhythm management devices in the pediatric population

Background

Pediatric patients with congenital or acquired heart lesions are surviving for longer periods of time thanks to placement of pacemakers, implantable cardioverter defibrillators, and cardiac resynchronization therapy and interventional electrophysiologic techniques. Patient size, growth, development, presence of CHD, and cardiac anatomy are considerations for unique pacemakers and ICD placement and electrophysiologic techniques in the pediatric population. As these patients present for cardiac and noncardiac surgery, anesthesiologists caring for this patient population must understand the patient's underlying heart pathophysiology and intended device function to optimize these patients in the perioperative period.

Pacemakers

A pacemaker basically consists of a generator capable of producing impulses and leads to convey the impulse to the myocardium. Modern pacemakers are small enough to be implanted in neonates as small as 2 kg in weight. All pacemakers use lithium battery sources that may have a lifespan of 5 to 10 years depending on cardiac output requirements. Infants and children have higher resting and peak heart rates than adults; therefore, increased battery utilization impact the longevity of pulse generators. Additionally, limits to maximum tracking rates from some devices may result in a significant decrease in exercise performance. Leads may be placed via a transvenous approach to the endocardium or via a surgical approach to the epicardium. The cephalic or left subclavian vein is normally used to place leads traveling to the right atrium and/or right ventricle with the transvenous approach. The pulse generator is then implanted in the left prepectoral region. In past years, transvenous pacemaker implantation in pediatric patients was limited by generator size and lead diameter compared to smaller vascular dimensions and capacitance. Initially, epicardial pacing was more common in smaller patients. More recently, with vast improvements in technology, generators are smaller and transvenous pacing systems are now being used in children with pacemaker therapy available to infants and neonates. Lead survival is

Essentials of Pediatric Anesthesiology, ed. Alan David Kaye, Charles James Fox and James H. Diaz. Published by Cambridge University Press. © Cambridge University Press 2015.

Table 8.1 NASPE/BPEG generic pacemaker code. Modified from reference 8

Positions/categories/additional information				
I/chamber(s) paced	**II/chamber(s) sensed**	**III/response to sensing**	**IV/rate modulation**	**V/multiple site pacing**
A = atrium	A = atrium	T = triggered	R = rate modulation	A = atrium
V = ventricle	V = ventricle	I = inhibited	O = none	V = ventricle
O = none	O = none	O = none		O = none
D = dual (A + V)	D = dual (A + V)	D = dual (T + I)		D = dual (A + V)

also noted to be superior in the transvenous pacing system. The major contraindication to transvenous pacing is presence of an intracardiac shunt. Presence of a shunt may allow paradoxical embolism.

Cardiac anatomy, age, and patient size determine the decision for surgical pacemaker placement. A minithoracotomy or subxiphoid approach is used to place leads on the epimyocardial surface. The leads are tunneled and connected to a pulse generator that is routinely implanted subcutaneously in the subdiaphragmatic fascia of the rectus abdominis. Low morbidity is associated with epicardial lead placement; however, the leads are more susceptible to fracture and displacement and are at increased risk of developing increasing pacing thresholds over time. Patient age at the time of implant and presence of CHD has proved to be the greatest risk factors to implanted leads.

Depending on the indication for pacemaker placement and patient size, pacemakers may pace a single chamber, two chambers, or multiple chambers (resynchronizing pacemakers). Commonly, leads are typically placed in both the right and left ventricle in resynchronization systems. The left ventricle lead is normally placed within the coronary sinus for endocardial systems, but patients with CHD may have different confirmations. For example, two epicardial leads are placed on a single ventricle for patients with single ventricle physiology.

>A revised NASPE/BPEG generic code describes a five- position ICHD code to communicate pacemaker fundamentals (Table 8.1). The first position describes the chamber(s) paced, the second position describes the chamber(s) sensed, and the third position describes the response to sensing. Position four describes the response or lack thereof to the patient's metabolic activity and the last position describes multisite pacing.

Indications and contraindications for pacemaker in the pediatric population

Abnormalities of the sinoatrial (SA) node to the atrioventricular node that result in insufficient heart rate are indications for pediatric pacemaker implantation. The American College of Cardiology, American Heart Association, and Heart Rhythm

Society updated guidelines for pacemaker implantation and included recommendations for pediatric patients (Table 8.2).

An expected survival of less than 6 months is a relative contraindication for pacemaker placement in terminally ill patients. Additionally, patients to return to normal conduction after transient postoperative heart block do not need permanent pacemaker therapy.

Implantable cardioverter defibrillators

An implantable cardioverter defibrillator is similar to a pacemaker; however, it has pacing and defibrillation capabilities. The ICDs sense atrial or ventricular activity, classify the activity into programmed "heart rate zones," deliver tiered therapy to terminate the tachyarrhythmia, and pace for bradycardia. Depending on the size of the patient, the coil of the ICD can be placed in the pericardial or subcutaneous space or implanted transvenously using a lead that allows for sensing, pacing, and defibrillation. The ICD functions by measuring each cardiac R–R interval. When the device detects a substantial amount of short R–R intervals, an antitachycardia event is noted. The device can respond by pacing or eliciting a shock depending on the program. Additionally, if the ICD detects numerous long R–R intervals, it has an antibradycardic function that allows it to pace the heart. An international generic code is used to describe ICD function and programs (Table 8.3).

Table 8.2 Indications for permanent pacemaker placement in children and adolescents. Modified from references 5, and 11

Class 1: Pacemaker implantation indicated - Advanced second-/third-degree AV block with symptomatic bradycardia, ventricular dysfunction, or low cardiac output that persists 7 days following cardiac surgery - Symptomatic age inappropriate sinus bradycardia - Congenital third-degree AV block with wide QRS, complex ventricular ectopy, or ventricular dysfunction - Congenital third-degree AV block in an infant with HR < 55 b/min or HR < 70 b/min or pauses > 3 s
Class 2a: Pacemaker implantation reasonable - Patients with CHD, sinus bradycardia, and intra-arterial re-entry tachycardia - Asymptomatic sinus bradycardia in a child with CHD with resting HR < 40 b/min or pauses > 3 s - Patient with CHD and impaired hemodynamics secondary to sinus bradycardia and loss of AV synchrony - Unexplained syncope in unrepaired CHD complicated by transient AV block with residual fascicular block
Class 2b: Pacemaker implantation may be considered - Transient postoperative AV block that reverts to sinus rhythm with bifascicular block - Congenital third-degree AV block in asymptomatic child/adolescent with acceptable rate, narrow QRS, and normal ventricular function - Asymptomatic sinus bradycardia after biventricular repair of CHD with resting HR < 40 b/min or pauses > 3 s
Class III: Pacemaker implantation not effective/ contraindicated - Transient postop AV block that reverts to normal AV conduction - Asymptomatic Type I AV block - Asymptomatic sinus bradycardia in adolescent with resting HR > 40 b/min and longest R–R interval < 3 s - Asymptomatic postoperative bifascicular block in the absence of transient complete AV block

Indications for ICD placement in the pediatric population

Children who suffer a sudden cardiac arrest or those at increased risk of malignant ventricular arrhythemias are candidates for implantable cardioverter defibrillators. Guidelines for placement of ICDs and similar devices in the pediatric population are derived from adult randomized clinical trials (Table 8.4).

In the perioperative period, it is imperative to keep in mind although ICDs are lifesaving there are a high number of inappropriate shocks and lead failures seen in the pediatric population. This evidence may be secondary to progressive growth and the activity of children stress the ICD leads.

Perioperative management of a CRMD in the pediatric population

A complete perioperative history and physical are indicated when preparing to care for any patient with a CRMD. It has been shown that an incomplete preoperative evaluation may lead to adverse outcomes. In adult patients, the HRS/ASA consensus statement concludes that most patients with CRs do not need a new preoperative evaluation by the CR management team because pertinent information will be available in the notes from the CR clinic.

Recommendations from the ASA practice advisory for the perioperative management of patients with a CR focus on three main areas:

1. Type of device
2. Dependency on device for antibradycardia pacing and underlying escape rhythm
3. Device function

In children, lead failure and fracture occur at higher rates than adults. Lead failure remains the single most common cause of inappropriate shocks and ICD complications in the pediatric population. Patients presenting for nonurgent surgery should have the

Table 8.3 NASPE/BPEG generic defibrillator code. Modified from reference 8

I/ Chamber(s) shocked	II/Antitachycardia paced chamber(s)	III/Tachycardia detection	IV/Antibradycardia pacing chamber(s)
A = atrium	A = atrium	R = rate modulation	A = atrium
V = ventricle	V = ventricle	E = electrogram	V = ventricle
O = none	O = none		O = none
D = dual (A + V)	D = dual (A + V)		D = dual (A + V)

Table 8.4 ICD placement indications in children and patients with CHD.

Class 1: ICD implantation indicated - Cardiac arrest secondary to VT/VF and reversible cause excluded - Spontaneous sustained VT in CHD patients - Symptomatic sustained VT in CHD patients who have had EPS - Unexplained syncope in CHD patients with EPS inducible sustained, hemodynamically significant VT
Class 2a: ICD implantation reasonable - recurrent unexplained syncope in CHD patients with LC dysfunction or EPS-induced ventricular arrhythmia - Sustained VT with near normal ventricular function - Long QT or catecholamine-induced VT with recurrent syncope or VT despite Beta blockers - HCM or arrythmogenic right ventricular dysplasia with one or more risk factors for sudden cardiac death - Brugada syndrome and syncope or VT that has not resulted in cardiac arrest - Nonhospitalized patients awaiting cardiac transplantation
Class 2b: ICD implantation may be considered - Complex CHD patients with recurrent syncope and advanced ventricular dysfunction where thorough investigations failed to identify etiology - Long QT syndrome and risk factors for sudden cardiac death - Familial cardiomyopathy associated with sudden death - Patients with LV noncompaction
Class 3: ICD implantation not effective/contraindicated - VT/VF from arrhythmia amenable to catheter ablation - Unexplained syncope with structurally normal heart and no inducible ventricular tachyarrythmia - Ventricular tachyarrhythmias because of reversible cause in absence of CHD - Incessant VT/VF - Patients without reasonable explanation of survival/functional status of 1 year

Modified from references 5 and 11

following information shared with the surgical, anesthesia and CR team.

A proper preoperative history consists of the indication for CR placment, coexisitng cardiovascular pathology, generator location, and any cardiac conditions that may influence defibrillator pad position.

Table 8.5 Information to be communicated to the perioperative team by the cardiovascular implantable electronic device (CIED) specialty team

1	Date of last device interrogation recommended within 6 months for ICD or cardiac resynchronization therapy (CRT) device, 12 months for pacemaker
2	Device type, manufacturer, and model
3	Indication for device placement
4	Battery longevity
5	Leads placed within the last 3 months
6	Current programming
7	Is the patient pacemaker-dependent?
8	Device response to magnet placement
9	Any alert status on device (such as manufacturing issues)
10	Lasting pacing threshold
11	Individualized perioperative recommendation/ prescription based on patient information, device characteristics, and surgical factors

Prior medical records, especially anesthesia and operative notes, and the most recent interrogation report contain relevant information. If old records are unavailable, imaging such as a chest X-ray is helpful in determining device type, number, position, and integrity of leads, configuration of lead/generator placement, and manufacturer. A 12-lead ECG should also be obtained to detect pacer use and determine which chamber(s) are being sensed and/or paced.

Pacemakers should be routinely interrogated once a year and ICDs every 3–4 months. However, it is recommendated that all devices should be assessed within 30 days of surgery. The most recent interrogation report should be obtained to assess the patient's underlying rate and rhythm, need for intraoperative back up pacing support, presence of magnet mode, and response to magnet placement. The following practice algorithm (Figure 8.1) can be used for device optimization in the perioperative period.

Electromagnet interference and reprogramming

Electromagnet interference (EMI) is radio-frequency waves in the 50–60 Hz range. It can cause inappropriate triggering or inhibition of paced output in addition to reversion to an asynchronous mode; and if it used within 6 inches, EMI may cause damage to the pulse generator. Asynchronous pacing can lead to an arrhythmia if the pacer competes with a spontaneous rhythm. Inappropriate triggering of an ICD may lead

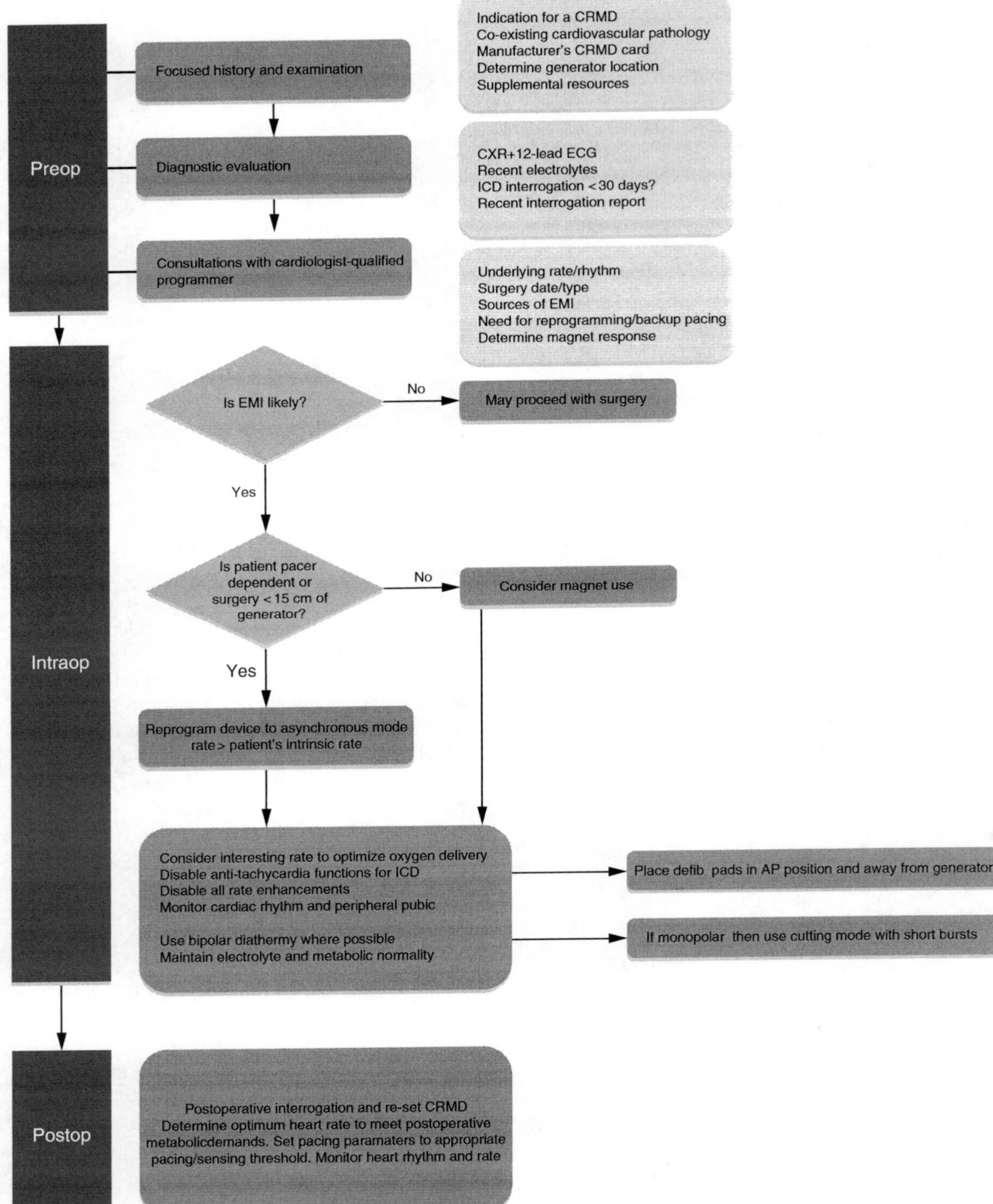

Figure 8.1 Algorithm for device optimization (modified from reference 1).

to unnecessary shock, antitachycardia therapy, or burn. Electrocautery, therapeutic radiation, extracorporeal shock wave lithotripsy, nerve stimulators, fasciculations, shivering, large tidal volumes, transthoracic defibrillation, radio-frequency ablation, electroconvulsive therapy, and MRI may result in EMI.

In patients who are pacemaker dependent and there is a significant risk of EMI, the ASA task-force recommends reprogramming the device to an asynchronous paced mode. An asynchronous mode at a higher rate than the patient's intrinsic rate will overcome oversensing or undersensing from EMI. In ICDs rate-adaptive functions and the antitachycardia function should be disabled. A magnet should not be routinely be used to disable an ICD; however, if the situation is an emergency, transthoracic defibrillator pads should be in place and a defibrillator in the OR.

In an attempt to reduce EMI, it is recommended that bipolar diathermy or an ultrasonic scalpel be used if the surgery is within 15 cm of the generator. If monopolar diathermy must be used, the minimal power setting and sort-intermittent irregular bursts of < 1 s duration should be used. The diathermy grounding pad should have appropriate skin contact and be placed so that the current flow will not intersect the pacing system.

Magnet use

Pacemakers contain magnet-activated switches to demonstrate remaining battery life and pacing threshold safety factors. Once a magnet is placed over the center of the pacemaker, no intrinsic cardiac activity is sensed and it will usually revert to an asynchronous pacing mode. However, the magnet rate varies with the make and model of the pacer. The preset magnet rate may not be sufficient to meet the metabolic demands of a pediatric patient and may vary according to the battery voltage of the generator.

When a magnet is placed over an ICD, most ICDs will suspend antitachycardia therapy. However, similar to pacemakers, the magnet response is variable and dependent on the manufacture and device program. Position for magnet placement also varies by manufacturer. Interrogation can reveal device magnet-response settings.

Intraoperative management

Intraoperative monitors must be able to detect packing spikes on ECG to verify pacmaker activity. An arterial line may be placed especially for long procedures with anticipated significant fluid shifts in patients with resynchronization devices, heart failure, or hypertrophic cardiomyopathy. Otherwise, other monitoring modalities, such as a pulse ox, with a waveform display that monitors peripheral pulse can be used. Temporary pacing and defibrillation equipment should be immediately available before, during, and after the procedure.

Current recommendations are placing transthoracic defibrillator pads in an anterior– posterior position and as far away from the pulse generator as possible. Damage to the circuit device, myocardial burns, and reprogramming of the pulse generator can occur following transthoracic defribillation. Device interrogation is necessary postoperatively to assess for proper function if an external defibrillator was used.

Anesthetic technique does not directly influence CR function; however, particular agents may have direct effects on myocardial activity. Use caution with agents that may cause depress SA or AV node activity as well as agents that can exacerbate long QT syndrome and result in arrhythmias.

Metabolic abnormalities and ischemia may cause pacemakers to exhibit acutely elevated lead thresholds and failure. Hyperkalemia, metabolic acidosis and alkalosis, hypothermia, and hyperglycemia all significantly increase the pacing threshold. Pacemaker function is influenced by dehydration, significant bleeding, and large fluid shifts. Hypoxemia and hypercarbia have been shown to increase the myocardial stimulation threshold.

Postoperative care

Following surgery, all devices should be reinterrogated if there were major fluid or blood components were administered, external defibrillation or monopolar diathermy was used. It is necessary to measure pacing and sensing thresholds and program the device to optimize hemodynamics postoperatively. Pacemakers that were reprogrammed for the surgery should be reset by the CR management team. Patients with ICDs in place should be monitored until antitachycardia therapy is reinstituted.

Diagnostic/interventional electrophysiologic techniques

In the pediatric population, most EP studies are done in patients with SVT.

Table 8.6 Radiofrequency catheter ablation complications. Modified from reference 18

Radiation e18xposure	40+/- 35 minutes Modern digital pulsed fluoroscopy and low-pulse fluoroscopic rates should not increase malignancy rate
Cardiac tamponade	Electrode catheter perforation
Pericarditis	Increased risk with posterior ablation sites
Groin hematoma	Rarely significant; retrograde arterial approach increases risk for femoral artery pseudoaneurysm
Arterial thrombus	Retrograde approach
AV block	Rare. Higher in procedures near the AV node/His bundle
Systemic embolization	Heparin used for all left-sided pathways intra- and postoperatively
Coronary artery dissection	Forceful use of ablation catheter into one of the coronary arteries. If energy is applied, result may be coronary artery thrombosis, late coronary artery stenosis
AV valve damage/ endocarditis	Rare; perforated mitral leavlet following energy application to the AV sulcus

Electrophysiologic studies are catheterization procedures that record intracardiac electrical signals using specialized catheters that record electrical activity and stimulate the heart. The mechanism of an arrhythmia, efficacy of pharmacologic therapy, location of an abnormal conduction pathway or automatic foci, and hemodynamic impact of the arrhythmia can be assessed through EP studies. Electrode catheters are positioned at various points of interest in the heart to examine the electrical activation of the heart in time and space. For example, right atrial pacing in the high right atrium is used to assess SA and AV node function, SVTs, and idiopathic ventricular tachycardia. Placing the catheter across the tricuspid valve at the medial and superior rim can be used to record local right atrial depolarization and local right ventricular depolarization along the bundle of His resulting in a His Bundle Electrogram (HBE). The HBE analyzes AV conduction disturbances and determines the origin of an arrhythmia. A catheter in the coronary sinus records both atrial and ventricular signals from the left heart and is mandatory for the evaluation SVT if an accessory pathway is suspected. The right ventricular apex is used also for SVE evaluation. It can also study ventricular arrhythmias and acts as an additional ventricular pacing site in the right ventricular outflow tract.

General anesthesia is used for most EP and ablation studies. The ASA NPO guidelines should be followed; however, prolonged NPO in patients with a single ventricle or shunt-dependent lesions, dehydration can increase viscosity. Most commonly used agents such as propofol and isoflurane have little effect on EP readings. Arterial line monitoring is essential to monitor for wide swings in blood pressure secondary to induced arrhythmias. Young age, low body weight, and cyanotic or complex CHD are the major risk factors for adverse events. Major complications of cardiac catherization in children are arrhythmias, hypoventilation, cardiac perforation, and hypothermia. In patients with long-term pulmonary arterial hypertension, paroxysmal pulmonary artery hypertension crisis can occur.

An ablation catheter is introduced to map the location once tachycardia has been induced and defined. The mechanism can be an accessory pathway with AV reentrant tachycardia, an ectopic focus in patients with atrial ectopic tachycardia, or a slow pathway in patients with AV nodal reentrant tachycardia. Transseptal or retrograde arterial techniques can be used to approach left-sided accessory pathways. Once the catheter tip is in the correct position, thermal injury to cardiac tissue is applied with 300–750 kHz energy. The arrhythmia should be abolished within 10 seconds of energy application.

Data were collected by the Pediatric RFCA Registry on 3653 procedures performed for SVT from 1991–1996. Absence of recurrence at 3 years was 71% for AV nodal reentrant tachycardias. Complications of the technique include those listed in Table 8.6. Overall success rate for the first attempt is roughly 70%.

Cardiopulmonary bypass in infants and children

Introduction

The use of cardiopulmonary bypass (CPB) for repair of congenital cardiac lesions in children dates back to the 1950s, with the first reported use by Gibbon (1954) who repaired an atrial septal defect. The initial survival rate was reported to be 60% or higher, but advancements in the field have led to decreasing mortality rates and the ability to repair complex lesions such as hypoplastic left heart syndrome (HLHS) and tetralogy of Fallot (TOF) possible.

Current trends in pediatric cardiac surgery are to repair congenital lesions as early as feasible to minimize the patient's adaptations to aberrant physiology. However, exposure to CPB is not without risk. Pediatric cardiac patients present with great variations in size and anatomy which can add complexity to the surgical procedure. Due to the variability existing in practices among congenital heart surgeons and perfusionists, it is difficult to describe a "standard of care" for every pediatric patient undergoing CPB. The purpose of this chapter is to define the physiologic effects of CPB in the pediatric population, components of the CPB circuit, and the main differences in management of CPB in pediatrics.

Physiologic effects of cardiopulmonary bypass in infants and children

The deleterious effects of CPB in neonates and infants are more pronounced than those seen in adults. Infants and children have smaller circulating blood volumes, higher oxygen consumption rates, highly reactive vascular beds, and at times altered physiology due to congenital abnormalities

The tissues and organ systems in neonates and infants are still immature. The developing myocardium may be at higher risk to CPB-related dysfunction due to relatively deficient contractile protein (compared to adult levels), increased calcium sensitivity, glucose substrate utilization, and altered enzyme activity. Congenital cardiac lesions may also place patients at risk for dysfunction after CPB. Congenital defects that yield collateral formation may also complicate cardioplegia delivery and myocardial protection. For example, hypertrophic and cyanotic lesions are more prone to ischemia–reperfusion injury. Aortopulmonary collaterals, often seen with cyanotic lesions, can cause a steal phenomenon from the arterial compartments to the lungs leading to low arterial perfusion and increased pulmonary perfusion. This increased pulmonary circulation can lead to pulmonary hypertension, decreased lung compliance and increased airway resistance which may worsen after CPB. Renal dysfunction is another significant source of morbidity after CPB, and it is not uncommon to see temporary oliguric renal dysfunction. The exact etiology is unknown, but may be related to the elevation of stress hormones and activation of the renin–angiotensin system. Most renal function gradually improves 24–48 hours post bypass.

The exposure to the CPB circuit and profound hypothermia leads to a systemic inflammatory response that is much more exaggerated in infants and neonates. This response can lead to capillary leakage, soft tissue edema, and end-organ dysfunction, which create challenges in fluid and hemodynamic management in the postoperative period. This inflammatory response includes neutrophils, complement and kallikrein-kinin systems, cytokines, and platelets all becoming activated. In addition, the huge disparity between the CPB circuit size and the patient amplifies this immune response. Often the bypass circuit volumes are 200% to 300% greater than the patient's circulating blood volume. To combat this response, high-dose corticosteroids are usually given before CPB.

As advancements in management of CHD improve, over 85% of infants are expected to survive to adulthood. This has shifted the focus on management of these patients not only on the mortality of CPB but on the morbidity associated with it, especially in regards to neurologic outcome. Neurologic sequela can vary from subtle to profound. The rate of devastating neurologic events has decreased from as high as 25% two decades ago to 2 to 11% today. There is currently more focus on neurodevelopmental and behavior deficits that may appear later in childhood. There are a number of factors that are associated with neurologic injury ranging from fixed factors and modifiable factors. Fixed factors include genetic syndromes, structural central nervous system malformations, prematurity, and CHD. Modifiable factors include preoperative events (hypotension, cyanosis), intraoperative/CPB circuit events (mainly emboli and reperfusion injury), and postoperative factors (low cardiac output, hyperthermia). Periventricular leukomalacia (PVL), the necrosis of white matter adjacent to lateral ventricles, is present in more than 50% of neonates after CPB by magnetic resonance imaging. The condition of PVL is not only seen in neonates, but has recently been described in term infants with CHD. Monitoring techniques with the use of cerebral oximetery and transcranial Doppler are becoming more widespread in clinical use for real-time monitoring of cerebral blood flow. Additionally improving techniques for deep hypothermic arrest or regional low-flow perfusion (to be discussed in a later section) have also decreased negative neurologic outcomes.

Optimizing high-risk infants, such as those with ductal-dependant heart defects with high pulmonary flow, in the pre- and postoperative period will attempt to decrease CPB-related morbidity. Also, patients who are septic, have depressed ventricular function, who have multiple congenital problems, and who are low birth weight (< 1800 g) are at increased risk for the deleterious effects of CPB.

Important differences in cardiopulmonary bypass in pediatrics

The CPB circuit must be adjusted to a wide range of sizes and age groups ranging from 1.5 kg neonates to obese adolescents. The normal cardiac index of a neonate is 3.5 to 4.0 l/min/m2 and because the body surface area is greater relative to weight, weight derived perfusion rates may be inadequate for perfusion. Therefore, higher flow rates on CPB may need to be considered than those calculated for adults based on weight. Also, neonates have metabolic rates which are 1.5 to 2.5 times higher than adults which may also require higher flow rates than their adult counterparts. This higher flow rate may result in higher shear stress on blood products. Another effect on blood products is that the large ratio of priming solution to blood volume results in significant dilution of red blood cells and clotting factors. Adding to the difficulty, many complex congenital cardiac operations require a bloodless field which may be difficult with intra- and extracardiac shunts, aortopulmonary collaterals or increased pulmonary venous return.

Considerations for extracorpeal circuitry in pediatrics

The extracorpeal circuit must allow isolation of the cardiopulmonary system and at a minimum allow for effective oxygenation, removal of carbon dioxide, and provide adequate perfusion to all vital organs. The CPB circuitry in infants in children is similar to that used in adults with some minor modifications mainly to account for the smaller size of the patient population, increased priming volume to blood volume ratio, increased metabolic rate of the neonate and infant, and different approaches to temperature regulation techniques than those seen in the adult population.

Due to the small size of the neonate and pediatric population, modifications must be made to the CPB circuit. For example, unlike in the adult population, tubing sizes vary due to the wide variety of patient sizes and one should be chosen that allows adequate flow rates, while decreasing the priming volume. The smaller the internal diameter of the tubing, the lower the priming volume, but the line pressure will increase with decreasing diameter and lead to increased shearing forces on blood products. The size of the arterial tubing is limited by maximal allowable outflow pressure. Venous lines can be placed on to vacuum which also allow for decreased internal diameters and therefore decreased priming volumes. Also, placement of the arterial and venous cannulae can vary in location in the pediatric population due to certain congenital lesions. For example, the aortic cannula is placed more distal in procedures involving the proximal aorta, such as transposition of great vessels. Irrespective of location, care must be taken during cannula placement, as small movements in cannula position can lead to venous obstruction leading to edema and poor distal perfusion. The increased metabolic demand of the neonate result in proportionally higher flow rates during normothermic CPB.

With miniaturization of CPB circuitry, improvements in blood salvage techniques, and the use of vacuum-assist venous drainage, priming methods have shifted to favor asanguinous. Conventional neonatal CPB requires large volumes of allogeneic blood to prevent hemodilution due to large priming volumes compared to neonatal blood volumes. It has been shown that use of a blood prime is associated with a lower postoperative cardiac index, higher pulmonary vascular resistance, and higher levels of tumor necrosis factor-α when compared to asanguinous prime. Weighing the risk vs. benefit of a decreased hematocrit (therefore decreased oxygen carrying capacity), the use of asanguinous prime continues to be difficult. The optimal hematocrit on CPB remains controversial. Studies have shown that patients with a hematocrit of 20% on CPB show no difference in lactate levels, oxygen delivery, and oxygen consumption compared to a group with a hematocrit of 25%. The formula to determine the final CPB hematocrit is the patient's initial hematocrit multiplied by the blood volume of the patient divided by the total priming volume (circuit plus the patient's blood volume). Another controversial issue is the type of blood prime. Some centers use whole blood and others favor packed red cells for their prime.

Temperature management in pediatric cardiopulmonary bypass

Temperature management is also typically different in the neonate and infant population compared to adults. The use of hypothermia is used more often in infant CPB and for complex repairs. Benefits of hypothermia include deceases in pump flow rates leading to increased surgical exposure and protection to the myocardium and other organs during periods of hypothermia. The degree of hypothermia depends on the exposure needed (15 to 18 °C core temperature for deep hypothermia, 22 to 28 °C for complex repairs, and 28 to 32 °C for ASD and VSDs.) Optimal flow rates are based on body surface area and adequate organ perfusion as determined by arterial blood gases and whole body oxygen consumption. Deep hypothermia is used with deep hypothermic circulatory arrest (DHCA) or when periods of low flow are desired. In recent years, there has been a shift toward avoidance of DHCA due to increasing evidence of associated neurologic injury. However, DHCA is still utilized in complex repairs. Research to develop strategies to decrease injury has led to modifications such as pretreatment with steroids, hyperoxygenation, adequate duration of cooling (at least 20 minutes), maintaining a higher hematocrit during cooling phase, using pH stat blood gas management, allowing for low-flow cerebral perfusion for 1 to 2 minutes at 15 to 20 minute intervals, using modified ultrafiltration, and ensuring adequate cerebral perfusion postoperatively.

During hypothermia the dissociation of water increases leading to decreased levels of hydrogen and hydroxyl ions. Additionally when blood cools, the oxyhemoglobin dissociation curve shifts to the left, resulting in a more alkaline state. This leads to reduced cerebral blood flow, increases in oxygen demand and decreases oxygen dissociation to ischemic tissues. To deal with acid–base management during hypothermia, two distinct strategies are employed. Alpha stat (temperature uncorrected) and pH stat (temperature corrected) are the two strategies. In alpha stat the pH is maintained at 7.4 and is not corrected for temperature (normal pH at all temperatures and the carbon dioxide is unchanged). This strategy is thought to preserve intracellular electroneutrality, cerebral autoregulation, and reduces cerebral blood flow and edema. In pH stat method, carbon dioxide is added to the system to achieve normal pH of 7.4 at the patient's actual temperature. This is at the expense of intracellular acidity and electrical balance. Despite this, pH stat appears to be superior to alpha stat with advantages including enhanced cerebral perfusion, more even cooling and increased oxygen offloading. Clinically, this benefit is highly debated and long-term outcomes with the different strategies appear to not be different. However, most institutions that do employ DHCA still use pH stat acid base management strategies.

Ultrafiltration techniques

Due to their small size, neonates and infants are a group that may accumulate excessive fluid during CPB. This edema can not only be seen in the periphery, but also effects vital organs such as the brain, heart, lungs, and intestines. This excessive fluid accumulation can be limited by limiting the volume of pump primes and replacing crystalloid administration with colloid. There have also been techniques developed to remove fluid during and after CPB and produce hemoconcentration. These devices consist of a semipermeable membrane that creates a hydrostatic pressure gradient across the device. Blood inflow is obtained from the arterial side and blood outflow is diverted to the cardiotomy or venous reservoir. The ultrafiltrate has the composition of glomerular filtrate.

Conventional ultrafiltration

Conventional ultrafiltration (CUF) occurs throughout CPB or whenever the venous reservoir is sufficient to allow filtration. The CUF method is difficult to undertake in infants and children as removal from miniaturized circuits demands replacement of filtered volume with fluid to maintain adequate reservoir levels.

Dilutional ultrafiltration (DUF) and zero-balance ultrafiltration (Z-BUF)

Dilutional ultrafiltration (DUF) and zero-balance ultrafiltration (Z-BUF) use the same concept as CUF, but involve replacement of the ultrafiltrate with high volumes of crystalloid solution, therefore maintaining reservoir volumes. The Z-BUF method uses ultrafiltration rates of 200 ml/kg/min whereas DUF uses rates of 40 to 80 ml/kg/min. These methods do not result in hemoconcentration but do result in decreased levels of inflammatory mediators.

The Z-BUF method has been reported to reduce postoperative blood loss, decrease time to extubation, and remove significant inflammatory mediators.

Modified ultrafiltration

Modified ultrafiltration (MUF) allows for filtration after weaning from cardiopulmonary bypass and before reversal with protamine. This can be accomplished in either arteriovenous or a venovenous system. To maintain adequate blood volume, the ultrafiltrate is replaced with blood from the CPB circuit, which results in better hemoconcentration. To minimize the deleterious effects of CPB, usually endpoints are set, which vary institutionally. The MUF process is usually terminated after a set time interval (15–20 minutes), a set hematocrit is obtained (40%), or a set volume removed (750 ml/m^2). The MUF and CUF processes are not mutually exclusive and are sometimes combined.

Future trends and developments

Continued miniaturization of extracorpeal circuits will hopefully lead to decreased exposure of the patient to circuit, therefore decreasing the systemic inflammatory response. Miniaturization would also lead to decreased hemodilution, and therefore also decrease the need to give allogeneic blood products in the pump prime.

Heparin-bonded circuits and circuits coated with poly-2-methoxyethylacrylate have been shown to reduce the inflammatory response, but they are not in widespread practice at this time mainly due to cost effectiveness.

Due to the massive inflammatory response seen in infants and children, additional strategies to combat this are under investigation. Administration of preoperative steroids, use of coated circuits, ultrafiltration techniques, and until recently aprotinin were all strategies to decrease the inflammatory response. New pharmacologic anti-inflammatory agents are under development that may assist in decreasing this response to CPB.

Adults with congenital heart disease

Introduction

In today's world, the majority of infants with CHD reach adulthood. Advances in knowledge and treatment are credited with seeing over 85% of these individuals reach this stage. It is now estimated that over one million adults with CHD exists in the USA and now more adults have surgery for primary repair, reoperation, or non-cardiac surgery than all neonates, infants, and children combined. These patients are often lost to follow-up and commonly appear only after symptoms occur. They can be extremely complex patients with high medical resource demands.

Many of these individuals are still being cared for by pediatric specialists in pediatric hospitals because of their familiarity with these defects. The majority of these individuals will need lifelong surveillance by a cardiologist and surgeons. Although knowledge of these heart defects has increased, institutions regularly caring for these individuals are somewhat limited. Because of present day numbers and the continued outcome success with today's infants and children, the appearance of these individuals at community hospitals will become commonplace. General practitioners and others will more commonly, in the future, deal with their complex issues. For the female adult with CHD, the issues surrounding pregnancy and relative risk related to the interplay between the mothers' cardiopulmonary system, her CHD, and the developing fetus are disease specific and frequently warrant tertiary or quaternary care facilities.

When caring for adults with CHD it is important to understand that only simple defects such as patent ductus arteriosus and secundum atrial septal defects, that are repaired early, are considered cured. Despite meticulous surgical technique, modern technology has revealed that most lesions are left with residual defects and/or sequelae from previous operations or interventions. These residual or sequelae create impairments with the cardiac electrophysiological, valvular, vascular, or ventricular functions. Due to this, the American College of Cardiology along with the American Heart Association has crafted a consensus opinion that outlines disease specific issues, treatment and diagnostic suggestions. It also provides the necessary requirements for institutions wishing to be labeled as "referral centers" for these patients.

The cardiac and pulmonary systems are stressed by anesthesia and surgery in patients with normal cardiac anatomy. So, the anesthesiologists caring for the adult with CHD must possess a basic understanding of the pathophysiology involved with each defect as well as their common residual or sequelae. Some lesions experience an increased perioperative morbidity and mortality and will require more complex evaluation and care.

Pathophysiology of congenital heart disease

Adults with CHD experience pathophysiology related to shunting, obstruction, mixing, and regurgitation lesions. These pathophysiologic changes result in ventricular volume or pressure overload and/or hypoxemia. Some adults with complex CHD may experience a combination of the above issues. Over time, these changes may cause dramatic perioperative effects for the patient. So, the anesthesiologist must develop a concise anesthetic plan based on the patient's specific pathophysiology.

Shunting lesions

In the normal heart, two circulatory systems exist in series each carrying either oxygenated or deoxygenated blood. These two systems are separated and reliant on one another. When shunting occurs, there is an abnormal connection between the two systems. These connections are either intracardiac between chambers or extra cardiac connections between the pulmonary and systemic arteries. The flow of blood is directed by the resistance involved between the two systems and the size of the shunt orifice. Examples of shunting lesions are atrial septal defects, ventricular septal defects (VSD), and a patent ductus arteriosus (PDA).

Right to left shunting

Right to left shunting is caused when resistance to flow in the pulmonary or right ventricular outflow tract exceeds the systemic vascular resistance. This forces deoxygenated blood into the systemic circulation and may cause hypoxemia. Two examples, which delineate this phenomenon, are persistent pulmonary hypertension and tetralogy of Fallot. In persistent pulmonary hypertension of the newborn right to left shunting occurs via a PDA when pulmonary vascular resistance (PVR) exceeds sytemic vascular resistance (SVR). The more frequent scenario for right to left shunting involves obstruction to flow. In tetralogy of Fallot, the right ventricular outflow obstruction results in increased flow across the VSD. In this scenario, the pulmonary vascular resistance (PVR) is low, but deoxygenated blood in forced into the systemic circulation.

Left to right shunting

Under normal conditions, pulmonary vascular resistance is lower than systemic vascular resistance, so when a shunt exists, as is the case with a VSD or ASD, the blood flow is directed to the lungs. This can cause a dramatic increase in pulmonary blood flow. The increase in pulmonary blood flow, over time, will cause a concomitant increase in PVR. The increased resistance will place more stress on the right ventricle and ultimately lead to diastolic dysfunction, ventricular dilation, and reduced ventricular compliance. If the shunt is not repaired, then irreversible damage to the pulmonary vascular bed will result. These fixed changes with pulmonary arterioles manifest into pulmonary hypertension.

Shunt volumes

The total flow in both the pulmonary and systemic circulations can be evaluated to assess shunt volumes. Comparing the two creates a ratio, which aids in determining shunt volume. The normal pulmonary blood flow (Qp) to systemic blood flow (Qs) ratio is 1:1 and this indicates no shunting. When the Qp:Qs ratio is $>$ 1:1, this indicates that blood flow is greater to the pulmonary circulation. This is the effect of a left-to-right shunt. If the Qp:Qs ratio is $<$ 1:1, then blood flow is being preferentially directed to the systemic circulation. This indicates a right-to-left shunt.

Obstructive lesions

Blood flows through either the right or left outflow tract with minimal resistance and is unobstructed. Certain CHD lesions cause narrowing in either the left or right ventricular outflow tracts. The lesion may be subvalvular, valvular or involve a great vessel. This obstruction results in an increased resistance to flow and ultimately impacts ventricular loading, pressure, and function. The ventricular chamber increases muscularity as a response to the increase in afterload resistance. The resultant hypertrophied ventricular walls require more blood flow and higher metabolic requirements. Over time, these chambers become noncompliant, dysfunctional, and unable to keep pace with exertional or daily demands. The more common stenotic lesions are: subvalvular pulmonary and aortic, valvar aortic and pulmonary, supravalvular aortic and pulmonary, branch pulmonary artery, and aortic coarctation.

Regurgitant lesions

Purely regurgitant lesions are uncommon. Regurgitant lesions usually result from associated structural valvular defects that occur as part of another defect such as a partial atrioventricular canal or truncus arteriosis. These defects can cause abnormalities with papillary muscle number and position, chordal attachment, and with leaflet size shape and thickness. Epstein anomaly is the most common purely regurgitant lesion, but it presents during infancy. Pulmonic, mitral, and aortic regurgitation occur as a progession of distal stenotic lesions such as coarctation of the aorta or branched pulmonary artery stenosis.

Mixing lesions

The pulmonary and systemic circulations usually exist in series. When certain congenital heart defects occur, it allows mingling of the two systems. For some of these lesions, the two systems exist in a common chamber, which permits significant mixing of the two circulations. These lesions are the most common cause of cyanotic heart disease. Flow is dictated by resistance, so if no outflow obstruction exists, then blood movement to the systemic or pulmonary system is directed by vascular resistance. In this case, blood is usually directed into the lower resistant pulmonary circulation.

Consequences of CHD

Preoperative evaluation of adults with CHD should determine if the patient has undergone an operation for their CHD. As mentioned earlier many lesions are repaired, but only a few are truly cured from the operation. Although surgical or interventional procedures exist for all CHD lesions, some are only palliative in nature. These patients are usually left with significant issues, which make noncardiac or cardiac surgery challenging. It is now known that the vast majority of CHD lesions are left with residual effects or sequelae from their previous surgery. The more common issues facing anesthesiologists caring for these patients are discussed below.

Pulmonary hypertension

Pulmonary hypertension results from numerous scenarios in adult patients with CHD. It is defined as a mean pulmonary pressure greater than 25 mmHg. It may be the result of left-to-right shunting, pulmonary venous obstruction, elevated left atrial end diastolic pressure or primary pulmonary hypertension. It is important to ascertain if the pulmonary hypertension is fixed or reversible. A right ventricle faced with these phenomena will hypertrophy from the workload. This can cause intracavitary pressure changes which influence coronary flow and may precipitate myocardial ischemia. It is important to investigate recent echocardiographic or catheterization reports and consult with the cardiologist to outline a perioperative course for the patient involved.

The anesthetic plan should eliminate all factors, which potentially exacerbate the existing pulmonary hypertension. Regional anesthesia is generally preferred if possible. If sedation is used with a regional technique, carbon dioxide levels should be kept as close to baseline as possible. Increases in carbon dioxide levels can greatly exaggerate pulmonary artery pressure. General anesthesia with endotracheal intubation requires strict control of ventilation. A carefully crafted induction plan can obviate the stimulatory effects commonly encountered with intubation and emergence.

Congestive heart failure

Some adult CHD patients with ventricles under siege from various physiologic assaults eventually face irreparable damage. Unable to function with normal ventricular compliance, these individuals are placed on a multitude of pharmacologic agents and eventually, if possible, listed for transplantation. Right ventricular failure is a common occurrence in adult patients with CHD. Careful preoperative investigation and consultation is advised before proceeding with any type of surgery. These individuals with poor ventricular function can require complex resource availability to navigate the perioperative process successfully.

Chronic hypoxemia

Cyanotic heart disease results from either inadequate pulmonary perfusion or from a lesion, which enables significant mixing of the deoxygenated and oxygenated blood. The most common causes are mixing lesions, shunt lesions, pulmonary hypertension, and arterial–venous malformations. Long-term hypoxemia causes hematologic, cardiac, and renal system issues.

Chronic hypoxemia results in increased red blood cell production as the body attempts to compensate for inadequate tissue oxygenation. This increased viscosity will need careful scrutiny preoperatively. These patients may experience headaches, fatigue, blurred vision, and in extreme cases cerebrovascular thrombosis and stroke. Phlebotomy is reserved for the symptomatic polycythemic patients, but routine preoperative fasting may exacerbate issues. Therefore, meticulous attention to perioperative hydration is warranted.

Platelet count, function, and coagulation factor production are affected by chronic cyanosis. Thrombocytopenia, increased prothrombin time and partial thromboplastin times, and clotting factor deficiencies are commonly found in chronically hypoxic patients. These patients should be considered high risk for perioperative bleeding. They should have preoperative bleeding studies and the availability of platelets and fresh frozen for transfusion if needed.

Cardiac and renal system abnormalities are common in this population. Chronic myocardial hypoxemia results in myocardial dysfunction, which results in decreased ventricular diastolic compliance. Chronic renal hypoxemia causes a reduction in renal glomerular filtration rate and increases plasma creatinine. Increased plasma urate levels are found due high red cell turnover.

Predictors of clinical outcome with congenital heart disease

1. **Pulmonary hypertension and Eisenmenger syndrome**: Without early surgical repair, about one-third of patients with CHD will develop pulmonary arterial hypertension. Eisenmenger's syndrome, characterized by reversed pulmonary-to-systemic (right-to-left) shunt, affects as many as 50% of those with pulmonary arterial hypertension and left-to-right shunts. In patients with suspected pulmonary vascular disease anticipating a two-ventricle repair, although preoperative testing via cardiac catheterization with vasodilators is reasonable, the preoperative parameters and the precise values of these parameters that best correlate with early and late outcome remain unclear.
2. **Vasodilator responders have a better outcome:** Krasuski *et al.* studied 215 patients with pulmonary arterial hypertension. The vasoreactivity of patients was assessed during inhalation of 40 parts per million nitric oxide (iNO) and vasodilator responders were defined as participants who achieved a mean pulmonary artery pressure (PAP) of $\leq$ 40 mmHg and a drop in mean PAP $\geq$ the median for the cohort (13%). There were 51 deaths (25.9%) over a mean follow-up period of 2.3 years. Vasodilator responders had significantly improved survival regardless of whether or not they had idiopathic or nonidiopathic pulmonary arterial hypertension or whether or not they had Dana Point class 1 or nonDana Point class 1 PAH. In multivariate modeling, advanced age, elevated right atrial pressure, elevated serum creatinine, and worsened functional class significantly predicted shorter survival, whereas vasodilator response predicted improved survival. It was concluded that vasodilator responsiveness to iNO is an important method of risk stratifying pulmonary arterial hypertension patients, with results that apply regardless of clinical etiology.
3. **Older age:** Older patients with CHD have higher morbidity and mortality rate if they undergo a surgical procedure. They are at increased risk of arrhythmia, valve regurgitation, pulmonary arterial hypertension, and heart failure. Data have demonstrated that the probability of pulmonary arterial hypertension increases with age in patients with cardiac defects.
4. **Gender:** Shapiro *et al.* investigated the gender differences in patients with CHD and pulmonary hypertension. 2318 female and 651 male patients were studied and a greater number of females had pulmonary arterial hypertension associated with connective tissue disease ($P < 0.001$). Further, more males had portopulmonary hypertension ($P < 0.001$); more females had CHD associated PAH ($P = 0.017$), thyroid disease ($P < 0.001$), and depression reported ($P \leq 0.001$). At diagnosis, males had higher mean pulmonary arterial pressure (53 ± 14 vs. 51 ± 14.3 mmHg; $P = 0.013$) and mean right atrial pressure (10 ± 6 vs. 9 ± 6 mmHg; $P = 0.031$). Females had better survival

estimates for 2 years from enrollment and for 5 years from diagnosis. However, Klitzner *et al.* showed the opposite results in mortality with the female gender associated with an 18% higher in-hospital and 30-day post-discharge mortality as compared with male gender. There was no difference in length of hospital stay between males and females. Thus, the role of gender on the short- and long-term survival of patients with CHD will require additional investigation.

In summary, surgical and technological advances in recent decades for patients with CHD have improved outcomes leading to longer lives and reduced morbidity. An appreciation of physiology and pathophysiological states in CHD go a long way to ensure good decision making and anesthetic considerations. Ongoing challenges will continue to press our brightest minds with regard to cardiopulmonary bypass techniques, implantable devices, and drug discovery into the future.

Further reading

1. Navaratnam M, Dubin A. Pediatric pacemakers and ICDs: how to optimize perioperative care. *Paediatr Anaesth* 2011; **21** (5); 512–21.
2. Fortescue EB, Berul C, Cecchin F *et al.* Patient, procedural and hardware factors associated with pacemaker lead failures in pediatrics and congenital heart disease. *Heart Rhythm* 2004; **1**: 150–9.
3. Cohen MI, Bush DM, Vetter VL *et al.* Permanent epicardial pacing in pediatric patients: seventeen years of experience and 1200 outpatient visits. *Circulation* 2001; **103**: 2585–90.
4. Mohamady H, Saleh M, Ahmed H. Disasters in pediatric cardiac catheterization laboratory. *Ain Shams J Anesthesiol* 2012; **5** (2): 121–5.
5. Chun T. Pacemakers and defibrillator therapy in pediatrics and congenital heart disease. *Future Cardiol* 2008; **4**: 469–79.
6. Shah MJ. Implantable cardioverter defibrillator-related complications in the pediatric population. *Pacing Clin Electrophysiol* 2009; **32**: S71–S74.
7. Mathony U, Schmidt H, Groger C *et al.* Optimal maximum tracking rate of dual chamber pacemakers required by children and young adults for a maximal cardiorespiratory performance. *Pacing Clin Electrophysiol* 2005; **28**: 378–83.
8. Bernstein AD, Daubert J-C, Fletcher RD *et al.* Naspe Position Statement. The revised NASPE/BPEG generic code for antibradycardia, adaptive-rate, and multisite pacing. *Pacing Clin Electrophysiol* 2002; **25**: 260–4.
9. Stone ME, Apinis A. Current perioperative management of the patient with a cardiac rhythm management device. *Semin Cardiothorac Vasc Anesth* 2009; **13**: 31–43.
10. Knight BP, Gersh BJ, Carlson MD *et al.* Role of permanent pacing to prevent atrial fibrillation. *Circulation* 2005; **111**: 240–3.
11. Epstein AE, Di Marco JP, Elenborgen KA *et al.* ACC/AHA/HRS2008 guide- lines for device-based therapy of cardiac rhythm abnormalities: a report of the American College of Cardiology/American Heart Association Task Force on Practice Guidelines (Writing Committee to revise the ACC/AHA/NASPE2002 guideline update for implantation of cardiac pacemakers and antiarrhythmia devices) developed in collaboration with the American Association for Thoracic Surgery and Society of Thoracic Surgeons. *Circulation* 2008; **117**: E350–E408.
12. Andrews RE, Tulloh RM. Interventional cardiac catheterization in congenital heart disease. *Arch Dis Child* 2004; **89** (12): 1168–73.
13. Bennet D, Marcus R, Stokes M. Incidents and complications during pediatric cardiac catheterization. *Paediatr Anaesth* 2005; **15**(12): 1083–8.
14. Schroeder VA *et al.* Surgical emergencies during pediatric interventional catheterization. *J Pediatr* 2002 **140**(5): 570–5.
15. Phodes JF *et al.* Impact of how body weight on frequency of pediatric cardiac catheterization complications. *Am J Cardiol* 2000 **86**(11): 1275–8.
16. Walsh E, Alexander M, Cecchin F. Electrocardiography and introduction to electrophysiologic techniques. In Keane J, Lock J, Fyler D, eds. *Nada's Pediatric Cardiology*, 2nd edition. Philadelphia, PA: Elsevier. 2006. pp.145–72.
17. Triredi K, Dubin A, Perry S, *et al.* Out of operating room procedures: pediatric catherizarion and electrophysiology. *Anesthesiologist's Manual of Surgical Procedures*, 4th edition. Philadelphia, PA: Lippincott Williams and Wilkins. 2009. Pp. 1493–5.
18. Lake C, Booker P *et al.* Pediatric electrocardiography and cardiac electrophysiology. *Pediatric Cardiac Anesthesiology* 2005; 138–51.
19. Dubin AM, Janousek J, Rhee E *et al.* Resynchronization therapy in pediatric and congenital heart disease patients: an international multicenter study. *J Am Coll Cardiol* 2005; **46**: 2277–83.

20. Stephenson EA, Batra AS, Knilans TK *et al.* A multicenter experience with novel implantable cardioverter defibrillator configurations in the pediatric and congenital heart disease population. *J Cardiovasc Electrophysiol* 2006; **17**: 41–6.
21. Rozner MA. The patient with a cardiac pacemaker or implanted defibrillator and management during anesthesia. Anesthesia and medical disease. *Current Opin Anaesthesiol* 2007; **20**: 261–8.
22. Berul CI, VanHare GF, Kertesz MJ *et al.* Results of a multicenter retrospective implantable cardioverter-defibrillator registry of pediatric and congenital heart disease patients. *J Am Coll Cardiol* 2008; **51**: 1685–91.
23. Silka MJ, Kron J, Dunnigan A *et al.* Sudden cardiac death and the use of implantable cardioverter defibrillators in pediatric patients. *Circulation* 1993; **87**: 800–7.
24. Alexander ME, Cecchin F, Walsh EP *et al.* Implications of implantable cardioverter defibrillator therapy in congenital heart disease and pediatrics. *J Cardiovasc Electrophysiol* 2004; **15**: 72–6.
25. Zaidan JR, Atlee JL, Belott P *et al.* Practice advisory for the perioperative management of patients with cardiac rhythm management devices: pacemakers and implantable cardioverter defibrillators: a report by the American Society of Anesthesiologists Task Force on Perioperative Management of Patients with Cardiac Rhythm Management Devices. *Anesthesiology* 2005; **103**: 186–98.
26. Mychaskiw G, Eichhorn JH. Interaction of an implanted pacemaker with a transesophageal atrial pacemaker: report of a case. *J Clin Anesth* 1999; **11**: 669–71.
27. Purday JP, Towey RM. Apparent pacemaker failure caused by activation of ventricular threshold test by a magnetic instrument during general anaesthesia. *Br J Anaesth* 1992; **69**: 645–6.
28. Kellow NH. Pacemaker failure during transurethral resection of the prostate. *Anesthesia* 1993; **48**: 136–8.
29. Joshi GP. Perioperative management of outpatients with implantable cardioverter defibrillators. *Curr Opin Anaesthesiol* 2009; **22**: 701–4.
30. Rozner MA. Review of electrical interference in implanted cardiac devices. *Pacing Clin Electrophysiol* 2003; **26**: 923–5.
31. Dohrmann ML, Goldschlager NF. Myocardial stimulation threshold in patients with cardiac pacemakers: effect of physiologic variables, pharmacologic agents, and lead electrodes. *Cardiol Clin* 1985; **3**: 527–37.
32. Schure AV. Cardiopulmonary bypass in infants and children: what's new? *South African Journal of Anesthesia and Analgesia* 2010; **16** (1): 25–7.
33. Hsia TY, Gruber PJ. Factors influencing neurologic outcome after neonatal cardiopulmonary bypass: what we can and cannot control. *Ann Thoracic Surg* 2006; **81**: S2381–S2388.
34. Shen I, Giacomuzzi C, Ungerleider RM. Current strategies for optimizing the use of cardiopulmonary bypass in neonates and infants. *Ann Thoracic Surg* 2003; **75**: S729–S734.
35. Davis PJ, Cladis FP, Motoyama EK. *Smith's Anesthesia for Infants and Children*, 8th edition. Elsevier, 2011.
36. Gravlee GP, David RF, Stammers AH, Ungerlider RM. *Cardiopulmonary Bypass Principles and Practice*, 3rd edition. Lippincott, Williams and Wilkins, 2008.
37. Lake CL, Booker PD. *Pediatric Cardiac Anesthesia*, 4th edition. Lippincott, Williams and Wilkins, 2005.
38. Hickey E, Karamlou T, You J, Ungerleider RM. Effects of miniaturization in reducing inflammatory response to infant cardiopulmonary bypass by elimination of allogeneic blood products. *Ann Thorac Surg* 2006; **81**: S2367–S2372.
39. Lovell A. Anaesthetic implications of frown-up congenital heart disease. *Br J Anaesth* 2004; **93**(1): 129–39.
40. Cannesson M, Collange V, Lehot JJ. Anesthesia in adult patients with congenital heart disease. *Curr Opin Anaesthesiol* 2009; **22**: 88–94.
41. Perloff JK, Warnes CA. Challenges posed by adults with repaired congenital heart disease. *Circulation* 2001: **103**: 2637–43.
42. Rhodes JF, Hijazi ZM, Sommer RJ. Pathophysiology of congenital heart disease in the adult, Part II: Simple obstructive lesions. *Circulation* 2008; **117**: 1228–37.
43. Sommer RJ, Hijazi ZM, Sommer RJ. Pathophysiology of congenital heart disease in the adult, Part I: Shunt lesions. *Circulation* 2008; **117**: 1090–9.
44. Deanfield J, Thaulow E, Warnes C *et al.* Management of grown up congenital heart disease. Task force of European Society of Cardiology 2003. *Eur Heart J* 2003*l*; **24**: 1035–84.
45. Warnes CA, Liberthson R, Danielson GK *et al.* Task force: the changing profile of congenital heart disease in adult life. *J Am Coll Cardiol* 2001; **37**: 1170–8.
46. Marelli AJ, Mackie AS, Ionescu-lttu R *et al.* Congenital heart disease in the general population; changing prevalence and age distribution. *Circulation* 2007; **115**: 163–2.
47. Giglia TM, Humpl T. Preoperative pulmonary hemodynamics and assessment of operability: is there a pulmonary

vascular resistance that precludes cardiac operation? *Pediatr Crit Care Med* 2010; **11**(2 Suppl): S57–S69.

48. Krasuski RA, Devendra GP, Hart SA *et al.* Response to inhaled nitric oxide predicts survival in patients with pulmonary hypertension. *J Card Fail* 2011; **17** (4): 265–71.

49. Mulder BJ. Changing demographics of pulmonary arterial hypertension in congenital heart disease. *Eur Respir Rev* 2010; **19**(118): 308–13.

50. Shapiro S, Traiger GL, Turner M *et al.* Gender differences in the diagnosis, treatment, and outcome of patients with pulmonary arterial hypertension enrolled in the Registry to Evaluate Early and Long-Term PAH Disease Management (REVEAL). *Chest* 2012; **141**(2): 363–73.

51. Klitzner TS, Lee M, Rodriguez S, Chang RK. Sex-related disparity in surgical mortality among pediatric patients. *Congenit Heart Dis* 2006; **1**(3): 77–88.

52. Warnes CA, Williams RG, Bashore TM *et al.* ACC/AHA 2008 Guidelines for the management of adults with congenital heart disease: executive summary. *Circulation* 2008; **118**: 2395–451.

Chapter 9

Central and peripheral nervous system

Jacqueline L. Tutiven, Lalitha V. Sundararaman, and Gabriel Sarah

Anatomy and physiology

Brain, fontanelles, cranial sutures, and spinal cord

The brain of the neonate weighs about 1/10 of the body weight. This is much larger than the adult, where it composes 1/50 of the body weight. The neonate's brain grows rapidly, tripling in size by age one year. The neural plate appears at 3 weeks gestation and by 8 weeks neurons begin their migration to form cortical layers. This migration is complete by the 24th week. The brain is only about 25% complete at birth in relation to neuronal development. This development is complete by around age 1 (1).

The central nervous system of the child is vastly different than the adult. The child's CNS undergoes tremendous structural and anatomic change in the first two years of life (1). Children have a relatively low intracranial pressure (ICP) and have a remarkable ability to maintain a normal ICP in the presence of a change in intracranial volume due to the highly compliant nature of their cranium. This is accomplished because of the presence of open fontanelles and cranial sutures. The cranial sutures represent the spaces in between the major bones enclosing the brain, and the fontanelles are the various intersections of these sutures. The sequence of fontanelle closures occurs from the beginning of the second to third month. The posterior fontanelle is the first to close followed by the sphenoidal fontanelle, which should be closed completely by the 6th month. The mastoid fontanelle closes at around the 6th–18th month and the last fontanelle to close is the anterior at around 1–3 years of age (2). These articulating surfaces allow for the extremely compliant pediatric skull to expand and maintain a relatively normal ICP in the presence of a slow-growing tumor or fluid collection. Children, however, are not as easily capable of compensating for a rapid increase of a space-occupying lesion (2). Once these sutures and fontanelles close, the pediatric patient is at an increased risk for elevated ICP compared to the adult and is at a higher risk for herniation secondary to factors including the presence of a higher ratio of brain content to intracranial capacity (3).

If an infant presents with enlarged fontanelle, common reasons may include:

- Intrauterine growth retardation
- Rickets
- Hydrocephalus
- Down syndrome
- Achondroplasia
- Apert syndrome
- Neonatal hypothermia
- Congenital rubella
- Osteogenesis imperfecta

If a brain herniation is present in a pediatric patient, the most common herniation is of the temporal lobe displaced infratentorially. This is called a transtentorial hernia. Other herniations to consider are the midline hernia, cerebellar hernia, and the subfalcine hernia (4).

The spinal cord of the fetus extends to the base of the spinal column at 8 weeks gestational age. By the 24th week, it has ascended to just below the S1 body. A newborn will present with the base of the conus medullaris at the L3 body and the dural sac terminating at S3, compared to the adult at L1 and S1 respectively (1).

Myelinization, autonomic nervous systems, and pain pathways

Myelinization and the growth of the dendritic cells continue into the third and fourth years of life. It is

Essentials of Pediatric Anesthesiology, ed. Alan David Kaye, Charles James Fox and James H. Diaz. Published by Cambridge University Press. © Cambridge University Press 2015.

the lack of myelin that accounts for the primitive reflexes seen in the infant such as the Moro and grasp (1). These serve as valuable assessments of the progression of myelinization with the eventual disappearance of these reflexes as the dendritic process proceeds. Many of the degenerative neurologic diseases discussed later are a result of demyelination.

The autonomic nervous system is relatively well developed in the newborn with the parasympathetic components of the cardiac system fully functional at birth while the sympathetic component lags behind by 4 to 6 months. This leads to the dominance of the sympathetic by the parasympathetic system that explains the ease with which children develop bradycardia during stimulation (i.e., vagal stimulation) (1).

It is believed that many, if not all, of the essential pain pathways involved in transmission, perception, and modulation of pain are present by 24 weeks gestational age (1). As mentioned above, myelinization is incomplete in the newborn and this leads to slowing of neural transmission; however, the main nociceptive neurons are unmyelinated (C fibers) or very mildly myelinated (A delta fibers). The presence of pain pathways at birth does not equal maturity, and the infant's physiologic response to pain varies from that of the adult. Compared to adults, children have exaggerated responses to pain. This has been described as being secondary to reduced inhibition of input from the dorsal horn of the spinal cord. Also, these dorsal horn neurons have a wider receptive field and lower threshold of excitation in infants when compared to older children (1). The treatment of pain in the newborn is essential, as animal studies have shown increased amplitude of pain perception in previously untreated subjects experiencing painful stimulus.

Neurophysiology

Normal cerebral blood flow

Normal cerebral blood flow (CBF) to a child's brain represents approximately 25% of cardiac output and is estimated at 100 ml/100 g of brain tissue per minute. This is almost double the adult CBF of 55 ml/100 g brain tissue per minute. The infant's CBF, however, is lower than the adult and child, measured at approximately 40 ml/100 g/min. This varies greatly secondary to sleep/awake cycles, feeding, and activity (5). Since cerebral blood flow is difficult to measure in a standard patient, attention should be paid to the cerebral perfusion pressure (CPP).

Autoregulation

Adults maintain a constant CBF in the presence of a MAP within the range of 60–150 mmHg. Despite moderate changes in MAP and CPP, the brain is able to compensate and maintain an adequate flow. Beyond the range of autoregulation, perfusion becomes pressure dependent, whether high or low (5).

The pediatric patient appears to have a left-shift of the cerebral autoregulation curve, being able to adequately perfuse at lower pressures while being less tolerant to elevated CPP.

Cerebral metabolic rate (CMR)

Cerebral metabolic rates for oxygen and glucose are higher in the child when compared to the adult patient. They are, however, similar to CBF and are lowest at birth and continue to rise until approximately the ninth year of life (6). The $CMRO_2$ peaks at 5.8 ml/100 g brain tissue per minute and CMRglu peaks at 6.8 ml/100 g brain tissue per minute (1).

Oxygen and carbon dioxide

Hypoxia is related to an exponential increase in cerebral blood flow in the adult and child. Hyperoxia has been shown to decrease CBF by up to 33% in infants (5). Carbon dioxide's relationship with CBF is proportional and linear.

- Clinical observations have shown that neonatal ischemic/hypoxic episodes results in a two-phase neuronal cell death. On the first initial insult, ATP levels decreased drastically with resultant increase in glutamate production. This is immediately followed with the intracellular movement of Ca2+, which further destroys the neuronal cell. Excitotoxicity will reflect the ultimate release of destructive enzymes, which includes the release of reactive oxygen species (ROS). Upon the resuscitation with 100% oxygen, studies have collected formidable evidence of a sudden hyperemic response with further release of ROS, lipooxygenase, cyclooxygenase, xanthine oxidase, etc. that would eventually bring upon further neuronal damage (7).

Intracranial pressure and blood flow

The intracranial compartment is a rigid structure with a fixed volume. The intracranial pressure (ICP) is determined by the interplay between its components namely:

- Brain parenchyma – 80%
- Cerebrospinal fluid (CSF) – 10%
- Blood – 10%

The relationship is predicted by the Monro–Kellie Doctrine which states that: *"As the overall volume of the cranial vault cannot change, an increase in the volume of one component, or the presence of pathologic components, necessitates the displacement of other structures, an increase in ICP, or both."* (8)

- ICP $\geq$ 20 mmHg is pathologic, although occasional transient elevations occur with physiologic events, including sneezing, coughing, or Valsalva maneuvers (9).
- The ICP changes in the first few months after birth. The changes in ICP in the newborn are both peculiar and unique to this stage of life and have monitoring and clinical implications. Newborn babies usually lose weight in association with a salt and water loss during the first few days after birth. That the brain participates in this loss is shown by the observation that the head circumference in the first few days of life is often less than the fetal diameter noted by ultrasound examination. The decrease in brain volume and salt and water creates low intracranial pressures which may be even sub atmospheric. These changes may be exaggerated in preterm babies and may be contributive to their increased risk of intracranial hemorrhage (10). As predicted from the Monro–Kellie doctrine, the decrease in brain volume is compensated for by an increase in CSF volume which often presents as a physiological hydrocephalus on the CT scan. This should not be mistaken as pathological hydrocephalus.
- In infancy too, the intracranial pressure (ICP) is normally maintained at a level that is very low by standards that apply later in life. At this stage, hydrocephalus may be masked or attenuated in severity and may come back in full force a few days later (10).

Causes of an elevated ICP

- Increase in volume of any or all of the intracranial components or presence of a new component such as a tumor, abscess etc.
- Uncoupling of CBF and metabolic activity (loss of autoregulation) which can lead to excessive CBF (10,11).
- Increased CSF production in response to cerebral hyperemia in trauma, tumor, seizures, fever etc.
- Hypercapnia or hypoxia in any setting, which may cause vasodilation and increased CBF.
- Herniation, brain swelling, or subarachnoid hemorrhage, which may obstruct the flow of CSF.
- Hematomas, cerebral contusions, or cerebral edema, which may increase intracranial volume.

Symptoms of increased intracranial pressure

Infants will demonstrate: Irritability, bulging fontanelles with widening of the cranial sutures and overall cranial enlargement. This can progress to altered state of consciousness, cranial nerve palsies with upward gaze of the eyes and papillary changes.

Children will complain of: Headaches, vomiting, and on exam will show papilledema with decreased consciousness, upward gaze of the eyes, papilledema, and eventually Cushing's triad with impending herniation of brain structures.

- Infants can develop macrocephaly, bulging fontanelles and split sutures.
- Altered sensorium, seizures, cranial nerve (VI) deficits.
- Hypertension, bradycardia, and respiratory depression (Cushing's triad) are late signs (12).

Neurophysiologic monitoring

Ventriculostomy: It is a reliable ICP monitor and considered the gold standard. It requires skill for placement, allows for therapeutic drainage of CSF, but may infer risks of hemorrhage and infection.

Subarachnoid bolts: Although these offer less risk of infection and hemorrhage, they can underestimate ICP in areas that are distant from the insertion site and are difficult to stabilize in very young craniums.

Epidural monitors: These monitors are placed outside the dura and do not require fluid interface. There is a decreased risk of CSF contamination and they can measure ICP via placement in the anterior fontanelles of infants but they cannot be recalibrated once inserted.

Camino: Fiber optic monitors with self-contained transducers are smaller in size and are easily inserted. These can measure the ICP from many sites, intraventricular, intra- and periparenchyma, but cannot be recalibrated after insertion and may give off false measurements if moved (13). This monitor is expensive, complex, and is not compatible for MRIs.

Cerebral blood flow

Cerebral blood flow (CBF) is a function of the pressure drop across the cerebral circulation divided by the cerebrovascular resistance (CVR).

CBF = mean arterial pressure (MAP) – central venous pressure (CVP) or intracranial pressure (ICP, whichever is higher) ÷ cerebral vascular resistance (CVR).

- Hypoxia does not affect the cerebral blood flow until the PaO2 < 50 mmHg. At this measure it causes vasodilatation in an attempt to maintain the oxygen delivery.
- $PaCO_2$ has an effect on CBF over a much broader range. Hypercapnia causes cerebral vasodilatation and increased CBF, whereas hypocapnea reduces CBF. Because the response to changes in $PaCO_2$ is rapid, hyperventilation can be a useful tool in the acute management of increased ICP complicated by transtentorial and tonsillar herniation of brain tissue.

Autoregulation

- CBF is normally maintained at a relatively constant rate by intrinsic cerebral mechanisms referred to as autoregulation. Autoregulation adjusts regional CBF to metabolic activity, primarily through changes in CVR. Thus, clinical conditions that increase metabolic activity (e.g., seizures, fever) result in increased CBF.
- Changes in CVR can maintain constant CBF at mean arterial pressures of 60 to 150 mmHg. Outside this range, the compensatory mechanisms break down and inadequate or excessive perfusion can occur (11).
- These set limits are shifted to the right in patients with chronic hypertension.
- In addition, autoregulation may be impaired in the setting of neurologic injury, particularly in young children, in whom rapid and severe brain swelling may result.

Cerebral perfusion pressure

- Cerebral perfusion pressure (CPP) is a clinical surrogate for the adequacy of cerebral perfusion. CPP is defined as mean arterial pressure (MAP) minus ICP (11).

  Normal CPP in adults ranges from 50 to 70 mmHg; normal CPP in children is probably lower than that in adults, since children have lower systolic blood pressures, but normal limits have not been well established. However, based upon a normal ICP < 20 mmHg and MAP > 60 to 80 mmHg, depending upon age (where MAP = 1.5 x age + 55 mmHg), normal CPP in children can be calculated to be at least 40 to 60 mmHg. When CPP falls below a critical level, either from hypotension or from a markedly elevated ICP, the brain receives inadequate CBF and ischemic injury can occur (14).

Pharmacology of diuretics, steroids, and anticonvulsants

The commonly used diuretics for the control of increased intracranial pressure are:

1. Osmotic diuretics: Mannitol
2. Hyperosmolar solutions: Hypertonic saline
3. Loop diuretics: Furosemide, bumetanide, ethacrynic acid
4. Carbonic anhydrase inhibitors: Acetazolamide

Mannitol

- Mannitol acts by establishing an osmotic gradient between plasma and parenchyma tissue, resulting in a net reduction in brain water content.
- Mannitol has a rapid onset of action within 10–15 minutes; its effect peaks in about an hour and maintains its effect for about 6 hours (15–17).
- It is used to decrease ICP and improve CPP.
- Mannitol is prepared as a 20 percent solution.
- The recommended dose is 0.25 to 1 g/kg IV bolus. Starting with the lower dose is recommended, since there is no proven benefit to the higher dose.
- Repeat doses can be administered every 6 to 8 hours to increase serum osmolarity to 300 to 310 mOsm/l.
- As with any osmotic agent, the use of mannitol should be carefully evaluated in patients who have renal insufficiency (16,17).

Potential side effects are hyperosmolarity, hypovolemia, electrolyte imbalance, and acute renal failure. These adverse effects are more common with chronic or high-dose administration, and patients who receive mannitol in this manner should be monitored carefully. Serum osmolarity, serum electrolytes, and renal function should be measured at least every 6 to 8 hours, preferably before administration of the next dose. In addition, when administered chronically and in high doses, mannitol may cross the injured blood–brain barrier at the site of the cerebral lesion and cause an exacerbation of cerebral edema (15,16).

Loop diuretics

- The loop diuretics, such as furosemide and ethacrynic acid, may reduce brain edema by inducing a systemic diuresis, decreasing CSF production, and improving cellular water transport.
- Although furosemide can reduce ICP without increasing cerebral blood volume or blood osmolality, it is not as effective as mannitol.
- The initial dose of furosemide should be 0.6–1 mg/kg if administered alone, or 0.3–0.4 mg/kg if administered with mannitol to children.
- It has been suggested that ethacrynic acid reduces secondary brain injury by decreasing glial swelling. Raising serum osmolality above 320 mOsm may precipitate acute renal failure and significant water retention causes a paradoxical decrease in serum osmolality.
- Periods of aggressive dehydration may be followed by rebound intracranial hypertension during the recovery or normalization period (18).

Acetazolamide

It inhibits carbonic anhydrase activity, which decreases CSF production.

Uses:

- In epilepsy, the main use of acetazolamide is in absence seizures and myoclonic seizures (19). It can be used in both episodic ataxia types 1 and 2.
- In catamenial epilepsy, an increase in seizure frequency around menses, acetazolamide can be an adjunct to an antiseizure medication regimen to aid in decreasing seizure frequency around menses.
- Acetazolamide is also used to decrease the production of cerebrospinal fluid in idiopathic intracranial hypertension as well as hydrocephalus to delay surgical intervention and has shown efficacy in some forms of periodic paralysis.
- Acetazolamide is administered in nuclear medicine before studies of the brain with the radioisotope technetium-99 m to increase the specificity of the study for brain death.
- It's been demonstrated in drug trials to relieve symptoms associated with dural ectasia in individuals with Marfan syndrome.
- Off-label uses include it as a conjunction drug to assist patients with *central* sleep apnea by lowering blood pH and encouraging respiration.
- In newborn infants with posthemorrhagic hydrocephalus, treatment with diuretics is generally not effective and is associated with complications.

Hypertonic saline

- Intravenous hypertonic saline, alone or in combination with dextran or hydroxyethyl starch, has been shown to decrease ICP and increase CPP in pediatric patients with elevated ICP that is refractory to conventional therapy (20,21).
- It is thought to act by establishing an osmotic gradient that reduces brain water content and appears to maintain efficacy with repeat dosing even in patients who have stopped responding to mannitol.
- Unlike mannitol, hypertonic saline does not cause profound osmotic diuresis, and the risk of hypovolemia as a complication is decreased.
- Additional proposed benefits include restoration of normal cellular resting membrane potential and cell volume, stimulation of atrial natriuretic peptide release, inhibition of inflammation, and enhancement of cardiac output (20–25).
- Rebound increased ICP has occurred after hypertonic saline administration.
- Theoretical complications, such as hyperosmolality, osmotic demyelination syndrome (formerly called central pontine myelinolysis), and heart failure have not been reported. However, renal insufficiency is associated with serum osmolality > 320 mOsm/l. The current pediatric TBI guidelines recommend that serum osmolality should be maintained < 360 mOsm/l.
- The optimal dose and form of administration have not been identified in controlled trials. Differing concentrations of hypertonic saline ranging from 3 to 29 percent have been used in adults and children. A commonly used dosing regimen consists of 3 percent saline administered as an initial bolus of 2 to 6 ml/kg. Continuous infusion of 3 percent saline at rates of 0.1 to 1 ml/kg per hour adjusted to maintain ICP < 20 mmHg have also been described (23–25).

Table 9.1 Drugs that affect sodium channels

Drug	Pharmacokinetic and pharmacodynamics profile	Adverse effects	Uses	Anesthetic implication
Carbamazepine	P450 inducer Highly protein bound	Hyponatremia myelosuppression, pancytopenia diplopia Steven–Johnsons syndrome	Bipolar disorder, partial seizures, GT-CS, trigeminal neuralgia	CP450 enzyme inducer, affects metabolism of opioids, neuromuscular blockers, increased sedation preop
Phenytoin Fosphenytoin	Highly protein bound	Gingival hypertrophy, diplopia, neurotoxicity bradycardia on injection, neuropathy	GTCS, status epilepticus	CP450 enzyme inducer.
Lamotrigine	Selective for aspartate, glutamate neurons. Increased clearance in pregnancy	Aseptic meningitis	Partial and generalized epilepsy, Lenox– Gastaut syndrome	
Oxcarbamezapine	Only minimally affects CP450	Sedation, headache, decreases thyroid hormones, hyponatremia	Partial and generalized seizures	Minimal interactions with anesthesia
Zonisamide	Carbonic anhydrase inhibitor	Somnolence, ataxia persistent cognitive deficits	Myoclonic epilepsy	Increased perioperative sedation
Lacosamide	Acts on sodium channels and collapsing response mediator protein involved in epileptogenesis	Vertigo, ataxia, second-degree atrioventricular block, atrial fibrillation. Contraindicated in cardiac disease	Lennox–Gastaut syndrome,	Watch out for perioperative atrial arrhythmias
Rufinamide	No effect on cytochrome P450, renally eliminated	Somnolence, vomiting, arrhythmias	Lennox–Gastaut syndrome	Increased half-life in ESRD, avoided in patients with short QT syndrome

Corticosteroids

- Corticosteroids are **not** useful in the management of elevated ICP from infarction, hemorrhage, or head trauma. However, because they have anti-inflammatory and membrane stabilization effects, they may be helpful in the management of vasogenic edema associated with mass lesions (e.g., tumors and abscesses).
- If indicated, d (0.25 to 0.5 mg/kg) is administered every 6 hours, with a maximum dose of 16 mg per day.
- Possible side effects include sodium and water retention, and gastric or peptic ulcer.
  An H2-blocker (e.g., ranitidine) should be prescribed concomitantly.
- Careful monitoring of the patient's glucose, electrolytes, blood pressure, hemoglobin, and stool for occult blood is necessary during systemic corticoid therapy (12).

Antiepileptic drugs

Antiepileptic drugs are broadly classified as generational or on their mode of action:

- Older generation antiepileptic drugs (AEDs): Phenobarbital, phenytoin, carbamazepine, and valproate.
- Newer generation AEDs: Felbamate and vigabatrin, gabapentin, lamotrigine, topiramate, levetiracetam, oxcarbazepine, pregabalin, lacosamide, zonisamide.

Table 9.2 Drugs affecting GABA activity

Phenobarbital	GABA A agonist, increases chloride ion flow	Sedation, GI upset, ataxia	GTCS, status epilepticus, partial seizures	
Tiagabine	GABA reuptake inhibitor	Somnolence, lack of energy, rare proconvulsive effect (?)	Partial seizures	Not to be used with seizure threshold lowering doses of ketamine, methohexital and remifentanil and sevoflurane
Vigabatrin	Inhibits GABA transaminase irreversibly	Possible vision loss, visual field deficits, MRI abnormalities, weight gain	Infantile spasms and seizures	
Benzodiazepines	Increase frequency of GABA chloride channel opening	Sedation, ataxia, irritability, paradoxical agitatation, withdrawal seizures	Status epilepticus, Lennox–Gastaut syndrome, partial seizures, clonazepam – myoclonic and atonic seizures	Decrease MAC, anxiolysis, sedation, favor parental separation, induction adjuvant

- Drugs that affect sodium channels: phenytoin, carbamazepine, valproic acid, lamotrigine, riluzole
- Drugs affecting calcium channels: Ethosuximide diminishes T-type currents, is used in the treatment of absence seizures and is known to produce nausea, sleep disturbances and hyperactivity. It can contribute to perioperative agitation (26–28).
- Drugs affecting GABA activity: phenobarbitol, tiagabine, vigabatrin, benzodiazepines
- Drugs affecting glutamate receptors:
  - Paramapanel is an orally active, noncompetitive AMPA-type glutamate receptor antagonist. It appears to inhibit AMPA-induced increases in intracellular calcium, reducing neuronal excitability.
  - Paramapanel is extensively metabolized by the liver, primarily via CYP3A4, CYP3A5, glucoronidation, and potentially other pathways. It has a prolonged and variable half-life (mean 105 hours), which may complicate dose titration and safety washout.
  - Clearance of paramapanel is increased in patients taking concomitant enzyme-inducing AEDs such as phenytoin and carbamazepine.
  - Can produce dizziness, weight gain, mood swings, and aggression (26,27).
- Drugs with multiple actions: topiramate, felbamate, valproate
- Drugs with other mechanisms of action: gabapentin, levetiracetam, pregabalin, ezogabine

Anesthetic implications of pervasive developmental disorder, developmental delay, and attention deficit hyperactivity disorder

Pervasive developmental disorders are those wherein there is abnormal development in social interaction and communication with restrictive, repetitive, and stereotyped behaviors manifesting before 3 years of age. The clinical picture changes with age with management of the preschool child difficult but amenable to intervention. There is improvement after 6 years of age with possible regression however at adolescence. Hence, age at presentation is important to the anesthesiologist. These patients often have diagnosed and undiagnosed attention deficit hyperactivity disorder and coexistent developmental delay. We shall hence consider the topics in an interrelated manner (29,30).

Preoperative assessment

A careful history from parents/care givers is necessary. Often these patients shy away from physical contact and sometimes examination under anesthesia may be

Table 9.3. Drugs with multiple actions

Drug	Pharmacological profile	Adverse effects	Uses	Anesthetic implications
Valproate	Increases GABA concentrations, blocks sodium channels, activates glutamic acid decarboxylase acts against T-type calcium currents. Highly protein bound	Alopecia, bruising, insulin resistance, metabolic syndrome, thrombocytopenia, hypothyroidism, Fanconi syndrome, teratogenic, hepatotoxicity, acute pancreatitis, parkinsonism, PCOS	Generalized and partial seizures	Sedation, carbapenem antibiotics decrease levels
Felbamate	NMDA antagonist, augments GABA	Fetal aplastic anemia, hepatic failure even after cessation of the drug	Partial seizures, Lennox–Gastaut syndrome	
Topiramate	NMDA antagonist, GABA A agonist. Action decreased by other enzyme inducers and valproate	Weight loss, cognitive deficits metabolic acidosis, teratogenic	Partial seizures, mixed seizures	

Table 9.4. Drugs with other mechanisms of action

Drug	Pharmacological profile	Adverse effect	Uses	Anesthetic implication
Gabapentin	Binds to aplha2delta2subunit of calcium channels, almost totally renally eliminated	Sedation, GI upset, serotonin syndrome	Partial epilepsy, treatment of neuropathy	Decreases MAC and perioperative opioid requirements, sedative, possible serotonin syndrome with other agents
Levetiracetam	Binds to synaptic vesicle 2 protein		Partial seizures, brain protection in head trauma, craniotomies, infantile spasms	Does not affect cytochrome P450, no interaction with immunosuppressants in transplantation. Rapid onset when given IV for brain protection
Pregabalin	Binds to alpha2delta2 calcium channel subunit. Modulates glutamate, noradrenalin, substance P. Renally eliminated, no hepatic effects	Dizziness, somnolence	Myoclonic epilepsy, partial seizures	Neuropathy treatment adjunct, possible adjunct to decrease opioid use
Ezogabine	Opens KCNQ2/3 voltage-gated potassium channels, activating M-current, excreted by kidney	Urinary retention ataxia, diplopia, confusion	Refractory partial epilepsy	Unknown

necessary for a diagnosis and further management. Care should be given to note the child's particular interests/dislikes, fetishes, and phobias as these often influence cooperation and ease of administration of anesthesia. Records of conduct of previous anesthesia and perioperative events must also be noted as these children often have repeated anesthetic exposures.

A careful history and physical examination to rule out associated comorbid conditions such as epilepsy, degree of cognitive impairment, recurrent respiratory tract infections, bipolar disorder, and obstructive sleep apnea is mandatory. Often other syndromic associations are present such as tuberous sclerosis, which can also present with hamartomas in the brain and spinal cord and focal neurological deficits, developmental delay, and epilepsy. Any other syndromic associations such as Prader–Willi syndrome that may have independent anesthetic implications should also be noted. Many of these patients are also dehydrated and have associated electrolyte abnormalities that have to be noted. Many inborn errors of metabolism are also associated with autism such as glucose 6-phosphate dehydrogenase deficiency, propionic academia, phenylketonuria, and others. These should also be identified (31).

These patients are often on medications for epilepsy that can interact with anesthetic drugs. Patients who have suffered one episode of convulsive status epilepticus, especially those with structural brain abnormalities and learning disability are often on long term prescribed benzodiazepines. Withdrawal can precipitate seizures and intraoperatively they may also exhibit tolerance and increased dose requirements (32).

- Phenobarbital, phenytoin, and carbamazepine are well- known inducers of cytochrome P450 and may affect the metabolism of benzodiazepines, opiates, and neuromuscular blockers.
- Valproate is an inhibitor of hepatic microsomal enzyme systems and may reduce the clearance of many concurrently administered medications, including other antiepileptics.
- Gabapentin, lamotrigine, levetiracetam, tiagabine, and vigabatrin do not induce hepatic enzymes (32).
- Macrolide antibiotics, particularly erythromycin, are potent inhibitors of CYP3A4, which is involved in carbamazepine metabolism and can lead to carbamazepine toxicity.
- Concomitant use of carbapenem antibiotics can lead to a significant decrease in serum valproate concentrations.
- Etomidate and propofol have been known to produce excitatory activity such as myoclonus, opisthotonus, and seizures though generalized seizures are seldom seen at induction of anesthesia.
- Ketamine at low doses can decrease the seizure threshold though at higher doses it is actually used for the treatment of status epilepticus. Nondepolarizing agents often mask the motor effects of seizures and should be used with caution in patients with refractory epilepsy (32).
- Patients with ADHD often are on methamphetamine derivatives on long-term use deplete norepinephrine at nerve endings and decrease response to indirect vasopressors. Chronic use can also decrease the minimum alveolar concentration (MAC) of concomitantly administered inhalational anesthetics.

Hence it is crucial to check the seizure history and if possible drug levels before anesthesia as well as the antibiotics indicated for the particular type of surgery.

Many of these patients often have genetic profiling. A defect in the methylene tetrahydrofolate reductase enzyme can cause impaired metabolism of nitrous oxide though this is controversial and may require multiple exposures for effect; though usually subclinical (33,34). Increased homocysteine levels and vitamin B12 deficiency have also been noted in these patients.

Intraoperative management:

- IV access is often challenging in these patients.
- Anxiolysis is usually achieved with oral midazolam on the day of surgery using 0.5 mg/kg up to a maximum of 20 mg.
- Intramuscular ketamine may be a good choice to achieve sedation without respiratory compromise and IV access may then be secured.
- Inhalational anesthesia may be used for induction and intravenous (IV) access placed thereafter. However, many patients object to the mask and in particularly agitated patients.
- Alternatively, if the child cooperates application of eutectic mixture of local anesthetics (EMLA) cream on the access site, it is an option to numb the skin and facilitate placement of IV access.
- Methemoglobinemia is a risk to be aware of when considering EMLA creams.
- Intravenous anesthesia can also be used as an alternative to inhalational agents. However it has been reported that an increased dose of propofol may be required in patients with autism (35,36).
- IV dexmedetomidine is also increasingly used for sedation for magnetic resonance imaging and CT scans in older patients as its lack of respiratory depression, anxiolysis, decreased requirement of perioperative opioids, and hemodynamic stability offer a favorable profile.

- Recovery agitation (emergence delirium) is common in autistic patients and should be anticipated. Emergence agitation, postoperative sedation, and dysphoric reactions have been shown to be decreased with the use of dexmedetomidine in autistic patients. This can be managed by small doses of propofol or awakening the patient on an IV dexmedetomidine infusion (37,38).
- Routine intravenous fluids and postoperative antiemetic prophylaxis have been shown to provide for a smoother transition from anesthesia to discharge (37,38).

Postoperative care

- Visual analog scores may not be an adequate indicator of pain scores in these patients as they often have poor affect.
- Maternal assessment of the patient as well as assessment of deviation from usual repetitive behaviors and agitation scores must be used in a comprehensive assessment of postoperative pain.

Some authors have ascertained that anesthetic exposure increases the risk of mitochondrial dysfunction and worsens autism in children. A recent study by Ing *et al.* suggested that early childhood anesthetic exposure may increase the risk of learning and reasoning deficits on a long-term basis (39). Whether this applies to children with autism is yet unproven.

A perioperative audit of anesthesia for patients with autism has proven the benefit of parental cooperation, dialogue and understanding of perioperative risks and benefits of anesthesia. This is crucial for the success of any anesthetic in patients with autism and developmental delay.

Tumors

Classification of central nervous system tumors in children

Brain tumors are the most common solid malignancy in children. 25–40% is supratentorial. The most common infratentorial tumors are medulloblastomas, cerebellar astrocytomas, brainstem gliomas, and ependymomas of the fourth ventricle.

Tumors in the midbrain include craniopharyngiomas, optic gliomas, pituitary adenomas, and hypothalamic tumors and account for approximately 15% of intracranial tumors. Hypothalamic tumors (hamartomas, gliomas, and teratomas) frequently appear with precocious puberty in children who are large for their chronological age (40,41).

Preoperative evaluation

Assessment of the following is of paramount importance:

- Intracranial pressure (ICP). Posterior fossa tumors block CSF outflow and cause an increase in ICP faster than supratentorial tumors which present late with an increase in ICP. The clinical presentation of patients with intracranial hypertension varies with the duration of increased ICP.
- Sudden massive increases in ICP often cause coma.
- In a less acute case, there may be a history of headache on awakening, suggestive of vasodilation caused by sleep, reflective of induced hypercapnia and reduced intracranial compliance.
- Vomiting is a common sign. Neonates and infants often present with a history of increased irritability, poor feeding, or lethargy. A bulging anterior fontanelle, dilated scalp veins, cranial enlargement or deformity, and lower extremity motor deficits are also common signs of increased ICP in this age group (42,43).
- Neurological deficits including cranial nerve palsies.
- Neurogenic pulmonary edema.
- Endocrine disturbances such as diabetes insipidus (DI), syndrome of inappropriate antidiuretic hormone secretion (SIADH), or cerebral salt wasting syndrome.
- Craniopharyngiomas often have pituitary dysfunction and should have a complete endocrine evaluation preoperatively.
- Steroid replacement (dexamethasone or hydrocortisone) is generally administered because the integrity of the hypothalamic–pituitary–adrenal axis may be uncertain.
- Symptoms often include growth failure, visual impairment, and endocrine abnormalities.
- Signs and symptoms of hypothyroidism should be sought and thyroid function tests measured (42).
- Coexistent arrhythmias may be present.
- Coexistent respiratory infections, electrolyte, and glucose abnormalities are present.

Premedication

The routine use of sedation in pediatric neurosurgical patients is best avoided as it may precipitate respiratory depression, hypercarbia, and hence increased cerebral blood flow and increased ICP. In patients with aneurysmal lesions, and no increase in ICP, mild sedation may be useful to decrease transmural pressure and decrease the risk of an aneurysmal rupture. The best form of anxiolysis would be careful patient communication parental presence and patient understanding and assent in older children.

Intraoperative conduct

- Standard ASA monitors, arterial line placement or a radial pulse Doppler, peripheral nerve twitch monitor, and a urinary catheter to monitor urine output are indicated.
- Preoperative IV access would be the best choice though it is often difficult to obtain in combative patients. In such patients inhalational induction and a smooth intubation may be a better choice than placing a difficult IV in an agitated combative patient. An alternative may be to place a small butterfly needle for induction followed by placement of a larger bore IV. All in all, care must be taken to ensure a smooth process of induction and intubation as often greater increases in ICP are achieved with agitation, coughing, crying than inhalational induction with hyperventilation.
- Large-bore IV catheters are a must as is availability of blood products in procedures where blood loss may be extensive. Hypo-osmolar and glucose containing maintenance fluids are best avoided except in very small infants wherein a glucose maintenance infusion intraoperatively may be indicated. Urine output may be misleading when osmotic diuretics are used and CVP monitoring may be indicated. Hypertonic saline while decreasing edema and ICU stay did not show a decrease in mortality or overall hospital stay. Mannitol and loop diuretics remain conventionally used in craniotomies.
- Surgical resection of a posterior fossa tumor presents a number of anesthetic challenges. Children are usually positioned prone, although the lateral or sitting positions are used by some neurosurgeons. In any case, the head will be flexed, and the position and patency of the endotracheal tube must be meticulously ensured.
- Hyperventilation, mannitol, loop diuretics, and corticosteroids are used to reduce the ICP intraoperatively. If ICP is markedly elevated or acutely worsens, a ventricular catheter may be inserted by the neurosurgeon prior to tumor resection to permit emergent drainage of CSF.
- A normothermic temperature goal of 35.5–36.5 °C should be used, with warming measures started below and cooling measures started above these temperature margins. Although hypothermia reduces the $CMRO_2$, it frequently delays drug clearance, slows reversal of muscle relaxants, decreases cardiac output, causes conduction abnormalities, attenuates hypoxic pulmonary vasoconstriction, alters platelet function, causes electrolyte abnormalities, and can induce postoperative shivering. Neonates and infants are at greatest risk of hypothermia because of their large surface area relative to body mass. Hyperthermia is particularly deleterious in patients with a history of ischemic stroke and closed head injury.
- Venous air embolism (VAE) can occur during morcellation of the cranial vault, craniectomy for craniosynostosis, and spinal cord procedures. The incidence is reduced by prone position for posterior fossa surgeries and mechanical ventilation.
- Transesophageal echo in older patients and precordial Doppler in younger patients best detect VAE. When venous air is detected during craniotomy in children, the patient should be repositioned to supine flat, the field immediately flooded with saline gauzes and air may be successfully aspirated from veins 38–60% of the time.
- Intravenous fluids, antiarrhythmic, and inotropic agents, or vasopressors may be necessary.
- Nitrous oxide must be discontinued. Some authors have proposed that a positive end-expiratory pressure (PEEP) of 10 cmH_2O might decrease the rate of air entry by increasing venous pressure, but less than 8 cmH_2O pressure is not adequate to do so. It is also possible that the use of PEEP may cause paradoxical air embolism as 27% of patients have an anatomically patent foramen ovale (43,44).

Perioperative complications

Fixation pins used in small children can cause skull fractures, dural tears, and intracranial hematomas. Elevation of the bone flap can result in sinus tears, massive blood loss, or VAE. Surgical resection of tumors in the posterior fossa can also lead to brainstem and cranial nerve damage. A VAE is a potentially serious complication that is not eliminated by the use of the prone or lateral position because head-up gradients of 10 to 20 degrees are frequently used to improve cerebral venous drainage. In infants and toddlers, large head size relative to body size accentuates this problem. Damage to the respiratory centers and cranial nerves can lead to apnea and airway obstruction after extubation of the patient's trachea.

Postoperatively

Prolonged ventilation, SIADH, DI, stroke, electrolyte abnormalities can be encountered and should be anticipated. Age-appropriate apnea monitoring may be necessary. Local anesthesia infiltration of incision site may be a good choice. Narcotics should be used with caution (43,44).

Anesthesia for hydrocephalus

Communicating (nonobstructive hydrocephalus) is caused by impaired cerebrospinal fluid resorption in the absence of any CSF-flow obstruction between the ventricles and subarachnoid space. This is due to functional impairment of the arachnoidal granulations, which are located along the superior sagittal sinus and is the site of cerebrospinal fluid resorption back into the venous system. Various neurologic conditions may result in communicating hydrocephalus, including subarachnoid/intraventricular hemorrhage, meningitis and congenital absence of arachnoid villi. Scarring and fibrosis of the subarachnoid space following infectious, inflammatory, or hemorrhagic events can also prevent resorption of CSF, causing diffuse ventricular dilatation (12).

- Normal pressure hydrocephalus (NPH) is a particular form of communicating hydrocephalus, characterized by enlarged cerebral ventricles, with only intermittently elevated cerebrospinal fluid pressure. The viscosity of the cerebrospinal fluid may play a role in the pathogenesis of normal pressure hydrocephalus.
- Hydrocephalus ex vacuo also refers to an enlargement of cerebral ventricles and subarachnoid spaces, and is usually due to brain atrophy as in post-traumatic brain injuries.

Noncommunicating hydrocephalus is caused by a CSF-flow obstruction ultimately preventing CSF from flowing into the subarachnoid space

- Foramen of Monro obstruction may lead to dilation of one or, if large enough (e.g., in colloid cyst), both lateral ventricles.
- The aqueduct of Sylvius, normally narrow to begin with, may be obstructed by a number of genetically or acquired lesions (e.g., atresia, ependymitis, hemorrhage, and tumor) and lead to dilation of both lateral ventricles as well as the third ventricle.
- Fourth ventricle obstruction will lead to dilatation of the aqueduct as well as the lateral and third ventricles (e.g., Chiari malformation).
- The foramina of Luschka and foramen of Magendie may be obstructed due to congenital failure of opening (e.g., Dandy–Walker malformation) (12).

Three types of ventricular shunts are in current use:

- Ventriculoperitoneal
- Ventriculoatrial
- Ventriculopleural

As the pediatric patient grows, the shunt must be revised. It must be replaced if it malfunctions or becomes infected. Placement or revision of shunts is common in both severely neurologically impaired children and in otherwise healthy patients. Patients who present for CSF shunting procedures may exhibit a broad spectrum of symptoms and clinical signs, ranging from an apparently healthy child with minimal disability to a seriously ill, comatose patient for whom surgery is urgent.

Preoperative evaluation

- Level of consciousness
- Presence of increased ICP
- Full stomach: Vomiting or delayed gastric emptying are indications to take precautions against aspiration of gastric contents (e.g., a rapid-sequence induction).

- Co-existing pathology: Does the child have evidence of other significant organ system compromise, such as the cerebral palsied child who frequently aspirates?
- Age-related pathophysiology: Is the patient likely to have apnea, poor pulmonary compliance or immature renal function?

Intraoperative conduct

- Routine monitoring is indicated. Arterial line placement is usually reserved for the patient with uncontrolled ICP and hemodynamic instability. A shunt scan helps to determine the site of malfunction.
- Increased ICP caused by shunt malfunction can be reduced acutely by tapping the proximal reservoir. Infiltration of the skin with local anesthetic allows the tap to proceed with minimal trauma to the patient. The needle can be left in place to monitor ICP during induction.
- In the patient at risk for emesis during induction of anesthesia, placement of a nasogastric tube may precipitate coughing and bucking and increase ICP. Severely neurologically compromised children often have gastrostomy tubes, and opening these tubes before induction of anesthesia is recommended. However, this does not guarantee that the patient will not vomit and aspirate gastric contents.
- If there is no clinical evidence of elevated ICP, anesthesia can be induced by mask or with IV drugs.
- In the presence of increased ICP and delayed gastric emptying, rapid sequence anesthesia induced with propofol, atropine, lidocaine, a narcotic, and a nondepolarizing muscle relaxant after preoxygenation may be in order. Cricoid pressure is applied and the patient is hyperventilated at low peak inspiratory pressures. Since laryngoscopy is a potent stimulus for increasing ICP, an oral tracheal tube is placed as smoothly as possible (12,45).
- Supine position with 30 degrees head up to promote venous drainage is used. Patients whose shunt tubing is placed posteriorly and those who are placed in a lateral position should have an axillary roll placed and all extremities padded. After the airway is secured, patients with increased ICP are hyperventilated to a $PaCO_2$ of between 25 and 30 mmHg. Patients with normal ICP are maintained at normocapnia.
- Spontaneous ventilation should be avoided in patients with ventriculopleural shunts to reduce the risk of pneumothorax and in those with ventriculoatrial shunts to avoid air embolism. Also, spontaneous ventilation should be avoided when the cranium is opened.
- Anesthesia is usually maintained with sevoflurane in oxygen. Muscle relaxation is usually maintained with a short- or intermediate-acting muscle relaxant.
- Ventricular shunt procedures are not usually associated with significant blood loss or third-space losses. Fluid management centers around replacement of intravascular volume associated with emesis or drug-induced diuresis.
- The body temperature may decrease during shunt procedures, despite their relatively short duration. Exposure of a large body surface area and cold preparation solution, particularly for ventriculoperitoneal shunting, may cause infants to cool rapidly and delay awakening.

Emergence from anesthesia

- Enough time for elimination of the anesthetic agents and adequate reversal of neuromuscular blockade should be ensured before extubation of the trachea.
- Although it does not provide absolute insurance against regurgitation, the stomach should be suctioned before extubation of the trachea in patients suspected of having increased gastric contents. The patient should be fully awake and have an appropriate gag reflex to protect their airway against emesis.
- Many patients coming for shunt procedures are severely neurologically impaired and have poor airway control. Extubation should therefore be planned electively in these patients when criteria are better met (12,43–45).

Postoperative management

As with any postsurgical patient, supplemental oxygen should be given and the respiratory pattern and adequacy assessed. Neurosurgical patients in general, and preterm infants who are less than 50 weeks

Table 9.5. Anesthetic medications interactions

Antiepileptic drug	Mechanism of Action	Anesthetic implication
Benzodiazepines (binds to BZ_2 receptors); tiagabine (prevents reuptake); gabapentin (prevents reuptake)	Increased GABA activity	Concomitant sedation and possible respiratory depression with other sedative hypnotics. Possible tolerance development, withdrawal seizures.
Barbiturates	Increased mean Cl channel opening duration	Concomitant sedation and possible respiratory depression with other sedative hypnotics. Protective against focal cerebral ischemia. Can induce burst suppression. Induces cytochrome P450 enzymes, alters drug metabolism.
Vigabatrin	Blocks GABA transaminase (blocking GABA catabolism within the neuron)	Gabapentin, lamotrigine, levetiracetam, tiagabine, and vigabatrin do not induce hepatic enzymes
Sodium valproate (K^+ channel)	Increased outward voltage-gated positive currents	CPY450 enzyme inhibitor. Carbapenem antibiotics can decrease levels.
Topiramate (at AMPA receptor)	Glutamate antagonist	Dose-dependent CYP450 enzyme inducer
Levatiracetam	Synaptic vesicle protein binder	Hemodynamically stable, minimal drug interactions
Oxcarbazepine, carbazepine and eslicarbazepine.	GABA agonist	Weak enzyme inducers

postconceptual age, in particular, are likely to have abnormal respiratory patterns or apnea after surgery and apnea monitoring may be necessary. Analgesics should be used judiciously in neurologically impaired patients.

Anesthesia and seizure disorders

Epilepsy is a tendency to have recurrent unprovoked seizures. It is the most common serious neurological disorder with a prevalence of 0.5–1% of the population. The highest incidence is at the extremes of age and in those with structural or developmental brain abnormalities. The International League against Epilepsy (ILAE) has classified seizures into:

- Focal (or partial) seizures, which arise from one hemisphere.
- Generalized seizures, which show electrographic seizure onset over both hemispheres.

Anesthetic management of patients with seizure disorders requires a thorough knowledge of antiepileptics and anesthetic drug interactions as well as management of status epilepticus (46).

A seizure can be seen as the result of imbalance between excitatory and inhibitory neuronal activity. This leads to the generation of hypersynchronous firing of a large number of cortical neurons. Traditional antiepileptics exert antiseizure activity by the following mechanisms:

- Reduce the inward voltage-gated positive currents (Na^+, Ca^{2+}).
- Increase inhibitory neurotransmitter activity (GABA).
- Decrease excitatory neurotransmitter activity (glutamate, aspartate).
- Synaptic vesicle 2 (SV2) binding (levatiracetam).
- Voltage-gated potassium channel activators (retigabine).
- Steroid binding on GABA A receptors (ganoxolone).

Preoperative assessment

- In addition to a thorough history and physical examination, a thorough history of medications the patient is on and careful assessment of the airway is mandatory.
- Special attention should be paid to the frequency of seizures and precipitating factors as well as associated syndromes and comorbid conditions

Table 9.6. Significance of anesthetic medication

Anesthetic medication	Significance in epilepsy
Nitrous oxide	Suppresses epileptiform activity, inhibits MTHFR gene, one-carbon metabolism, induces myoclonus that can mimic seizures
Etomidate	Myoclonus, decreases seizures
Sevoflurane	Can cause excitatory activity, especially in high concentrations with hypocapnea
Alfentanil Remifentanil	Enhances seizures in abnormal neurons, depresses seizure activity in normal neurons
Fentanyl	No antiseizure effects
Propofol	Can increase seizure activity, least potential to induce seizures among induction agents
Ketamine	Low doses can increase and high doses decrease seizures
Benzodiazepines	Decrease seizures, increase threshold
Nondepolarizing agents	Prevent motor manifestations of seizures
Atracurium	Metabolite laudanosine can increase seizures
Meperidine	Not given in conjunction with other norepinephrine uptake inhibitors and serotoninergic agents. Accumulation of metabolite in renal failure patients can cause seizures

such as cerebral palsy, pervasive development disorder, Gervais syndrome etc.

- Antiepileptic medications must be continued on the morning of surgery.
- Assessment of preoperative conscious status is also necessary as often the patients are sedated due to antiepileptic medications. In these patients additional preoperative sedatives must be avoided (47).
- Preoperative electrolyte and drug levels are also important as they are often altered in patients with epilepsy and may affect the seizure threshold and the development of seizures perioperatively.
- Preoperative intravenous (IV) access is important in patients with poorly controlled seizures but often may be difficult to obtain.
- Inhalational induction may be an acceptable method to obtain access.
- Ketamine use for sedation to obtain IV access is controversial as ketamine at low doses can lower the seizure threshold though at the higher doses typically used for anesthesia, it has definite anticonvulsant properties (47).

Intraoperative management

In addition to standard ASA monitors, BIS with raw EEG display may be used. There is controversial evidence as to the use of BIS to diagnose seizures intraoperatively in the presence of paralysis; albeit, typical spike wave pattern in the presence of certain seizures may be easily recognized.

Use of anesthetic medications must be tailored to the patient and the case (26,27,48). Many anesthetic medications interact with antiepileptics:

Care should be taken not only to have a smooth emergence but also recovery period as seizures can also occur in the postoperative period. Prompt renewal of anticonvulsive medications must be initiated in the postoperative period.

Status epilepticus

Continued convulsions beyond 30 minutes are called status epilepticus. The brain initially compensates by increasing blood flow to decrease ischemic damage but compensatory mechanisms start to fail beyond 30 minutes and permanent damage can result unless prompt action is taken (see Figure 9.1) (49).

Cerebrovascular disorders

Arteriovenous malformations (AVMs)

Intracranial hemorrhage is the most common presentation of young patients with AVM and it carries an associated mortality of 25% (5). Large malformations may, however, present as congestive heart failure in the infant and may require vasopressor support (1).

Treatment of large AVMs are focused on multiple interventional intravascular embolization procedures to shrink the malformation but ligation can be associated with severe hypertension which must be treated with vasodilators such as labetalol or nitroprusside (1).

Status epilepticus: Treatment algorithm

Stage I: 0–10 minutes
1. Confirm diagnosis: Examine patient, cranial nerves, motor tone, and level of conciousness. Observe/identify seizure activity
2. ABCs: Stabilize Airway, maintain Breathing (intubate if required), give oxygen, check Circulation (BP, pulse), start CPR if indicated
3. Place 1 (preferably 2) large-bore IV catheters. Start normal saline infusion
4. Draw bloods: glucose,electrolytes,CBC, serum anti-epileptic drug and toxicology screen if indicated
5. Thiamine 100 mg IV followed by 1 amp D50

↓

Stage II: 10–30 minutes
1. Phenytoin 20 mg/kg at 50 mg/min (20–30') IV (precipitates in glucose solution; give in NS; can cause hypotension and local toxicity) OR
Fosphenytoin: Note: To ensure the correct dose of fosphenytoin, this drug should always be prescribed in Phenytoin Equivalents (PE). 15–20 mg PE/kg at 100–150 mg PE/min IV preferred (can cause hypotension, paresthesias).
2. While phenytoin infuses, begin IV lorazepam, 0.1 mg/kg in 2 mg boluses, no faster than 2 mg/min
3. Monitor BP, respiration closely; intubate if necessary (benzodiazepines depress respiration)
4. If seizures persist, give additional 5 mg/kg phenytoin and send STAT phenytoin level
5. If seizures persist, call EEG technologist, re-assess all lab data, and prepare for Stage III.
6. If new seizures or focal findings noted, obtain brain CT and LP (if not contraindicated) once seizures stop

↓

Stage III: 30–60'
1 Intubate patient if not already intubated
2 Phenobarbital 10–20 mg/kg at 100 mg/min IV
3 Watch for hypotension, myocardial depression
Midazolam or propofol may be used as alternatives to phenobarbital (doses below)

↓

- **Seizures stop, patient alert** → Continue phenytoin and phenobarbital, adjusting dosage to maintain therapeutic drug levels
- **Seizures stop but patient remains comatose** →
  - Obtain STAT EEG to exclude electrographic status
  - Evaluate patient carefully for signs of subtle, generalized status, including twitching, myoclonus, or rhythmic eye movements

  → EEG or clinical evidence of persistent seizures? → Stage IV (or alternative agents)
- **Seizures persist** → Assess all laboratory data, CBC, chemistry, toxicology screen, anti-epileptic drug levels, arterial blood gas. Prepare for Stage IV → Stage IV

alternative agents

Stage IV: > 60'
Begin continuous EEG monitoring.
Start Pentobarbital Coma: 5 mg/kg or until burst suppression induced on EEG.
Maintain at 0.5–2.0 mg/kg/hr to continue burst suppression pattern.
Monitor BP, ECG, ABG, renal function. Pressor agents may be needed.

↓

If EEG or clinical evidence of persistent seizures, try alternatives below:

- Midazolam 0.2 mg/kg load, then maintain at 0.1–2.0 mg/kg/hr. Maintain Phenytoin level > 20 and/or phenobarb level > 40. Wean when seizure free > 12 H
- Propofol 3–5 mg/kg load, then 1–15 mg/kg/hour
- Lidocaine 1.5–2.0 mg/kg IV at 50 mg/min. Repeat if seizures recur. Can cause arrhythmias, paresthesias
- Consider IV valprote for a DNR patient in status or for patients failing standard 1st and 2nd line agents. Dose: 25 mg/kg, dilute 1:1 D5W at 3–6 mg/kg/min (25–50 mg/min),then 10–15 mg/kg/d. If IV, start maintenance dosing 1-hour post load (q 6h dosing). If oral- start maintenance immediately after load. Monitor BP/ECG, ✓peak level 20 min post infusion.

Chang CWJ, Bleck TP. Status Epileptius. Neurologic clinics 13 (3):529–48, 1995.
Treiman DM. Generalized convulsive status epilepticus in the adult. Epilepsia 34 (Suppl1), S2–11,1993
Leppick IE. Status epilepticus: the next decade. Neurology 40 (Suppl2): 4–9, 1990

Figure 9.1 Status epilepticus: treatment algorithm.

These embolic procedures carry unique issues for the anesthesiologist. Fluid overload may occur secondary to increasing amounts of IV contrast and this may exacerbate the CHF already present. The major complication, vessel rupture, should always be anticipated and the anesthesiologist must always be prepared for an emergency craniotomy. Special attention should be paid to the femoral artery cannulation site, as it may be a source of a potential hemorrhage.

Aneurysms

Aneurysms are rather rare in children, with most being congenital malformations often associated with coarctation of the aorta or polycystic kidney disease. Surgery is indicated and surgical treatment focuses mainly on surgical resection or clipping (1,5). Surgery is often associated with massive blood loss and the anesthesiologist should anticipate the need for adequate vascular access and blood products should be readily available. Detailed attention should be paid to prevent hypertension secondary to induction, laryngoscopy, or emergence. Deep preoperative sedation and deep induction of anesthesia are necessary. One must, however, be diligent as hypotension can lead to decreased cerebral perfusion pressure, especially in the setting of an increased intracranial pressure secondary to a bleeding malformation (5).

Moyamoya disease

Moyamoya disease is a chronic syndrome of occlusive crisis of the internal carotid arteries that manifests as recurrent and worsening transient ischemic attacks or strokes. The Japanese name, translated as "puff of smoke," refers to the appearance of the abnormal angiographic appearance of the network of collateral vessels that develop from these diseased carotid arteries.

Patients may have coexisting disease, including Down syndrome, sickle cell anemia, neurofibromatosis, or prior history of radiation to the cranium (1). Sometimes, systemic arteries, especially renal, can also be involved in this process (5). Patients may develop worsening strokes with subsequent worsening of neurologic status.

The mainstay of medical treatment is antiplatelet therapy, including aspirin or calcium channel blockers (5). Surgical correction may be obtained with a pial synangiosis, the surgical implantation of a scalp artery on to the pial surface of the brain to enhance revascularization (5).

Anesthetic management revolves around:

- Maintaining normal blood pressures with adequate cerebral perfusion pressures. Adequate and aggressive preoperative hydration can aid in this.
- EEG monitoring should be initiated.
- Maintenance of normothermia and normocapnea is of the utmost importance.

It appears that most postoperative complications center around strokes secondary to dehydration and hyperventilation episodes (5).

Open and closed head injuries

Special consideration must be paid to the child with a traumatic head injury, as trauma is the primary cause of death in children and head injuries the cause of major morbidity and mortality. While intracranial hematomas (epidural, subdural, or intraparenchymal) can happen in children, diffuse cerebral edema after blunt head trauma occurs more often in children than adults (5). The most common head injury associated with mechanical force is the concussion. Concussion is associated with immediate and transient alteration of mental status and disturbance of vision, hearing, and equilibrium.

Initial evaluation of a child with head trauma may provide few clues to the patient's impending neurologic status. This evaluation must have a two-stepped approach: the first being in relation to the actual trauma itself along with presenting symptoms, while the second must focus on the impending insult subsequent to the initial trauma. This may manifest as parenchyma damage from hypotension, hypoxia, cerebral edema, or intracranial hypertension (5).

Scalp injuries can lead to a large amount of blood loss as a larger fraction of the child's cardiac output perfuses the scalp when compared to adults. This blood loss may be enough to lead to significant hemodynamic instability and a closed scalp injury can contain more blood than appears, so preoperative treatment of hypovolemia should be aggressive prior to the induction of anesthesia. Always be vigilant, as a scalp injury, open or closed, may hide coexisting intracranial pathology and a head CT should be considered in a child with significant scalp injury (5).

Major childhood physical trauma commonly affects the head. Proper resuscitation in the emergency room with immediate Glasgow assessment helps define the treatment route to a surgical or medical management. A pediatric trauma assessment is indicated to determine transfer of care and immediate treatments. Children who have received prehospital resuscitation may arrive intubated after various attempts, and may still need proper airway and cardiopulmonary care during in-hospital resuscitation. The question of whether to intubate can be triaged with the following indications:

- Unconsciousness
- Apnea and hypoventilation
- A compromised airway
- Controlled ventilation to decrease intracranial hypertension treatment should consist of ICU management

If intubation is imminent:

- Rapid sequence induction entails provision of 100% oxygenation
- The head positioned with in-line stabilization
- Minimal manipulation of the head and spine during intubation
- Care in not augmenting further trauma by the use of muscle relaxants which will reduce resistance
- Succinylcholine 1–2 mg/kg is used and may be followed by a non-depolarizing agent and an anticholinergic (50,51)

Early CT scans should help define mass lesions, midline shifts and/or spinal compromise. Midline shifts greater than 5 mm form the basis for early surgery.

Anesthesia for head injuries that need to go into the surgical suite entails complete monitoring. Aside from the required ASA recommended monitors:

- An arterial line needs to be established for continuous blood pressure reading and resuscitation profiles off of blood samples.
- A central line is appropriate for restitution of blood loss, rapid infusion of fluids and or infusions of medications given centrally.
- Catheterization of the bladder permits several objectives:
  - Perioperative monitoring of urinary output throughout
  - Assesses renal perfusion
  - Sampling for physical/chemical properties
- Temperature is monitored throughout the perioperative period as the pediatric thermoregulatory center is immature and may be very compromised in head injuries.
- Cerebral tissue oxygen utilization monitors has been used in older children and young adults to guide therapy, but it has not shown to have an effective correlation with cerebral blood flow (51,52).

An elevated ICP requires methods to decrease intracranial pressure without compromising optimal perfusion pressures. Intracranial pressure management may be targeted when pressures begin to exceed 25 cmH_2O, but every case is treated differently depending on the site of the insult and the presence of compromised cerebral perfusion pressure. The use of ICP monitoring is required for those who have abnormal CT findings secondary to trauma and a Glasgow score less than 8.

The methods used to decrease intracranial pressure include:

- Positioning and maintaining the head of the patient elevated will facilitate venous drainage from the cranium to the spinal area.
- Hemodynamic support and providing normovolemia will assure CPP.
- Sedation and analgesia assures a decrease in the release of catecholamines secondary to pain and injuries accompanying the trauma. The $CMRO_2$ is attenuated in the face of this treatment. Judicious use of sedation requires the utilization of short acting sedatives so as to not confuse the neurological assessment throughout therapy. Propofol is often used because of its pharmacology profile and its little effect on cerebral vessels; however propofol may affect MAP by systemic vasodilation.
- Neuromuscular blocking agents have been used as temporizing agents to lower dangerous levels of ICP. They do interfere with neurological assessments and should be used judiciously with appropriate nerve monitoring to gauge effect.
- Maintain euvolemia and match diuretic losses with appropriate fluid resuscitation. Consider adding mannitol to the regimen. Mannitol has long been the choice for acute ICP elevation because it acts as an osmotic diuretic and a cerebral arterial vasoconstrictor (51–53).

Skull fractures will commonly present in children with head trauma but the vast majority of these are linear fractures not requiring surgical repair. The concern should be focused on the damage to the underlying cerebral structures, as the force required to fracture the skull can cause diffuse intracranial damage, including damage to a major blood vessel or dural sinus that may lead to intracranial hemorrhage.

- Depressed skull fractures, with or without scalp laceration, should prompt quick evaluation of the intracranial contents for underlying damage.
- While one-third of depressed skull fractures are uncomplicated, one-third are associated with dural tearing, and the final third may present as cortical damage. Emergently proceed to the operating room for surgical evaluation.
- Basilar skull fractures are rare in children but are associated with a good prognosis. Consider basilar skull fracture in any patient with altered mental status or seizures associated with trauma.
- Physical signs include:
  - Battle's sign (retroauricular ecchymosis)
  - "Raccoon eyes" (periorbital ecchymosis)
  - Hemotympanum, or clear rhinorrhea (5)
- Usually, nasal intubation or passage of a nasogastric tube is contraindicated in these patients to avoid inadvertent passage of instruments into the cranium.

Hematomas

Hematomas can present as intracerebral, epidural, or subdural. Intracerebral contusions can present with focal symptoms at the site of injury (coup) or the area geometrically opposite the injury (contracoup). These injuries are often associated with skull fractures (2). These injuries have a poor prognosis and extensive cortical contusions can lead to deep parenchymal hematomas associated with severe neurologic injury and high morbidity and mortality. These are treated with prophylactic anticonvulsant therapy early and we avoid medications that interfere with coagulation (5).

Epidural hematomas

- Epidural hematomas are rapidly accumulating insults that occur between the dura and the cranium.
- Eighty-five percent are associated with skull fracture and the most serious arise from damage to the middle meningeal artery.
- The neurologic pattern consists of loss on consciousness followed by an awake interval usually associated with severe headache (2).
- Children may not demonstrate altered mental status initially (5).
- Death can occur rapidly, as fast as 15–30 minutes. Rapid surgical evacuation is indicated.
- The deterioration phase is associated with:
  - Expansion of the hematoma and
  - May present with loss of consciousness
  - Hemiparesis
  - Pupillary dilatation
- Focus on anesthetic techniques to reduce intracranial pressure. Prognosis is good with evacuation but prolonged morbidity is usually indicative of underlying cerebral damage (5).

Subdural hematomas

Subdural hematomas occur when arteries or bridging veins are torn between the dura and brain parenchyma. They frequently occur in children playing sports and are the most common cause of sports-related head injury (2). In younger children, concern should be focused to the shaken baby syndrome, where infant shaking is so vigorous that significant neuronal rupture and vein tearing can occur.

Newborns with subdural hematomas should be promptly evaluated for:

- Vitamin K deficiency
- Congenital coagulopathies
- Disseminated intravascular coagulopathies

Patients should be aggressively resuscitated with focus on maintenance of appropriate hemodynamic parameters while simultaneously being prepared for emergent surgical treatment. Postoperatively, these patients manifest cerebral edema with uncontrolled ICP and persistent neurologic deficits.

Spinal cord disorders

Spina bifida (myelodysplasia)

These disorders are defects in the spine that require surgical intervention. Lesions containing CSF without the presence of neural tissue are called meningoceles. When neural tissue is also present, it is called a meningomyelocele. Neural tissue open to air that is not contained in a sack is known as rachischisis.

Surgery is performed urgently to reduce the risk of permanent neurologic devastation and infection.

Anesthetic considerations include attention to patient positioning and the presence of hydrocephalus.

- Infants are brought into the operating room in the prone position and sterile moist dressings protect the spinal defect.
- Patients with this bulging meningomyelocele or rachischisis are unable to be placed supine on the operating room table. The only moment a neonate is placed supine is for induction and intubation. Here the spine and area of defect can be placed on a gel or foam roll "donut" for protection of the sack contents and neural structures.
  If the sac ruptures, lactated Ringer's solution may be given intravenously to reconstitute the losses at a rate of 4–6 ml/kg/h or 1 ml for 1 ml of CSF loss.
- They may also be placed in the lateral decubitus position for intubation, if required. These patients may present with concomitant hydrocephalus and attention must be paid to a possible inability to mask ventilate or intubate.
- These patients are at a high risk for development of latex allergy and should be introduced to a latex free environment as early as possible.
- Spinal anesthesia may be used together with a general anesthetic. Once the infant is asleep and positioned prone for surgery, hyperbaric tetracaine 0.5–0.7 mg/kg can be placed into the inferior portion of the meningomyelocele by the surgeon to decrease the general anesthesia requirements for the surgery (5).

Neurodegenerative disorders

Neurodegenerative disorders of childhood encompass a large, heterogeneous group of diseases that result from specific genetic and biochemical defects, chronic viral infections, and varied unknown causes (2). These diseases are characterized by a progressive regression and deterioration of neurologic function with loss of speech, vision, hearing, or locomotion, often associated with seizures, feeding difficulties, and impairment of intellect (2). White matter disorders present with upper motor neuron signs and progressive spasticity. Grey matter disorders present with convulsions, intellectual, and visual impairment that occur early in the disease (2).

Sphingolipidoses are disorders of catabolism of sphingolipids resulting in intracellular storage of lipid substrates that compromise cell membranes. These include Niemann–Pick disease, Gaucher disease, Tay–Sachs disease, Krabbe disease, and metachromatic leukodystrophy. Patients with these diseases may present with a myriad of disorders of the liver, spleen, and hematologic systems (5). Patients may present with disorders of bleeding or early atherosclerotic disease secondary to dyslipidemia. Careful attention must be given to hematological and coagulation parameters. The main anesthetic concern, however, lies in the progressive neurologic devastation encountered by these patients and perianesthetic morbidity secondary to need for reintubation and the development of postoperative pneumonia, hypothermia, and seizure (6).

Cerebral palsy and spasticity

Multiple causes during the development of the CNS, either antenatal fetal events or post-natal events may result in damage of the CNS that result in the disorder of motion and posture, or cerebral palsy (CP). It occurs in two per 1000 live births and neonatal asphyxia is not a common cause. Premature infants are likely to present periventricular hemorrhage that commonly progresses to leukomalacia with subsequent CP. Infections, surgical complications in the neonatal ICU, and endocrinopathies have also contributed to CP. Additional systemic disabilities are relative to the degree of spasticity involving the trunks and limbs. These may be seen as sensorial loss, cognitive deficiencies, seizures, GI disorders, etc.

Anesthetic considerations for these children involve recognition of the clinical problems, their treatment modalities, medications that may affect how our anesthetics affect their systems to better serve their perioperative period (51).

Chiari malformations

These malformations are almost always seen in concert with spina bifida. Chiari malformations are disturbances in the posterior fossa and upper cervical spine that lead to downward movement of the cerebellar vermis, fourth ventricle, and lower brainstem below the foramen magnum (1). The pathogenesis is the underdevelopment of the occipital bone with intracranial overcrowding.

- Type I malformations can present in children without spina bifida who are otherwise healthy. These tend to be mild presentations mainly manifesting with headache and neck pain as adults. Type I displays a herniation of the cerebellar tonsils.
- Type II malformations (Arnold–Chiari) are associated with myelomeningocele and these children can be quite neurologically damaged. This herniation compromises the fourth ventricle and the medulla oblongata along with the caudal part of the cerebellum. The pediatric type mainly belongs to type II and babies born with this malformation present with myeloschisis, brainstem dysfunction, and hydrocephalus.
- Type III Chiari is the downward displacement of the cerebellum into the posterior encephalocele, whose clinical manifestations include hydrocephalus with brain stem dysfunction.
- Type IV Chiari manifests as cerebellar hypoplasia and is accompanied by ataxia (54,55).
- Presentation includes:
  - Progressive vocal cord paralysis
  - Respiratory distress
  - Apnea
  - Abnormal swallowing and aspiration

  All of these considerations present a challenge to the anesthesiologist. The basic operation is one of uncrowding the area at the base of the cerebellum. Avoiding extreme head flexion during intubation or positioning, it will decrease the risks of exacerbating or worsening a preexisting problem.

Anesthesia for neurosurgical procedures

Seizure surgery:

- Antiepileptic drugs should be measured for appropriate plasma levels preoperatively; they should be given on the day of surgery and restarted soon after surgery.
- LFTs and coagulation status should also be reviewed preoperatively.
- A preoperative sedative is often given to reduce anxiety and avoid the child hyperventilating. Hyperventilation decreases the seizure threshold.
- Sevoflurane in O_2 with or without N_2O is still the preferred inhalation induction for children knowing that it may give epileptiform changes on the EEG. Epileptiform changes on EEG can also be seen with low doses of propofol. High doses will suppress activity. Phenytoin, phenobarbital, and carbamazepine induce hepatic enzymes and increase the metabolism of our inhalation agents and opioids; Most inhalation agents will depress the sensitivity of the neurophysiologic monitors needed to map out the foci.
- We should avoid anesthetics or adjuvants whose metabolites.
- Are epileptogenic (ketamine, atracurium, alfentanil, meperidine) (56,57).

The various types of seizure surgeries include:

- Ressective surgery, which removes the part of the brain where the seizure is originating.
- A corpus collosotomy that severs the connections between the two hemispheres. Risk of bleeding and VAE is high. These patients are somnolent and lethargic postoperatively and will need ICU observation.
- Placement of the vagal nerve stimulator, which discharges currents to stimulate the vagus nerve. This is inserted behind the left clavicle and may incite bradycardia or a transient asystole during initial charges.
- Awake craniotomies can be performed on very cooperative older children with MAC and local anesthesia. A remifentanil infusion may be used to support the procedural sedation (56).

Seizures under anesthesia:

- Convulsions under general anesthesia are difficult to diagnose
- Subtle signs are: Increase in $etCO_2$, tachycardia, muscle rigidity, HTN, pupillary dilatation.
- Treatment entails 100% O_2, deepening the anesthetic, anticonvulsant medications, and resolving any precipitating factors.

Craniofacial reconstruction/ cranioplasty

Congenital and acquired deformities of the cranium and facial bones are the most challenging of pediatric cases. The disorders encountered often are:

- Cleft lip and palate
- Pierre Robin association
- Craniofacial dysostosis
- Treacher Collins syndrome

Table 9.7. The Glasgow Coma Scale

	Eye-opening response		
	> 1 year		< 1 year
4	Spontaneous		Spontaneous
3	To verbal command		To shout
2	To pain		To pain
1	None		None
	Motor response		
	> 1 year		< 1 year
6	Obeys commands		Displays spontaneous response
5	Localizes pain		Localizes pain
4	Withdraws from pain		Withdraws from pain
3	Displays abnormal flexion to pain (decorticate rigidity)		Displays abnormal flexion to pain (decorticate rigidity)
2	Displays abnormal extension to pain (decerebrate rigidity)		Displays abnormal extension to pain (decerebrate rigidity)
1	None		None
	Abnormal response		
	> 5 years	2–5 years	0–23 months
5	Is oriented and converses	Uses appropriate words and phrases	Babbles, coos appropriately
4	Conversation is confused	Uses inappropriate words	Cries, but is consolable
3	Words are inappropriate	Cries or screams persistently to pain	Cries or moans to pain
2	Sounds are incomprehensible	Grunts or moans to pain	Grunts or moans to pain
1	None	None	None

Range: 3–15
Severe: less than or equal to 9
Moderate: 9–12
Mild: 13–15

Pediatric Care Online 2011 American Academy of Pediatrics
Modified from: Teasdale G, Jennett B. Assessment of coma and impaired consciousness: a practical scale. *Lancet* 1974; 304(7872): 81–4.

- Klippel–Feil syndrome
- Beckwith-Weiderman syndrome
- Trisomy 21
- Freeman–Sheldon syndrome
- Fibrodysplasia ossificans progressive
- Mucopolysaccharidoses

Perioperative issues:

These children will tend to have obstructive type breathing with a history of snoring and repeated respiratory infections. All their medications should be reviewed prior to surgery along with a complete lab work-up (58). Before a child is ready to undergo craniofacial surgery:

- The Hgb should be at least 10 gms%
- Normal coagulation profile
- Electrolytes with BUN to gauge perioperative diuretic therapy
- 3 units of cross-matched pRBCs available
- Avoid preoperative sedation in unsupervised environments to reduce risks of airway obstruction and increasing ICP

We follow the basic principles to avoid any further increases in ICP during surgery:

- Reducing brain bulk with meds
- 30 degrees of head lift for positioning
- Hyperventilation to control $PaCO_2$
- Diuretics (mannitol, lasix)
- Lumbar CSF drainage

Venous air embolism

This complication can occur frequently due to the open venous channels of the skull while the head is positioned above the level of the heart predisposing the patient to air entrapment. This event is defined with intense pulmonary vasoconstriction, ventilation/perfusion mismatch, pulmonary edema, and a decrease in cardiac output. Children < 5 years of age may still have a patent foramen ovale, which can place them at an additional risk for a paradoxical air embolism (12).

Monitors for detection of VAE:

- TEE
- Precordial Doppler
- Pulmonary artery catheter (increase in PAP)
- Capnography (decrease in $etCO_2$)
- Mass spectrometry (increase in etN_2) most specific

At the moment an air embolism is suspected:

- The field should be flooded with saline soaked gauzes/bone wax
- Change the position of the patient to horizontal
- Discontinue N_2O and assure 100% O_2
- Hemodynamic support and increase CVP
- Jugular venous compression
- Attempt aspirating air from the CVP line in the right atrium

References

1. Vavilala M, Soriano S. Anesthesia for neurosurgery. In Davis PJ, Cladis FP, Moyotama EK, eds., *Smith's Anesthesia for Infants and Children*, 8th Edition. Philadelphia PA: Elsevier Mosby, 2011, pp. 713–44.
2. Zitelli BJ, Davis HW. *Atlas of Pediatric Physical Diagnosis*, 5th Edition. Philadelphia PA: Elsevier, 2011.
3. Keasly W. The intracranial pressure in infants; *J Neurosurg* May 2012; **116** (5): 693–9.
4. Feigelman S. Overview and assessment of variability. In Kliegman R M, Stanton B, St. Geme J, Schor N, Behrman R, *Nelson's Textbook of Pediatrics*, 19th Edition. Philadelphia PA: Elsevier, 2011, pp. 26–36.
5. Loepke AW, Davisdson AJ. Surgery anesthesia and the immature brain. In Cote JC, Lerman J, Anderson B, eds., *A Practice of Anesthesia for Infants and Children*, 5th Edition. Saunders, 2013, pp. 492–509.
6. Miao N, Lu X, O'Grady NP, Yanjanin N. Niemann–Pick disease type C: Implications for sedation and anesthesia for diagnostic procedures. *J Child Neurol* 2012 Dec; **27**(12): 1541–6, epub 2012 Feb 28 PMID: 22378675.
7. Zimmermann A, Dumoki F, Bari F. Seizure-induced alterations in cerebrovascular function in the neonate. *Dev Neurosci* 2008; **371**(2): 691.
8. Monro, A. *Observations on the structure and Functions of the Nervous System*. Edinburgh, Creech and Johnson, 1783.
9. Allen CH, Ward JD. An evidence-based approach to management of increased intracranial pressure. *Crit Care Clin* 1998; **14**(3): 485.
10. Welch K. The intracranial pressure in infants. *J Neurosurg* 1980; **52**: 693.
11. Bouma GJ, Muizelaar JP, Fatouros P. Pathogenesis of traumatic brain swelling: role of cerebral blood volume. *Acta Neurochir Suppl* 1998; **71**: 272.
12. Bissonette B, Brady K, Easley B. *Gregory's Pediatric Anesthesia*, 5th Edition. Blackwell Publishing, 2012.
13. Raboel PH, Bartek J Jr, Anderson M. Intracranial pressure monitoring: Invasive vs. non-invasive methods – a review. *Crit Care Res Pract* 2012; **2012**: 950393.
14. Haque IU, Zaritsky AL. Analysis of the evidence for the lower limit of systolic and mean arterial pressure in children. *Pediatr Crit Care Med* 2007; **8**(2): 138–44.
15. Chestnut RM. Medical managmeent of severe head injury: Present and future. *New Horiz* 1995; **3**: 581.
16. Hartl R, Barat TF, Kiening KL, *et al.* Mannitol decreases intracranial pressure but does not improve brain tissue pO_2 in severely head-injured patients with intracranial hypotension. *Acta Neurochir Suppl* 1997; **70**: 40.
17. Mendelow AD, Teasdale GM, Russell T, *et al.* Effect of mannitol on cerebral blood flow and cerebral perfusion pressure in human head injury. *J Neurosurg* 1985; **63**: 43.
18. Milson C, James HE, Shapiro HM, *et al.* Intracranial hypertension and brain edema in albino rabbits,

part 2: Effects of acute therapy with diuretics. *Acta Neurochir (Wein)* 1981: **56**: 167.

19. Perucca E. NICE: Guidance on newer drugs for epilepsy in adults. *BMJ* 2004; **328**: 1273.
20. Hartl R, Ghajar J, Hochleuthner H, Mauritz W. Hypertonic/ hyperoncotic saline reliability reduces ICP in severely head-injured patients with intracranial hypertension. *Acta Neurochir Suppl* 1997; **70**: 126.
21. Khanna S, Davis D, Peterson B, *et al.* Use of hypertonic saline in the treatment of severe refractory post-traumatic intracranial hypertension in pediatric traumatic brain injury. *Crit Care Med* 2000; **28**: 1144.
22. Fisher B, Thomas D, Perterson B. Hypertonic saline lowers raised intracranial pressure in children after head trauma. *J Neurosurg Anesthesiol* 1992; **4**: 4.
23. Munar F, Ferrer AM, de Nadal M, *et al.* Cerebral hemodynamic effects of 7.2% hypertonic saline in patients with head injury and raised intracranial pressure. *J Neurotrauma* 2000: **17**: 41.
24. Suarez JI, Qureshi AI, Bhardwaj A, *et al.* Treatment of refractory intracranial hypertension with 23.4% saline. *Crit Care Med* 1998; **26**: 118.
25. Horn P, Munch E, Vajkoczy P, *et al.* Hypertonic saline solution for control of elevated intracranial pressure in patients with exhausted response to mannitol and barbiturates. *Neurol Res* 1999; **21**: 758.
26. Perks A, *et al.* Anesthesia and epilepsy. *Br J Anaesth* 2012:**108** (4): 562–71.
27. Sanders J, Sharvon S. The incidence and prevalence of epilepsy. *Br J Anaesth* 1987; **108**: 4: 562–71.
28. Allman K, McIndoe A, Wilson L, *et al. Emergencies in Anesthesia.* Oxford, UK: OUP, 2005.
29. Stam A, Schothorst P, Vortsman J, *et al.* The genetic overlap of attention deficit hyperactivity and autistic spectrum disorder. *Appl Clin Genet* 2009 **10**; 2: 7–13.
30. Shuvarikov A, *et al.* Recurrent HERV-H mediated 3q13.2-q13.31 deletions cause a syndrome of hypotonia and motor, language and cognitive delays. *HUM Mutat* 2013; **34**(10): 1415–23.
31. Ghaziuddin, M. Autism spectrum disorders and inborn errors of metabolism: an update. *Pediatr Neurol* 2013; **49**(4): 232–6.
32. Perks A, Cheema S, Mohanraj R, *et al.* Anaesthesia and epilepsy. *Br J Anaesth* 2012; **108**(4): 562–71.
33. Perry J, *et al.* The effect of nitrous oxide-induced activation of Vit B12 on the activity of formyl-methenyl-methylenetetrahydrofolate synthase-transferase. *Biochem Biophys Res Commun* 1980; **97**(4): 1329–33.
34. Sanders RD, Weinmann J, Maze M. Biologic effects of nitrous oxide, a mechanistic and toxilogic review. *Anesthesiol* 2008; **109** (4):707–22.
35. Asahi Y, Kubota K, Omichi S. Dose requirements for propofol anesthesia for dental treatment for autistic patients compared with intellectualy impaired patients. *Anesth Intensive Care* 2009; **37**(1): 70–3.
36. Miyawaki T, Kohijtani A, Maeda S, *et al.* Intravenous sedation for dental patients with intellectual disability. *Intellect Disabil Res* 2004; **48**(8): 764–8.
37. Shirakami G, Tanimotok K, Matsuura S, Fukuda K. Ambulatory anesthesia for an adult patient with autism and epilpepsy: Sedation using oral and intravenous dexmedetomidine. *Masui* 2008; **57**(6): 735–8.
38. Mason K, Zurakowski D, Zgleszewski S, *et al.* High dose dexmedetomidine as the sole sedative for pediatric MRI. *Paediatr Anaesth* 2008; **18**(5): 403–11.
39. Caleb I, Dimaggio C, Whitehouse A, *et al.* Long-time differences in language and cognitive function after childhood exposure to anesthesia. *Pediatrics* 2011; **130**: e476.
40. Kleihues P, Burger PC, Scheithauer BW. The WHO classification of brain tumours. *Brain Path* 1993; **3**: 255–68.
41. Lopes MBS, Vandenberg SR, Sheithauer BW. The WHO classification of nervous system tumors in experimental neuro-oncology. In Levine AJ, Schmidek HH, eds., *Molecular Genetics of Nervous System Tumors.* New York: Wiley-Liss, 1993, pp.1–36
42. Berger TM, Kistler W, Berendes E. Hyponatremia in a pediatric stroke patient: Syndrome of innappropriate anti-diuretic hormone secretion or cerebral salt wasting? *Crit Care Med* 2002; **30**: 792–5.
43. Francis L, Mohamed M, Patino M. Intraoperative neuromonitoring in pediatric surgeries. *Int Anesthesiol Clin* 2012; **50**(4): 130–43.
44. Liang BA. Blood, bone and dura: Anesthesia responsibility and pediatric neurosurgery *J Clin Anesth* 1997; **9**(7): 597–601.
45. Davis PJ, Cladis FP, Moyotama EK. *Smith's Anesthesia for Infants and Children*, 8th Edition. Philadelphia PA, Elsevier Mosby, 2011.
46. National Institute for Health and Clinical Excellence (UK). Newer drugs for epilepsy in adults: full guidance. *Technology Appraisal Guidance* **76**, Mar 2004, www.nice.org.uk/guidance/ TA076.
47. French JA, Leppi E. *New Anti-Epileptic Drug Development: Pre-clinical and Clinical Aspects.* Amsterdam: Elsevier, 1993.

48. Andrew P, Gratrix I, Enright S. Epilepsy in anesthesia and intensive care. *Contin Educ Anaesth Crit Care Pain* 2005; **5**(4): 118–21.
49. Chang CWJ, Black TP. Status epilepticus. *Neurol Clin* 1995; **13** (3): 528–48.
50. Teasdale G, Jennett B. Assessment of coma and impaired consciousness: A practical scale. *Lancet* 1974; **304**(7872): 81–4.
51. Morrow SE, Nakayama DK, Davis PJ. Anesthesias for trauma. In Davis PJ, Moyotama EK, eds., *Smith's Anesthesia for Infants and Children*, 6th Edition. St Louis, MO: Elsevier, 1996, pp. 991–1012.
52. Jimmy W, Raghupathi R. New concepts in treatment of pediatric traumatic brain injury. *Anesth Clin* 2009; **27**(2): 213–40.
53. Holzman R, Mason K. Anesthesia for trauma in pediatric patients.In Gregory GE, ed., *Pediatric Anesthesia*, 3rd Edition. Wiley, 2012, pp. 896–918.
54. Nolan J, Chalkiadis GA. Anesthesia and pain management in cerebral palsy; review article. *Anesthesia* 2000: **55**: 32–41.
55. Niskawa M. Pathogenesis of Chiari malformation: A morphometric study of the posterior cranial fossa. *J Neurosurg* 1997; **86**: 40–7.
56. Ahmed R, Barakat A, Mallory S. Anesthesia and childhood epilepsy: continued education. *Anesth Crit Care* 2011; **11**(3): 93–8.
57. Soriano SG, Eldridge EA. Pediatric anesthesia. *Anesthesiol Clin North America* 2002; **20**(2): 389–404.
58. Norgozian C. The airway in patients with craniofacial abnormalities. *Paediatr Anaesth* 2004; **14**(1): 53–9.

Chapter

10 Development of the gastrointestinal tract and associated conditions

Louise K. Furukawa

Developmental anatomy of the foregut

The foregut extends from the pharynx to include the esophagus, stomach, liver, pancreas, and first and second portions of the duodenum to just beyond the entry of the pancreatic duct. The celiac artery supplies blood to the foregut. At 4 weeks of development, two buds develop from the ventral wall of the foregut. The proximal diverticulum branches and forms the trachea, bronchi, and lungs, and the distal diverticulum forms the hepatobiliary tree. Between these two diverticula the endodermal tube forms the stomach. The respiratory diverticulum becomes separated from the esophageal portion of the foregut by formation of the esophagotracheal septum. As development of the embryo proceeds, the stomach tube rotates 90° along its longitudinal axis so that the left side is anterior and the right side is posterior. The left vagus nerve therefore innervates the anterior wall and the right vagus innervates the posterior wall. Differential growth of the stomach results in the formation of the greater curvature and accounts for positioning of the pylorus to the right and upward. The pancreas derives from endodermal buds originating in the lining of the duodenum during the 5th week of gestation. Dorsal and ventral pancreatic buds then develop within respective mesenteries. Fusion of the pancreatic buds occurs during rotation of the duodenal loop. The dorsal bud becomes the body of the pancreas and the ventral bud becomes the uncinate process. The duodenum is part of both the foregut and the midgut given that the junction of the two is at the level of the ampulla. The proximal duodenum receives blood supply from the celiac artery and the distal portion from the SMA. The duodenal lumen goes through a solid phase due to rapid endolumenal proliferation with recanalization by week 8–10.

Congenital anomalies of the foregut

Tracheoesophageal fistula (TEF) and esophageal atresia (EA)

Tracheoesophageal fistula and esophageal atresia result from incomplete formation of the esophagus with or without connection to the trachea. The fistulous connection is a remnant of the common origin of the respiratory and digestive system whereas the atresia may represent unbalanced septation. The mechanism of this embryopathologic process is unknown although animal models suggest a displacement disorder of the notochord. (1) Five anatomic variants (Fig. 10.1) are described in the Gross classification (2). Type C, proximal EA with distal TEF, is the most common presentation affecting 84% of patients. A Type F is also described consisting of esophageal stenosis without fistula and will not be discussed. The prevalence of TEF is approximately 1:5000 live births with a slight male predominance. In the most common variant, the location of the fistula is in the distal tracheal close to the carina. Prenatally, failure of the fetus to swallow amniotic fluid results in maternal polyhydramnios. After birth the initial presentation depends on the anatomic variant and presence of esophageal atresia, fistula, or both. The classic presentation of an infant is a triad of coughing, choking, and cyanosis after the first feed due to accumulation of fluid in the blind esophageal pouch. Infants may present with gastric distention or pneumonia if a fistula is present. A diagnosis is often made by failure to pass a feeding tube further than 10–12 cm and chest radiograph confirming coiling of the tube in the blind

Essentials of Pediatric Anesthesiology, ed. Alan David Kaye, Charles James Fox and James H. Diaz. Published by Cambridge University Press. © Cambridge University Press 2015.

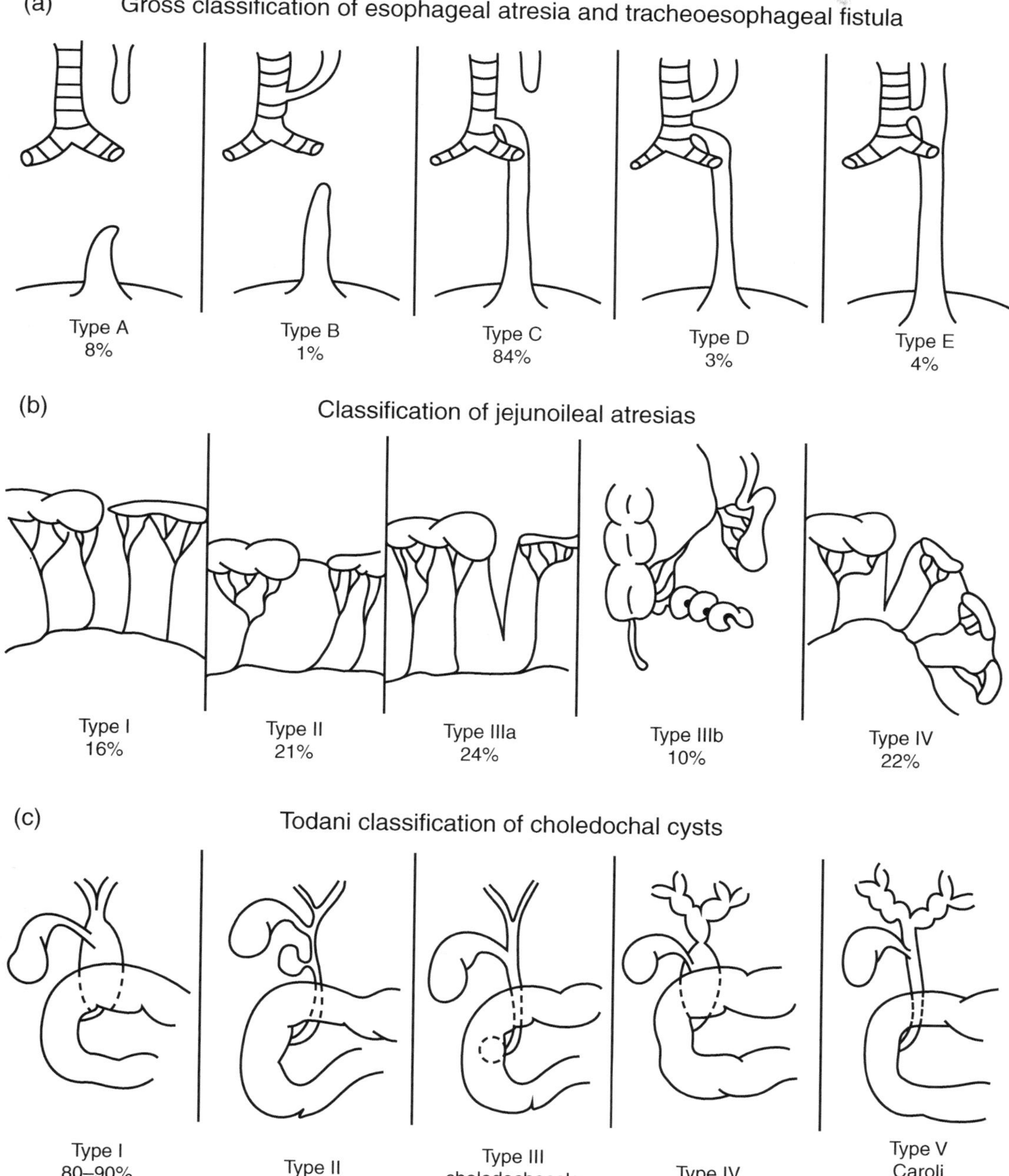

Figure 10.1 Classification of GI anomalies.

esophageal pouch. Associated anomalies are common, most notably cardiac, renal or urinary anomalies, or Trisomy 13, 18, or 21. These may exist as isolated lesions or as part of the VATER/VACTERL association (anomalies of **V**ertebrae, **A**norectum, **C**ardiac, **TEF**, **EA**, **R**enal, **L**imb). Associated anomalies are most common with Type A and least common with Type E. All infants must be evaluated for associated anomalies. Mortality is higher in patients with associated cardiac and/or chromosomal anomalies. **Surgical and anesthetic considerations**: Prior to repair the surgeon may perform rigid or flexible bronchoscopy to determine location of the fistula. A Fogarty catheter may be placed through the fistula at this time to facilitate exterior identification of the fistula as well as to enhance ventilation. Even without Fogarty catheter placement, this information is helpful to the anesthesiologist in determining optimal placement of the endotracheal tube (ETT). Surgery commences in the lateral position through either open or thoracoscopic technique. The anesthetic management of TEF is challenging, particularly if the patient has pneumonia or a complex cardiac lesion. In the most common presentation, the fistula is located just above the carina. Placement of the long end of the ETT over the fistula yet above the carina should favor lung ventilation over fistula ventilation. Practically speaking, after intubation, positioning, and surgical retraction, the tube may migrate. The anesthesiologist should always be mindful of potential ventilatory problems prior to ligation of the fistula including inspissation of secretions within the tube, migration of the tube into the bronchus of the operative side, fistula ventilation, and surgical compression of the trachea. Right-lung isolation with a bronchial blocker may be difficult in cases of very proximal take-off or tracheal location of the right upper lobe bronchus. Ventilation may be intermittent and hypercarbia can be profound. Ventilation usually becomes much easier after the fistula is ligated. If reintubation is required in the days following surgery, great care must be taken to avoid hyperextension of the neck and traction on the esophageal anastomosis. An epidural may be placed for postoperative analgesia if not contraindicated by vertebral pathology. A wide esophageal gap is typical of Type A EA, and definitive repair is typically delayed. Initial surgery consists of gastrostomy tube placement and bolus feeding so that the stomach and distal esophagus can grow and lengthen. Common problems postoperatively include gastroesophageal reflux (GERD), tracheomalacia, and esophageal anastomotic stricture.

Foregut duplications

Intestinal duplications are tubular or cystic structures defined as having three characteristics: (1) a well-defined smooth muscular coat, (2) an epithelial lining containing at least one tissue type found in the gastrointestinal tract, and (3) an intimate association to the gastrointestinal tract. The developmental etiology of this disorder is unknown with theories ranging from a split notochord to partial twinning. The presentation of a duplication depends on its location. Some cause symptoms by compression, others contain acid-producing mucosa and cause bleeding or perforation, still others can cause volvulus or intussuception, and some are asymptomatic. Duplications tend to be located on the mesenteric side of the viscus. Prevalence data are derived from autopsy findings with duplications found in 1:4500 autopsies. The most common site of duplication is in the small intestine. Synchronous duplications are found in 15% of cases. Malignant transformation has been reported, therefore, when detected, duplications should be resected. Associated anomalies are common with duplications.

Esophageal duplication

Duplication in the cervical region is very rare. The thoracic location represents 4% of duplication cysts. These cysts can present with airway compression and respiratory distress or reflux symptoms owing to presence of heterotopic gastric mucosa in 1/3 of cases. In 75% of patients with thoracic or thoracoabdominal duplications of the esophagus there are vertebral anomalies. **Surgical and anesthetic considerations**: The surgical approach is excision through either open or thoracoscopic incisions.

Gastric duplication

Seven percent of duplications are gastric. Most are cystic, located on the greater curve, and have no luminal connection with the stomach. Many patients present before the age of one due to difficulties feeding associated with mass effect. The mucosa of the duplication is typically gastric in origin therefore bleeding and perforation are risks. **surgical and anesthetic considerations**: Excision is the goal but if hazardous, partial excision with mucosal stripping is acceptable.

Pyloric atresia

Pyloric atresia is an extremely rare condition found in 1 in 100 000 live births with no sex predilection. It is associated with epidermolysis bullosa simplex, junctional epidermolysis bullosa, aplasia cutis congenita and can be associated with other intestinal atresias (3).

The presence of epidermolysis bullosa does not necessarily preclude surgical repair. Polyhydramnios is a common prenatal finding and infants are often small for gestational age. Clinical findings are apparent shortly after birth with nonbilious vomiting after feeds. **Surgical and anesthetic considerations**: The patient must be stabilized with intravenous hydration and gastric decompression. If epidermolysis bullosa (EB) exists, the anesthetic preparation is extensive and cannot be covered in this chapter. Absolutely no adhesives may be used including a bovie pad. The patient must be treated with full stomach precautions. Surgical repair commences with either excision of a web and pyloroplasty, pyloroplasty alone or gastroduodenotomy. Although the surgical repair is straightforward, mortality is related to the associated disorders.

Duodenal atresia and stenosis

Faulty recanalization of the duodenum results in stenoses, webs, and atresias. The atretic area is typically located at the level of the ampulla of Vater. Duodenal atresia is classified as follows. Type I involves only a translumenal membrane within a normal muscular wall. Type II is described as fibrous cord connecting two atretic segments. Type III involves complete separation of atretic segments and includes a mesenteric defect. Associated biliary anomalies are common with Type III defects. Type I defects are the most common. The prevalence of duodenal atresia is 1:6000 live births with males and females equally affected. Associated anomalies are common with Trisomy 21 occurring in 20–40% of patients. Many other patients have anomalies of the GI tract (malrotation, heterotaxy, biliary atresia, annular pancreas), cardiac, renal, vertebral anomalies. These infants tend to be born at term but are small for gestational age. There is often a maternal history of polyhydramnios and a prenatal diagnosis is frequently established. Infants present with bilious vomiting within hours of birth. A classic radiographic finding is the double bubble sign representing air within the stomach and air within the duodenum proximal to the atresia. Preoperative work-up includes echocardiogram, evaluation for vertebral anomalies and renal ultrasonography. Duodenal stenosis is usually diagnosed later in life when oral intake changes to more solid foods. **Surgical and anesthetic considerations**: Surgical repair of Type I duodenal atresia involves membrane resection alone or membrane resection and duodenoduodenostomy. Repair of Type II and III defects typically involves duodenoduodenostomy. If the affected infant has Trisomy 21 the surgeon may wish to take rectal biopsies to rule out Hirschprung disease. Associated anomalies, particularly cardiac must be known to the anesthesiologist and the anesthetic plan formed accordingly. The patient has a full stomach by definition and will require rapid sequence induction and intubation (RSII). In the presence of Trisomy 21 the possibility of atlanto-occipital instability must be assumed.

Duodenal duplication

See previous section on duplications. 15% of duodenal duplications contain heterotopic gastric mucosa and can lead to ulceration and bleeding. Some can extend into the liver or transdiaphragmatically. **Surgical and anesthetic considerations**: Surgical treatment can involve resection, or in cases where the location is not amenable to resection, partial excision and mucosal stripping, or drainage.

Annular pancreas

Annular pancreas results from failure of the ventral pancreatic bud to completely migrate posterior to the duodenum resulting in encasement of the duodenum. Symptoms are related to duodenal constriction although it is estimated that 2/3 of cases are asymptomatic. Annular pancreas either presents very early in life with bilious vomiting, gastric distension, and feeding intolerance, or it remains asymptomatic until middle age, when pain becomes the most common presenting symptom (4). Of the population presenting in infancy, over 70% have associated anomalies including trisomy 21, cardiac anomalies, malrotation, duodenal atresia, and other GI abnormalities. **Surgical and anesthetic considerations:** In addition to managing transitional circulation and possible cardiac anomalies, the infant presenting with annular pancreas has a full stomach and warrants RSII. Surgical repair typically includes either a duodenoduodenostomy or duodenojejunostomy.

Acquired conditions of the foregut

Foreign bodies in the esophagus and stomach

Foreign body (FB) ingestion occurs predominantly in children 18 months to 4 years of age. The FB tends to be an object rather than food. The cricopharyngeus is the most common site of obstruction in children although pre-existing esophageal stricture, diverticula or achalacia can predispose to entrapment at other sites (5). Once reaching the stomach, a FB has a 90% chance of passing through the GI tract. Ingestion of foreign bodies can cause abrasions, punctures, and perforation with mediastinitis, or abscess. Batteries can erode through the esophagus and fistulize to the trachea or aorta. The toddler presenting with an esophageal FB displays drooling, vomiting, dysphagia, pain, or stridor. Of particular concern are ingestion of lithium disk batteries ("button batteries") commonly found in children's toys. Liquefaction necrosis can occur when these batteries lodge in the esophagus and can occur within 2 hours after ingestion. If button battery ingestion is suspected by history or X-ray, urgent evaluation and removal is warranted if the battery is lodged in the esophagus. Coins are the most frequently swallowed FB. Pennies of US origin are currently minted from copper-clad zinc which can cause esophageal or gastric ulceration if they fail to pass. **Surgical and anesthetic considerations**: Patients unable to manage oral secretions, those with airway symptoms, signs of sepsis, perforation or bleeding must present for urgent rigid or endoscopic foreign body removal. A button battery lodged in the esophagus is also considered an indication for urgent removal because of erosion risk. Most patients are intubated using RSII to protect against aspiration as well as accidental deposition of the FB into the airway. Surgical extraction can occur via rigid esophagoscopy, flexible endoscopy, or foley catheter balloon extraction. Balloon extraction is not appropriate for disk batteries given the need for mucosal evaluation.

Esophageal strictures

The majority of literature written about pediatric esophageal stricture is related to repaired esophageal atresia (EA), epidermolysis bullosa (EB), or the sequelae of caustic ingestion. Of EA patients, this complication is more frequent in those with longer gap EA, presumably due to tension in the repair and/or ischemia. A second population of patients presenting frequently with esophageal strictures are those with epidermolysis bullosa (EB). Epidermolysis bullosa is a rare genetic condition in which patients are deficient in one or more proteins important in anchoring skin layers. Minimal contact or trauma results in blister formation and scarring. Recessive dystrophic EB (RDEB) is one of the most severe types and is very frequently associated with esophageal stricture due to mucosa involvement. Approximately 80% of all patients with RDEB will undergo treatment for esophageal stricture. Caustic ingestion also results in esophageal stricture. Other more uncommon causes of esophageal stricture in children include, GERD, nonreflux esophagitis (radiation, infectious, eosinophilic) and graft-versus-host-disease (GVHD) involving the gut. Children with esophageal strictures have symptoms of dysphagia and an inability to manage oral secretions. **Surgical and anesthetic considerations**: The esophagus can be dilated through use of serial dilators or by endoscopically guided hydrostatic balloon dilation. In the case of caustic ingestion, endoscopy may be advantageous since there is an increased risk of developing esophageal cancer. In cases of extensive pharyngeal scarring, it may be possible to approach the stricture in a retrograde fashion from the gastrostomy site. The anesthesiologist must be aware of any coexisting conditions or anomalies in the EA population and adjust the anesthetic plan accordingly. Anesthesia for patients with EB is extremely challenging and involves extensive preparation of the procedure area and an expected difficult airway. Children who have survived a caustic ingestion may also have a difficult airway due to oropharyngeal or laryngeal scarring.

Pyloric stenosis

Pyloric stenosis (PS) is one of the most common disorders of the neonatal/infantile GI tract occurring in approximately 2–4:1000 live births. Whether this disorder is acquired or develops in utero is still debated. It is most commonly believed to be inherited by a multifactorial threshold model. Classic age at presentation is from 2 weeks to 2 months with a 4:1 male:female ratio. The baby displays nonbloody, nonbilious vomiting yet does not appear ill. The child may appear hungry immediately after emesis. Frequency and intensity of vomiting increases over time to projectile vomiting. Typical laboratory findings include hypochloremic, hypokalemic metabolic alkalosis but delays in diagnosis can result in severe dehydration with prerenal azotemia. **Surgical and anesthetic considerations**: Pyloric stenosis is not a surgical emergency. Treatment consists initially of volume and electrolyte correction along with gastric decompression followed by surgical pyloromyotomy.

The surgical approach may be open or laparoscopic. Regardless of surgical technique, the primary anesthetic concern revolves around the risk of aspiration. Respiratory depression can occur given the metabolic alkalosis resulting from hydrogen ion loss through emesis.

Development of the midgut and associated conditions

Developmental anatomy of the midgut

The midgut extends from the second portion of the duodenum distal to the pancreatic duct caudally to the area of the splenic flexure of the colon. During the 6th to 12th week of development rapid midgut growth occurs. By week 8 of gestation the intestines cannot be contained within the abdominal cavity and herniate through the umbilical ring pulling the superior mesenteric artery (SMA) along its mesentery. The apex of this primitive intestinal loop initially retains connection with the yolk sac. The bowel undergoes an initial 90° counterclockwise rotation followed by further counterclockwise rotation to a total 270° upon return of the intestines to the abdominal cavity. Return of the midgut to the abdomen commences with the small bowel and ends with the colon. This rotation results in a broad-based mesentery extending from the ligament of Treitz to the cecum in the right lower quadrant.

Congenital anomalies of the midgut

Intestinal atresias and stenoses

Midgut atresias (jejunoileal) and stenosis are believed to result from disruptions in vascular supply. Maternal conditions predisposing to thrombosis and maternal use of vasoconstrictors is associated with increased risk of these disorders (6). Atresias are more common than stenoses. Four configurations of jejunoileal atresia are described (Figure 10.1b). Patients present in the first few days of life with bilious vomiting, abdominal distension, and failure to pass meconium. Prenatal diagnoses are rare. Infants are often premature and small for gestational age. **Surgical and anesthetic considerations:** Surgical repair typically consists of resection of the atretic segment and primary anastomosis. In type IIIb and IV, a staged approach may be necessary and the patient is at risk for short bowel syndrome (SBS). Given the uncommon occurrence of associated anomalies in jejunoileal atresias, the anesthesiologist merely has to prepare for a large abdominal case in a small or premature neonate. Vascular access must be sufficient to keep pace with significant third space losses and potential transfusion, allow for arterial or venous blood gas sampling, and possible future need for intravenous hyperalimentation. An epidural may be used to decrease postoperative narcotic requirements in a patient population prone to apnea and bradycardia.

Small intestinal duplication

The small intestine is the most frequent location of duplications (44%) with the ileum most commonly involved (7). Small cystic duplications can act as a lead point for intussuception or volvulus. Larger tubular duplications can cause obstruction. Presence of heterotopic gastric mucosa can cause bleeding, pain, ulceration or perforation. Intestinal atresia is associated with small bowel duplication. **Surgical and anesthetic considerations**: Anesthetic management depends upon the presentation whether it be obstructive symptoms, volvulus, intussusception, or gastrointestinal bleeding and/or perforation. Surgical management is typically excision.

Meckel's diverticulum

During physiologic midgut herniation the primary intestinal loop is composed of a cranial and a caudal loop, the apex of which initially retains connection with the yolk sac by the vitelline (omphalomesenteric) duct. Persistence of this structure results in a Meckel's diverticulum. This is a true diverticulum as it contains all three layers of the bowel wall. The rule of 2s reminds us that this disorder occurs in 2% of the population, the diverticulum is located in the ileum within 2 feet of the ileocecal value, is usually 2 inches long, occurs in males twice as often as females and typically contains two types of heterotopic mucosa: gastric and pancreatic. Many patients are asymptomatic, but those who develop symptoms are usually under the age of 2. Presenting symptoms include painless melena, obstruction, volvulus, intussusception or perforation and may mimic acute appendicitis. The diagnosis can often be made by CT scan or technetium 99m pertechnetate scan which detects ectopic gastric mucosa. **Surgical and anesthetic considerations**: Surgical treatment is resection performed through an open or laparoscopic approach. The anesthetic plan and preparation is related to the patient's presenting symptoms and stability.

Rotational anomalies

Malrotation/nonrotation

Rotational anomalies can present at any time in life or remain asymptomatic. Malrotation, symptomatic or not, is estimated to occur in 1: 500 live births. Symptomatic malrotation occurs in 1: 6000 live births. Physiologic midgut herniation occurs during the 6th to 12th week of gestation. Conditions in which the gut fails to return to the abdominal cavity (gastroschisis, omphalocele, CDH) are by definition malrotated. Intestinal contents which return to the abdomen but completely fail to rotate (nonrotation) result in the small bowel located on the right side of the peritoneal cavity and colon on the left. This configuration results in a short mesenteric base at risk for volvulus. Malrotation is defined as nonrotation of the duodenal limb and partial rotation of the cecocolic limb. The cecum is fixed in the right mid abdomen by thick Ladd's bands. Presenting symptoms of patients with malrotation can be related to obstructive symptoms or ischemia. Obstruction occurs due to duodenal compression caused by Ladd's bands or intermittent volvulus. Ischemia occurs in midgut volvulus when the hypermobile small bowel twists about a short mesenteric base. Midgut volvulus is a life-threatening emergency of closed-loop obstruction and ischemic compromise of the entire small intestine (see below). Approximately 50% of infants with malrotation present within the first month of life with volvulus. Initial signs include abdominal pain and vomiting. Peritonitis, sepsis, and cardiovascular instability are ominous signs of necrotic bowel. Other neonates may present with signs of duodenal obstruction. Older children and adults present with volvulus much less frequently and are more likely to present with abdominal pain and obstructive symptoms (8). **Surgical and anesthetic considerations**: Surgical treatment involves the Ladd procedure which divides the obstructive bands and results in a broader mesenteric base placing the bowel in the position of nonrotation. Placement in the normally rotated position is anatomically impossible. Appendectomy is also performed since appendicitis would present in an atypical manner. The Ladd procedure may be performed via laparoscopy or laparotomy. Patients with suspected midgut volvulus need cardiovascular stabilization and urgent surgery (see midgut volvulus). Patients with incidentally noted malrotation are advised to have corrective surgery to decrease the risk of subsequent volvulus (9).

Situs inversus/situs ambiguus (heterotaxy)

Situs inversus refers to a mirror image arrangement of truncal organs. Situs ambiguus (Heterotaxy) is defined as abnormal development of the truncal organs around the left–right axis of the body. Isomerism refers to the symmetric development of organs which are normally asymmetric and exists along a spectrum with the two extremes being left isomerism (polysplenia syndrome), and right isomerism (asplenia syndrome). Cardiac manifestations occur in 90% of patients with left isomerism and include two morphologic left atria with hypoplastic SA and AV nodes. Extracardiac anomalies in left isomerism include bilobed lungs, interrupted IVC, malrotation, abdominal venous anomalies, extrahepatic biliary atresia, midline liver, and polysplenia. Extrahepatic biliary atresia is strongly associated with polysplenia (10). In 99% of right isomerism cases, patients have severe cardiac lesions including HLHS, TAPVR, and DORV. Extracardiac anomalies include trilobed lungs, malrotation, asplenia, right-sided stomach, and primary ciliary dyskinesia (11). Left–right asymmetry in visceral organ development requires proper motile ciliary function very early in development as cells migrate toward the primitive node (11,12). Many patients with heterotaxy have primary ciliary dyskinesia (PCD). Lateralization defects occur in 1:10 000 live births with a male to female ratio of 2:1. Situs inversus occurs in 67%, right isomerism in 24%, and left isomerism in 9% (13). Survival of heterotaxy patients is related to severity of heart disease and presence of PCD, which can cause severe respiratory compromise (12). Surgeries relating to extracardiac manifestations are complicated from both a surgical perspective due to anatomic challenges and from an anesthetic perspective stemming from management of the cardiac lesion.

Acquired conditions of the midgut

Midgut volvulus

Midgut volvulus is the most feared complication of malrotation and nonrotation. The malrotated gut has a short mesenteric base and lack of cecal fixation. This combination favors clockwise rotation around the axis of the superior mesenteric artery resulting in a high closed loop obstruction and insufficiency of arterial inflow and venous outflow. This leads to ischemia and necrosis of the entire midgut. Infants form 70% of patients presenting with midgut volvulus and most cases of volvulus will present in the first 2 months of life. Initial presentation in infants is vomiting, which may or may not be bilious. Signs of peritonitis, sepsis, and cardiovascular instability are ominous for necrotic bowel. If the diagnosis of volvulus is suspected in the setting of hemodynamic instability, the patient must undergo emergent surgical evaluation and treatment. **Surgical and anesthetic considerations**: Time is of the essence in getting the patient with suspected midgut volvulus to the operating room. Surgical treatment is detorsion followed by a Ladd procedure. Detorsion causes reperfusion of the ischemic gut and can result in hemodynamic decompensation or cardiac arrest. Frankly necrotic bowel must be resected and may result in short bowel syndrome. If the viability of the bowel is in question, the patient may require a second-look laparotomy. Factors increasing mortality from midgut volvulus include presence of necrotic bowel, younger age, and associated anomalies (14). The anesthesiologist must be prepared to conduct RSII due to obstruction. The patient may be hemodynamically decompensated so sufficient vascular access is necessary to be prepared for massive volume resuscitation, arterial blood gas sampling, and infusion of inotropes and vasopressors. Treatment of cardiac arrest due to acidosis and hyperkalemia may become necessary during detorsion of the volvulus. It is helpful for the anesthesiologist to have precalculated code doses of epinephrine, bicarbonate, calcium, insulin, and glucose for expeditious treatment. Blood and blood products should be available given the possibility of disseminated intravascular coagulopathy.

Intussusception

Intussusception refers to the condition in which one portion of the bowel invaginates into itself. Intussusception is the most common cause of bowel obstruction in children between the ages of 6 months to 3 years. Sixty percent of patients present under the age of 1 and 30% present between the ages of 1 and 3 (15). Sixty percent of patients are male. Most cases are considered idiopathic but viral factors likely play a role. Viral and bacterial gastroenteritis can cause hypertrophy of Peyer's patches in the ileum which act as a lead point for the intussusception. Other cases of intussusception can result from lymphoma, Meckel's diverticula, polyps, tumor, hematoma, intestinal duplications, or inspissated bowel contents. Intussusception occurs primarily in the ileocolic region although others areas have been described. The intussusceptum is the proximal bowel which invaginates into the intussuscipiens, the more distal portion of bowel. The mesentery is pulled along resulting in venous and lymphatic obstruction and edema which can cause ischemia and necrosis. The patient presents with intermittent severe crampy abdominal pain increasing in frequency and severity over time. The patient may experience vomiting and pass a bloody mucoid "current jelly" stool. A sausage-shaped mass may be palpable in the right lower quadrant. The diagnosis is made based on clinical suspicion as well as a variety of radiologic studies including barium enema. A classic ultrasonographic sign is the bullseye or target sign representing the layers of bowel within bowel. **Surgical and anesthetic considerations**: Reduction of ileocolic intussusception can occur with hydrostatic pressure during contrast enema with 80% success in patients felt not to have perforation. Recurrence rate is 10%. Operative reduction is reserved for those who have either failed hydrostatic reduction, are unstable with suspected necrosis or perforation, have a nonileocolic intussusception, or suspicion exists for a pathologic leadpoint. The anesthesiologist must be prepared for the patient with possible bowel ischemia with adequate IV access, inotropes, vasopressors, and the possibility of transfusion of blood or blood products. Patients with intussusception are obstructed and require RSII. Surgical reduction consists of manual reduction or resection of the ileocolic segment. Recurrence is extremely low after surgical reduction.

Necrotizing enterocolitis

Necrotizing enterocolitis (NEC) is an inflammatory bowel condition with multifactorial etiology. It is most commonly found in premature neonates but can occur in term babies as well. Contributory factors include ischemia, immunologic immaturity, infection, and an immature mucosal barrier. The typical presentation is a premature formula fed infant who develops symptoms in the second to third week of life. Incidence is inversely related to gestational age and birth weight. Term babies with NEC tend to present earlier in postnatal life than premature infants. Presenting symptoms include vomiting, diarrhea, feeding intolerance associated with abdominal distension, and blood in the stool. As the disease progresses the infant can become lethargic, apneic, hypotensive, and display temperature instability, which can progress to cardiovascular collapse and DIC. Abdominal wall erythema and edema are advanced signs. Abdominal radiographs reveal dilated loops of bowel, thickening of the bowel wall, pneumatosis intestinalis, portal venous gas, ascites, or abdominal free air. Pneumatosis intestinalis is seen in 70–80% of patients with NEC. The terminal ileum and proximal colon are most commonly involved. Disease staging is graded according to the Bell system. Stage I being mild disease treated with conservative measurement and Stage III encompassing severe disease and need for surgical intervention. **Surgical and anesthetic considerations**: Infants requiring surgical intervention are Bell stage III patients. Surgical management includes peritoneal drain under local anesthesia or laparotomy. During laparotomy, the bowel is examined for signs of ischemia and necrosis. Frankly necrotic and perforated areas are resected and either undergo anastomosis or ostomy. If the infant is found to have less than 25% viable bowel treatment options are limited. The mortality rate of NEC totalis is approximately 42–100%. Resection would lead to short bowel syndrome. A recent multicenter randomized trial compared survival in preterm infants with perforated NEC receiving either primary peritoneal drainage or laparotomy with bowel resection. No difference in outcome was found between the two groups (16,17). Anesthetic management of these babies is extremely challenging. Most premature infants have chronic lung disease and many have a patent foramen ovale or patent ductus arteriosus. Vascular access is difficult yet these infants require central lines for both TPN and vasoactive infusions. An arterial line is necessary to monitor hemodynamics, and for titration of vasoactive infusions. Arterial blood gas sampling is necessary to monitor acidosis, adequacy of ventilation, hemoglobin, and coagulation status as well as potassium and calcium, which can be significantly affected by transfusion. The infant also requires IV access adequate for rapid replacement of blood and coagulation factors. Surgery may commence in the ICU for unstable patients or those on HFOV. Long-term complications of NEC include short bowel syndrome, TPN-induced liver disease, stricture formation, fistulae, and intra-abdominal abscess. Overall mortality from NEC is approximately 25% with substantially higher mortality in patients with perforated NEC, NEC totalis, or extremely low birth weight infants (18).

Development of the hindgut and associated conditions

Developmental anatomy of the hindgut

The hindgut is comprised of the splenic flexure of the colon, descending colon, sigmoid, rectum, and upper half of the anal canal. Blood supply originates from the inferior mesenteric artery. In development, the cloaca abuts a shallow depression where endoderm and ectoderm are joined termed the cloacal membrane. The anal canal is composed of both endodermal and ectodermal components which meet at the dentate line, the site of cloacal membrane rupture. The urorectal septum is a mesenchymal structure which grows downward resulting in division of the cloaca to form the bladder anteriorly and the anus posteriorly. The upper half of the anus is formed from endoderm of the cloaca with blood supply from the IMA and the lower half is formed from proctoderm (ectoderm) receiving its blood supply from the internal iliac vessels.

Congenital anomalies of the hindgut

Colonic duplication

See section on duplications. Colonic duplications represent 15% all duplications and tend to be asymptomatic or present with an abdominal mass (7). Cystic duplications can present with fistulous communication to skin, urinary tract, or normal colon. Prevalence of ectopic gastric mucosa is relatively low. Tubular colonic duplications can be associated with duplication of the anus, vagina, penis, or the colon itself. **Surgical and anesthetic considerations**: Surgical excision is typically recommended for duplications but if the colon is normal and the duplication drains well internally, no treatment may be necessary.

Hirschprung disease

Hirschprung disease results from failure of neural crest cells to migrate into the colon to form Meissner's and Auerbach's plexus, typically occurring by the 12th week of gestation. Without these neural elements, smooth muscle is unable to relax and results in colonic spasm causing constipation or obstipation. The missing neural elements extend from the anal sphincter proximally. Most commonly, the aganglionic segment extends to the rectosigmoid, but can involve the entire colon in approximately 5% of cases, or include extension into the small bowel. At least eight genetic mutations have been associated with Hirschprung disease, the most common mutation is in the RET proto-oncogene which encodes a receptor tyrosine kinase involved in growth and differentiation signals. Hirschprung disease occurs in approximately 1–2:10 000 children. In 20–25% of patients with Hirschprung disease there are associated anomalies including trisomy 21, Bardet–Biedel, Smith–Lemli–Opitz, and MEN-2. Kidney and GU anomalies are also common. While short-segment Hirschprung disease occurs with a 3:1 male to female ratio, long-segment Hirschprung disease is associated with a ratio closer to 1:1. Infants present within the first few days of life with failure to pass meconium and signs of distal bowel obstruction. Prolonged retention of colonic contents can cause enterocolitis. The diagnosis is made histologically on a rectal biopsy specimen although supportive radiologic studies can also help elucidate the level of aganglionosis. **Anesthetic and surgical considerations**: Surgical management involves resection of the aganglionic segment and reanastomosis. This may be accomplished as a two-stage procedure; colostomy followed by resection and establishment of continuity, or completed in one single stage. The anesthesiologist should be aware of any associated syndromes and adjust the anesthetic plan accordingly. Additionally the infant may have a full stomach due to bowel obstruction and the presence of a distended abdomen can decrease FRC considerably. Muscle relaxation should be avoided if perineal muscle stimulation testing is planned.

Rectal duplication

Rectal duplications represent 5% of all duplications and are the most common of colonic duplications (7). Presenting symptoms may include constipation or obstipation. **Surgical and anesthetic considerations**: Surgical excision through a transanal, posterior saggital or transcoccygeal approach with drainage and mucosal stripping is the preferred treatment.

Imperforate anus

Imperforate anus results from incomplete separation of the cloaca by the urorectal septum and failure of the cloacal membrane to rupture. This disorder occurs in 1:5000 live births and is slightly more common in boys. Males typically present with a rectourethral fistula and girls with a rectovestibular fistula. Imperforate anus without a fistula is rare (5%) though many of these patients have trisomy 21. In general, higher fistulas are associated with a less well-developed anorectal muscle complex and sacral anomalies and patients without fistulas and those with perineal fistulas typically have a well-developed anorectal muscle complex. More than 50% of patients with imperforate anus have associated anomalies. In general, the higher the fistula, the greater the incidence of associated anomalies. **Surgical and anesthetic considerations**: The goal in repair of imperforate anus is to establish anorectal continuity with continence. A muscle stimulator is used to identify the anorectal muscle complex. Most surgeons favor a posterior saggital approach in which the rectum is mobilized and placed in the center of the muscle complex but patients with very high fistulas may need a combined abdominal–perineal approach and colostomy. The anesthesiologist must be aware of any associated anomalies which may alter anesthetic management. Patients without fistulae will demonstrate intestinal obstruction and will likely have a very distended abdomen causing decreases in FRC. Muscle relaxants must not be used so that surgical electrostimulation may guide the dissection of the muscle complex.

Acquired anomalies of the hindgut

Meconium ileus

Meconium ileus is a condition of distal ileal obstruction due to inspissated meconium. Eighty to ninety percent of these patients have cystic fibrosis (CF) (19). Affected infants present within the first 3 days of life with failure to pass meconium, vomiting, and abdominal distention. Simple meconium ileus consists of obstruction but no complications or associated intestinal pathology. Meconium ileus is complex if associated with volvulus, atresia, perforation, or peritonitis. The diagnosis is made with contrast enema in the absence of perforation. The colon is classically small (disuse microcolon) and the ileum proximal to the plug is dilated. **Surgical and anesthetic considerations**: Hyperosmolar contrast can break up the meconium plug in at least 50% of patients, however perforation is a risk. Patients failing contrast enema resolution or who have complex meconium ileus present for surgery involving enterotomy, irrigation, possible resection of nonviable bowel or repair of perforation. Although most patients have CF, pulmonary manifestations are not yet evident. Anesthetic concerns during surgery deal largely with fluid shifts accompanying bowel surgery, peritonitis, and loss of fluid into the intestinal lumen after attempted hyperosmolar enemas.

Inflammatory bowel disease

Inflammatory bowel disease (IBD) consists of ulcerative colitis (UC) and Crohn's disease (CD). The IBD peak incidence is between the ages of 15–25. Ulcerative colitis involves only the colon continuously from rectum proximally and is confined to the mucosa. Histopathologic findings of UC include crypt abscesses, cryptitis, and mucosal and submucosal inflammation. Ulcerative colitis can be associated with primary sclerosing cholangitis (PSC). Crohn's disease can involve any part of the intestine, may skip areas, and is a full-thickness inflammatory process. Fistula formation is only found in CD. The terminal ileum is the most commonly affected site in CD. Histopathologic findings of CD include transmural lymphoid aggregates, and noncaseating granulomas. Patients with IBD have a history of loose, sometimes bloody stools, abdominal pain, slowing of growth, delayed puberty, fatigue, anemia, and occasionally extraintestinal manifestations. Extraintestinal manifestations occur in approximately 10% of patients with IBD and include uveitis, aphthous ulcers, rash, or arthritis. The diagnosis of IBD can be made from endoscopy and biopsy or endoscopy plus imaging studies. Medical treatment of UC depends on the severity of disease but includes oral or rectal steroids and/or 5-aminosalisylic acid, and in severe cases, immunosuppression with cyclosporine or antiTNF agents. Treatment of CD is similar but involves additional use of 6-MP, azathioprine, methotrexate as well as antiTNF drugs. Risk of colorectal cancer is elevated in both groups after 10 years of disease. **Surgical and anesthetic considerations.** Diagnoses can be made from tissue specimens obtained during endoscopy. Many centers routinely perform upper and lower endoscopy even in the absence of upper gastrointestinal symptoms as CD can present in any area of the GI tract. Colonoscopy performed during acute inflammation of the colon carries a higher risk of perforation. The endoscopist, desires a complete examination including biopsy of the terminal ileum and of each segment of the colon as ileal involvement can exclude UC. See section below on gastrointestinal endoscopy for anesthetic considerations. Patients with UC may present for total proctocolectomy and ileoanal J-pouch. Long-term use of steroids will warrant stress dose steroid administration and can impact wound healing. Patients with CD may present for a variety of surgeries including need for central vascular access, repair of strictures, and obstruction as well as exams under anesthesia for the diagnosis and subsequent treatment of fistulas. These patients also tend to have a history of long-term steroid use and will need stress dosing.

Development of the hepatobiliary system and spleen and associated conditions

Developmental anatomy of the hepatobiliary system

During the fourth week of gestation two buds appear on the ventral wall of the foregut. The more distal bud is termed the hepatic diverticulum. These rapidly proliferating cells penetrate the septum transversum. The connection between the hepatic diverticulum and the foregut narrows into what eventually becomes the common bile duct and the bile duct generates a small diverticulum forming the gallbladder and cystic duct. The ventral mesentery within which the hepatic diverticulum formed and grew becomes the falciform ligament and the area of the septum transversum in direct contact with the liver is known as the bare area of the diaphragm. Every cell within the foregut endoderm has the potential to differentiate into liver tissue but this is inhibited by factors secreted by neighboring tissues. Bone morphogenic protein and fibroblast growth factor 2 act to inhibit inhibitors in hepatic tissue allowing development.

Congenital anomalies of the hepatobiliary system

Biliary atresia

Biliary atresia is a disorder characterized by inflammation and obliteration of the extrahepatic biliary ducts. It can be categorized as isolated nonsyndromic

(84%) or as part of a syndrome, either the heterotaxy/polysplenia syndrome (10%) or associated with cardiac, gastrointestinal, and renal anomalies(6%) (20). The etiology of nonsyndromic biliary atresia remains unknown although histopathologic evidence suggests that a viral, toxic, or immune dysregulatory process is likely. The prevalence is 1:10 000 with females affected more often than males and Asians more than other ethnic groups. Babies are typically born at term. Infants present with jaundice within the first 2 months of life. Laboratory studies reveal conjugated hyperbilirubinemia, increased serum aminotransferases and a disproportionate increase in ductal markers such as GGT or alkaline phosphatase. The work-up and diagnosis includes ultrasound, hepatobiliary scintigraphy revealing failure of excretion, and liver biopsy. Suggestive findings prompt intraoperative cholangiography, liver biopsy, and possible Kasai procedure. **Surgical and anesthetic considerations**: The Kasai portoenterostomy represents the only possibility of surgical cure to restore bile flow for this disorder although it must be performed prior to the establishment of cirrhosis, optimally in the first 2 months of life. A Kasai procedure consists of dissection of the obliterated biliary system to the level of the porta hepatis and placement of a roux limb at this location to restore bile flow. In 60–80% patients there is initial bile flow; however, even if biliary flow is re-established, progressive liver disease may still occur. Timing of portoenterostomy is important with greater success achieved if the intervention occurs within the first month of life. Ultimately more than 50% of patients will fail portoenterostomy and require liver transplantation before the age of 2. Complications seen after portoenterostomy include initial or late failure of bile drainage, cholangitis, and development of portal hypertension. From an anesthetic perspective, Kasai portoenterostomy is performed in the infant or neonate, so all aspects of providing anesthesia to this age group are important. Considerations unique to infants with hepatic dysfunction include a greater propensity to hypoglycemia, and an increased likelihood of bleeding and subsequent need for transfusion. Regional anesthesia is an appealing option however pre-existing coagulopathy may preclude its use and dissection around the liver typically leads to further abnormalities of the coagulation profile. Indications for liver transplantation in patients with biliary atresia include primary failure of bile drainage, failure to thrive, complications of portal hypertension, and refractory coagulopathy.

Alagille syndrome

Alagille syndrome is an autosomal dominant disorder characterized by paucity of intralobular bile ducts causing chronic cholestasis. Patients with Alagille syndrome have been shown to have abnormal villin expression in bile canaliculi and this is felt to be the pathogenetic mechanism of the disease. The prevalence is 1:100 000 live births with females affected slightly more than males. Associated anomalies are very common and include cardiac anomalies (peripheral pulmonic stenosis), vertebral anomalies, dysmorphic facies, other vasculopathies (including CNS) and ocular findings. Treatment is symptomatic and Kasai portoenterostomy is not effective. Twenty percent of children develop progressive liver disease and require transplantation. **Surgical and anesthetic considerations**: Patients with Alagille syndrome may present for interventions related to their associated anomalies such as cardiac catheterization, balloon dilation of pulmonary arteries, and cerebral angiograms. The extent of vasculopathy should be well known prior to referral for liver transplantation (see below) and treated.

Progressive familial intrahepatic cholestasis

Progressive familial intrahepatic cholestasis (PFIC) is a group of three related conditions of chronic cholestasis inherited in an autosomal recessive manner. They present in infancy and childhood with progressive liver disease. The PFIC 1 and PFIC2 conditions are caused by mutations in a protein required for bile formation and export although GGT levels tend to be low. Pruritis is profound and out of proportion to the degree of jaundice. All patients have malabsorption and growth retardation. Patients with PFIC2 can develop hepatocellular carcinoma in childhood. Patients with PFIC3 have abnormalities in hepatocyte phospholipid export resulting in absence of phospholipid in the ductal lumen and damage to the bile ducts. The GGT is elevated in PFIC3. **Surgical and anesthetic considerations**: Medical treatment is generally unhelpful. Some patients undergo partial cutaneous biliary diversion via gallbladder ostomy. It is ineffective if cirrhosis has already developed. Patients with cirrhosis or failed diversion may be candidates for liver transplantation.

Caroli syndrome

Caroli syndrome is a disorder of large intrahepatic ductal ectasia and congenital hepatic fibrosis and is associated with autosomal recessive polycystic kidney disease (ARPKD). Caroli disease refers to intrahepatic ductal dilation without hepatic disease. Mutations in the gene PKHD1 result in defective proteins expressed on the surface of renal tubular cells and cholangiocytes. Pathologic features include hyperplastic biliary epithelium and underdeveloped intrahepatic portal veins. Predominance of renal and/or hepatic disease is variable. Patients can present at any age depending on severity. Common hepatic presentations include multiple bouts of cholangitis due to bile stasis, sequelae of portal hypertension, pruritis, abdominal pain or hepatomegaly. Caroli syndrome is rare affecting 1:100 000 with females affected more often than males. It is inherited in an autosomal recessive fashion. The diagnosis is easily made with ultrasonography, ERCP or MR cholangiography. Treatment is based on relieving symptoms but progressive decline in hepatic function is an indication for liver transplantation. Patients with Caroli syndrome are at an increased risk of cholangiocarcinoma. **Surgical and anesthetic considerations**: Infants and children with Caroli syndrome may require anesthesia for diagnostic studies such as MRI, ERCP or liver biopsy. They may need central venous access for long-term antibiotic therapy or hemodialysis, may require biliary drain placement, nephrectomy, or liver transplantation. The anesthetic plan must take into consideration severity of liver disease and renal disease. Poor hepatic synthetic function results in coagulopathy, low serum albumin, impaired metabolism of drugs metabolized by the P450 system, hypoglycemia, thrombocytopenia due to splenic sequestration, ascites, and reductions in FRC. Excessively large kidneys resulting from ARPKD can also lead to dramatic respiratory impairment. Other sequelae of renal dysfunction include hyperkalemia, anemia, metabolic acidosis, volume overload, impaired excretion of certain drugs, and changes in total body water.

Choledochal cysts

Choledochal cysts are dilatations of the biliary tree of unknown etiology which can present in infancy or adulthood. Five variants have been described (Fig10.1c) by Todani (21). Type I is the most common, affecting 80–90% of patients and consists of a dilatation in the common bile duct. Reported prevalences are variable due to the rarity of the disease. The prevalence is as low as 1:150 000 but is much more common in Asia. Females are affected more often than males with a ratio of 4:1. Choledochal cysts can be associated with a number of other anomalies including ARPKD, biliary atresia, duodenal atresia, colonic atresia, imperforate anus, and absent portal vein. Affected individuals usually present in infancy or childhood. Presenting signs depend on the type of cyst, but symptoms related to obstruction are common such as jaundice, pancreatitis, cholangitis, and a palpable mass. Long- standing or severe disease can result in hepatic damage or cholangiocarcinoma. **Surgical and anesthetic considerations**: The surgical treatment of choledochal cysts is excision with formation of a biliary–enteric anastomosis depending on the type of cyst. Type V (Caroli disease) cannot be excised. Partial excision is not recommended due to increased risk of cholangiocarcinoma. Infants or children with choledochal cysts will often present for central venous catheter placement, diagnostic studies or temporary drainage procedures as well as surgical excision. It is felt that surgery early in life is advantageous in reducing the amount of hepatic damage. Anesthetic concerns deal mostly with associated disorders, impairment of hepatic function, and abdominal surgery in the infant.

Acquired disorders of the hepatobiliary system

Pediatric acute liver failure (**PALF**) is the rapid-onset of hepatic failure in patients with unknown pre-existing liver disease. It is the end result of a variety of disorders resulting in severe hepatic dysfunction and causes dramatic and life-threatening physiologic derangements. Ten to fifteen percent of pediatric patients receiving liver transplants have PALF; 50% of these patients are transplanted without having a readily identified etiology. Virtually every organ system is affected by acute liver failure. The cardiovascular system is hyperdynamic with low systemic vascular resistance often requiring use of vasopressors. Hepatic manifestations include severe jaundice and profound coagulopathy often requiring continuous infusion of plasma and blood. Metabolic derangements include acidosis, hypoglycemia, and other electrolyte abnormalities that may be due to concomitant renal failure. Renal failure occurs in approximately half of all patients with PALF and renal replacement therapy is helpful not only for hemofiltration but also for the volume overload accompanying blood and blood product replacement and intravenous hyperalimentation as well as to reduce serum ammonia levels. Patients with PALF are extremely susceptible to infections which can lead to a systemic inflammatory response syndrome. Neurologic sequelae of acute liver failure can lead to long-term morbidity and death. Hepatic encephalopathy (HE) occurs in at least 50% of patients with PALF. Hyperammonemia results in the development of HE but levels of ammonia do not correlate directly with degree of HE. Cerebral edema complicates severe HE and can lead to hypoxic brain injury, herniation, and death. Current management principles include elevation of the head, avoidance of hypo-osmolarity, hypoxia, hypotension, and control of hyperammonemia (22). In developed countries neonatal hemochromatosis, hepatitis, and metabolic disorders are the most common cause of PALF in the youngest patients whereas autoimmune hepatitis and acetaminophen overdose are the most common causes in older children (23).

Pediatric liver transplantation

Over 500 pediatric liver transplants are performed each year in the USA in patients ranging from neonates to young adults. This population constitutes approximately 10% of all liver transplant candidates. With a critical shortage of donor organs, a new allocation system based on objective data of disease severity was created in 2002 called PELD (pediatric end-stage liver disease). The PELD is used for candidates under the age of 11 and the disease severity score includes bilirubin, INR, serum albumin, age less than 1 year, and growth failure (24). Candidates older than 11 are scored using the adult scoring system called MELD. Candidates are then stratified within PELD for blood type; however, patients with PALF may be listed for all blood types and receive an ABO-incompatible liver. Exceptions to PELD and MELD are Status IA and Status IB. Status IA indicates severe acute liver failure with the likelihood of death in hours or days without transplant. Status IB indicates patients with chronic liver disease and life-threatening complications. Patients with severe metabolic disease but normal liver synthetic function are usually listed as IB since their PELD score would be very low. Children can receive livers from both adult and pediatric deceased donors, liver segments from living donors, or organs procured after circulatory death. Because of size discrepancies, livers often need to be split or reduced in size. 1-year survival rates for children receiving liver transplants are in the range of 80–90%. Indications for liver transplantation include cirrhosis, metabolic disorders, malignancy, and acute liver failure. Disorders causing cirrhosis include biliary atresia, Caroli syndrome, progressive familial intrahepatic cholestasis, primary sclerosing cholangitis and TPN-induced cholestasis. Metabolic disorders include urea cycle defects, amino acidemias and acidurias, glycogen storage disease, hyperoxaluria, familial hypercholesterolemia, Wilson's disease, and alpha 1-antitrypsin deficiency. Malignancies include hepatoblastoma and hepatocellular carcinoma. Biliary atresia is the preoperative diagnosis in 50% of children requiring liver transplantation.

Surgical and anesthetic considerations: Prior to transplantation, the donor liver may need to be split or reduced in size. Liver transplantation progresses through distinct phases including the **preanhepatic phase** in which dissection and ligation of the hepatic artery, portal vein, suprahepatic vena cava, infrahepatic vena cava, and bile duct (or hepatic portoenterostomy) takes place. Removal of the native liver commences the **anhepatic phase**. Use of partial veno–veno bypass during the anhepatic phase is helpful in maintaining preload and limiting bleeding but remains limited to children of approximately 40 kg or larger due to cannula size constraints. After bicaval and portal vein anastomosis the donor liver is **reperfused**. In the **postreperfusion phase** the hepatic artery is anastomosed and the bile duct reconstructed either by a duct-to-duct technique over a T-tube, or through a Roux-en-Y hepaticojejunostomy. Liver segments procured from living donors or left segments from a split liver do not contain a vena cava. In these cases the native vena cava is left intact and the anhepatic phase consists only of anastomosis of the hepatic vein (s) and portal vein. This type of transplant is called a "piggy-back" liver transplant. In cases of retransplantation for hepatic artery thrombosis or in the case of an abnormal or extremely small hepatic artery, the surgeon may choose to perform a supraceliac aortic cross-clamp and proceed with a jump graft to the hepatic artery. Significant vascular anatomic variability exists in patients with biliary atresia and those with heterotaxy including a replaced right hepatic artery, preduodenal portal vein, absent portal vein, and interrupted inferior vena cava. Anesthetic concerns are considerable and vary depending on the recipient's underlying disease process. The anesthesiologist must have a thorough understanding of the preoperative diagnosis and management of the disorder. The surgical team must transmit information about the donor including whether the donor liver is of the same blood type as the recipient, whether the organ was procured after circulatory death, or if the donor liver has had significant warm or cold ischemic time. General goals of the preanhepatic phase include a safe induction, securing the airway, adequate ventilation, and plentiful vascular access. Central venous access is necessary for infusion of vasoactive infusions and concentrated dextrose solutions as well as for measurement of central venous pressure. Reliable large-bore short intravenous catheters are essential for administration of crystalloid, blood, and blood products. The anesthesiologist must be prepared with enough intravenous access to keep pace with massive and sudden blood loss which can occur at any time during the transplant. Lower extremity access is suboptimal given that the vena cava will be clamped periodically throughout the case and is subject to surgical trauma. Arterial catheters are necessary for pressure monitoring as well as frequent arterial blood gas sampling. Femoral catheters are more resistant to dampening during extreme vasoconstriction but are useless during aortic clamping. Radial arterial lines may be used alone or in conjunction with femoral arterial access. The anesthesiologist should strive for normothermia, euvolemia, normoglycemia, correction of acidosis, adequate urine output, and serum potassium less than 4 mEq/l in preparation for reperfusion. The anhepatic phase is characterized by fibrinolysis and the accrual of acidosis. The patient's core body temperature will drop between one and two degrees centigrade with placement of the iced organ in the peritoneal cavity. With the exception of exsanguinating hemorrhage, reperfusion represents the phase in which the patient is most likely to suffer the greatest hemodynamic perturbation. Even if the liver has been flushed, reperfusion will result in wash-out of cold fluid which may contain end products of ischemia including organic acids and potassium, particularly if the liver was procured from a donor after circulatory death. Donor livers with a cut edge can bleed profusely. Preparations must be made for high-volume resuscitation and treatment of hyperkalemia and acidosis both of which can cause cardiac arrest and can be exacerbated by rapid transfusion. Steroids are frequently given prior to or after reperfusion. The combination of steroids and a properly functioning liver can result in profound hyperglycemia. The post-reperfusion phase can be characterized by ongoing coagulopathic bleeding combined with high insensible and third-space losses. In replacing blood loss and third-space fluids care must be taken to avoid volume overloading the liver. This can result in a tight abdominal closure causing ischemic necrosis of the liver and ventilatory impairment. Osmotic diuresis due to glycosuria coupled with third-space losses can result in dramatic hemoconcentration. Hemoconcentration and overzealous correction of coagulopathy in the absence of pathologic bleeding can predispose to hepatic artery thrombosis (HAT). Hepatic artery thrombosis is a major potential complication of pediatric liver transplantation and rapid normalization of INR as well as polycythemia may predispose to a prothrombotic state. These general anesthetic management principles hold for most pediatric liver transplants. Given the diverse population of liver transplant candidates, certain conditions warrant unique and special management techniques. **Cirrhosis:** The patient with cirrhosis and portal hypertension will have difficulty maintaining normoglycemia and require a continuous dextrose infusion. One can expect coagulopathic bleeding and great care must be taken during invasive line placement. Clamping of the vena cava may precipitate variceal bleeding and may necessitate placement of a Blakemore tube. Octreotide infusion may help to decrease portal hypertension. **Metabolic disorders of the urea cycle** include carbamyl phosphate synthetase 1 deficiency, ornithine transcarbamylase deficiency, argininosuccinate synthetase deficiency, argininosuccinate lyase deficiency, and *N*-acetyl glutamate synthetase deficiency. All are characterized by defective breakdown of nitrogen into urea for excretion and result in hyperammonemia. Hyperammonemia causes profound neurologic damage in proportion to the degree of elevated ammonia and time spent in hyperammonemic crisis. These patients have no coagulopathy since liver synthetic function is normal with the exception of the genetically missing enzyme. Key elements include continuous infusion of ammonia scavenging drugs and strict avoidance of catabolism by continuous dextrose infusion and lipids. Catabolism results in muscle breakdown and increased nitrogen production. Ammonia scavenging drugs are dessicants with multiple incompatibilities, which can impact the degree of central access required. **Metabolic disorders of amino acid metabolism** result from either accumulation of amino acids in the plasma or accumulation of organic acid metabolites and increased excretion of amino acids in the urine (maple syrup urine disease, methylmalonic aciduria, proprionic acidemia). Patients tend to have anion gap acidosis, hyperammonemia, and ketosis. The intraoperative anesthetic management of these disorders is very similar to management to the urea cycle defects in avoidance of catabolic states and provision of glucose substrate but require correction of metabolic acidosis. The specialty physician primarily managing the disorder will have specific recommendations for appropriate ammonia-scavenging drugs, correction of acidosis, and optimal glucose infusion rates. **Primary hyperoxaluria** results from defects in glyoxylate metabolism and overproduction of oxalate which results in calcium oxalate deposition, most notably in the kidneys. Patients may require either liver transplantation alone to correct the defect or combined liver–kidney transplantation if significant renal oxalosis is present. Anesthetic management requires consideration of intraoperative renal replacement therapy, concern for volume overload, and hyperkalemia. Delay in diagnosis of primary hyperoxaluria can result in widespread systemic deposition of oxalate causing cardiac conduction defects and vasculopathy. Some patients require aggressive preoperative dialysis to reduce systemic oxalate levels. **Hepatoblastoma** patients sometimes present for liver transplantation if the tumor is nonmetastatic and unresectable or resistant to chemotherapy. Such patients are often thrombocytopenic and anemic as a result of chemotherapy. Cisplatin, the primary chemotherapeutic agent, can cause nephrotoxicity. **Pediatric acute liver failure** requires many of the same anesthetic management techniques as described above but with extra attention given to the management of cerebral edema. Dextrose infusions are necessary but after administration of steroids and reperfusion, one must avoid hyperglycemia given the deleterious effects it may have on the potentially ischemic brain and insulin infusion may be necessary. Ketamine should be avoided due to its increase in cerebral metabolic oxygen demand. The anesthesiologist should avoid placing the patient in steep Trendelenburg position for any extended period of time. Placement of central venous lines in bilateral jugular veins may increase cerebral venous pressure and should be avoided if possible. Patients in renal failure may require continuous renal replacement therapy during transplant surgery though vascular access sites are limited and challenging due to edema. **Special transfusion considerations**: Many components of blood are given during a liver transplant. Rapid transfusion of packed red blood cells can result in profound hyperkalemia and hemodynamically significant hypocalcemia in young children. Several factors contribute to higher potassium levels in banked blood including prolonged storage and irradiation. Potassium-reducing strategies include utilization of washed units of blood or nonirradiated freshest blood (less than 5 days old). Limitations of washed units include time required to wash the unit, inability to return the washed unit, and the fact that after 6 hours, washed units contain higher levels of potassium than prior to washing (25). In cases of PALF, in which patients may be open to all blood groups, preoperative use of AB-negative plasma may be useful to avoid antibodies directed against the donor liver. In the operating room plasma compatible with both donor liver and recipient blood type must be used. Infectious disease considerations usually require CMV-negative blood products although red blood cells which have been filtered and designated "leukoreduced" are a proxy for CMV negative products. Irradiation of blood destroys the ability of passenger leukocytes to proliferate, which can cause transfusion-associated graft-versus-host disease (TA-GVHD). TA-GVHD is of greatest concern in premature infants and patients with stem cell transplants. The risk of TA-GVHD is more theoretical in children immunosuppressed for solid organ transplant and chemotherapy.

Complications of liver transplantation

Complications of liver transplantation include technical issues, drug-related problems, and complications related to immunosuppression. Technical complications include biliary leak and stricture and hepatic artery thrombosis (HAT). Acute HAT is the most serious complication often leading to immediate relisting as IA. Thrombolysis and anticoagulation are usually unsuccessful in treating HAT. Hepatic artery anastomoses of diameter < 3mm are at greatest risk. Drug-related complications of calcineurin inhibitors (tacrolimus) include nephrotoxicity and seizures.

Immunosuppression related complications include infection, rejection, and cancer. Fungal infections are common in the immediate post-transplant period, but thereafter viral infections predominate. Epstein–Barr virus (EBV) in particular is worrisome since it is associated with post-transplant lymphoproliferative disease (PTLD). This is a form of B-cell hyperproliferation which affects 6–20% of transplant patients. It is seen most commonly in the first few years after transplantation and is strongly related to EBV seroconversion combined with immunosuppression. Treatment is aimed at reducing immunosuppression. The prognosis is varied but is worse with CNS PTLD, nonEBV PTLD, and late-onset PTLD. Graft loss is a risk of treatment.

Development of the abdominal wall and body cavities

Developmental anatomy of the abdominal wall

The embryonic mesoderm appears in the 3rd week of development after formation of the embryonic ectoderm and endoderm. Embryonic ectodermal cells from the primitive knot migrate between the ectoderm and endoderm extending anteriorly, posteriorly, medially, and laterally from the notochord. Two areas devoid of mesodermal infiltration are the buccopharyngeal membrane cranially and the cloacal membrane caudally. The embryonic mesoderm then differentiates into a paraxial mesoderm from which somites are derived and a lateral mesoderm which splits to form somatic and splanchnic layers. These layers enclose the body cavity and eventually become the pleural and peritoneal cavities. Somites derived from the paraxial mesoderm further differentiate into skin, subcutaneous tissues, and muscle. Between the 6th to 12th week of development the primary intestinal loop undergoes physiologic herniation into the umbilical cord. Subsequent expansion of the peritoneal cavity permits the intestinal loops to return to the abdomen.

Congenital anomalies of abdominal wall development

Gastroschisis

Gastroschisis is a full-thickness defect in the abdominal wall to the right lateral side of the umbilicus with evisceration of intestine. The most commonly accepted etiologic hypothesis is a vascular event interrupting blood flow through either the umbilical vein or omphalomesenteric artery. Other theories exist including mesodermal failure in the anterior abdominal wall, rupture of the amnion around the umbilical ring, abnormal involution of the right umbilical vein, and abnormal infolding of the body wall (26). The defect through which the bowel is herniated is typically small posing a significant risk of ischemia. Malrotation/nonrotation exists and associated intestinal atresias and stenoses can occur in 10–25% of infants (27). Gastroschisis is classified as simple or complex based on the presence or absence of atresias and stenoses, volvulus, compromised bowel, or perforation. Exposure to amniotic fluid causes the bowel to become thickened, edematous, and display delayed motility. Exclusive of gastrointestinal abnormalities, other associated anomalies are rare. Babies with gastroschisis tend to be small for gestational age and are frequently premature. Reported prevalence of gastroschisis is highly variable depending on the source, but occurs roughly in 1:2000 live births with increasing incidence (28). **Surgical and anesthetic considerations:** This condition warrants urgent protection and coverage of abdominal contents to reduce third-space and evaporative losses. Evaporative losses can be profound and lead to hypovolemia, hypothermia, and acidosis. The gut is also at high risk for vascular compromise from volvulus or incarceration. Reduction of abdominal contents can occur immediately after birth or as a delayed primary closure after silo reduction. Anesthetic concerns include management of transitional circulation, control of aspiration risk requiring RSII, and fluid management. Vascular access must be sufficient to keep pace with the 10–100 cc/kg/h insensible loss which is associated with this disorder. Invasive blood pressure monitoring may be warranted and allow frequent sampling of acid–base status, hemoglobin level, and blood glucose. Delayed function of the thickened edematous bowel occurs and central access is necessary for administration of parenteral nutrition. In both gastroschisis and omphalocele, the notion of lost abdominal domain may be significant and preclude complete reduction of abdominal contents. Small amounts of extruded bowel may be closed primarily but larger reductions may warrant placement of a spring-loaded silastic silo. This allows gradual reduction of abdominal contents as permitted by expansion of the abdominal cavity and definitive closure can commence as an elective procedure. Primary closures under tension can lead to abdominal compartment syndrome, renal compromise, bowel necrosis, and pulmonary insufficiency. Clinicians must be aware of volvulus risk and bowel compromise. Several multicenter studies of primary closure vs. silo reduction and closure have failed to show significant differences in time on ventilator, time to reach full enteral feeds, length of stay, and complications (29,30). Survival rates overall are greater than 90% with most morbidity and mortality in those with complex gastroschisis.

Omphalocele

Omphalocele results from failure of the intestinal loops to return to the peritoneal cavity in embryonic development. The prevalence of this disorder is 1:5000 live births and is associated with other anomalies in over 50% of cases. Most common associated anomalies include cardiac defects, other midline defects, chromosomal abnormalities (trisomy 13, 18, and 21), and Beckwith–Wiedemann syndrome (macrosomia, macroglossia, visceromegaly, neonatal hypoglycemia). Males are affected more often than females. The majority of cases are diagnosed prenatally and the infant presents with herniated bowel covered by the two-layered amnionic–peritoneal membrane (unless ruptured) with insertion of the umbilical at the apex of the sac. By definition, the gut is nonrotated. As only the midgut undergoes physiologic herniation, liver should not be present in the sac. If, however, the embryologic lateral folds fail to close, the liver may be present. This is termed giant omphalocele. The size of the omphalocele defect is not directly related to presence of associated anomalies; in fact, the converse is true. **Surgical and anesthetic considerations**: Surgical treatment consists of immediate closure, staged closure, or delayed closure. As long as the omphalocele sac is not ruptured, urgent surgical intervention is not indicated and the infant can be evaluated for associated anomalies. The omphalocele sac acts as a silo and if the amount of herniated bowel is small, immediate reduction is possible. The anesthetic management is highly dependent on the management of coexisting anomalies, particularly complex cardiac anomalies. Infants with Beckwith–Wiedemann syndrome can have difficult airways due to macroglossia and require close monitoring of serum glucose.

Prune belly syndrome (PBS)

Also known as Eagle–Barrett syndrome, PBS is a congenital disorder named for its characteristic wrinkled-appearing abdominal wall consisting of abdominal wall muscle deficiency, urinary tract abnormalities, and undescended testicles (in males). This condition occurs with a frequency of 3.8:100 000 live births and occurs almost exclusively in males. The etiology is largely unknown but a genetic basis is likely. The histopathology of the abdominal wall suggests mesodermal developmental arrest. Oligohydramnios is common during the pregnancy causing a restrictive uterine environment with resultant lung hypoplasia and orthopedic abnormalities (scoliosis and congenital hip dysplasia). Trisomy 18 and 21 are common as well as GU, GI (malrotation, stenoses, and atresias) and cardiac anomalies (TOF and VSD) (31). Of the urinary tract anomalies, obstruction is most common and occurs as distal as the urethra or as proximal as the UPJ. Megaurethra and megacystis is common. Renal dysplasia can occur due to reflux nephropathy. Some patients develop end-stage renal disease, requiring dialysis or transplantation. Complications of deficient abdominal wall musculature include poor pulmonary hygiene due to ineffective cough and constipation related to the inability to elevate intra-abdominal pressure during defecation. **Surgical and anesthetic considerations**: PBS has a relatively high mortality rate, particularly in the neonatal period so the decision to aggressively treat associated conditions is predicated on the patient's stability and overall prognosis (32). Children with PBS may present for correction of cryptorchidism, abdominal wall reconstruction, percutaneous nephrostomy, pyeloplasty, vesicostomy, ureteral reimplantation, peritoneal or hemodialysis access, or to correct other associated anomalies. Anesthetic concerns will be related primarily to respiratory care in the operative and immediate postoperative period given the lack of effective cough mechanism. Use of regional anesthesia is possible if not contraindicated and can help reduce postoperative respiratory depression and constipation.

Inguinal hernias

Virtually all inguinal hernias in children are indirect hernias. Inguinal hernias are extremely common and affect 1–5% of all babies. Males are affected much more often than females and premature infants are

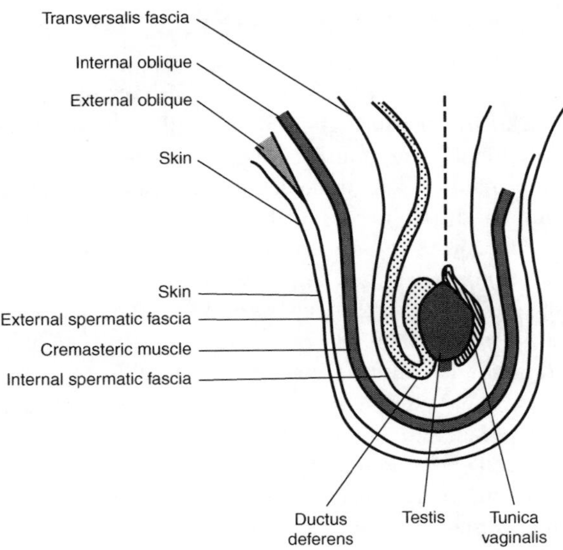

Figure 10.2 Scrotal anatomy.

affected more often than term babies. In embryonic development the testes are attached to the posterior abdominal wall. The gubernaculum guides descent of the testes through the muscles of the abdominal wall and into the scrotum through an evagination of the peritoneal cavity called the processus vaginalis. Because the processus vaginalis traverses the abdominal wall layers, the testes are sheathed by tissues that correspond directly to these layers. The testes first are covered by reflected peritoneal folds called the tunica vaginalis. The transversalis fascia becomes the internal spermatic fascia, the internal oblique becomes the cremasteric fascia and muscle, and the external oblique forms the external spermatic fascia (see Figure 10.2). The testes retain their blood supply from the abdominal aorta. The connection between the processus vaginalis and the abdominal cavity is normally obliterated before birth but, if patent, intestinal contents may descend into the inguinal canal and scrotum. In females the gubernaculum guides descent of the ovaries. The lower portion of the gubernaculum forms the round ligament and traverses the inguinal canal ending in the labia majora. In both males and females the left canal closes first. It is logical, then, that hernias are more common on the right, in premature infants, and in males. Inguinal hernias present with a bulge in the inguinal region or as scrotal swelling which appears during straining and reduces when relaxed or recumbent. Hernias are not painful unless incarcerated. Incarcerated hernias are an indication for urgent surgery since the bowel is at risk for necrosis. Incarceration risk is higher in the first 6 months of life, in premature infants, girls, and on the right side. **Surgical and anesthetic considerations**: Inguinal hernias in children do not spontaneously resolve, therefore elective repair is scheduled once the diagnosis is made. Risk of incarceration and strangulation always exist. Herniorraphy can be accomplished as an open or laparoscopic procedure. Laparoscopy mandates intubation whereas open repair can be accomplished with caudal or spinal anesthesia alone. The patient presenting for reduction and repair of an incarcerated hernia will likely require intubation due to bowel obstruction. If signs of strangulation are present the anesthesiologist must be prepared to resuscitate the patient. Hemodynamic compromise can occur due to third- space fluid losses from edematous bowel and bowel obstruction as well as wash-out of ischemic bowel upon reduction and reperfusion. The family should be counseled appropriately preoperatively for the chance of delayed extubation and hemodynamic instability.

Developmental Anatomy of the diaphragm

The diaphragm derives in large part from the embryonic septum transversum during the 7th to 10th week of gestation. The septum transversum originates from cervical myotomes 3,4, 5, which explain the innervation of the diaphragm and location of referred diaphragmatic irritation to the shoulder. Growth of the septum transversum and medial migration of the pleuroperitoneal membranes fusing with the septum transversum and the dorsal mesentery of the esophagus (crura) leads to separation of the pleuroperitoneal canal and formation of the intact diaphragm.

Congenital anomalies of the diaphragm

Congenital diaphragmatic hernia (CDH)

The condition of CDH results from incomplete fusion of the pleuroperitoneal membranes with the septum transversum leading to persistence of the pleuroperitoneal canal and subsequent herniation of abdominal contents into the developing thorax. Congenital diaphragmatic hernia occurs either posterolaterally through the foramen of Bochdalek or anteriorly in the parasternal location, through the foramen of Morgagni. Ninety percent of cases involve herniation posterolaterally on the left. Varying amounts of abdominal contents are displaced into the affected thorax. Herniation occurs during a critical period of pulmonary arterial and bronchoalveolar branching, therefore the lung on the affected side can be severely hypoplastic and the pulmonary arteries have muscular hyperplasia (33). The contralateral lung may also be underdeveloped due to mediastinal shift. One very rare variant of diaphragmatic hernia is the pentalogy of Cantrell consisting of a cleft sternum, ectopia cordis, epigastric omphalocele, parasternal diaphragmatic hernia, and intrinsic cardiac anomalies. The prevalence of CDH is approximately 2.6:10 000 live births with a slight male preponderance. In 50% of cases there are associated anomalies including congenital heart disease, neural tube defects, and chromosomal abnormalities. A prenatal diagnosis is often made. Newborns display respiratory distress with absent breath sounds over one hemithorax. The infant has a barrel-shaped chest and a scaphoid abdomen. Chest X-ray confirms the presence of abdominal contents in the thorax. Initial treatment includes immediate intubation and gastric decompression. Positive-pressure mask ventilation can result in gastric distention which further impairs oxygenation and ventilation. Arterial and venous access should be obtained to support blood pressure with inotropic support if necessary. Ventilator strategies aimed at reducing barotrauma favor peak pressures less than 25 cmH_2O and physiologic levels of PEEP. Although alkalosis, hypocapnia, and avoidance of hypoxia are normally employed to reduce pulmonary hypertension, the primary ventilatory strategy is to avoid barotrauma. Permissive hypercapnea, use of nitric oxide, and alternative ventilator strategies such as HFOV and ECMO are often employed (34). Indications for ECMO vary between institutions, but typically include the inability to maintain adequate oxygenation with gentle ventilation strategies, refractory hypotension, and hypoxia associated with acidosis. **Surgical and anesthetic considerations**: The timing for correction of CDH is deferred until the patient is stabilized on a regimen of gentle ventilation and control of pulmonary hypertension. Surgical reduction of CDH and repair/reconstruction of the diaphragm can be accomplished on or off ECMO. The diaphragm may be approached from either a thoracic incision or abdominal incision utilizing open or laparoscopic/thoracoscopic technique. Loss of abdominal domain can be problematic and the use of silo has been reported (35). Anesthetic management is challenging from the perspective of ventilation and control of pulmonary hypertension. Neuromuscular blockade is helpful and an opioid-based technique can be helpful in controlling pulmonary hypertension. Preductal and postductal oxygen saturation should be monitored. Epidural anesthesia, if not contraindicated, can be useful postoperatively. Great care must be taken to avoid bubbles in the IV since a patent foramen ovale or ductus arteriosus is at high risk for right-to-left shunting. Continuing gentle ventilation can be difficult when laparoscopy is used due to increases in CO_2 induced by laparoscopy or thoracoscopy. The anesthesiologist should never attempt to "reinflate" the hypoplastic lung. Pneumothorax of the more well-developed lung is possible and should be considered in cases of acute decompensation. Pulmonary hyptertensive crisis is another cause of acute decompensation. Postreduction ventilation can be compromised by tight abdominal closure. Overall survival rate is 65% but prognostic factors predicting lower survival rates include presence of the liver in the left thorax, low lung to head ratio, right-sided diaphragmatic defects, and presence of abnormal karyotype or severe cardiac defects (36,37). Long-term complications include neurologic deficits, hearing impairment, and gastrointestinal complications such as GERD.

Morbid obesity

Obesity in children is defined using the BMI growth curve since growth patterns change the height to weight ratio. Children are considered overweight if they are between the 85th to 95th percentile on the BMI growth curve. Obesity is defined as greater than the 95th percentile on the BMI growth curve. Any value greater than the 99th percentile is termed extreme obesity, which correlates with adult standards of a BMI greater than 40. The adult BMI scale is sometimes applied to older teens considering bariatric surgery since it correlates with conservative selection. A recent survey revealed that from 2009–2010 31.8% of children ages 2–19 were overweight or obese, 16.9% were obese, and 12.3% had a BMI greater than the 97th percentile (38). Comorbidities of obesity are significant including obstructive sleep apnea, metabolic syndrome and Type II diabetes, hypertension, hypertrophic cardiac disease, non-alcoholic fatty liver, and depression. Bariatric surgery in adults has demonstrated success in producing significant reductions in BMI and decreases in obesity-related comorbidities (39). Behavioral therapies and dietary modifications are relatively ineffective for long-term weight loss in severely obese teens. **Surgical and anesthetic considerations**: Selection of teens appropriate for bariatric surgery should be based on evaluation by a multidisciplinary team. Rapid weight loss can inhibit statural growth so selected patients should be within 95% of their predicted adult height based on bone age. Other criteria include BMI greater than 40 kg/m^2 with minor comorbidities or BMI of 35 kg/m^2 and severe comorbidities such as type II diabetes, pseudotumor cerebri, AHI $>$ 15 or severe fatty liver (40). The most commonly used surgical approaches are either restrictive procedures such as the laparoscopic adjustable gastric band or sleeve gastrectomy, combined restrictive and malabsorptive techniques such as the Roux-en-Y gastric bypass or creation of a malabsorptive environment via biliopancreatic diversion. Laparoscopic surgery has great benefit in minimizing postoperative discomfort and recovery time. Anesthetic concerns are significant. Intravenous access can be difficult. Contrary to popular belief, most obese individuals are not difficult to intubate provided they are positioned properly on a ramp (41). Intraoperative use of PEEP and recruitment maneuvers can help prevent atelectasis. Use of insoluble and short-acting anesthetics such as desflurane and remifentanil may help to achieve prompt awakening after surgery. Alpha-2-agonists can also reduce anesthetic requirements with minimal respiratory depression postoperatively. Maximizing nonopoid analgesics such as ketorolac and acetaminophen may reduce the need for long-acting narcotics (42). Drug dosing in the morbidly obese is complex and depending on the drug, dosing should be based on lean body weight, total body weight, or ideal body weight (43). Various comorbidities will dictate the conduct of anesthesia but the presence of OSA warrants close monitoring in the immediate postoperative period. Use of CPAP in OSA patients postoperatively has been postulated to increase the risk of anastomotic leak; however, numerous studies have not shown this complication (44,45).

Gastrointestinal endoscopy

Gastrointestinal endoscopy is used for a variety of diagnostic and therapeutic procedures. Esophagogastroduodenoscopy (EGD) is used to diagnose conditions of the esophagus, stomach, and proximal small bowel and biopsies are frequently taken. Therapeutic procedures include removal of foreign bodies from the esophagus or stomach, dilation of esophageal strictures, banding, and injection of esophageal varices, control of upper GI bleeding, botulinum toxin injection, and placement of gastrostomy tubes. Endoscopic retrograde cholangiopancreatography (ERCP) is similarly used for diagnosis of biliary and pancreatic disorders as well as therapeutic sphincterotomy and placement of biliary stents. The ERCP is usually used in conjunction with fluoroscopy. Colonoscopy is used to diagnose disorders of the anus, rectum, colon, and distal small bowel. Therapeutic procedures include polypectomy, control of GI bleeding, banding of varices, and occasionally reduction of sigmoid volvulus. **Anesthetic considerations**: Anesthesia for endoscopic procedures varies tremendously depending on the patient's underlying condition and age encompassing moderate sedation to general anesthesia. The EGD requires sharing the airway with the endoscopist but does not always require intubation. Patients and procedures warranting intubation include severe GERD, severe OSA or lung disease, procedures requiring protection of the airway such as control of upper GI bleeding, placement of gastrostomy tubes, extraction of foreign bodies, achalacia, procedures requiring unusual positioning which may render the airway inaccessible, and patients with severely compromised FRC such as neonates, infants, and the morbidly obese. Cardiorespiratory problems are the most common complication during upper endoscopy in both children and adults most notably hypoxia (46). The anesthesiologist must be very vigilant about the airway when administering sedation or general anesthesia for upper endoscopy. Intravenous anesthesia in the nonintubated patient may be more desirable to avoid anesthetic vapor contamination. A thorough examination of the mouth for loose teeth, dental or orthodontic appliances, and oral piercings is warranted as the procedure can cause dislodgement. Passage of the upper endoscope through the cricopharyngeus is the most stimulating part of diagnostic upper endoscopy. Inexperienced endoscopists can cause massive gastric distention with air which severely impacts spontaneous as well as mechanical ventilation particularly in patients with marginal pulmonary reserve. Elevation of the diaphragm can cause an endotracheal tube to migrate into the right mainstem bronchus or abut

Table 10.1 Table of gastrointestinal anomalies

Condition	Etiology	Prevalence (live births)	M:F	Associated anomalies	Other
TEF	Faulty formation of esophagotracheal septum	2:10 000	$M \geq F$	Trisomy 13,18,21, VATER/VACTERL, CHARGE, cardiac, renal/GU	Mortality related to underlying anomalies
Duplications	Split notochord vs. partial twinning	1:4500	$M > F$	Esophageal: vertebral anomalies Small bowel: atresias Colonic: GU duplications	Small bowel is the most common site
Pyloric atresia	Recanalization failure	1:100 000	$M = F$	EB Simplex, JEB, aplasia cutis congenital, other intestinal atresias	Often SGA. Prognosis related to other diagnoses
Duodenal atresia	Recanalization failure	1:10 000	$M \geq F$	Trisomy 21, annular pancreas, malrotation, cardiac anomalies	Mortality related to cardiac disease
Annular pancreas	Failure of ventral pancreatic bud rotation	Rare	$M < F$	> 70% trisomy 21 Duodenal atresia, GI, Cardiac anomalies	
Pyloric stenosis	Unknown	2–4:1000	4:1	None	
Jejunoileal atresia	In utero vascular events	1:3000		Gastroschisis, malrotation	Infants premature and SGA
Meckel's diverticulum	Persistence of vitelline duct. True diverticulum	2:100	2:1	Rare	
Intestinal malrotation	Faulty return of intestinal contents during physiologic midgut herniation	1:500 1:6000 symptomatic	2:1 in infancy	30–60% associated anomalies. Abdominal wall defects, CDH, atresias, Meckel's, Hirschprung, imperforate anus, EA/TEF, biliary atresia, PBS, cardiac, situs anomalies	Many asymptomatic
Heterotaxy syndrome	Errors in lateralization of endodermal and mesodermal structures	1:10 000	2:1	L: 90% cardiac. Biliary atresia, malrotation, polysplenia R: 99% cardiac, malrotation, asplenia	Mortality related to cardiac lesions
Hirschprung disease	Migrational failure of neural crest cells	2:10 000	3:1 short 1:1 long	20–25% have associated anomalies: Trisomy 21, Smith–Lemli-Opitz, Bardet Biedel, kidney/GU anomalies, MEN-2, Waardenburg syndrome	
Imperforate anus	Faulty separation of cloaca by urorectal septum. Failed rupture of cloacal membrane	1:4000	$M \geq F$	50% associated anomalies. Trisomy 21, VATER/VACTERL, cardiac, GU	Rectourethral fistula in boys Rectovestibular fistula in girls Higher fistula = more anomalies

Table 10.1 *(cont.)*

Condition	Etiology	Prevalence (live births)	M:F	Associated anomalies	Other
Gastroschisis	Failure of body wall closure. Possible vascular accident	5:10 000	M ≥ F	10–20% have associated anomalies, mostly GI tract atresias	Many premature and SGA. Survival > 90% in the absence of catastrophic bowel loss
Omphalocele	Failure of intestines to return to abdomen	2:10 000	M > F	50% have chromosomal defects. 80% with normal karyotype have anomalies	Mortality dependent on associated anomalies
Prune belly syndrome (PBS)	Abnormal mesodermal development of abdominal wall	3.8:100 000	M >>>F	Renal dysplasia & cryptorchidism. Lung hypoplasia, Trisomy 18, 21. GI 30%, cardiac 10%, orthopedic 50%	Mortality 30%
Indirect hernia	Patent processus vaginalis	1–5:100	4–8:1		R > L. Preemies > term
CDH	Failure of pleuroperitoneal membranes to close	2.6:10 000	M > F	50% have associated anomalies. Neural tube defects, cardiac defects, Beckwith–Wiedemann syndrome	Mortality 30–40%. Worse prognosis: R defect, liver in defect, cardiac and chromosomal anomalies, low lung: head ratio
Biliary atresia	Inflammatory destruction of extrahepatic bile ducts. Toxic, viral	1:10 000	M < F	None in nonsyndromic. Syndromic: cardiac, GU, heterotaxy polysplenia	More common in Asians
Alagille syndrome	Genetic absence of villin expression in bile canaliculi	1:100 000	M < F	Peripheral pulmonic stenosis, butterfly vertebrae, ocular findings, dysmorphic facies, vasculopathy	
Caroli syndrome	Mutation of PKHD1: defective proteins on renal tubular cells & cholangiocytes	1:100 000	M < F	ARPKD	
Choledochal cysts	Unknown	1:150 000	1:4	ARPKD, biliary atresia, duodenal atresia, colonic atresia, imperforate anus, absent portal vein	More common in Asians

the carina resulting in severe bronchospasm and desaturation. If a significant amount of gastric air migrates past the pylorus, postoperative respiratory status may be compromised. Balloon dilation of esophageal strictures can be very stimulating while the balloon is inflated and is associated with post-operative nausea and vomiting (PONV). The ERCP typically requires intubation in children due to prone positioning and the anesthesiologist may be physically distant from the child during fluoroscopy. Sphincterotomy is also associated with PONV. Lower endoscopy is usually well tolerated but looping of the endoscope can result in vagal responses.

References

1. T.L. Spilde, A.M. Bhatia, J.K. Marosky, *et al.* Fibroblast growth factor signaling in the developing tracheoesophageal fistula. *J Pediatr Surg* 2003; **38**: 474–7.
2. R.E. Gross. *The Surgery of Infancy and Childhood.* Philadelphia, PA: WB Saunders, 1953, p.76.
3. M.J.G Andriessen, L.E. Matthyssens, H.A. Heij. Pyloric atresia. *J Pediatr Surg* 2010; **45**: 2470–2.
4. N.J. Zyromski, J.A. Sandoval, H.A. Pitt, *et al.* Annular pancreas: Dramatic differences between children and adults. *J Am Coll Surg* 2008; **206**: 1019–25.
5. B. Rybojad, G. Niedzielska, A. Niedzielski, E. Rudnicka-Drozak, R. Rybojad. Esophageal foreign bodies in pediatric patients: A thirteen-year retrospective study. *Sci World J* 2012; 102642. doi:. Epub 2012 Apr 19.
6. J.H. Hersh, Angle B, Fox TL, *et al.* Developmental field defects: coming together of associations and sequences during blastogenesis. *Am J Med Genet* 2002; **110**: 320–3.
7. S.T. Ildstad, D.J. Tollerud, R.G. Weiss, *et al.* Duplications of the alimentary tract. Clinical characteristics, preferred treatment and associated malformations. *Ann Surg* 1998; **208**: 184–9.
8. D. Nehra, A.M. Goldstein. Intestinal malrotation; varied clinical presentation from infancy through adulthood. *Surgery* 2011; **149**: 386–93.
9. P. Prasil, H. Flageole, K.S. Shaw, *et al.* Should malrotation in children be treated differently according to age? *J Pediatr Surg* 2000; **35**: 756–8.
10. G.D. Williams, A. Feng. Heterotaxy syndrome: Implications for anesthesia management. *J Cardiothorac Vasc Anesth* 2010; **24**: 834–44.
11. I. Shiraishi, H. Ichikawa. Human heterotaxy syndrome – from molecular genetics to clinical features, management, and prognosis. *Circ J* 2012; **76**; 2066–74.
12. N. Nakhleh, R. Francis, R.A. Giese, *et al.* High prevalence of respiratory ciliary dysfunction in congenital heart disease patients with heterotaxy. *Circulation* 2012; **125**: 2232–42.
13. S.E. Lee, H.Y. Kim, S.E. Jung, *et al.* Situs anomalies and gastrointestinal abnormalities. *J Pediatr Surg* 2006; **41**: 1237–42.
14. A. Messineo, J.H. MacMillan, S.B. Palder. Clinical factors affecting mortality in children with malrotation of the intestine. *J Pediatr Surg* 1992; **27**: 1343–5.
15. K. Mandeville, M. Chien, F.A. Willyerd, *et al.* Intussusception. Clinical presentations and imaging characteristics. *Pediatr Emerg Care* 2012; **28**: 842–4.
16. R.L. Moss, R.A. Dimmitt, D.C. Barnhart, *et al.* Laparotomy versus peritoneal drainage for necrotizing entercolitis and perforation. *N Engl J Med* 2006; **354**: 2225–34.
17. C.D. Downard, E. Renaud, S.D. St Peter, *et al.* Treatment of necrotizing enterocolitis: an American Pediatric Surgical Association Outcomes and Clinical Trials Committee systematic review. *J Pediatr Surg* 2012; **47**: 2111–22.
18. S.C. Fitzgibbons, Y Ching, D Yu *et al.* Mortality of necrotizing entercolitis expressed by birth weight categories. *J Pediatr Surg* 2009; **44**: 1072–5.
19. K. Fakhoury, P.R. Durie, H. Levison, G.J. Canny. Meconium ileus in the absence of cystic fibrosis. *Arch Dis Child* 1992; **67**: 1204–6.
20. K.B. Schwartz, B.H. Haber, P. Rosenthal, *et al.* Extra-hepatic anomalies in infants with biliary atresia: results of a large prospective North American multi-center study. *Hepatology* 2013; **23**. Doi: 10.1002/hep26512.
21. T. Todani, Y. Watanabe, M. Narusue, *et al.* Congenital bile duct cysts: classification, operative procedures, and review of thirty-seven cases including cancer arising from choledochal cyst. *Am J Surg* 1977; **134**: 263–9.
22. D.L. Shawcross, J.A. Wendon. The neurological manifestations of acute liver failure. *Neurochem Int* 2012; **60**: 662–71.
23. R.H. Squires, E.M. Alonso. Acute liver failure in children. In Suchy F.J., Sokol R.J., Balistreri W.F., eds. *Liver Disease in Children*, 4th edn. Cambridge: Cambridge University Press, 2012, pp. 32–50.
24. R.B Freeman Jr., R.H Weisner, J.P. Roberts, *et al.* Improving liver allocation: MELD and PELD. *Am J Transplant* 2004; **4**; 114–31.

25. R. B. Weiskopf, S. Schnapp, K. Rouine-Rapp, A. Bostrom, P. Toy. Extracellular potassium concentrations in red blood cell suspensions after irradiation and washing. *Transfusion* 2005; **45**: 1295–301.

26. M.L. Feldkamp, J.C. Carey, T.W. Sadler. Development of gastroschisis: review of hypotheses, a novel hypothesis, and implications for research. *Am J Med Genet A* 2007; **143**: 639–52.

27. E. Christison-Lagay, C. Kelleher, J. Langer. Neonatal abdominal wall defects. *Semin Fetal Neonatal Med* 2011; **16**: 164–72.

28. L.T. Vu, K.K. Nobuhara, C. Laurent, G.M. Shaw. Increasing prevalence of gastroschisis: population-based study in California. *J Pediatr* 2008; **152**: 807–11.

29. A.C. Pastor, J.D. Phillips, S.J. Fenton, *et al.* Routine use of a SILASTIC spring-loaded silo for infants with gastroschisis: a multicenter randomized controlled trial. *J Pediatr Surg* 2008; **43**: 1807–12.

30. E.D. Skarsgard, J. Claydon, S. Bouchard, *et al.* Canadian Pediatric Surgical Network: a population-based pediatric surgery network and database for analyzing surgical birth defects. The first 100 cases of gastroschisis. *J Pediatr Surg* 2008; **43**: 30–4.

31. J.R. Wright, R.F. Barth, J.C. Neff, *et al.* Gastrointestinal malformations associated with prune belly syndrome: three cases and a review of the literature. *Pediatr Pathol* 1986; **5**: 421–48.

32. K.A. Burbige, J. Amodio, W.E. Berdon, *et al.* Prune belly syndrome: 35 years of experience. *J Urol* 1987; **137**: 86–90.

33. R.S. Bloss, J.V. Aranda, H.E. Beardmore. Congenital diaphragmatic hernia: pathophysiology and pharmacologic support. *Surgery* 1981; **89**: 518–24.

34. J. Boloker, D.A. Bateman, J.T. Wung, C.J. Stolar. Congenital diaphragmatic hernia in 120 infants treated consecutively with permissive hypercapnea/spontaneous respiration/elective repair. *J Pediatr Surg* 2002; **37**: 357–66.

35. A.R. Rana, J.S. Khouri, D.H. Teitelbaum, *et al.* Salvaging the severe congenital diaphragmatic hernia patient: is a silo the solution? *J Pediatr Surg* 2008; **43**: 788–91.

36. D. Mullassery, M.E. Ba'arth, E.C. Jesudason, P.D. Losty. Value of liver herniation in prediction of outcome in fetal congenital diaphragmatic hernia: a systematic review and meta-analysis. *Ultrasound Obstet Gynecol* 2010; **35**: 609–14.

37. V. Datin-Dorriere, S. Rouzies, P. Taupin, *et al.* Prenatal prognosis in isolated congenital diaphragmatic hernia. *Am J Obstet Gynecol* 2008; **198**: 80e1–5.

38. C.L. Ogden, Carroll, B.K. Kit, K.M. Flegal. Prevalence of obesity and trends in body mass index among US children and adolescents, 1999–2000. *JAMA* 2012; **307**: 483–90.

39. S. Bolen, H. Chang, J. Weiner, *et al.* Clinical outcomes after bariatric surgery: a five-year matched cohort analysis in seven US states. *Obes Surg* 2012; **22**: 749–63.

40. D.S. Hsia, S.C. Fallon, M.L. Brandt. Adolescent bariatric surgery. *Arch Pediatr Adolesc Med* 2012; **166**: 757–66.

41. P.J. Neilgan, S. Porter, B. Max, *et al.* Obstructive sleep apnea is not a risk factor for difficult intubation in morbidly obese patients. *Anesth Analg* 2009; **109**: 1182–6.

42. R. Schumann. Anaesthesia for bariatric surgery. *Best Pract Res Clin Anaesthesiol* 2011; **25**: 83–93.

43. A. Mortensen, K. Lenz, H. Abildstron, T.L. Lauritsen. Anesthetizing the obese child. *Paediatr Anaesth* 2011; **21**: 623–9.

44. T.N Weingarten, M.L. Kendrick, J.M. Swain, *et al.* Effects of CPAP on gastric pouch pressure after bariatric surgery. *Obes Surg* 2011; **21**: 1900–5.

45. A. Ramirez, P.F. Lalor, S. Szomstein, R.J. Rosenthal. Continuous positive airway pressure in immediate postoperative period after laparoscopic Roux-en-Y gastric bypass: is it safe? *Surg Obes Relat Dis* 2009; **5**: 544–6.

46. K. Thakker, H.B. El-Serag, N. Mattek, M.A. Gilger. Complications of pediatric EGD: a 4-year experience in PEDS-CORI. *Gastrointest Endosc* 2007; **65**: 213–21.

Chapter

11 Renal maturation

Kasia Rubin and John Stork

Embryologic development of the renal system begins in the 5th week of gestation. By 20 weeks, there is a functioning kidney with collecting system, although throughout fetal development, the placenta remains the major excretory organ.[1] There are 33% of nephrons present at 20 weeks and all are present by 36 weeks estimated gestational age. During intrauterine life, the kidneys are of minor importance in the regulation of salt and water balance, as the placenta is the primary homeostatic organ. Prenatally, the kidneys produce large amounts of hypo- or isotonic urine; a reduction may cause a low amniotic fluid volume (oligohydramnios). Urine output begins at 10 weeks, and increases to about 35 to 50 ml/h at 40 weeks. The fetal urine is hypotonic, less than 250 mOsm/kg, and correlates directly with gestational age. After birth renal function begins to mature, but this function in preterm and term infants is less than in adults. This is due to incomplete glomerular development, a lower perfusion pressure and a decreased ability to handle an osmotic load.

Renal blood flow (RBF) in the fetus and term infant are low, with only 4% and 6% of cardiac output, respectively, compared with about 20 to 25% of the adult cardiac output.[2] The hemodynamic factors involved in the increase in renal blood flow during develop include an increase in cardiac output and perfusion pressure and a decreasing renal vascular resistance.[3] Even in neonates, RBF is autoregulated over a wide range of arterial pressures, due to changes in the resistance of the afferent arterioles. The renal vascular resistance (RVR) is high in infants. It is inversely proportional to gestational age, and falls after birth, but it is still higher than in adults.

The glomerular filtration rate (GFR) is determined by the permeability of the glomerular capillary barrier and the net ultrafiltration pressure. The GFR is about 25% of the adult value at birth. It doubles by two weeks postnatal life, and triples by 3 months. It is at near maturity by 20 weeks, and adult GFR values are reached by 2 years.[2] The increase in the GFR initially is due to an increase in glomerular perfusion pressure; subsequent increases are due to increases in renal blood flow and the maturation of superficial cortical nephrons, increasing the glomerular filtration surface area. The neonate's decreased ability to excrete a water load is related primarily to this decrease in GFR, as well as a possible decreased sensitivity of the tubules to arginine vasopressin, which increases water reabsorption in the collecting duct.[4] The ability to excrete a water load increases after 3 to 4 days in term infants and preterm infants born at 35 weeks of gestation or more.[5] The neonate is less able to conserve or excrete water, making this age group vulnerable to sodium and osmolar fluctuations.

Renal elimination of drugs is via glomerular filtration and/or tubular secretion.[6] Dexmedetomidine, morphine, and acetaminophen clearance follows GFR maturation. Water soluble drugs are excreted unchanged; elimination follows kidney maturation. Maturation of GFR and other aspects of renal function occur at varying rates, so infants must be individually evaluated in terms of pharmacologic drug dosing.[5]

Tubular function is also decreased in the neonate. The decreased RBF and decreased GFR decrease the volume of solutes the tubules must handle per unit time. While sodium reabsorption is greater than 99% of the filtered load in an adult, and this occurs throughout the nephron, the term neonate has a tubular reabsorptive surface area, fewer solute transporters, and lower tubular thresholds for reabsorption of solutes, and is thus more likely to lose sodium.[7] The neonate is unable to concentrate urine beyond 600–800 mOsm/l; adult values are approximately

Essentials of Pediatric Anesthesiology, ed. Alan David Kaye, Charles James Fox and James H. Diaz. Published by Cambridge University Press. © Cambridge University Press 2015.

1200 mOsm/l. Preterm infants are more likely to be in negative sodium balance with difficulty conserving sodium during the first few weeks after birth.[5] The altered tubular reabsorption with decreased proximal tubular reabsorption, decreased loop of henle reabsorption, and increased tubule load results in increased fractional sodium excretion.[5]

Decreased tubule function also affects the ability of the neonate to modify urinary acidity. Acid excretion can be upregulated in the collecting duct, but urinary pH cannot be lowered below 4.5. The renal tubules resorb bicarbonate, with 85% absorbed in the proximal tubule and 15% in the ascending loop of Henle. The neonate has an impaired ability to resorb bicarbonate, leading to a relative renal tubular acidosis.

Infants with kidney disease

Major malformations of the renal system and urinary tract are often able to be diagnosed in utero. Prenatal ultrasound is able to identify the presence of bilateral small or enlarged kidneys, renal cysts, hydronephrosis, bladder enlargement, or oligohydramnios, all of which may indicate the presence of renal or urologic abnormalities. An abdominal mass of renal origin is most commonly hydronephrosis, followed by multicystic dysplastic kidney.[2] A constellation of findings, consisting of clubbed feet, pulmonary hypoplasia and cranial anomalies, known as Potter sequence, may be seen in infants with bilateral renal agenesis, a condition which is uniformly fatal. Abdominal laxity may indicate Eagle–Barrett, or prune belly syndrome, which is characterized by a urethral obstruction leading to bladder distention, urologic abnormalities, and cryptorchidism. Poor cough is noted due to the abdominal muscular deficiency. Other characteristics that may alert a physician to the possibility of underlying renal defects include: abnormal ears, aniridia, microcephaly, meningomyelocele, pectus excavatum, hemihypertrophy, persistent urachus, bladder or cloacal exstrophy, abnormalitiy of the external genitalia, cryptorchidism, imperforate anus, and limb deformities.[2]

Acute kidney injury

Acute kidney injury (AKI) is a sudden decline in kidney function, manifested by a decrease in GFR (Table 11.1). While creatinine clearance is used as an estimate of GFR in adults, it is a poor indicator in neonates and small children as it is reflective of muscle mass. The GFR may be decreased by 50% before the creatinine begins to rise. RIFLE criteria are used to classify acute kidney injury (Table 11.2). RIFLE is an acronym for Risk for renal dysfunction, Injury to the kidney, Failure of kidney function, Loss of kidney function, and End-stage renal disease. These criteria are for adult and pediatric patients. There are attempts to implement the RIFLE score with neonatal modification, as neonatal AKI is frequently complicated by unfavorable outcomes.[9]

Table 11.1 GFR in acute kidney injury

STAGE	GFR description	ml/min
Stage 1	Kidney damage with normal or increased GFR	> 90
Stage 2	Kidney damage with mildly decreased GFR	60–89
Stage 3	Moderately decreased GFR	30–59
Stage 4	Severely decreased GFR	15–29
Stage 5	End-stage kidney disease (ESRD)	< 15

Table 11.2 RIFLE: Risk for renal dysfunction, Injury to the kidney, Failure of kidney function, Loss of kidney function, and End-stage renal disease[8]

	Estimated CrCl	Urine output
Risk	eCrCl decrease by 25%	< 0.5 ml/kg/h for 8 h
Injury	eCrCl decrease by 50%	< 0.5 ml/kg/h for 16 h
Failure	eCrCl decrease by 75% or eCrCl < 35 lL/min/1.73 m^2	< 0.3 ml/kg/h for 24 h or anuric for 12 h
Loss	Persistent failure > 4 weeks	
ESRD	Persistent failure > 3 months	

Kidney injury as described in terms of GFR:

Acute kidney injury can be due to three mechanisms: prerenal, renal, or postrenal. Prerenal injury is characterized by decrease in intravascular volume, either real (i.e., hemorrhage, gastrointestinal loss, sepsis) or via a decreased effective intravascular volume (i.e., congestive heart failure). Renal injury may be due to acute tubular necrosis, caused by ischemic injury, drugs, or nephrotoxins. Uric acid nephropathy and tumor lysis syndrome may also damage the kidney. Kidney disorders such as interstitial nephritis and glomerulonephritis are other causes of intrinsic renal damage. Postrenal damage is obstructive, due to either ureteral or urethral obstruction.

Calculation of a fractional excretion of sodium (FE_{Na}) may be beneficial in differentiating prerenal AKI from intrinsic AKI. Neonates with a FE_{Na} of more than 2.5% to 3.0% generally have intrinsic AKI, while those with a FE_{Na} less than 1.0% have prerenal AKI.[2]

$$FE_{Na} = 100\% \times \frac{[Na_{urine}] \times [Cr_{plasma}]}{[Na_{plasma}] \times [Cr_{urine}]}$$

Treatment for AKI is dependent on prerenal vs. intrinsic vs. postrenal causes. Prompt resuscitation of prerenal AKI typically has an excellent prognosis, while those with intrinisic AKI have a poor course. Risk factors for the development of ESRD include: multisystem organ failure, prolonged hypotension with need for vasopressors, need for mechanical ventilation, and need for dialysis. Infants who have survived an episode of significant AKI should be followed for development of chronic kidney disease as they grow older.

Anesthesia for common pediatric urology cases

Most children presenting for urologic surgery are otherwise healthy with singular urinary tract defects.[10] It is out of the scope of this chapter to discuss the numerous congenital syndromes found in children, but the presence of any congenital malformation should alert the anesthesiologist of the possibility of malformation of other organs, particularly cardiac malformations (see Table 11.1). In children with known chronic renal failure, preoperative assessment must focus on the cardiorespiratory function, volume status, and the presence of any electrolyte imbalances or coagulation disorders.[11] A particular note of caution during the preanesthetic evaluation and room set-up is the classic association of latex allergy in pediatric urological patients. Sensitization often occurs in patients with several previous operations, spina bifida, or urinary malformations.[11] Type 1 hypersensitivity reactions often 20–30 minutes after exposure, with delayed type IV hypersensitivity occurring 6–48 hours after exposure.[10] Providing a latex-free environment will prevent these life-threatening reactions.

Circumcision

Circumcision is one of the most common pediatric urologic surgeries. Many circumcisions are done in the awake neonate in the first few days of life. The use of local anesthesia is superior to either placebo or simple analgesics and sucrose.[12] The use of a dorsal nerve block is likely the most effective pain management modality. Circumcision in infants and older children is typically performed as an outpatient surgery, under general anesthesia, utilizing an LMA or endotracheal tube for airway management. Analgesia is provided with a caudal or dorsal nerve block; both provide an equivalent efficacy in the early postoperative period.[12] The ideal agent, dose, or concentration of a caudal block has not been determined; our practice has been to utilize 0.125% bupivacaine with 1:600 000 epinephrine, 1 ml/kg.

Hypospadius

A hypospadias is a birth defect in which the urinary meatus is displaced. The incidence is 1:350 male births.[13] The meatus may be anywhere along the urethral groove, from the ventral aspect of the shaft to the perineum.[14] Multiple hypotheses exist to explain the etiology of hypospadias, including maternal environmental exposure and endocrine disruptors that prevents the development of the normal circumferential prepuce.[15] Factors associated with hypospadias include advanced maternal age, maternal diabetes mellitus, and exposure to smoking and pesticides.

Picture of surgical repair

The surgical repair is usually performed in children 12–24 months of age. Anesthetic management is usually general anesthesia, performed with LMA or oral endotracheal tube. Postoperative is most commonly management with caudal local anesthesia. This technique demonstrates high efficacy, low failure, and it reduces the need for postoperative opioids.[12] Practice patterns, however, vary greatly for these common pediatric urology procedures.[16]

Orchidopexy

Cryptorchidism is the absence of one or both testes from the scrotum. It is the most common birth defect affecting the male genitalia.[14] The testis can be found anywhere from the high in the retroperitoneal abdomen, near the kidney, to the inguinal ring. The undescended tests leads to two significant consequences: infertility and conversion of neonatal gonocytes into carcinoma-in-situ and then invasive seminoma in early adult life, due to the increased intra-abdominal temperature.[17] Orchidopexy involves surgical dissection and exploration of the inguinal region to mobilize the testis, followed by fixation of the testis in its normal scrotal position.

Picture of surgery

Anesthetic management depends on the location of the undescended testis, as the surgical approach will vary. An open orchidopexy or a laparoscopic orchidopexy is performed for an palpable testis. A nonpalpable testis is managed with laparoscopy, and a retractile testis can be managed with a simple scrotal orchidopexy.[18] If surgery is performed via the inguinal approach a general anesthetic with spontaneous respiration using an LMA is most commonly preferred. In cases of laparoscopy, the airway is generally secured with an oral endotracheal tube. Postoperative pain is best managed with a caudal block, with low rates of complications and side effects, and greater efficacy measured by less supplementary analgesic use, when compared with ilioinguinal nerve block plus local infiltration.[12]

Pyeloplasty

Pyeloplasty is performed to relieve an obstruction of the ureter at the junction of the renal pelvis. This blockage causes hydronephrosis that, if untreated, may lead to permanent loss of renal function. Ureteropelvic junction (UPJ) obstruction is often a prenal detection that is found on ultrasound. Boys are typically affected more than girls, and the left kidney is more commonly affected than the right. The open surgical approach allows a pediatric surgeon to access the kidney via an extraperitoneal approach, providing excellent exposure of the UPJ, and it is associated with minimal morbidity to the child. Laparoscopic pyeloplasties have become the standard of care for adult patients, and the technique is being rapidly adopted by pediatric urologists, with three ports in a retroperitoneal approach allowing access to the kidney with minimal mobilization, cosmetically acceptable scars, and reduced perioperative morbidity.[18]

Most children at the time of surgery are healthy with normal renal function and a normal renal function panel. Associated conditions may, however, include spina bifida, renal artery stenosis, polycytic kidney disease, or chronic renal failure, which may affect the anesthetic technique.[10] General anesthesia is maintained with tracheal intubation and controlled ventilation, often in the lateral position. When performed laparoscopically, the procedure is less painful: local anesthetic infiltration combined with acetaminophen and opioids are often adequate. Open procedures typically require multimodal analgesia using parenteral opioids or epidural analgesia, plus systemic NSAIDs and acetaminophen should be utilized unless specifically contraindicated in the postoperative pain management of these patients. Intravenous opioids or epidural infusion are acceptable and well-tolerated options, with side-effect profiles dependent on dose and particular opioid which is used.[12]

Vesicoureteral reflux

Vesicoureteral reflux (VUR) is an abnormal flow of urine from the bladder into one or both ureters and, in some cases, to one or both kidneys.[19] It may be caused by a valve pressing against the bladder wall that does not close properly, or there may be an abnormal fold of tissue in the urethra that prevents urine from flowing freely out of the bladder. The condition is often seen as hydronephrosis on prenatal ultrasound. In infants and young children, a urinary tract infection (UTI) is the most common presentation of the pathophysiology. Thirty percent of children and 70% of infants with a UTI are found to have VUR.[20] The VUR may spontaneously resolve as the child grows older. Continuous antibiotics are recommended for children younger than 1 year of age and older children with bowel/bladder dysfunction. Surgery is considered when the kidneys show evidence of inflammation, or if the reflux shows no improvement in the course of a year. Surgical approaches include open reimplantation or endoscopic correction via a deflux procedure, in which a gel-like liquid containing complex sugars is injected into the submucosal plane creating a flap-valve to prevent reflux.

Deflux injection allows for anesthetic management to remain similar to a cystoscopy. This is a relatively short procedure and is commonly performed under general anesthesia using an LMA and spontaneous ventilation. Application of a local anesthetic gel to the urethra may be useful for pain relief after cystoscopy.[10]

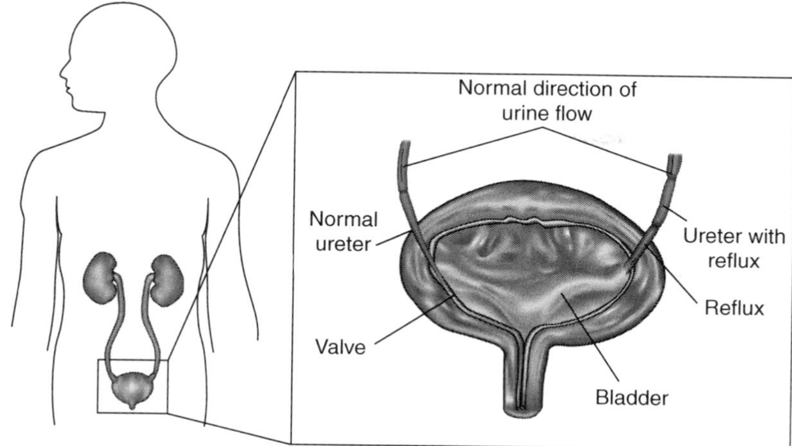

Figure 11.1 Vesicoureteral reflux

Open ureteric reimplantation requires general anesthesia with controlled ventilation via an endotracheal tube. A caudal or epidural should be considered for postoperative pain control. Ketorolac has been found to significantly reduce bladder spasms after reimplantation.[21]

Bladder exstrophy

Bladder exstrophy is a rare congenital malformation involving an exposed or open dorsal urethra. It is often a component of a spectrum of manifestations ranging from cloacal exstrophy, involving the bladder and intestines, to isolated epispadias. Classic bladder extrophy involves an epispadias, the absence of the anterior wall of the bladder, and a separation of the pubic symphysis. Cloacal exstrophy involves bladder exstrophy, a varying degree of pelvic diastasis, exstrophy of the terminal ileum, and an omphalocele. Multiple surgical options exist for treatment of this condition. A staged repair may involve neonatal closure of the bladder, posterior urethra, and abdominal wall defect with the epispadius repair between 6 months to 1year of age, and a bladder neck reconstruction with bilateral ureteral reimplantation at 4–5 years of age. A complete primary repair is possible, but these patients typically still experience multiple procedures during their lifetime. Urinary incontinence and sexual dysfunction are common.

These are typically long procedures with significant blood loss due to the pelvic osteotomies. Anesthetic management with general anesthesia, oral endotracheal intubation, multiple large-bore intravenous access, and an arterial line are recommended. Barring contraindications, a continuous epidural/caudal with local anesthetic is recommended for postoperative analgesia.

Kidney transplantation

Kidney transplantation is typically performed when children reach Stage 5 of end-stage renal disease (ESRD). The GFR is typically less than 15 ml/min/1.73 m2. Most common etiologies for pediatric ESRD are focal segmental glomerulosclerosis, hereditary nephropathies, such as polycystic kidney, and congenital disorders, including congenital anomalies of the kidney and urinary tract (CAKUT).[22] See Table 11.3 below for breakdown of primary diagnoses in all transplant recipients, as of 2010.

Progression of chronic kidney disease (CKD) is variable and depends on the underlying disease and the presence of additional risk factors, with a mean time to ESRD of 4.5 years when initially followed at stages 2–4.[22] The ESRD is treated with renal replacement therapy (RRT) in the form of hemodialysis (HD) and peritoneal dialysis (PD). Hemodialysis may be more difficult due to vascular access issues and smaller intravascular volumes. All children reaching ESRD should be considered for renal transplantation. Pediatric kidney transplantation is the optimal treatment for children with ESRD. The Nephrologists of the Pediatric Committee of the American Society of Transplant Physicians have defined indications for transplantation in children as follows:[23]

Table 11.3 Primary diagnoses in transplant recipients

Recipient primary diagnosis	N	%
Aplasia/hypoplasia/dysplasia	1681	15.8
Obstructive uropathy	1630	15.3
Focal segmental glomerulosclerosis	1246	11.7
Reflux nephropathy	549	5.2
Chronic glomerulonephritis	340	3.2
Polycystic kidney disease	323	3.0
Medullary cystic disease	287	2.7
Congenital nephrotic syndrome	277	2.6
Hemolytic uremic syndrome	273	2.6
Prune belly	268	2.5
Familial nephritis	241	2.3
Membranoproliferative glomerulonephritis	186	1.7
SLC nephritis	159	1.5
Henoch–Schönlein nephritis	113	1.1
Other	1310	16
Unknown	663	6.2

Reference 24: North American Pediatric Renal Trials and Collaborative Studies.

1. Symptoms of uremia not responsive to standard therapy
2. Failure to thrive due to limitation is total caloric intake
3. Delayed psychomotor development
4. Hypervolemia
5. Hyperkalemia
6. Metabolic bone disease due to renal osteodystrophy

Absolute contraindications to transplantation include infection, ongoing or disseminated malignancy, ABO incompatibitily, positive lymphocytotoxic cross-match, progressive neurologic disorders, and multi-organ failure. Relative contraindications include a history of malignancy, HIV infection, Hepatitis B or C, age younger than 6 months, severe mental retardation, and likelihood of nonadherence to antirejection medication regimen.[25] Approximately 800 kidney transplants are performed per year in children under the age of 18 years in the USA.[26] Modern immunosuppression regimens have provided outstanding success rates with both cadaveric and living donor transplantation. The 5-year patient survival after pediatric renal transplantation is 91.7%, compared with 78.6% with HD and 80.6% with PD.[26]

Surgical techniques for kidney transplantation are similar in adults, teenagers, and children weighing more than 30 kg, with retroperitoneal exposure and anastomosis to the external iliac artery and vein. In children weighing less than 20 kg, the renal vessels are anastomosed to the aorta and vena cava. Between 20–30 kg, the common iliac artery and vena cava are used for anastomoses.[25]

Preoperative assessment of the patient is mandatory, as this is an urgent, but often not emergent surgery. Postdialysis electrolytes should be obtained, with correction of abnormalities, including hyperkalemia. Hypo- or hypervolemia may be present, depending on timing of transplantation relative to hemodialysis. Patients with ESRD often have multiple comorbidities that need to be evaluated prior to induction of anesthesia (Table 11.3). Children may need a hypercoagulability work-up, including anticardiolipin antibodies, factor VIII and homocysteine levels, and an analysis of protein S, C, and anti-thrombin III activity.

Common conditions associated with ESRD

Pericardial effusion
Arrhythmias
Hypertension
Cardiomyopathy
Congestive heart failure
Anemia
Abnormal platelet function
Peripheral neuropathy
Somnolence
Developmental delay
Memory loss

General anesthesia with oral endotracheal intubation is standard intraoperative management for a renal transplant. Induction may be intravenous or inhalation, depending on patient NPO status. Drugs without renal elimination (cisatracurium, remifentanil) or metabolism (propofol) and inactive metabolites (midazolam, fentanyl) should be utilized. In addition to standard monitors, use of a Foley catheter and central line may be considered. Invasive arterial pressure monitoring is not required, unless dictated by the patient's cardiovascular status. Smaller children often show significant fluid shifts, in which case an upper extremity arterial line may be beneficial.

Maintenance of anesthesia often consists of a balanced anesthetic with volatile agent and opioid. Fluid management in these patients is guided by volume status, with many institutions utilizing specific protocols. Blood pressure should be maintained within 10% of preinduction values. Lactated Ringer's solution is typically avoided due to the potassium concentration (4 mEq/l), and red blood cells must be washed prior to administration.[27] Volume status is often supplemented with fluid boluses, especially in small children who are receiving a large kidney. The blood volume required to fill an adult kidney is approximately 250 ml, a significant proportion of the child's total intravascular volume. Appropriate fluid resuscitation is required to avoid low-flow states that could lead to vascular thrombosis or acute tubular necrosis in the allograft.[28] Correction of acute hypotension and avoidance of graft hypoperfusion is critical to postoperative graft survival. Intraoperative and postoperative anticoagulation is often necessary in the child under 20 kg who is receiving an adult size kidney in order to prevent vascular thrombosis.[25]

Immunosuppressant medications are typically begun in the operating room. In conjunction with the managing nephrologist, an individual protocol should be developed, delineating the drugs, doses, and the appropriate time to administer the drugs. Therapy varies by institution; the most popular regiment at this time is prednisone, tacrolimus, and mycophenolate mofetil, with use in 55% of living donor and 63% of deceased donor organ transplants since 2005.[26]

Epidural anesthesia in combination with general anesthesia may be beneficial for providing postoperative pain relief. Though there is more data being published regarding the safety and efficacy, its use does remain controversial due to (i) a theoretically increased risk of epidural hematoma and abscess formation, (ii) perceived risks of vascular instability resulting in reductions in graft perfusion, and (iii) limited data on the profile of minor adverse events.[29]

Acknowledgments

Thank you to Lynn Woo, Assistant Professor of Pediatric Urology, Rainbow Babies & Children's Hospital/ University Hospitals of Cleveland for providing the urology images in this chapter.

References

1. Reddy, P., & Khoury, A. (2011). Genitourinary tract: surgical considerations. In B. Bissonnette, ed., *Pediatric Anesthesia*. PMPH-USA, p. 1476.
2. Kenagy, D., & Vogt, B. (2012). The kidney. In M. Klaus, ed., *Kalus and Fanaroff's Care of the High-risk Neonate, Expert Consult – Online and Print.* . Elsevier Health Sciences.
3. Jose, P., Fildes, R., Gomez, A., Chevalier, R., & Robillard, J. (1994). Neonatal renal funciton and physiology. *Current Opinion in Pediatrics*, **6**, 172–7.
4. Linshane, M. (2012). Concentration and dilution of the urine. In R. Polin, W. Fox, & S. Abeman, eds., *Fetal and Neonatal Physiology*. Philadelphia, PA: Saunders.
5. Blackburn, S. T. (2012). Renal system and fluid and electrolye homeostasis. In Susan Tucker Blackburn, ed., *Maternal, Fetal, & Neonatal Physiology*, 3rd edn. Elsevier.
6. Anderson, B., & Allegaert, K. (2010). The pharmacology of anaesthetics in the neonate. *Best Practice & Research Clinical Anaesthesiology*, **24**, 419–31.
7. Costanzo, L. (2009). *Physiology* (4th edn.). Philadelphia, PA: Saunders.
8. Akcan-Arikan, A., Zappitelli, M., Loftis, L., Washburn, K., Jefferson, L., & Goldstein, S. (2007). Modified RIFLE criteria in critically ill children with acute kidney injury. *Kidney International*, **71**, 1028–35.
9. Ricci, Z., & Ronco, C. (2013). Neonatal RIFLE. *Nephrology Dialysis & Transplantation*, **28**(9), 2211–14.
10. Gandhi, M., & Vashisht, R. (2010). Anaesthesia for paediatric urology. *Critical Care & Pain*, **10**(5), 152–7.
11. Von Unger-Sternberg, B., & Habre, W. (2007). Pediatric anesthesia – potential risks and their assessment: part II. *Paediatric Anaesthesia*, **17**, 311–20.
12. Howard, R., Carter, B., Curry, J., *et al.* (2008). Postoperative pain. *Paediatric Anaesthesia*, **18**(s1), s36–63.
13. Tekgul, S., Riedmiller, H., Gerharz, E., *et al.* (2008). Guidelines on paediatric urology. *European Society of Paediatric Urology*, **1**(78), 6.
14 en.wikipedia.org. (n.d.).

15. Baskin, L., & Ebbers, M. (2006). Hypospadias: anatomy, etiology, and technique. *Journal of Pediatric Surgery*, **41**, 463–72.

16. Morrison, K., Herbst, K., Corbett, S., & Herndon, C. (2014). Pain management practice patterns for common pediatric urology procedures. *Pediatric Urology*, **83**, 206–10.

17. Hutson, J. (2009). *Pediatric Surgery: Diagnosis and Management*. Berlin Heidelberg: Springer.

18. Bissonnette, B. (2011). *Pediatric Anesthesia*. PMPH-USA.

19. National Institute of Diabetes and Digestive and Kidney Diseases. (n.d.). *Vesicoureteral Reflux*. Retrieved from National Kidney and Urologic Diseases Information Clearinghouse: kidney.niddk.nih.gov/kudiseases/publs/vesoureteralreflux/.

20. Khoury, A., & Bagli, D. (2007). Reflux and megaureter. In A. Wein, ed., *Campell-Walsh Urology*, 9th edn. Philadelphia, PA: Saunders Elsevier. pp. 3423–81.

21. Park, J., Houck, C., Sethna, N., *et al.* (2000). Ketorolac suppresses postoperative bladder spasms after pediatric ureteral reimplantation. *Anesthesia & Analgesia*, **91**(1), 11–15.

22. Harambat, J., vanStralen, K.. (2011). Epidemiology of chronic kidney disease in children. *Pediatric Nephrology*, **27**(3), 507–30.

23. Davis, I., Bunchman, T., Grimm, P., *et al.* (1998). Pediatric renal transplantation: indications and special considerations. A position paper from the Pediatric Committee of the American Society of Transplant Physicians. *Pediatric Transplantation*, **2**(2), 117–29.

24. McEnery, P., Stablein, D., Arbus, G., & Tejani, A. (1992). Renal transplantation in children. A report of the North American Pediatric Rental Transplant Cooperative Study. *New England Journal of Medicine*, **326**, 1727–32.

25. Sharma, A., Ramanathan, R., Posner, M., & Fisher, R. (2013). Pediatric kidney transplantation: a review. *Dovepress Journal*, **5**, 21–31.

26. North American Pediatric Renal Trials and Collaborative Studies. (n.d.). NAPRTCS 2010 Annual Transplant Report. Retrieved November 1, 2013, from https://web.emmes.com/study/ped/annlrept/2010_Report.pdf.

27. Uejima, T. (2004). Anesthetic management of the pediatric patient undergoing solid organ transplantation. *Anesthesiology Clinics of North America*, **22**, 809–26.

28. Salvatierra, O. J., Singh, T., Shifrin, R., *et al.* (1998). Successful transplantation of adult-sized kidneys into infants requires maintenance of high aortic blood flow. *Transplantation*, **66**, 819–23.

29. Coupe, N., O'Brien, M., Gibson, P., & DeLima, J. (2005). Anesthesia for pediatric renal transplantation with and without epidural analgesia – a review of 7 years' experience. *Paediatric Anaesthesia*, **15**, 220–8.

Chapter

12 Endocrine/Metabolic

Nicole C. P. Thompson and Rosalie F. Tassone

Introduction

Pediatric anesthesiologists are tasked with taking care of patients with endocrine disorders. Many of these patients present to us for elective procedures that require perioperative management. In this chapter, we will review endocrine anatomy, physiology, and pathophysiology. We will review the preoperative, intraoperative, and postoperative concerns for disorders commonly encountered by anesthesiologist. The endocrine system is comprised of multiple organs and glands. It is composed of the pituitary gland, thyroid gland, parathyroid, islets cells of the pancreas, adrenal gland, and gonads. These glands communicate broadly with other organs through the nervous system, hormones, cytokines, and growth factors (1). These endocrine functions are regulated by positive and negative feed back loops. To fully understand the disease states that we are tasked with treating we must first understand the integrated hormonal pathways that cause most biologic responses.

Prenatal and postnatal development

Pituitary gland

The pituitary gland begins developing in utero as early as 8 weeks. During the first trimester, the role of the fetal pituitary is negligible with most development directed by hCG. Maturation occurs in the second trimester that coincides with increased secretion of anterior pituitary hormones (2). The pituitary gland is composed of the adenohypophysis (anterior) and the neurohypophysis (posterior). The adenohypophysis originates from the upward evagination of ectoderm lining the oral cavity. It is composed of glandular epithelial cells separated by capillary sinusoids. The adenohypophysis is directly innervated by the autonomic nerves from the carotid plexus.

It is subdivided into the pars distalis, pars tuberalis, and the pars intermedia. These subdivisions are responsible for secreting luteinizing hormone (LH), follicle stimulating hormone (FSH), growth hormone (GH), thyroid stimulating hormone (TSH), adrenocorticotropic hormone (ACTH), melanotrophs (MSN), and prolactin (2). The LH stimulates ovarian follicles and cause follicle maturation. The FSH stimulates ovarian follicles or seminiferous tubules resulting in follicle development or spermatogenesis. The GH stimulates the liver and epiphyseal cartilage and enhances growth rate of most cells.

The TSH stimulates thyroid follicular cells that cause synthesis and release of thyroxine (T4) and triiodothyronine (T3). The ACTH targets the zona glomerulosa of the adrenal gland to maintain production of mineralocorticoids to cause sodium reabsorption by renal tubules. It targets the zona fasciculata of the adrenal cortex to stimulate the synthesis and secretion of glucocorticoids, which inhibits corticotropin releasing hormone (CRH) secretion by the hypothalamus. It also targets the zona reticularis of the adrenal cortex to stimulate the synthesis and secretion of adrenal androgens (2).

The MSN stimulate melanocytes to increase melanin production. Prolactin stimulates the mammary glands and the brain. It causes the mammary glands to secrete milk. In the brain it increases maternal behavior and maintains progesterone secretion. It also increases dopamine secretion by the hypothalamus that inhibits prolactin secretion by decreasing prolactin releasing factor (PRF) (3).

The neurohypophysis originates from the downward growth of neural ectoderm of the hypothalamus. It is composed of abundant axons whose cell bodies are located mainly in supraoptic and paraventricular nuclei of the hypothalamus. It is subdivided into the median

Essentials of Pediatric Anesthesiology, ed. Alan David Kaye, Charles James Fox and James H. Diaz. Published by Cambridge University Press. © Cambridge University Press 2015.

eminence, infundibular stem, and pars nervosa (3). The pars nervosa is responsible for secreting antidiuretic hormone (ADH) and oxytocin. The ADH targets the collecting ducts of the kidneys to absorb water, thus producing hypertonic urine. It also targets vascular smooth muscle to cause vasoconstriction to increase blood pressure. Oxytocin targets myoepithelial cells of the mammary glands and uterine smooth muscle to cause cell contraction. The cell contraction causes milk ejection and induction of labor respectively.

Thyroid gland

The fetal thyroid gland develops initially in the absence of detectable TSH. By 12 weeks the thyroid is capable of iodine-concentrating activity and thyroid hormone synthesis, but prior to this time the maternal thyroid appears to be the primary source for T4. During the second trimester, TRH, TSH, and free T4 all begin to rise. Fetal T3 is detectable during the third trimester and also begins to rise. About five days after birth TSH, T4, and T3 decline to normal levels. The thyroid gland originates from the evagination of floor of the pharynx (4).

The T4 and T3 hormones target the heart, adipose tissue, muscle, bone, nervous system, gastrointestinal system, and lipoprotein. They increase chronotropy and inotropy, stimulate lipolysis, and increase protein breakdown. In addition, T4 and T3 promote normal skeletal and brain growth, increase carbohydrate absorption, increase LDL receptor formation, and stimulate oxygen consumption (4).

Parathyroid gland

The fetal parathyroid develops in the fifth week. It develops from the third and fourth brachial pouches. The gland from the third pouches descend caudally, while the glands from the fourth pouches remain stationary (5). The parathyroid hormone (PTH) increases osteoclastic activity in bone, increases the renal tubular reabsorption of calcium, and stimulates the synthesis of 1, 25- dihydroxycholecalciferol by the kidney. It also inhibits the absorption of phosphate and bicarbonate by the renal tubule (6). Collectively these actions cause an increase in serum calcium.

Pancreas

The pancreas is a mixed exocrine and endocrine gland. Endocrine function has been measured as early as 9 weeks. The exocrine function of the pancreas is measurable after birth. The pancreas develops from endoderm of dorsal and ventral buds found on either side of the duodenum (7). The pancreatic islets contain many cell types with beta cells the most commonly found. Beta cells produce insulin and alpha cells produce glucagon while somatostatin is produced by delta cells. The pancreatic hormones insulin and glucagon are central to regulating glucose homeostasis by affecting glycogen breakdown, gluconeogenesis, glucose absorption, uptake, and disposal (8).

Adrenal glands

The adrenal glands primary role is steroid synthesis. The fetal adrenal cortex is identifiable as early as 4 weeks of fetal age (2). The adrenal gland consist of the adrenal cortex and the adrenal medulla. The adrenal cortex is derived from mesodermal tissue and synthesizes the adrenal steroids (glucocorticoids, mineralocorticoids, and androgens) (9). The adrenal medulla is derived from neural crest cells and synthesizes catecholamines (epinephrine and norepinephrine) in response to direct sympathetic stimulation (9).

Gonads

Testis differentiation begins around 8 weeks gestation and ovaries become morphologically recognizable during this time (2). Testicular function is primarily due to the Sertoli and Leydig cells. Sertoli cells work to develop spermatozoa and Leydig cells are responsible for testosterone production. Both the testis and ovaries have reproductive and endocrine functions. Ovaries are responsible for releasing estrogen and progesterone that work to regulate embryo development from conception to birth.

Diabetes mellitus

Introduction

Diabetes mellitus is characterized by increased blood glucose levels that consist of two types. Patients present with polydipsia, polyuria, and polyphagia. Diabetes mellitus has increased morbidity and mortality rates, with comorbidities arising from microvascular and macrovascular damage. Type 1 arises from autoimmune destruction of islet cells resulting in absolute insulin deficiency. Type 1 patients are insulin dependent and exhibit more fluctuations in blood glucose and may develop diabetic ketoacidosis (10). Type 2 diabetes results from insulin secretory deficit in the setting of high insulin resistance with beta cell defect (10). They have more pronounced signs of insulin resistance, greater BMI, higher lipid levels, and lower HBA1c. Type 2 diabetics experience fewer blood glucose fluctuations and are less likely to develop diabetic ketoacidosis, but may develop hyperosmolar hyperlglycemic state (HHS).

As reported by Tieh *et al.*, Type 2 diabetes mellitus (DM) is on the rise worldwide. Increasingly, more children have been diagnosed with DM. Many of these cases can be attributed to childhood obesity. However, there has also been an increase of diagnosis in normal weight children. Diagnosis can be made by measuring blood glucose levels or HbA1c level. Fasting glucose levels greater than or equal to 200 mg/dl or HbA1c greater than or equal to 6.5 is consistent with a diagnosis of diabetes mellitus. Diagnosis of DKA can be made if glucose levels are greater than 600 mg/dl, in the presence of ketones and acidosis. Diagnosis of hyperosmolar hyperglycemia can be made if serum glucose is greater than 600 mg/dl, serum osmolality is greater than 330 mosm/l, and no acidosis with mild ketosis (11). The conditions of DKA and the HHS are serious acute decompensations of type 1 and type 2 diabetes mellitus due to various degrees of insulin deficiency and increased levels of counter-regulatory hormones (12).

Preoperative considerations

When these children require surgery it is imperative that glycemic control be maintained perioperatively. They may present for a variety of outpatient or inpatient procedures. Whenever possible, surgery on children and adolescents with diabetes should be performed in centers with appropriate personnel and facilities to care for children with diabetes. A team approach including the parent, child, anesthesiologist, surgeon, and endocrinologist is best established preoperatively to guide the patient's care. Elective surgery should be scheduled as the first case of the day and should be performed when the diabetes is under the best possible control (13). The patient should be given instructions to hold or reduce their morning dose of medication and be reminded to continue clear liquids until two hours before surgery.

Adjustments to morning medications should be made based on the type of insulin or oral medications that the patient is taking. Betts *et al.* suggest omitting or decreasing by 50% the morning dose of intermediate-acting insulin while eliminating the short- or rapid-acting insulin. If patients exhibit signs of hyperglycemia short- or rapid-acting insulin can be given to obtain glucose control. It is also recommended that patients discontinue metformin 24 hours before the procedure and stop sulfonylureas and thiazolidinediones the morning of the procedure. All attempts should be made to make this experience as stress free as possible because increased stress causes increase glucose levels in all patients. A baseline blood glucose should be measured preoperatively and IV access obtained as early as possible.

Intraoperative management

Glucose levels can be controlled during surgery by obtaining frequent blood glucose levels, starting a basal insulin infusion and 5% glucose infusion if there are concerns for hypoglycemia. Adequate hydration during the surgical procedure is essential. Dexamethasone is best avoided in diabetic patients as it causes an increase in glucose. If glucose levels are greater than 250 mg/dl the 5% glucose infusion can be omitted. The goal is to maintain the blood glucose levels between 90–180 mg/dl (13). Blood glucose should be closely monitored as frequently as every 30 to 60 minutes during surgery. Any elevations or decreases of the blood glucose levels can be managed with an insulin infusion or dextrose infusion. For most minor procedures of short duration blood glucose levels can be monitored immediately pre- and postoperatively.

Postoperative considerations

Patients that quickly resume a preoperative diet may be able to resume their treatment regimen. The patients that remain NPO or have undergone major surgery may continue to need insulin and/or dextrose infusions. Close monitoring will still be required to maintain glucose hemostasis. At discharge, patients need to be given specific instructions on medications and insulin, including treatment options for diet disruption, encouragement of blood glucose testing, and a responsible physician to contact with questions about their glucose management (10). Metformin should be restarted 48 hours after surgery.

Diabetes insipidus

Introduction

Diabetes insipidus is characterized by the inability to resorb free water. Patients present with polyuria, polydipsia, and dilute urine. Hypernatremia may also be present especially in young infants.

Diabetes insipidus may be central or nephrogenic (14). Central diabetes insipidus may be congenital or acquired. Congenital central diabetes insipidus is very rare and maybe caused by structural malformations affecting the hypothalamus. Acquired central diabetes insipidus is more common and can result from primary tumors or metastases, infection, histiocytosis, granulomatous diseases, autoimmune disorders, trauma, surgery, or may be labeled as idiopathic. Nephrogenic diabetes insipidus may also be congenital or acquired (15,16). Nephrogenic congenital diabetes insipidus may be a result of mutations on the AVPR gene, located on the X chromosome or from mutations of the AQP-2 gene located on chromosome 12 (17). Nephrogenic diabetes insipidus that is acquired maybe caused by several conditions including primary renal disease, obstructive uropathy, hypokalemia, hypercalcemia, sickle cell disease, and some medications including lithium and demeclocycline (15,16).

Regardless of the cause diabetes insipidus is most often diagnosed with laboratory tests that reveal serum hyperosmolality with concurrent with inappropriately dilute urine. Often, the diagnosis can be made when the serum osmolality rises above 300 mOsm/kg and the urine osmolality remains below 300 mOsm/kg.

Preoperative considerations

Preoperative evaluation of the patient with known diabetes insipidus is paramount. Additionally, identification of the patient who may develop diabetes insipidus in the perioperative period is also important. These patients often include patients who undergo neurosurgical procedures, especially those involving the hypothalamus and pituitary glands. Evaluation of the patient's current fluid status and the patient's current medical regimen should be reviewed. Laboratory studies to evaluate electrolyte disturbances should be considered. Consideration should also be given to scheduling these patients as the first case of the day so that fluid restriction during fasting does not exacerbate symptoms. Discussion with the patient's surgeon and endocrinologist should occur to provide a cohesive plan of intraoperative fluid management and postoperative disposition, as some patients may require admission for postoperative fluid and electrolyte management.

Intraoperative management

Intraoperative management of the patients who has or may develop diabetes insipidus intraoperatively requires vigilance with respect to fluid and electrolyte treatment. Faberowski *et al.* developed and prospectively evaluated a multidisciplinary approach to the perioperative management of DI with a standard protocol. A continuous intravenous infusion of aqueous vasopressin was initiated and titrated until antidiuresis was established, and intravenous fluids were given as normal saline and restricted to two-thirds of the estimated maintenance rate plus amounts necessary to replace blood losses and maintain hemodynamic stability. The authors found that in the children managed with the protocol, perioperative serum sodium concentrations were generally maintained between 130 and 150 mEq/l, no adverse consequences of this therapy developed, less fluctuations in serum sodium were noted, and hyponatremia occurred less frequently compared with the historical controls (18).

Postoperative considerations

Postoperative considerations of the patient who has or develops diabetes insipid should be focused on fluid and electrolyte management. These patients may require continued administration of desmopressin or vasopressin. Strong communication between the surgical team endocrinologist, and perioperative physician is important in creating a comprehensive management plan for the patient with diabetes insipidus.

Syndrome of inappropiate antidiuretic hormone (SIADH)

Introduction

The syndrome of inappropriate antidiuretic hormone secretion (SIADH) is characterized by hyponatremia and serum hypo-osmolality with inappropriately concentrated urine and excretion of sodium in the urine. Etiologies of SIADH include neurological and psychiatric disorders, medications, lung diseases, non-CNS tumors with ectopic production of arginine vasopressin, and miscellaneous causes (14).

Neurologic and psychiatric disorders that cause SIADH include infections like meningitis, encephalitis, and brain abscess. Vascular disorders such as thrombosis subarachnoid or subdural hemorrhage, temporal arthritis, cavernous sinus thrombosis, and stroke have also been identified as causes of SIADH. Central nervous system neoplasms, both primary and metastatic, skull fractures, and traumatic brain injury have also been identified as etiologies (19). Other neurologic and psychiatric disorders include psychosis, delirium tremens, Guillain–Barré syndrome, acute intermittent porphyria, autonomic neuropathy, postpituitary surgery, multiple sclerosis, epilepsy, hydrocephalus, and lupus erythematosus. Several medications have been implicated in causing SIADH. These include intravenous cyclophosphamide, carbamazepine, vincristine, haloperidol, amitriptyline, monoamine oxidase inhibitors, bromocriptine, general anesthetics and narcotics, desmopressin overtreatment of diabetes insipidus, or enuresis (14). Pulmonary etiologies of SIADH include pneumonia, tuberculosis, lung abscesses and empyema, acute respiratory failure and, positive-pressure ventilation. Noncentral nervous tumors with ectopic production of arginine vasopressin include carcinoma of the lung (especially small cell bronchogenic), duodenal, pancreatic, thymus, olfactory neuroblastoma, bladder, prostate, and uterine cancer. Additionally, lymphomas, sarcomas, and leukemia have also been implicated (19,20).

Preoperative considerations

Preoperative identification and evaluation of the patient with SIADH is geared toward optimizing the underlying condition and creating a plan for optimal intraoperative fluid management. Classification as to whether the SIADH is acute or chronic is also important. History and physical examination may identify causes and current treatment regimen as well as symptoms. Laboratory studies should also be carried out to best guide fluid management intraoperatively. It is important to be aware that the infant is much more sensitive to hyponatremia than older children and adults and may manifest symptoms earlier. Outside of the operating room, treatment for SIADH includes treatment of the underlying disorder and fluid restriction. In severe cases, hyponatremia may be associated with seizures or other central nervous system abnormalities. It is also important to understand whether the SIADH is acute (< 48 h) or chronic (> 48 h), as aggressive correction of sodium in the patient with SIADH over 48 hours may precipitate central pontine myelinolysis or other brain damage (19).

Intraoperative considerations

As mentioned above treatment of SIADH includes treatment of the underlying disorder and fluid restriction. In severe cases treatment may require hypertonic intravenous sodium chloride, and possibly use of a diuretic. In patients with chronic SIADH, it is important to not correct serum sodium levels too aggresively. It has been generally suggested that plasma sodium be corrected to a "safe" level of approximately 120 – 125 eEq/l at a rate of no greater than 0.5 mEq/l/h with an overall correction that does not exceed 12 mEq/l in the initial 24 hours and 18 mEq/l in the initial 48 hours of treatment (20).

Postoperative considerations

Postoperatively, patients may require continued intensive therapy of correction of the serum sodium over time. Discussion with the surgeon and endocrinologist or primary care physician with respect to postoperative disposition and treatment plan is important as the patient transitions from the operating room environment. Continued correction of sodium may be necessary for several days. Assessment of neurologic status should be documented and compared pre- and postoperatively, especially when corrections may be aggressive.

Pheochromocytoma

Introduction

Pheochromocytomas are tumors that arise from the chromaffin cells of the adrenal medula or extra adrenal periganglionic tissue. These tumors synthesize metabolize and secrete catecholamines. Pheochromocytomas are rare in children; they are more frequently familial, extra-adrenal, bilateral, and multifocal compared to those in adults (21).

Preoperative considerations

Preoperative evaluation with the patient who has pheochromocytoma should include proper genetic testing with appropriate locations for future follow-up and treatment options. These patients may be at increased risk for developing a moment to seize depending on the underlying mutation.

Additionally, adequate preoperative treatment with alpha-adrenergic blockade is mandatory for all pheochromocytomas, those that synthesize and secrete, and those that do not secrete but only synthesize catecholamines (22). Preoperative medical treatment to block the effects of catecholamines should occur for at least 10 to 14 days before surgery. Goldstein *et al.* demonstrated that adequate preoperative alpha blockade reduced the number of perioperative complications from 69% to 3% (23). Only after adequate alpha blockade (often to the point of orthostatic hypotension) has been carried out, should beta blockade for residual symptoms be started, as this will reduce the risk for unopposed alpha receptor stimulation (24).

Intraoperative considerations

Intraoperative management of the patient with pheochromocytoma is often challenging. Despite adequate preoperative alpha- and beta- blockade, the anesthesiologist should be prepared for catecholamine surges, especially during manipulation of the tumor. This may result in wide swings of the blood pressure with extreme hypo- or hypertension. Vasopressor and vasodilator infusions should be part of the anesthetic regimen. Additionally, these patients are often volume contracted and their intracellular volume may be low despite adequate blood pressure control preoperatively. It should be noted however that children are at increased risk for catecholamine-induced pulmonary edema compared to adults (25). The last fluid replacement should not be excessive. Placement of adequate IV access and invasive monitoring including intra-arterial catheterization are very helpful in the management of patients with pheochromocytoma. Perioperative monitoring of potassium and glucose level should be considered as patients may be at risk for postoperative hypoglycemia (25).

Postoperative considerations

The perioperative team should consider the postoperative disposition of the patient with pheochromocytoma in the intensive care unit. As mentioned above the risk for postoperative hypoglycemia is especially high in children. Additionally other electrolyte abnormalities including potassium disturbances may become manifest in the perioperative period. In the case of open surgery, placement of an epidural catheter may be helpful in providing additional pain relief. Additionally genetic testing should be performed on every child with pheochromocytoma, as some children may be at increased risk for lifelong development of recurrent disease contralateral disease or malignant dedifferentiation (21).

Thyroid disorders

Introduction

Surgical diseases of the thyroid in children represent both benign and malignant conditions. Benign conditions include Graves disease, toxic adenoma, and congenital goiter. Graves disease is an autoimmune condition that causes hyperthyroidism or thyrotoxicosis secondary to the production of auto antibodies to the thyroid stimulating hormone (TSH) receptor. Toxic adenomas are autonomously functioning benign tumors that cause symptomatic hyperthyroidism. Another benign disease is congenital goiter. Goiters may be large, uninodular, or multinodular. Malignant thyroid nodules do occur rarely in children, but it should be noted that the incidence of malignancy is higher in children and adults (26,27).

Preoperative considerations

Regardless of the etiology of the fibroid disease, preoperative evaluation of the patient should include a thorough history and physical examination with special attention on the thyroid and the surrounding structures. Large goiters may cause mass-effect symptoms including dysphasia, dyspnea, dysphonia, or orthopnea. The symptomatic patients should have additional imaging studies to evaluate compression and distortion of the trachea. Additionally assessment of the presence of mediastinal extension is paramount, as complete airway collapse may occur on induction of anesthesia. Asleep or awake fiberoptic intubation may be necessary to secure the airway, and assessment and counseling of the patient and family should occur at the preoperative visit.

Patients with Graves disease may be undergoing pretreatment with methimazole and calcium (26). Laboratory studies, especially calcium levels, should be reviewed. Side effects of methimazole include skin rash, joint and muscle pain, fever, and agranulocytosis (26). If side effects occur, consultation with the surgeon and endocrinologist and discontinuation of methimazole should be considered.

Intraoperative considerations

The first intraoperative consideration is that of securing the airway. There is a significant spectrum of airway deviation with respect to thyroid disease. This can result in absolutely no airway compromise, or severe airway compromise. In the patient with symptoms of dysphasia or shortness of breath especially while lying down, one should assume airway compression and possible hemodynamic compromise upon induction of anesthesia. Maintenance of spontaneous breathing either with and awake fiberoptic or inhalation induction may be the safest choice of induction of anesthesia in patients with mediastinal mass effect. Once the airway has been secured with an endotracheal tube, progressive assisted ventilation and control ventilation may be considered. Standby with extracorporeal bypass (ECMO) may be considered if ventilation becomes impossible.

Postoperative considerations

Common complications of thyroid surgery include injury to the recurrent laryngeal or superior laryngeal nerves. This may result in partial or complete airway obstruction and care should be taken when debating these patients. Postoperative bleeding is another cause of airway compromise. In this instance bleeding may not only deviate the trachea but obstruct venous drainage, and thus promote airway edema. Often evacuation of the hematoma restores patency of the airway, and this maneuver may improve visibility of the airway with direct laryngoscopy in an emergency.

Hypocalcemia is another common complication of thyroid surgery. Serial laboratory studies should be performed postoperatively. The disposition of patients undergoing thyroid surgery often includes intensive care monitoring because of the concerns surrounding the airway and hypocalcemia.

DiGeorge syndrome

Introduction

DiGeorge syndrome is a condition characterized by outflow tract defects of the heart, hypoplasia of the thymus gland, parathyroid hypoplasia, hypocalcemia, and T-cell immunodeficiency (28). It is a result of a hemizygous deletion of 22q11.2. This deletion presents with variable phenotypes including DiGeorge syndrome, velocardiofacial syndrome, and cotruncal anomaly face syndrome (29).

Preoperative considerations

As the main manifestations of children with DiGeorge syndrome are related to cardiac cotruncal defects, hypoplasia of the thymus gland, parathyroid hypoplasia, hypocalcemia, and T-cell immunodeficiency, the preoperative evaluation should be focused, but not limited to these areas. A comprehensive cardiac work-up including a thorough cardiac history, cardiology consultation, and echocardiogram reports, is often helpful in anesthetic planning. Patients with thymic hypoplasia may be at increased risk for recurrent infections, and patients with hypoparathyroidism may present with hypocalcemia. Often these children are followed by a team of specialists, and preoperative consultation is often helpful in optimizing the care of these patients preoperatively. Airway examination is important in these patients, as often they do exhibit characteristic facial features including short forehead, hooded eyelids with upslanting palpebral fissures, malar flatness, bulbous nasal tip with hypoplastic alae nasi, and protuberant ears (29,30).

Intraoperative considerations

With respect to intraoperative care of the patient with DiGeorge syndrome, care must be tailored to the specific constellation findings. Children with DiGeorge syndrome are often familiar with the medical environment and premedication to allay preoperative anxiety may prove helpful. Increased airway management may present in the form of vascular rings or laryngeal webs as these patients often exhibit some set of dysmorphic features. As these patients may present with cardiac anomalies and various stages of palliation or repair, consideration of SBE prophylaxis may be warranted in addition to consideration of invasive monitoring if the surgical case may involve significant bleeding or fluid shifts. It is important to note that these patients may also be prone to arrhythmias. Aseptic technique should be emphasized for all patients, and especially for those with immunodeficiency.

Postoperative considerations

Postoperative care of the DiGeorge patient focuses on the specific needs of the patient. Appropriate postoperative disposition should take into consideration both the procedure and the patient, especially if the patient has a considerable cardiac history.

References

1. Jameson JL. Principles of endocrinology. In Longo DL, Fauci A, Kasper D, *et al.*, eds., *Harrison's* (18th edition). McGraw-Hill Professional; 2011.
2. Taylor RN, Badell M. The endocrinology of pregnancy. In Shanahan JF, Boyle PJ, eds., *Greenspan's Basic and Clinical Endocrinology* (9th edition). McGraw-Hill Medica; 2011.
3. Paulsen DF. Pituitary gland and hypothalamus. In Paulsen DF, ed., *Histology and Cell Biology: Examination and Board Review* (5th edition); 2010.
4. Barrett KE, Boitano S. *Ganong's Review of Medical Physiology* (24th edition). McGraw-Hill Medical; 2012.
5. Lalwani A. *Current Diagnosis and Treatment in Otolaryngology – Head and Neck Surgery* (3rd edition); 2012. Retrieved from http://accessmedicine.com.
6. Singer MC, Terris DJ. *Current Diagnosis and Treatment in Otolaryngology – Head and Neck Surgery* (3rd edition); 2012. Retrieved from http://accessmedicine.com.
7. Radi M, Gaubert J, Cristol-Gaubert R, *et al.* A 3-D-reconstruction of pancreas development in the human embryos during embryonic period (Carnegie stages 15–23). *Surg Radiol Anat* 2010; **32**: 11–15.
8. Molina PE. Endocrine Pancreas. In Molina PE, ed., *Endocrine Physiology* (4th edition); 2013. Retrieved from http://accessmedicine.com.
9. Molina PE (2013). Adrenal gland. In Molina PE, ed., *Endocrine Physiology* (4th edition). McGraw-Hill Medical; 2013.
10. Vann MA. Perioperative management of ambulatory surgical patients with diabetes mellitus. *Curr Opin Anesthesiol* 2009; **22**: 718–24.
11. Tieh P, Dreimane D. Type 2 diabetes mellitus in children and adolescents. *Indian J Pediatr* 2013; **81**(2): 165–9.
12. Yared Z, Chiasson JL. Ketoacidosis and the hyperosmolar hyperglycemic state in adult diabetic patents. Diagnosis and treatment. *Minerva Med* 2003; **94**(6): 409–18.
13. Betts P, Brink SJ, Swift PGF, *et al.* Management of children with diabetes requiring surgery. *Pediatr Diabetes* 2007; **8**: 242–7.
14. Sayali A, Ranadive SM, Rosenthal S. Pediatric disorders of water balance. *Endocrinology and Metabolism Clinics of North America* 2009; **38**: 663–72.
15. Baylis PH, Cheetham T. Diabetes insipidus. *Arch Dis Child* 1998; **79**: 84–9.
16. Verbalis JG. Diabetes insipidus. *Rev Endocr Metab Disord* 2003; **4**: 177–85.
17. Maghnie M, Cosi G, Genovese E, *et al.* Central diabetes insipidus in children and young adults. *N Engl J Med* 2000; **343**: 998–1007.
18. Wise-Faberowski L, Sulpicio SG, L. Ferrari, *et al.* Perioperative management of diabetes insipidus in children. *J Neurosurg Anesth* 2004; **16**: 14–19.
19. Verbalis JG, Goldsmith SR, Greenberg A, *et al.* Hyponatremia treatment guidelines 2007: expert panel recommendations. *Am J Med* 2007; **120** (11 Suppl 1): S1–S21.
20. Baylis PH. The syndrome of inappropriate antidiuretic hormone secretion. *Int J Biochem Cell Biol* 2003; **35**: 1495–9.
21. Havekes B, Romijn JA, Eisenhofer G, *et al.* Update on pediatric pheochromocytoma. *Pediatr Nephrol* 2009; **24**: 943–50.
22. Pacak K, Eisenhofer G, Ahlman H, *et al.* Pheochromocytoma: recommendations for clinical practice from the First International Symposium. *Nat Clin Pract Endocrinol Metab* 2007; **3**: 92–102.
23. Goldstein RE, O'Neill JA Jr, Holcomb GW III, *et al.* Clinical experience over 48 years with pheochromocytoma. *Ann Surg* 1999; **229**: 755–64.
24. Pacak K. Preoperative management of the pheochromocytoma patient. *J Clin Endocrinol Metab* 2007; **92**: 4069–79.
25. Hack HA. The perioperative manangement of children with phaeochromocytoma. *Paediatr Anaesth* 2000; **10**: 463–76.
26. Breuer C, Tuggle C, Solomon D, Sosa JA. Pediatric thyroid disease: when is surgery necessary, and who should be operating on our children? *J Clin Res Pediatr Endocrinol* 2013; **5** (Suppl 1): 79–85.
27. Josefson J, Zimmerman D. Thyroid nodules and cancers in children. *Pediatr Endocrinol Rev* 2008; **6**: 14–23.
28. Scambler PJ, Carey AH, Wyse RK, *et al.* Microdeletions within 22q11 associated with sporadic and familial DiGeorge syndrome. *Genomics* 1991; **10**: 201–6.
29. Chen CP, Huang JP, Chen YY, *et al.* Chromosome 22q11.2 deletion syndrome: prenatal diagnosis, array comparative genomic hybridization characterization using uncultured amniocytes and literature review. *Gene* 2013; **527**: 405–9.
30. Bassett AS, McDonald-McGinn DM, Devriendt K, *et al.* Practical guidelines for managing patients with 22q11.2 deletion syndrome. *J Pediatr* 2011; **159** (2): 332–9.

Chapter 13

Hematology/Oncology

Stacey Watt, Helen Nazareth, Ravinder Devgun, and Navyugjit Virk

Anatomy and physiology

Prenatal and postnatal development

In the prenatal period of development, hematopoiesis takes place in the yolk sac, liver, and preterm bone marrow. These can be broken down into three stages of development: mesoblastic, hepatic, and myeloid. Mesoblastic development mainly occurs in the yolk sac between the 10th and 14th gestational days and continues until the 10th–12th week of gestation. Hepatic blood cell production starts at week 6–8 and continues throughout gestation. The hepatic stage remains the dominant source until gestational weeks 20–24. After this point the third stage of hematopoiesis – the myeloid proliferation – within preterm bone marrow takes over. All hematopoietic cells originate from pluripotent stem cells and these progenitor cells differentiate based on the effects of various fetal growth factors.

Lymphopoiesis begins at the ninth week of gestation within the spleen and thymus. Cells originating from the thymus are named T-lymphocytes and those originating from the bone marrow are called B-lymphocytes.

Granulocyte colony-stimulating factor (G-CSF) expression has been found as early as week 8 of gestation and postnatally at week 6. Thus, neutrophils are the most common granulocytic cell found in fetal bone marrow by week 14. There are low neutrophil levels prenatally as there is little need for them. However, the production capacity is present so that postnatal granulocytic production is adequate to meet the needs of the developing neonate.

Erythropoietin (EPO) is a glycoprotein and is the primary stimulus for fetal and infant RBC (red blood cell) production. The mechanism of its action involves binding to specific erythroid precursor receptors thus stimulating maturation. Both hypoxia and anemia trigger the EPO production cascade. Erythropoietin does not cross the placenta. Therefore, neither maternal EPO stimulation nor inhibition has any effect on fetal erythropoiesis. Monocyte and macrophage precursors in the fetal hepatic system produce EPO during the first and second trimesters. Renal production of EPO dominates only after birth. Hence, the kidneys are not significantly involved in fetal erythropoiesis.

After birth, RBC mass declines in response to the increased availability of oxygen and concurrent downregulation of EPO. The RBC counts continue to decrease until oxygen delivery is insufficient, thus stimulating EPO production. Of note, term infants experience a phenomenon known as physiologic nadir that is a resultant of postnatal life and not indicative of a hematologic disorder. It results in a hemoglobin of 9–11 g/dl which occurs at 8–12 weeks of age.

Erythrocyte and granulocyte indices increase during the second and third trimesters, while hematocrit levels rise from 30–40% at the second term to 50–63% by the end of the third trimester. In contrast, platelet concentrations hold constant to a normal adult range (of 150 000–450 000/μl) from the 18th week of gestation onwards. The MCV of RBCs decrease from > 180 fl in embryonic development to 110 fl by 40 weeks gestation. In a full term infant the mean hemoglobin level seen in cord blood is between 13.5 and 20 g/dl. These numbers vary due to variables such as asphyxia, blood transfer from the placenta to the infant at delivery, and delay of cord clamping. The longer the delay in cord clamping the greater the blood volume of the newborn. The hemoglobin value rises in the first several hours after delivery due to the movement of plasma from the intravascular to extravascular space.

Essentials of Pediatric Anesthesiology, ed. Alan David Kaye, Charles James Fox and James H. Diaz. Published by Cambridge University Press. © Cambridge University Press 2015.

Table 13.1 Anesthetic considerations when caring for a patient with coagulation abnormalities

Preoperative	• Hematology consultation • Discontinuation of appropriate medications (ASA) • Determination of appropriate factor levels • Timely administration of treatment therapy
Intraoperative	• Caution with regional, IVs, IM drug administration, NGT, nasal intubations • Coag profiles for major surgeries • Consider blood products or antifibrinolytics prn
Postoperative	• Monitor for bleeding • Availability of blood products • Monitor for thromboembolism

Neonatal RBCs have a life span of 60–90 days. Adult RBCs have a life span of approximately 120 days. Premature neonates have RBC life spans near 30–50 days. The decreased life span can be attributed to decreased ATP, lipid membrane concentration differences, and decreased levels of intracellular carnitine.

Clinical science

Hematology

Caring for patients with hematological disorders is especially challenging in the perioperative period. A familiarity with these diseases is imperative in providing optimal care during the stress of surgery. Anesthetic management of the patient with coagulation abnormalities extend from the preoperative well into the postoperative period. (Table 13.1) Preoperative concerns require adequate history and physical examination, discontinuation of appropriate medications, determinations of preoperative hemoglobin concentration or specific factor levels, and timely administration of therapy. These concerns are often addressed in consultation with a hematologist. Intraoperative concerns for the anesthesiologist necessitate caution in regard to many procedures, including regional anesthesia, insertion of vascular access catheters including intravenous lines, intramuscular drug administration, nasogastric tube insertion, or traumatic airway insertion (e.g., nasal intubation). Postoperative concerns include vigilance for surgical site bleeding, ensuring availability of blood products, as well as monitoring for paradoxical thromboembolism.

Table 13.2 Systemic effects of sickle cell disease

Organ system	Symptoms
Musculoskeletal	Bone and joint pain, avascular necrosis
Kidneys	Hematuria, inability to concentrate urine, chronic renal failure
Central nervous system	Cerebral infarction, hemorrhagic stroke
Spleen	Recurrent infarcts lead to loss of splenic function
Pulmonary	Chronic inflammation, acute chest syndrome, hypoxemia
Hematologic	Hemolytic anemia, aplastic anemia

Anemias

Disorders in hemoglobin structure may lead to anemia which reduces the oxygen carrying capacity of blood. Illness secondary to altered hemoglobin may result from anemia as well as systemic tissue infarction, inflammation, and immunocompromise.

Sickle cell disease

Sickle cell disease is an inherited hemoglobinopathy resulting from a mutant gene which replaces glutamate with valine in the beta chain of hemoglobin. The resulting hemoglobin molecule is more unstable when deoxygenated, causing it to take a sickled shape, eventually causing sludging and microvascular occlusion. Heterozygous individuals are usually asymptomatic, whereas homozygous individuals have sickle cell disease affecting many organ systems. Patients may present with hemolytic anemia and end-organ damage early in life. Vasoocclusive crisis secondary to sickle cell disease may affect nearly all organ systems in the body (Table 13.2).

Avoidance of vasoocclusive crisis is key in managing patients with sickle cell disease during the perioperative period. Preoperative preparation of the patient should be done in consultation with a specialist. Risk factors for perioperative complication include age greater than 30 years, history of acute coronary syndrome, chronic lung disease causing chronic hypoxemia, pulmonary hypertension, history of cerebrovascular occlusion, and frequent painful crises. Preoperative laboratory testing should include hematocrit as well as BUN, creatinine, and electrolytes to evaluate multiorgan system involvement.

Avoiding conditions which may favor sickling is also essential in managing patients with sickle cell disease. Patients should be well hydrated. Normothermia should be maintained. Preoperative oxygen supplementation via nasal cannula or face mask may be advised. Use of a tourniquet or sequential compression devices should be used cautiously due to the increased risk of sickling in the affected extremity. Transfusion to hematocrit of greater than 30 may be advised for patients undergoing surgery. Anesthetic drugs are not associated with a higher risk of sickling. Both general anesthesia and regional anesthesia have been used successfully in patients with sickle cell disease without complication. Postoperatively, achievement of adequate pain control may be challenging to the anesthesiologist due to the fact that many patients with sickle cell disease have a history of chronic sickle crisis and may have developed tolerance to opioid pain medication. The NSAIDs should be used with caution due to risk of renal impairment.

Thalassemia

Thalassemia is a genetic disorder which causes inadequate synthesis of either the alpha or beta globin chain of the hemoglobin molecule, resulting in hemolysis. Patients of Middle Eastern, south Asian, and Mediterranean descent are more likely to be affected. Symptoms of thalassemia are variable and are related to severity of the disease. Lifelong transfusions may be necessary in patients with severe disease. Transfusion to hemoglobin of 9–10 g/dl suppresses thalassemic erythropoiesis. Chelation therapy may also be necessary to prevent complications of iron overload. Diffuse hemolysis results in chronic inflammation which has multiorgan system involvement manifesting as cardiomyopathy, pulmonary hypertension, cirrhosis, and splenomegaly. Bone marrow hyperplasia may cause extramedullary deposits in the pleura, paranasal sinuses, and epidural space.

Anesthetic management of the patient with thalassemia involves maintenance of adequate hemoglobin concentrations using RBC transfusion and supplementation with folate. Iron supplementation should be avoided due to risk of iron overload. In addition, bone marrow hyperplasia causes skeletal hyperplasia which may affect craniofacial structures and be cause for potential difficult intubation. In addition, extramedullary bone marrow deposits in the epidural space may complicate neuraxial anesthesia.

Coagulation disorders

Disorders of hemostasis are exceptionally challenging to the anesthesiologist during the perioperative period. Many coagulation abnormalities alter the mechanism of normal hemostasis, causing either hemorrhagic or thrombotic complications. Both hemophilia A and B are hereditary x-linked recessive disorders caused by decreased or abnormal factor VIII or IX, respectively. von Willebrand disease is the most common hereditary bleeding disorder characterized by decreased or abnormal von Willebrand factor.

Hemophilia A

Patients with hemophilia A have decreased or defective factor VIII:C and occurs in approximately 1 in 10 000 males. Symptoms may include hemarthroses and hematuria and are related to factor VIII levels. Laboratory findings include prolonged aPTT, normal PT and bleeding times, deficiency in factor VIII activity, and normal levels of vWF, factor IX, and factor XI.

In the perioperative period, treatment is aimed at increasing factor VIII concentrations. This may be achieved with plasma-derived factor VIII concentrates or with recombinant factor VIII concentrates. Elective surgical procedures require factor VIII levels of 100%. Patents may develop inhibitors to factor VIII:C, requiring increased amounts of procoagulant to be administered to reach desired levels. There is an inherent risk of viral transmission when administering factor concentrates, even when heat-treated. Use of DDAVP is an additional treatment which increases factor VIII levels by improving concentrations of vWF and by causing release of factor VIII:C from liver endothelial cells. Additional treatments used to mitigate bleeding episodes include the use of antifibrinolytics such as tranexamic acid and aminocaproic acid.

Hemophilia B

Hemophilia B is an x-linked recessive disorder which causes a deficiency in factor IX occurring in 1 in 25 000 males. Clinical presentation is similar to hemophilia A. Patients have normal PTT and prolonged aPTT, similar to hemophilia A. Surgery

Table 13.3 Classification of von Willebrand disease

vWD Type	Deficiency	Treatment
Type 1	Partial quantitative	DDAVP
Type 2a	Qualitative	FVIII concentrate
Type 2b	Qualitative	FVIII concentrate
Type 2n	Qualitative	FVIII concentrate
Type 3	Complete absence of vWF	DDAVP and FVIII concentrate

requires factor IX levels of 50–100%. Perioperative management includes administration of recombinant factor IX to reach desired levels. Caution must be taken when administering factor IX-prothrombin concentrates, however, as there is an increased risk of thromboembolic complications. Factor IX dosing is nearly double that of factor VIII due to decreased availability. Doses may need to be continued into the postoperative period secondary to the ongoing risk of surgical site bleeding.

von Willebrand disease

von Willebrand disease (VWD) is the most common hereditary bleeding disorder, resulting from either decreased concentration or abnormally functioning von Willebrand factor. Normal von Willebrand factor is produced by endothelial cells, megakaryocytes, and platelets. The condition of vWF causes platelet adhesion to the subendothelial surface in platelet plug formation. In addition to its role in primary hemostasis, von Willebrand factor also functions as a carrier for factor VIII.

Severity of von Willebrand disease varies depending on subtype. (Table 13.3) Patients with VWD often present with a history of abnormal mucosal bleeding, such as epistaxis or gingival bleeding. Additional symptoms may include menorrhagia, easy bruising or hematoma formation.

Type I vWD (70–80% of cases) is a quantitative defect caused by reduced amounts of normal von Willebrand factor. Type II vWD is caused by a qualitative deficiency in the amount of vWF. Type IIB causes abnormal platelet aggregation, and complexes of abnormal vWF and platelets cause thrombocytopenia. Bleeding abnormalities in type IIN (Normandy) VWD are caused by decreased affinity for vWF to factor VIII. Type III VWD is very rare and is characterized by a complete deficiency of von Willebrand factor.

von Willebrand disease may be present in patients despite normal results of common coagulation tests such as platelet count, aPTT, and PT. Bleeding time is prolonged in von Willebrand disease. Platelet function assay (PFA-100) is dependent on von Willebrand factor activity and platelet function and has a 90% sensitivity and specificity for diagnosing von Willebrand disease. Specialized laboratory tests may be necessary to distinguish disease subtype, which is important in determining appropriate treatment. Markers used in distinguishing disease subtype include vWF factor antigen (vWF:Ag), vWF ristocetin cofactor activity (vWF:RCo), or vWF collagen binding activity (vWF: CB). Diagnosis of specific subtype often requires expert consultation with a hematologist.

Treatment of von Willebrand disease is specific to the disease subtype. Generally, treatment consists of specific factor concentrates and desmopressin (DDAVP). The use of DDAVP promotes the release of vWF from endothelial cells and is first-line therapy for most subtypes of von Willebrand disease. When used at a dose of 0.3 mcg/kg, DDAVP is effective for 6–8 hours; DDAVP is available in intranasal or IV forms. Side effects of DDAVP administration include hypotension and tachyphylaxis. For patients who do not respond to DDAVP, administration of virally inactivated factor concentrates may be necessary. DDAVP is contraindicated in patients with type IIB von Willebrand disease as it may cause thrombocytopenia secondary to enhanced aggregation. Adjunctive treatments which may be used perioperatively include the use of antifibrinolytics such as tranexamic acid or aminocaproic acid to aid in preventing breakdown of formed clots. Additional considerations important for the anesthesiologist caring for the patient with von Willebrand disease include the potential for bleeding in the postoperative period. Until wound healing is complete DDAVP may need to be continued, depending on the type of surgery performed.

Oncology

Leukemias

Acute leukemia accounts for approximately 25% of newly diagnosed cancers in patients less than 15 years of age, and is the most common type of cancer in children. The incidence peaks at 2 to 5 years of age. Acute lymphoblastic leukemia accounts for 75% of cases, while acute myelogenous leukemia accounts for 20% of cases.

Acute lymphoblastic leukemia (ALL)

The majority of ALL stems from B-cell progenitors, while T-cell progenitors account for 15% of cases. Children may present with fatigue, irritability, anorexia, pallor, tachycardia, and more rarely evidence of CHF. Patients may also have a low-grade fever. Signs of marrow invasion include anemia, thrombocytopenia, leukopenia, and neutropenia. Bleeding secondary to thrombocytopenia may result in petechiae, bruising, gingival oozing, and epistaxis. Life-threatening hemorrhage is rare. Signs of bone pain include refusal to walk and irritability. Patients may also present with pathologic fractures.

T-cell ALL is more common in males, and the incidence of CNS leukemia is higher in T-cell than for B-cell ALL. Patients are more likely to present with a mediastinal mass or a white blood cell count above 100 x 10^9. An anterior mediastinal mass may cause airway or cardiovascular compromise. Involvement of CNS occurs in less than 5% of patients at presentation. In these cases, the patient may present with evidence of increased intracranial pressure or parenchymal involvement, hypothalamic syndrome, or diabetes insipidus. Rare complications include chloromas causing compression of the spinal cord or CNS hemorrhage. Two to five percent of boys present with involvement of the testes and this presents as painless enlargement.

Laboratory investigations in ALL may reveal elevated LFTs and LDH. Tumor lysis may result in hyperuricemia, hyperkalemia, and hyperphosphatemia with hypocalcemia. Other investigative studies generally include a CBC with differential, bone marrow aspirate, metabolic panel, blood culture if the patient is febrile, chest radiography to evaluate for mediastinal mass, and plain films of long bones. Evaluation of CSF should be performed prior to initiation of therapy. Patients may require platelet transfusions prior to spinal tap. An echocardiogram and ECG should be ordered for patients who will be treated with anthracyclines, as acute and delayed cardiotoxicity may occur. Viral serologies for Hepatitis B and C, CMV, HSV, and VZV are also obtained for baseline information.

The goal of treatment for ALL is to induce a permanent remission. Approximately 85% of children with ALL will be cured. Therapy involves chemotherapy with cranial radiation in select groups.

Acute myelogenous leukemia

Acute myelogenous leukemia (AML) does not have a peak incidence in children, and patients have a poorer prognosis than ALL. Therapy is highly toxic, and long-term survival is approximately 50–60%. Children with Down syndrome have a 10–20 times greater risk of developing AML than other children.

Both AML and ALL are indistinguishable at presentation. Children with extreme leukocytosis (WBC $> 200 \times 10^9/l$) may present with metabolic abnormalities and tumor lysis syndrome. These patients are also at risk of hypoxia in the small vessels of the brain and lungs, as a result of increased blood viscosity. Unique features of AML include leukemia cutis in infants and chloromas. Life-threatening bleeding may also occur.

The diagnostic work-up for AML is similar to ALL. The goal of induction therapy is to induce remission by rapidly reducing the number of malignant cells. Therapy involves chemotherapy with cranial irradiation for those children with refractory CNS involvement. Complications of treatment include cytopenias, mucositis, liver toxicity, need for parenteral hyperalimentation, and severe prolonged marrow suppression. Infection is also common.

Neuroblastoma

Neuroblastoma is a neoplasm of the sympathetic nervous system and it the most common solid tumor of early childhood. The incidence of neuroblastoma peaks at 2 years of age.

Neuroblastoma most commonly presents as an abdominal mass. The primary tumor is in the adrenal gland, often with metastatic disease via lymphatic and hemotogenous spread. Tumors may be found in the neck, thorax, and pelvis. Common sites of metastasis include the lymph nodes, bone marrow, bone, liver, and skin.

Signs and symptoms of neuroblastoma depend on the tumor size and degree of spread. Abdominal tumors are usually palpable, hard, fixed masses. The liver may be enlarged, and there may be signs of anemia, coagulopathy, and bone pain. Paraneoplastic syndromes are also associated with neuroblastoma.

The diagnosis is elucidated by a history of constitutional symptoms, abdominal pain, bowel, or bladder control problems, bleeding, bone pain, and limping. Physical examination may reveal fever, hypertension, abdominal mass, and spinal cord compression. Other more specific findings may include subcutaneous nodules in infants, enlarged liver or lymph nodes, and evidence of anemia or coagulopathy. Laboratory investigations should include CBC with differential, serum chemistries, ferritin, urine for catecholamines including homovanillic acid (HVA) and vanillylmandelic acid (VMA). Patients with confirmed neuroblastoma should have bilateral bone marrow aspiration and biopsy performed to assess for bone marrow involvement. Lumbar puncture should be avoided, as this procedure may increase the risk of CNS metastasis. Imaging studies should be performed to assess the degree of tumor involvement.

Localized tumors should be removed, if possible. Further treatment includes observation, chemotherapy and high-dose chemotherapy with autologous stem cell rescue and adjuvant therapy with immunomodulation.

Retinoblastomas

Retinoblastoma is the most common malignant ocular tumor in childhood. It has a strong genetic component related to a mutation in the RB1 gene located on chromosome 13. The genetic form is inherited in an autosomal dominant manner.

In many cases, the loss of the normal papillary red reflex is replaced by leukoria, which is often noticed by family members. Strabismus is the second most common ocular presenting sign. Metastatic spread may occur through infiltration of the optic nerve, dissemination into the subarachnoid space, invasion into the choroid plexus, and anteriorly into the conjunctiva. The brain and spinal cord may be involved. Vascular spread may also occur, as well as regional lymph node involvement. A patient with bilateral retinoblastoma may present with an intracranial neuroblastic tumor, which is referred to as trilateral retinoblastoma, with a poor prognosis.

Imaging studies including ultrasound, CT, and MRI are typically used in addition to the ophthalmologic exam to further characterize the tumor.

Treatment for retinoblastoma includes enucleation, which is indicated for large tumors filling the vitreous and in those with little or no likelihood of vision preservation. Focal treatments such as laser photocoagulation, cryotherapy, and thermotherapy may be used for very small tumors. Chemotherapy may be used for localized tumors. Radiation is reserved for patients with refractory or recurrent disease.

Secondary malignancies are common after treatment for retinoblastoma, which include head and neck cancers, osteosarcoma, soft tissue sarcoma, and melanoma.

Sarcomas/osteosarcomas

Rhabdomyosarcoma is the most common soft tissue sarcoma in younger children. Other soft tissue sarcomas include synovial sarcoma, leiomyosarcoma, liposarcoma, fibrosarcoma, alveolar soft part sarcoma, and malignant peripheral nerve sheath tumor. The most common bone sarcomas in children are osteosarcoma and Ewing sarcoma.

Soft tissue sarcomas (STS) may occur anywhere in the body. Presenting symptoms are highly variable, but STS often present as a painless growing mass. To evaluate the tumor, open surgical biopsy is required, as well as a complete history and physical, laboratory studies, and radiographic studies including chest CT and radioisotope bone scan to assess for potential lung metastases and bone metastases. Bilateral bone marrow aspirate is suggested, and lumbar puncture may be performed in patients with parameningeal head and neck primary lesions.

Treatment of rhabdomyosarcoma includes systemic treatment of micrometastatic disease with adjuvant chemotherapy and aggressive local control with definitive surgery and addition of radiation as necessary. For nonrhabdomyomatous soft tissue sarcoma, surgery is the main therapy, although patients with high-grade tumors with positive tumor margins may receive adjuvant irradiation.

Bone sarcomas are the 6th most common malignant neoplasm in children. They are the third most common malignancy in adolescents and young adults. The two most common bone sarcomas are osteosarcoma and Ewing sarcoma.

Bone sarcomas generally present as a mass in the involved area with pain. Symptoms may precede diagnosis by several months. Systemic symptoms such as weight loss or dyspnea may present in late disease.

Osteosarcomas primarily occur in the metaphysis of the most rapidly growing bones. Most Ewing sarcomas occur in different locations from osteosarcomas, such as the flat bones of the axial skeleton.

Evaluation of bone sarcomas should include a complete history and physical and routine labs. Alkaline phosphatase may be elevated, as well as serum lactate dehydrogenase, which may correlate with tumor burden. Imaging studies should include plain radiographs, MRI, and CT. Technetium-99 m bone scan may also be required. Bilateral bone marrow aspirate with biopsy should be performed in patients with Ewing sarcoma. A baseline audiogram and echocardiogram should be obtained prior to chemotherapy, due to the toxic nature of treatment.

Multiagent chemotherapy is required prior to and following radical excision of the tumor. In patients unable to undergo complete resection, radiation therapy may be used. Cure in Ewing sarcoma requires a multimodal approach using surgery with or without radiation therapy for eradication of the primary tumor, and chemotherapy for treatment of subclinical micrometastases. Late effects of chemotherapy include a lifelong risk of cardiomyopathy.

Wilms tumor

Wilms tumor is a tumor of the developing kidney, and is the second most common retroperitoneal tumor in children. It presents as an abdominal enlargement or mass. Other symptoms and signs include abdominal pain, malaise, fever, hypertension, and microscopic hematuria. If there is bleeding within the tumor the patient may present with anemia. If tumor thrombus extends into the vena cava, partial obstruction, hypertension and distention of abdominal veins may occur. Polycythemia, acquired von Willebrand disease, as well as reduced factor VIII and ristocetin cofactor levels may also be associated with Wilms tumor.

Evaluation of Wilms tumor should include history and physical exam, and laboratory studies including von Willebrand panel. Imaging studies should include abdominal ultrasound, abdominal CT or MRI to evaluate for evidence of bilateral involvement, as well as vessel involvement or extension to the IVC, lymph node involvement, and liver metastases. Chest radiography and CT should be performed to assess for lung metastases. If the tumor is a clear cell sarcoma, a bone scan should be performed to assess for metastases, as well as for patients with Wilms tumor and lung or liver metastases, and also bony symptoms. An MRI of the brain should be performed for metastases if the tumor is a rhabdoid or clear cell tumor. Echocardiography should be performed for detecting tumor extension from the IVC to the right atrium, and in patients requiring anthracycline therapy.

Eight-five percent of children are cured of the disease. Many tumors may be fully resected and these tumors are particularly sensitive to chemotherapy and radiation. Relapse is uncommon. Patients who are treated with anthracyclines or lung irradiation are at risk for cardiac complications. Patients with right-sided tumors who receive flank irradiation and those receiving whole abdomen irradiation are at increased risk for hepatic carcinoma.

Chemotherapeutic agents and side effects

There are many chemotherapeutic agents that potentially will impact the care of a pediatric patient undergoing anesthesia (see Table 13.4). It is important to know the potential risks involved with each agent your patient has been exposed to prior to induction of anesthesia.

Radiotherapy

Radiotherapy is used against many childhood malignancies including malignant brain tumors, acute lymphoblastic leukemia, acute myelogenous leukemia, retinoblastoma, sarcomas, osteosarcomas, and Wilms tumor. The dose of radiation used is generally dependent on the type of tumor and the location and volume to be irradiated. Adverse side effects of radiation therapy are most significant before the age of six, and include marked impairment of intellectual and physical development (see Table 13.4 for additional toxicities). There is also concern for the development of secondary malignancies. New therapies have been developed to minimize the side effects of radiation, including 3-D conformal planning techniques and intensity-modulated radiation therapy, as well as proton beam therapy.

Table 13.4. Chemotherapeutic agents and side effects

Drug	Mechanism	Treats	Side effects
Asparaginase	Depletes L-asparagine from leukemic cells by catalyzing the conversion of L-asparagine to aspartic acid and ammonia	Acute lymphoblastic leukemia, acute myelogenous leukemia, nonHodgkin lymphoma	Allergic reaction, coagulopathy secondary to decreased synthesis of antithrombin III, fibringogen, and other clotting factors
Bleomycin	Leads to the formation of oxygen-free radicals that cause single-strand and double-strand DNA breaks	Germ cell tumors, Hodgkin lymphoma	Infusional fever and chills, mucositis, pruritus, and excoriation leading to hyperpigmentation, Raynaud's phenomenon, rash, dysgeusia, anorexia, dose-dependent pneumonitis, and rarely pulmonary fibrosis, rare anaphylactoid-type reaction
Cisplatin/ Carboplatin	Cause interstrand DNA cross-linking and bind to replicating DNA causing single-strand breaks	Brain tumors, germ cell tumors, hepatoblastoma, Hodgkin lymphoma, neuroblastoma, osteogenic sarcoma, soft tissue sarcomas, Wilms tumor	Infusional nausea and vomiting, myelosuppression, electrolyte abnormalities, hypokalemia, hypomagnesemia, hypocalcemia, hyponatremia, Fanconi syndrome, nephrotoxicity, ototoxicity
Cyclophosphamide/ Ifosfamide	Require conversion by the hepatic P_{450} system to their active form that ultimately leads to the intracellular release of two compounds, acrolein and phosphoramide mustard. Phosphoramide mustard causes interstrand DNA cross-linking	Acute lymphoblastic leukemia, acute myelogenous leukemia, brain tumors, Ewing sarcoma, germ cell tumors, Hodgkin and nonHodgkin lymphoma, neuroblastoma, osteogenic sarcoma, soft tissue sarcoma, Wilms tumor	Nausea, vomiting, anorexia with drug infusion, myelosuppression, immunosuppression, alopecia. Sterility is dose dependent. Nephrotoxicity, SIADH, hemorrhagic cystitis
Cytarabine (ara-C)	Inhibits DNA polymerase, and is cell-cycle specific, killing cells during synthesis. Therefore, targets rapidly dividing cells	Acute lymphoblastic leukemia, acute myelogenous leukemia, Hodgkin and nonHodgkin lymphoma	Nausea, vomiting, anorexia, myelosuppression, stomatitis, alopecia. Ara-C syndrome includes fever, myalgias, bone pain, malaise, conjunctivitis, maculopapular rash, occasional chest pain, flu-like syndrome with fever, chills, rash. Intrathecal cytarabine can cause fever, nausea, vomiting, headache, arachnoiditis, somnolence, meningismus, convulsions, paresis
Dactinomycin (actinomycin–D)	Intercalates with DNA, inhibiting RNA and DNA synthesis. Also interacts with topoisomerase which is	Soft tissue sarcomas, Wilms tumor	Infusional nausea and vomiting, alopecia, myelosuppression. Anorexia, fatigue, diarrhea, mucositis, radiation recall in

Table 13.4. *(cont.)*

Drug	Mechanism	Treats	Side effects
	required for DNA replication, and leads to single-strand DNA breaks.		patients who previously received radiation
Daunorubicin/ Doxorubicin/ Idarubicin	Nucleotide base intercalation and cell membrane lipid-binding activity. Nucleotide intercalation inhibits replication as well as DNA and RNA polymerases. Anthracyclines also interact with topoisomerase II, which is vital for DNA replication. Electron reduction of the anthracyclines produces free radicals leading to DNA damage and lipid peroxidation.	Acute lymphoblastic leukemia. acute myelogenous leukemia, hepatoblastoma, Hodgkin and nonHodgkin lymphoma, neuroblastoma, osteogenic sarcoma, soft tissue sarcomas, Wilms tumor	Nausea, vomiting. Urine, saliva, tears, and sweat may all have a pink or red coloring. Myelosuppression, alopecia, mucositis. Dose-dependent cardiotoxicity occurs as a late finding. Radiation recall is a potential rare complication of anthracyclines when given after radiation therapy
Etoposide	Binds to topoisomerase II, which is vital for DNA replication, leading to DNA strand breakage. Acts mainly on G_2 and S phases	Acute myelogenous leukemia, brain tumors, Ewing sarcoma, germ cell tumors, Hodgkin and nonHodgkin lymphoma, hemophagocytic lymphohistiocytosis, neuroblastoma, osteogenic sarcoma, Wilms tumor	Infusional nausea and vomiting, myelosuppression, alopecia, possible hypotension, and anaphylaxis
Imatinib (Gleevec)	Selective inhibitor of the tyrosine kinase activity of the BCR–ABL fusion protein, a product of the Philadelphia chromosome seen mainly in CML and rarely with AML	Acute lympoblastic leukemia (Philadelphia chromosome positive), chronic myelogenous leukemia	Fluid retention, nausea, diarrhea, fatigue, muscle cramps, rash, arthralgias, myelosuppression
Irinotecan	Potent inhibitor of topoisomerase I, which inhibits replication and leads to DNA damage	Brain tumors, hepatoblastoma, soft tissue sarcomas	Cholinergic symptoms including intestinal hyperperistalsis, that can lead to abdominal cramping and early diarrhea. Other cholinergic symptoms include rhinitis, increased salivation, miosis, lacrimation, diaphoresis and flushing. Later side effects include diarrhea, alopecia, transaminitis, neutropenia, mucositis, hyperbilirubinemia
Mercaptopurine (6-MP)	Converted into several active metabolites that inhibit RNA and DNA synthesis. Can also	Acute myelogenous leukemia, nonHodgkin lymphoma	Myelosuppression, anorexia, nausea, vomiting

Table 13.4. *(cont.)*

Drug	Mechanism	Treats	Side effects
	interfere with purine biosynthesis. 6-MP is converted to nucleotide metabolities, some of which can lead to DNA toxicity.		
Methotrexate	Inhibits folic acid by preventing the reduction of folic acid by the enzyme dihydrofolate reductase, which limits the synthesis of purines and DNA	Acute myelogenous leukemia, acute lymphoblastic leukemia, brain tumors, nonHodgkin lymphoma, osteogenic sarcoma	Transaminitis, nausea, vomiting, anorexia. Intrathecal methotrexate often causes nausea and headache, occasional arachnoiditis, occasional long-term cognitive dysfunction and learning disabilities. Rarely causes leukoencephalopathy and progressive cognitive deterioration. Neurotoxicity includes seizures, confusion, ataxia, cranial nerve palsies, speech disorders, paraparesis
Steroids	Destroy lymphoblasts by binding to the cortisol receptor found on lymphoid cells and specifically in large numbers on lymphoblasts. Immunosuppressive, targets T-lymphocytes, monocytes, and eosinophils. May also halt DNA synthesis.	Acute lymphoblastic leukemia, hemophagocytic lymphohistiocytosis, Hodgkin and nonHodgkin lymphoma, Langerhans cell histiocytosis	Hyperphagia, insomnia, personality changes, adrenal suppression, acne, immunosuppression, and Cushings syndrome. Occasional gastritis, hyperglycemia, poor wound healing, facial erythema, striae, thinning of the skin, muscle weakness, osteopenia and cataracts. Rare avascular, necrosis of joints, hypertension
Temozolomide	DNA interstrand cross-linking	Brain tumors	Anorexia, nausea, vomiting, constipation, myelosuppression, occasional abdominal pain, diarrhea, headache, and mucositis
Thioguanine (6-TG)	Interferes with purine synthesis and DNA replication, DNA strand breaks	Acute lymphoblastic leukemia, acute myelogenous leukemia, nonHodgkin lymphoma	Myelosuppression, occasional fatigue, nausea, vomiting, diarrhea, anorexia, rare transaminitis, veno-occlusive disease (sinusoidal obstructive syndrome), and hepatic fibrosis
Topotecan	Inhibits topoisomerase I, inhibiting replication and leads to DNA damage	Brain tumors, neuroblastoma	Nausea, vomiting, diarrhea or constipation, fever, pain and later myelosuppression, fatigue, and alopecia. Occasional headache, rash, hypotension, transaminitis, and mucositis.

Table 13.4. *(cont.)*

Drug	Mechanism	Treats	Side effects
Vincristine/Vinblasti	Binds to microtubules especially in the mitotic spindle leading to metaphase arrest, thus targeting rapidly dividing cells	Acute lymphoblastic leukemia, brain tumors, Ewing sarcoma, hepatoblastoma, Hodgkin and nonHodgkin lymphoma, Langerhans cell histiocytosis, neuroblastoma, soft tissue sarcomas, Wilms tumor	Vinblastin: myelosuppression Vincristine: neurotoxicity, including constipation and loss of deep tendon reflexes. Both: alopecia. Also, jaw pain, peripheral paresthesias, wrist and foot drop, and abnormal gait occur, especially with vincristine. Ptosis, vocal cord dysfunction and damage to 8th cranial nerve rare

Adapted from: C.A. Hastings, Joseph C. Torkildson, A.K. Agrawal . Chemotherapy basics. *Handbook of Pediatric Hematology and Oncology,* 2nd edition. Wiley-Blackwell. 2012.

Table 13.5 Malignant conditions potentially benefiting from allogenic transplant

Acute lymphoblastic leukemia (ALL) in first remission and high risk for relapse
Relapsed ALL in second remission
Acute myelogenous leukemia (AML)
Juvenile myelomonocytic leukemia (JMML)
Hodgkin or nonHodgkin lymphoma in second or subsequent partial or complete remission
Myelodysplastic syndromes (MDS)
Relapsed, refractory, or familial hemophagocytic lymphohistiocytosis

Table 13.6 Malignant conditions potentially benefiting from autologous transplant

High-risk neuroblastoma
High-risk brain tumors (medulloblastoma/PNET)
Metastatic retinoblastoma
Recurrent high-risk germ cell tumors
Relapsed Hodgkin or nonHodgkin lymphoma
Relapsed Wilms tumor
Abbreviation: PNET, primitive neuroectodermal tumor

Bone marrow and stem cell transplants

Hematopoetic stem cell transplantation (HSCT) is a therapy used for malignant and nonmalignant conditions. It involves ablation of the recipient's bone marrow with high doses of chemotherapy, as well as radiation therapy, in order to allow engraftment of the donor's stem cells. Collected stem cells can be either allogenic (separate donor) or autologous (patient). In pediatrics, allogenic transplantation is used for hematologic malignancies due to bone marrow involvement (see Tables 13.5–7).

Stem cells for allogenic transplantation are taken from the bone marrow, peripheral blood, or umbilical cord blood. Stem cells for autologous transplantation are collected most commonly from peripheral blood. Pretransplant, high-dose chemotherapy with or without radiation is used to prepare for the transplant (see Table 13.8). Evidence of donor replacement of the recipient's bone marrow is evident with an increase in the white blood cell count, and decreasing transfusion requirement. Engraftment syndrome, which includes fever, rash, pulmonary symptoms, and weight gain, may appear during the initial replacement phase.

Complications from stem cell transplants include drug toxicity from the pretransplant preparative regiments (see Table13.11). Other complications include veno-occlusive disease (VOD) of the liver, also known as sinusoidal obstructive syndrome (SOS). Patients are at high risk for infection, and may develop graft versus host disease (GVHD).

Graft versus host disease

Graft versus host disease (GVHD) occurs due to proliferation of donor T- cells that recognize host antigen as foreign. The direct effects of the T-lymphocytes and cytokine response lead to the signs and symptoms of GVHD. Acute GVHD occurs within weeks of transplantation and chronic lasts beyond 100 days after transplant (see Tables 13.9 and 13.10)

Table 13.7 Nonmalignant conditions benefiting from allogenic transplant

Congenital syndromes	
Immunodeficiency syndromes	SCID, congenital agammaglobulinemia (Bruton's), DiGeorge syndrome, Wiskott–Aldrich syndrome, chronic mucocutaneous candidiasis, lymphproliferative syndromes
Hematologic disorders	Sickle cell disease, β-thalassemia, Fanconi anemia, Shwachman–Diamond syndrome, Diamond–Blackfan anemia, dyskeratosis congenital, chronic granulomatous disease, Chediak–Higashi syndrome, leukocyte adhesion deficiency
Metabolic disorders	Storage diseases, lysosomal diseases, mucolipidosis, mucopolysaccharidoses
Acquired syndromes	
Severe aplastic anemia	
Paroxysmal nocturnal hemoglobinuria	
Abbreviation: SCID, severe combined immunodeficiency syndrome	

Immunologoic disorders (congenital and acquired)

The basic function of the immune system is to recognize and attack foreign antigens, for which it is armed with a complex network of cells. First and foremost, is the dominant innate (nonspecific) immune system. It acts as the first line of defense and, as the name implies, attacks recognized foreign proteins in a generic manner. There is no memory conferred in this system. Essentially, cytokines are recruited to the site of infection thus activating the complement cascade and phagocytes remove the antigen.

The second and more sophisticated line of defense is known as the adaptive or specific immune system. It is made up by the B and T lymphocytes. Binding sites on each of the two cells (immunoglobulins for B-cells and T-cell receptors for T-cells) function to recognize foreign proteins which in turn cause the release of cytokines and activate the complement cascade of the innate system. The adaptive system differs in that activation of the two cells confers memory of the antigen by the B- and T-cells, thus donning them the name of memory cells. The memory is stored as a "database" of antigens and leads to a more rapid and fast immune response.

There are five classes of immunoglobulins which are secreted into the systemic circulation: IgG, IgM, IgA, IgD, and IgE. In the case of IgG it is present in the highest concentration and helps to prevent deep tissue infections. It is the only immunoglobulin to cross the placenta; IgM is the largest as it can combine to form a pentameric structure and it is produced as a part of the primary immune response. Both IgM and IgG can activate the complement cascade;IgA is found in the serum in low concentrations but is more commonly found in the secretory form, accounting for the mucosal immunity it provides; IgD has an unclear role in the immune system; IgE, present in the smallest concentration, plays a role in allergic diseases.

There are four categories of primary immune deficiency disorders characterized by the nonfunctioning step/cell in the system. The most common type involves a defect in antibody (B-cell or immunoglobulin) production.

B-cell or immunoglobulin deficiencies

Recurrent sinopulmonary infections are the hallmark of immunoglobulin deficiencies. The X-linked agammagloublinemia or Bruton's agammaglobulinemia is a B-cell deficiency. It is characterized by recurrent pyogenic infections of the skin, respiratory tract, blood, and deep tissues. At 4–8 months of age, most of the maternal IgG dissipates from the infant and it is at this time that the disease presents. Serologic testing results show low immunologic levels across the board and very few B-cells are found in the bloodstream. Bruton tyrosine kinase or BTK is the specific gene that has been identified as the cause. The treatment is with regular interval treatment with intravenous (IV) administration of γ-globulin (IVIG), which replaces IgG.

Table 13.8 Common agents used in pretransplant preparative regimens

Agent	Mode of action	Common potential risks
Antithymocyte globulin	Alteration of function and elimination of T-cells	Fever and chills, pruritus, anaphylaxis, serum sickness
BCNU (Carmustine)	Alkylation leading to DNA damage	Nausea and vomiting, pulmonary infiltrates and fibrosis, transaminitis, nephrotoxicity
Busulfan	Alkylating agent	Nausea and vomiting, electrolyte abnormalities, seizures, mucositis, alopecia, hyperpigmentation, sterility
Carboplatin	Inhibits DNA synthesis by forming DNA cross-links	Nausea and vomiting, type I hypersensitivity, renal impairment and electrolyte wasting, ototoxicity
Cyclophosphamide	Alkylating agent, elimination of T regulatory cells, immunosuppressant	Fluid retention (SIADH), hemorrhagic cystitis, nausea, vomiting, and anorexia, cardiomyopathy, sterility
Etoposide	Inhibits topoisomerase II causing DNA strand breakage	Hypotension, nausea, skin blisters or erythema, nephropathy, hemorrhagic cystitis, alopecia, stomatitis, transaminitis
Fludarabine	Purine analog inhibiting DNA synthesis, immunosuppressant	Nausea, vomiting, and anorexia, mucositis, hemolytic anemia
Melphalan	Alkylating agent	Nausea and vomiting, mucrositis
Thiotepa	Alkylating agent	Nausea, vomiting, and anorexia, sterility, excretion through the skin
Topotecan	Inhibits topoisomerase I causing DNA strand breakage	Nausea, vomiting and anorexia, diarrhea, mucositis, peripheral neuropathy
Total irradiation	Antitumor activity, immunosuppressant	Fever, myelosuppression, mucositis, alopecia, diarrhea, skin reactions and hyperpigmentation, parotitis, pancreatitis, multiple late effects including risk of secondary malignancy

Abbreviation: SIADH, syndrome of inappropriate antidiuretic hormone

IgA deficiency

The most common inherited immunodeficiency is selective IgA deficiency, affecting 1 in 700 to 1000 individuals. Patients do not usually exhibit symptoms as long as levels are > 10 mg/dl. Below that, patients develop recurrent infections. Similar to Bruton's and CVID, patients are susceptible to chronic sinopulmonary infections caused by pyogenic bacteria. However, they are less severe in selective IgA deficiency. Systemic infections are rare in this setting. Notably, these patients are at risk for the development of anti-IgA antibodies. Replacement therapy with γ-globulin is ineffective as IVIG preparations contain only trace amounts of IgA.

Disorders of T-lymphocytes or cell-mediated immunity

T lymphocytes perform numerous functions including enhancing B-cell production of immunoglobulin, killing cells directly, rejecting incompatible/graft tissue.

Cell-mediated immunodeficiency presents within the first 3 months. It results in recurrent infections, usually by opportunistic pathogens. Fatal graft versus

Table 13.9 Signs and symptoms of acute and chronic graft-versus-host disease

Acute GVHD	Skin	Mild macrolpapular rash to generalized erythroderma; can be nonspecific
	GI	Secretory diarrhea, nausea, vomiting, anorexia, stomatitus, hepatic dysfunction
	Hematologic	Anemia, thrombocytopenia
	Ocular	Photophobia, hemorrhagic conjunctivitis
	Pulmonary	Interstitial pneumonitis, alveolar hemorrhage
Chronic GVHD	Skin	Sclerodermatous changes, contractures, alopecia
	GI	Xerostomia, oral atrophy with depapillation of tongue, oral erythema and/or lichenoid lesions, esophagitis, cholestasis, malabsorption, hepatic dysfunction
	Hematologic	Thrombocytopenia
	Ocular	Dry eyes, keratoconjunctivitis sicca (conjunctival and/or corneal inflammation caused by dryness)
	Pulmonary	Interstitial pneumonitis, bronchiolitis obliterans
	Other	Arthritis, immunologic abnormalities
Abbreviations: GVHD, graft-versus-host disease; GI, gastrointestinal		

Table 13.10 Agents used for prophylaxis and treatment of graft-versus-host disease

Agent	Mode of action	Common potential risks
Cyclosporine	Inhibits T-cell activation	Hypomagnesemia, bicarbonate wasting, renal insufficiency, nausea, vomiting, hyperglycemia, gingival hypertrophy, hirsutism, hypertension, seizures, paresthesias, tremors
Methotrexate	Cell-cycle specific; inhibits T-cells as they divide	Transaminitis, mucositis, renal insufficiency, effusions, nausea, vomiting, anorexia, bone marrow suppression
Tacrolimus	Inhibits T-cell activation	Hypomagnesemia, hyperkalemia, renal insufficiency, hypertension, seizures, paresthesias, nausea, vomiting, hyperglycemia
Methylprednisolone	Immunosuppressant; mechanism not well understood	Hypertension, increased blood sugars, increased appetite, insomnia, mood swings, acne, truncal obesity
Mycophenolate mofetil (MMF)	Inhibits T-cell proliferative response	Nausea, vomiting, anorexia, bone marrow suppression, multiple others
Antithymocyte globulin (ATG)	Alteration of function and elimination of T-cells	Fever and chills, pruritus, anaphylaxis, serum sickness
Etanercept/Infliximab	TNF-α inhibitors; consideration in refractory GVHD	Severe immunosuppression
Abbreviations: TNF, tumor necrosis factor; GVHD, graft-versus-host disease		

Table 13.11 Late effects of hematopoietic stem cell transplantation

Late effect	Underlying cause
Endocrine disorders (gonadal failure, delayed pubescence, growth hormone deficiency, hypothyroidism)	TBI
Sterility	TBI, busulfan, cyclophosphamide, thiotepa
Secondary malignancy	TBI, busulfan, ATG, cyclophosphamide, etoposide, genetic factors
Cataracts	TBI
Renal insufficiency	Cyclosporine, other nephrotoxic drugs
Pulmonary disease	Chronic GVHD, BCNU
Cardiomyopathy	Anthracycline therapy, TBI, chronic GVHD
Avascular necrosis	Steroid therapy
Leukoencephalopathy	IT methotrexate
Immunological dysfunction	Chronic GVHD, immunosuppressive therapy
Post-transplant lymphoproliferative disorder	Immunosuppressive therapy
Poor dentogenesis (in young children)	TBI
Decreased bone mineral density	Multiple factors
Abbreviations: GVHD, graft-versus-host disease; TBI, total body irradiation; ATG antithymocyte globulin; IT, intrathecal	

host disease resulting from the transfusion of nonirradiated blood products containing small numbers of lymphocytes from the donor is a risk.

DiGeorge syndrome

DiGeorge syndrome is caused by embryonic dysmorphogenesis of the third and fourth branchial pouches resulting in thymic absence or hypoplasia and absence of the parathyroid glands. Furthermore, the aortic arch and heart are also affected structurally. Neonatal hypocalcemia, congenital heart disease (aortic arch anomaly such as interrupted aortic arch, truncus arteriosis, or right-sided aortic arch), and infection especially mucocutaneous candidiasis characterize the presentation. The clinical severity varies depending on the amount of thymic tissue present. In many patients, the disorder has been traced to a deletion in chromosome 22. Patients with severe DiGeorge anomalies should undergo some form of immune reconstitution, such as bone marrow transplantation or possibly fetal thymus transplantation. Most patients have a partial variant that often requires careful observation but usually no specific therapy.

Severe combined immunodeficiency

Severe combined immunodeficiency (SCID) or "bubble boy" disease is characterized by the absence of functional T lymphocytes. It is the most severe form of the primary immunodeficiencies. Children are susceptible to virtually all infectious agents, with early intractable diarrhea, candidiasis, cytomegalovirus infection, and *Pneumocystis carinii* pneumonia. As maternal IgG wanes, severe bacterial infections can develop. Patients have lymphopenia, marked thymic hypoplasia, and hypogammaglobulinemia. Graft versus host disease and malignancy are commonly seen and most patients die within the first 2 years of life.

Patients with SCID require bone marrow transplantation for long-term survival.

Further reading

1. P. G. Barash, B. F. Cullen, and R. K. Stoelting. *Clinical Anesthesia*. Philadelphia, PA: Lippincott Williams & Wilkins, 2009.
2. F. A. Bonilla and R. S. Geha. Primary immunodeficiency disease. *J Allergy Clin Immunol* 2003; **111**: S571–81.
3. R. H. Buckley. Primary immunodeficiency diseases due to defects in lymphocytes. *N Engl J Med* 2000; **343**: 1313.
4. D. A. Calhoun and D. A. Christensen. Human developmental biology of

granulocyte colony-stimulating factor. *Clin Perinatol* 2000; **27**: 559–76.

5. C. J. Coté, J. Lerman, and I. D. Todres. *A Practice of Anesthesia for Infants and Children*. Philadelphia, PA: Saunders/ Elsevier, 2009.
6. C. Dame and S. Juul. The switch from fetal to adult erythropoiesis. *Clin Perinatol* 2000; **27**: 507–26.
7. V. R. Deutsch and A. Toner. Megakaryocyte development and platelet production. *Br J Haematol* 2006; **134**: 453–66.
8. L. A. Fleisher. *Anesthesia and Uncommon Diseases*. Philadelphia, PA: Elsevier/Saunders, 2012.
9. C. A. Hastings, J. C. Torkildson, and A. K. Agrawal. *Handbook of Pediatric Hematology and Oncology*, 2nd Edition. Oxford: Wiley Blackwell, 2012.
10. K. Kaushansky. Lineage-specific hematopoietic growth factors. *N Engl J Med* 2006; **354**: 2034–45.
11. R. M. Kliegman, R. E. Berhman, and H. B. Jenson. 2007. *Nelson Textbook of Pediatrics e-dition*, 18th Edition & *Atlas of Pediatric Physical Diagnosis*, 5th Edition package, 1e; Chapter 446.
12. R. D. Miller and R. F. Cucchiara. *Anesthesia*. Philadelphia, PA: Churchill Livingstone, 2010.
13. R. K. Ohls, Y. Li, A. Abdel-Mageed, *et al*. Neutrophil pool sizes and granulocyte colony-stimulating factor production in human mid-trimester fetuses. *Pediatr Res* 1995; **37**: 806–11.
14. J. M. Puck. Primary immunodeficiency diseases. *JAMA* 1997; **278**: 1835.
15. W.T. Shearer, R. H. Buckley, R. H. Engler, *et al*. Practice parameters for the diagnosis and management of immunodeficiency. *Ann Allergy Asthma Immunol* 1996; **76**: 282–94.
16. M. C. Sola, C. Dame, and R. D. Christensen. Toward a rational use of recombinant thrombopoietin in the neonatal intensive care unit. *J Pediatr Hematol Oncol* 2001; **23**: 179–84.
17. R. K. Stoelting, R. L. Hines, and K. E. Marschall. *Stoelting's Anesthesia and Co-existing Disease*. Philadelphia, PA: Churchill Livingstone/Elsevier, 2012.
18. S. J. Szilvassy. Haematopoietic stem and progenitor cell-targeted therapies for thrombocytopenia. *Expert Opin Bio Ther* 2006; **6**: 983–92.
19. A. Vats, R. C. Bielby, N. S. Tolley, *et al*. Stem cells. *Lancet* 2005; **366**: 592–602.

Chapter 14

Genetics

Jacob Hummel and Scott Friedman

This section is dedicated to outlining several genetic mutations and their associated syndromes seen in the pediatric population while discussing their relevance to the practice of anesthesiology. Many subgroups of genetic disorders are described below with the focus on the more commonly tested items. This long list may seem daunting to review, but their application to anesthesia can be simplified into some common complications/challenges. Please use the charts at the end of each section to use as a quick, focused review. Most of the anesthetic complications involve the potential for a difficult intubation, an increased risk for malignant hyperthermia, an abnormal response to paralytics or a potential drug interaction (particularly neuromuscular agents and opioids) with anticonvulsant medication. In addition, preoperative cardiac evaluation should always be considered because of increased risk of congenital heart defects and the risk for respiratory complications should always be discussed preoperatively with the pediatric patient and their family.

Mitochondrial myopathies

This is a group of disorders that are characterized by mitochondrial disease leading to muscle weakness and neurologic symptoms. These disorders are caused by genetic defects in the proteins that aid aerobic metabolism. The body has to rely more on anaerobic metabolism which is less efficient and requires more energy sources, like glucose. Muscle and nerve cells are most affected by mitochondrial disease because of their high energy requirements. The list of mitochondrial myopathies includes:

- Kearns–Sayre syndrome (KSS)
- Leigh syndrome and maternally-inherited Leigh syndrome (MILS)
- Mitochondrial DNA depletion syndrome (MDS)
- Mitochondrial encephalomyopathy, lactic acidosis and stroke-like episodes (MELAS)
- Mitochondrial neurogastrointestinal encephalomyopathy (MNGIE)
- Myoclonus epilepsy with ragged red fibers (MERRF)
- Neuropathy, ataxia and retinitis pigmentosa (NARP)
- Pearson syndrome
- Progressive external ophthalmoplegia (PEO)

The symptoms associated with these myopathies include muscle weakness, drooping eyelids, spasms, seizures, cardiomyopathy, myoglobinuria from muscle breakdown and diabetes. All volatile anesthetics have been shown to have a depressant effect on mitochondrial function.

Preoperatively, patients suspected of having a mitochondrial myopathy should be screened with lactate/pyruvate ratios, muscle biopsies ("ragged red" fibers) or other assessments of glucose metabolism. Those with known disease should have routine blood and urine testing done to evaluate lactate and glucose levels. Also, patients should not be subject to long fasting times.

Intraoperatively, these patients may benefit from the administration of glucose containing fluids intravenously. In addition, malignant hyperthermia precautions should be followed.

Postoperatively they are at increased risk for stroke, deteriorating neurologic status, coma, seizures, respiratory failure, arrhythmias, and death. Notice how these symptoms are related to nerve and muscle tissues as the body may not be able to keep up with the increased energy requirements from the stress of surgery.

Essentials of Pediatric Anesthesiology, ed. Alan David Kaye, Charles James Fox and James H. Diaz. Published by Cambridge University Press. © Cambridge University Press 2015.

Mitochondrial myopathies	Nine different types characterized by muscle pain/ weakness and neurologic symptoms	MH precautions, higher risk of postoperative complications, +/- arterial line for glucose and lactate monitoring, dextrose IV fluids
Myotonias	Three main types characterized by muscle stiffness	MH precautions, higher risk of postoperative complications, abnormal response to succinylcholine, be aware of heart block/ arrhythmias

Myotonias

This is a group of disorders characterized by the symptom of delayed relaxation of a muscle after voluntary contraction. Most of the genetic mutations involve distortions of the ion channels leading to irregular depolarization. The distortions in ion channels can also affect the conductance in the heart and the motility of the gut. In addition, neurologic manifestations, such as mental retardation, can be present. The list of myotonias includes:

- Myotonia congenita (Becker's and Thomsen's)
- Paramyotonia congenita
- Myotonic dystrophy

Preoperatively an ECG may be warranted to help elicit any conduction abnormalities in the heart.

Intraoperatively, these patients are at increased risk for aspiration given their irregular gut motility. However, if a rapid sequence intubation is planned, succinylcholine should not be used as it causes prolonged contractures that can last several minutes. If nondepolarizing muscle relaxants are used, they should be short acting as the use of neostigmine to reverse motor blockade can result in a myotonic contracture. The avoidance of any muscle relaxation is the best choice. Volatile anesthetics or hypoxia may precipitate conduction blocks in the heart and should be avoided. In addition, antiarrhythmic medications should be immediately available.

Postoperatively, like all patients with muscle disease, these patients are more likely to have respiratory complications and are at higher risk for malignant hyperthermia. The alternative of regional anesthesia should always be considered.

Muscular dystrophies

This is a group of disorders characterized by progressive muscle weakness. Genetic mutations involve the dystrophin protein that is a key component of the muscle cell and key for stabilizing the membrane during muscle contraction. The most common of these disorders is Duchenne muscular dystrophy. Manifestations of these dystrophies include abnormal gait, difficulty walking up steps due to proximal muscle weakness, along with frequent falling. A cardiomyopathy also develops as an increased intracellular calcium load leads to inflammation and destruction of heart tissue.

Preoperatively these patients need an ECHO to assess the severity of the cardiomyopathy. In addition to heart function, their pulmonary status needs to be evaluated as there is increased risk of respiratory complications secondary to respiratory weakness. Oxygenation saturation $< 95\%$ on room air, forced vital capacity $< 50\%$ of predicted and a cough strength of < 60 maximum expiratory pressure or < 270 l/min peak flow are warning signs of increased risk for postoperative complications.

Intraoperatively, volatile anesthetics and succinylcholine should be avoided because of increased risk of malignant hyperthermia and additionally the risk for hyperkalemia with succinylcholine administration. Patients will have prolonged recovery from administration of paralytics.

Postoperatively, try to avoid respiratory depressants like opioids as respiratory complications are common. Regional anesthesia may be a safer alternative.

Muscular dystrophies	Characterized by progressive muscle weakness, mutation in dystrophin gene	MH precautions, cardiomyopathy, prolonged recovery from paralytics
Duchenne muscular Dystrophy	X-linked muscular dystrophy, lack of dystrophin	Preoperative cardiac evaluation for cardiomyopathy; hyperkalemia with succinylcholine; no increased risk of malignant hyperthermia; possible increased risk of aspiration secondary to respiratory muscle weakness and delayed gastric emptying
Becker Muscular Dystrophy	Abnormality in size or amount of dystrophin, milder course than Duchenne	Hyperkalemia with succinylcholine, low risk of malignant hyperthermia, risk of aspiration, preoperative cardiac evaluation for cardiomyopathy

Neurological disorders

Several different hereditary neurological disorders fall under this category and are further classified into hereditary peripheral neuropathies and hereditary sensory and autonomic neuropathies. Most of these disorders are due to a defect in peripheral nerve myelination. The most notable of peripheral neuropathies group is Charcot–Marie–Tooth disease. The nerve demyelination eventually leads to muscle wasting. This muscle wasting can create respiratory weakness and the risk of hyperkalemia with succinylcholine use.

Similar to the peripheral neuropathies, the hereditary sensory and autonomic neuropathies are due to a defect in myelination. The most notable of this group is familial dysautonomia. Seen almost exclusively in people of Ashkenazi Jewish descent, the anesthetic risks involve respiratory complications as these patients may have recurrent pneumonias secondary to aspiration. Rapid sequence induction is usually indicated. Also, there is a risk of decreased cardiac output secondary to the hypotonia and lack of compensatory sympathetic response that can occur under anesthesia.

Charcot–Marie–Tooth syndrome	Hereditary peripheral neuropathy and muscle atrophy	May have hyperkalemia with succinylcholine; may have perioperative respiratory complications

Overgrowth syndromes

This is a group of disorders characterized by overgrowths of the body or a body part. The body part can be nerves as is seen with neurofibromatosis or several body parts as is seen with Beckwith–Wiedeman syndrome. In Beckwith–Wiedeman, there is exopthalmos, macroglossia and generalized gigantism.

Intraoperatively, neurofibromas may involve airway and make intubation difficult. Intubation of patients with Beckwith–Wiedeman syndrome can also be challenging because of the macroglossia. Also, neurofibromatosis patients have an increased sensitivity to succinylcholine and nondepolarizing muscle relaxants.

Osteochondrodysplastic syndromes

In contrast to the overgrowth syndromes, this is a group of disorders of stunted or absent growth with the focus on bone and cartilage. The most notable of these disorders are achondrogenesis, achondroplasia and osteogenesis imperfecta.

Achondroplasia is a form of dwarfism that results from abnormal cartilage formation and the effect on epiphyseal growth plates leads to short limbs. This disease is caused by a mutation in the fibroblast growth factor receptor (FGF 3) and is an autosomal dominant disorder. Achondrogenesis is a more severe disease with very few surviving past infancy. Several different mutations account for the many types of this disease, but most involve dysfunction in protein transport within the cell between the endoplasmic reticulum and the Golgi apparatus.

Beckwith–Wiedemann syndrome	Generalized overgrowth of body and organs	May have significant upper airway obstruction because of macroglossia; preoperative cardiac evaluation as they may have congenital heart disease; monitor blood glucose
Neurofibromatosis (von Recklinghausen disease)	Neurofibromas of central and peripheral nervous system, café-au-lait spots and bone lesions, association with pheochromocytoma	Neurofibromas may involve airway, increased sensitivity to succinylcholine and nondepolarizing muscle relaxants
Osler–Weber–Rendu syndrome(hereditary hemorrhagic telangiectasia)	Vasculopathy with multiple telangiectases	Preoperative CBC because of bleeding risk; avoid nasal instrumentation; care with laryngoscopy to avoid bleeding; paradoxical emboli can occur; consider avoiding neuraxial blocks

Osteogenesis imperfecta results in "brittle bones" as a result of genetic mutation in a structural collagen. Patients are prone to many fractures and therefore patients must be moved with care. The lack of structural collagen and multiple fractures leads to structural abnormalities.

Preoperatively, patients with these disorders should have an ECG, chest X-ray and ECHO as the structural abnormalities include kyphosis or scoliosis, which can alter cardiopulmonary physiology. In addition, patients should be evaluated for atlantoaxial instability and may need CT or MRI of the head and neck before surgery.

Intraoperatively, these patients should be treated as difficult airways as the disproportionate or misshapen body structure can make intubation a challenge. Consideration should be given to video laryngoscopy, awake fiberoptic or an intubating LMA as these devices not only help aid intubation, but minimize any extra torque on the mandible and neck, which are prone to injury in these patients. Osteogenesis imperfecta patients should be well padded around all of their joints.

Postoperative issues are similar to many of the genetic disorders as respiratory complications are more common.

Connective tissue disorders

There are over 200 disorders that affect the connective tissue, but the major ones are Ehler–Danlos and Marfan Syndrome. Ehler–Danlos syndrome is characterized by the hyperextendable joints and stretchy skin and is due to dysfunctional collagen. Unlike the osteochondrodysplastic disorders, the dysfunctional collagen leads to more elasticity. Marfan syndrome is characterized by the long, thin body habitus with multiple organ systems affected. This syndrome is

Achondrogenesis	Types 1 and 2 result in severe defect in the development of bone and cartilage	May be difficult airway because of micrognathia; care with positioning
Achondroplasia	Premature fusion of the bones, fusion, small stature, obesity, normal intelligence	May be difficult airway; may have cervical spine compression with positioning; altered lung mechanics secondary to chest wall deformity; regional anesthesia has been performed
Osteogenesis imperfecta	Mutation in a gene for collagen	Fractures may occur with any manipulation

the result of a mutation in the gene encoding for the fibrillin-1 protein. The most serious complication of Marfan's is an aortic dissection which carries a high fatality rate.

All of these disorders should have a cardiac evaluation done preoperatively as the structural integrity of the vasculature and the valves may be affected. Premature onset of ischemic heart disease is also seen.

Intraoperatively, positive-pressure ventilation should be closely managed as they are at increased risk for pneumothorax. In addition, arterial line placement can cause arterial rupture and significantly compromise blood flow distally to the site of insertion.

Ehlers–Danlos syndrome	Defect in gene encoding collagen, ten types, more elastic structures	May bleed significantly from vascular aneurysm; preoperative cardiac evaluation for congenital defects, premature ischemic heart disease and conduction abnormalities; risk for pneumothorax; risk for arterial rupture with cannulation
Marfan syndrome	Connective tissue disorder, defect in fibrillin, recurrent joint dislocations	Preoperative cardiac evaluation for aortic and valvular pathology, aortic dissection possible, pneumothorax possible with positive-pressure ventilation

Craniofacial syndromes

Craniofacial anomalies refers to an abnormality of the face and/or the head. A craniofacial condition may include disfigurement brought about by birth defect, disease or trauma and can be either acquired or congenital. Although rare, they make up a considerably diverse group of defects and this diversity makes the classification of these syndromes extremely difficult. According to the Committee on Nomenclature and Classification of Craniofacial Anomalies of the American Cleft Palate Association, these disorders are classified into five groups:

- Clefts
- Synostosis
- Hypoplasia
- Hyperplasia
- Unclassified

More details about these disorders are being discovered all the time and as developments occur, so does the advancement of the surgical corrections. This field of surgery has grown to include the surgical expertise from multiple fields and is an ongoing challenge for anesthesiologists as well.

The preoperative assessment of children with craniofacial anomalies is the most important step in managing the patient. Once the anomaly is discovered, it must be determined if the child has an associated syndrome, which can complicate the picture even more due to the associated airway involvement, other organ involvement and intricacies of surgical repair. The airway on these children can be altered significantly and a thorough airway examination must be completed. Complications with the airway can arise with ventilation and/or intubation. The incidence of a difficult airway is higher in patients with congenital craniofacial syndromes, as well as those patients who have already undergone reconstruction. Other major preoperative assessments include checking for heart conditions and brain conditions as these are two well-known complications associated with these syndromes and can have a serious affect on the anesthesia.

Due to the multitude of complications that are associated with patients with craniofacial syndromes, it is imperative for the anesthesiologist to be fully prepared intraoperatively. The proper equipment is important to have on hand and readily available. It is also important to have a pediatric ENT available for emergencies. Intraoperatively, there is a lot to consider associated with these anomalies. Most of the procedures can last for long periods of time and can be associated with hypovolemia, hypothermia, significant blood loss, and venous air emboli. It is recommended to have adequate IV access, baseline hemoglobin/hematocrit, and arterial blood pressure monitoring available.

Postoperatively, mask ventilation can remain difficult due to the surgical site involved as well as any bandaging or devices left in place by the surgical team. It is important to keep proper airway management devices close by following extubation. It is also extremely important to monitor patients' vitals and resuscitation following these surgeries. If there is ever concern for the adequacy of resuscitation or the post-extubated airway, patients may benefit from a delayed extubation in a controlled setting once stabilized properly.

Pierre Robin	Micrognathia, glossoptosis, may also have cleft palate	May be very difficult to intubate due to micrognathia, glossoptosis; successful intubation described with fiberoptic scopes and LMA, prone positioning, and tongue suture to displace tongue forward
Treacher Collins syndrome	Mandibulofacial dysostosis, malar hypoplasia, downsloping palbebral fissures, micro-ophthalmia, low-set ears, small mouth, micrognathia	May be extremely difficult airway; fiberoptic endoscopy and LMA for airway; preoperative cardiac evaluation for congenital heart defects

Endocrine disorders

There are a number of diseases associated with the endocrine system. One of the biggest factors for anesthesiologists when dealing with disorders of the endocrine system is to focus not only on the organ of interest, but also the end-organ consequences of the endocrine dysfunction and possible rare syndromes. The endocrine system can directly and indirectly alter many critical functions of the body. Due to the vast nature of the endocrine system and its ability to alter many areas of the human body, it is imperative for the anesthesiologist to also understand the surgery about to be performed and be cognizant of the potentially dramatic pathophysiological effects of altering the specific targeted endocrine organ. The endocrine system consists of the parathyroid glands, thyroid gland, pituitary gland, adrenal cortex, adrenal medulla and pancreas. The most prominent of the genetic disorders affecting these glands is congenital adrenal hyperplasia (CAH). This disorder is due to a defect in the synthesis of cortisol with overproduction of an androgen cortisol precursor leading to virilization. The clinical features depend on enzyme deficiency and can involve salt wasting from the deficiency of mineralcorticoids and hypoglycemia from a deficiency in glucocorticoids.

Preoperatively, when dealing with endocrine disorders, two main themes guide the anesthesia provided for patients. First, the cardiovascular system is the organ system that most influences the anesthetic management. Second, if possible, stabilizing or correcting the endocrine abnormality that is affecting the patient preoperatively may improve patient outcomes. For CAH, electrolytes should be evaluated with a basic metabolic panel before surgery.

Intraoperatively, it is extremely important to monitor closely for fluid shifts, electrolyte imbalances, cardiac dysrhythmias and dysfunction and other endocrine related abnormalities. Dextrose or potassium-containing fluids may be needed intraoperatively to help correct imbalances in glucose and potassium. A stress dose of a corticosteroid-like hydrocortisone is often given before surgery. Be aware that dexamethasone is a potent glucocorticoid and effective for preventing postoperative nausea and vomiting, but has minimal mineralcorticoid effect and is not effective for treating these patients.

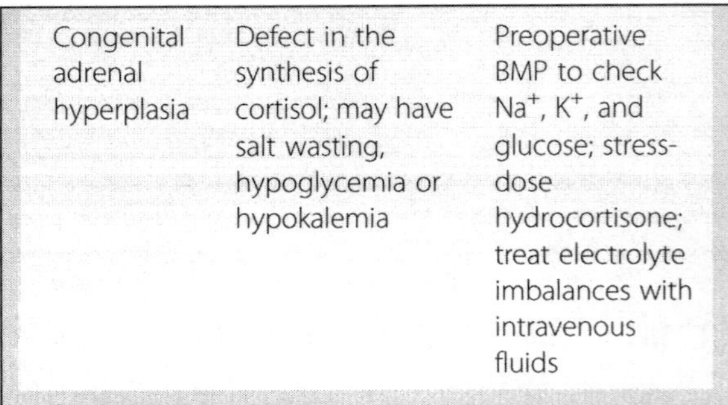

Congenital adrenal hyperplasia	Defect in the synthesis of cortisol; may have salt wasting, hypoglycemia or hypokalemia	Preoperative BMP to check Na^+, K^+, and glucose; stress-dose hydrocortisone; treat electrolyte imbalances with intravenous fluids

Inborn errors of metabolism

This class of disorders consists of a large number of genetic disorders (approximately 550) in which single genes that usually code for enzymes are disrupted and lead to metabolic disorders. The disruption of the metabolic pathway can lead to a buildup of substrates which can be potentially toxic. These disorders are associated with multisystem complications in the pediatric population that often can develop into severe neurologic disorders, mental retardation, premature death and/or a poor quality of life.

Due to the large number of inborn errors of metabolism and the large number of presenting symptoms, it may be hard for the anesthesiologist to prepare for cases involving these diseases. Inborn errors of metabolism manifest as a variety of metabolic diseases, all of which may complicate the anesthetic technique. Most of the time these diseases are clinically asymptomatic and some may only be noticed in response to certain triggering factors (food or certain drugs). There are a number of metabolic diseases and over time they have been categorized into many different classes. These include, with examples, disorders of:

- Carbohydrate metabolism
- Glycogen storage disease
- Amino acid metabolism
- Phenylketonuria, Maple syrup urine disease
- Urea cycle
- Carbamoyl phosphate synthetase 1 deficiency
- Organic acid
- Alcaptonuria
- Fatty acid oxidation and mitochondrial metabolism
- Medium-chain-acyl-coenzyme A dehydrogenase deficiency (MCADD)
- Porphyrin metabolism
- Acute intermittent porphyria
- Purine or pyrimidine metabolism
- Lesch–Nyhan syndrome
- Steroid metabolism
- Lipoid congenital adrenal hyperplasia, congenital adrenal hyperplasia
- Mitochondrial function
- Kearns–Sayre syndrome
- Peroxisomal function
- Zellweger syndrome
- Lysosomal storage
- Gaucher's disease
- Niemann–Pick disease

Preoperatively, it is important for the anesthesiologist to examine for any cardiopulmonary compromise. If a particular inborn error is known or suspected, laboratory testing should be individualized to that exact inborn error.

Intraoperatviely, the main complications that can arise in patients with these disorders are seizures and generalized respiratory insufficiency. It is suspected that patients with a number of these disorders can have respiratory complications because of the possible hypotonia, poor suckling ability and overall underdevelopment of the cardiopulmonary system.

Postoperatively, these patients must be watched and observed very closely. They often have respiratory insufficiency and a delayed extubation (or a nonrushed extubation) could be beneficial to these children. These children also have a high risk of postoperative metabolic decompensation and clinical deterioration. It has been shown that early pharmacologic and dietary management is beneficial for these children.

Lesch–Nyhan syndrome	Hyperuricemia, developmental delay, hypertonia, spasticity, self-mutilation	Check CBC preoperatively and renal function preoperatively because of risk of megaloblastic anemia and recurrent kidney stones, respectively
Porphyria	Defect in heme synthesis; precipitating factors include infection, starvation, drugs, and pregnancy	Preoperative fasting should be minimized; can administer glucose-containing solution; premedication may decrease stress; avoid barbiturates; safe anesthetics include opioids, propofol, nitrous oxide, newer generation volatile anesthetics and muscle relaxants; neuropathy may cause respiratory muscle weakness and aspiration

Malignant hyperthermia

Malignant hyperthermia (MH), also known as malignant hyperpyrexia, is an extremely rare and life-threatening condition that must be recognized and treated quickly in order to prevent fatal outcomes.

Susceptibility to MH is an autosomal dominant disorder and commonly involves the gene encoding for the ryanodine receptor. Volatile anesthetic agents and succinylcholine are the two main agents used by the anesthesiologist that can trigger MH in susceptible patients. The mechanism behind MH is through the dramatic release of stored calcium from the sarcoplasmic reticulum, causing a drastic increase in intracellular calcium and muscle contraction. When triggered, there is an uncontrolled increase in skeletal muscle oxidative metabolism. As a result, the body loses its ability to regulate body temperature, remove carbon dioxide and supply oxygen. This can eventually lead to death secondary to circulatory collapse. Malignant hyperthermia develops rapidly after exposure in susceptible patients.

Preoperatively, all patients should be screened for MH. This is accomplished by asking if they or any of their direct family members have ever experienced any problems with anesthesia in the past. If the patient is susceptible to developing MH, all providers should be made aware of this and the patient should avoid inhaled anesthetics and succinylcholine when possible.

Intraoperative awareness of MH is a feature that all anesthesiologists should learn. The signs and symptoms of MH are secondary to a hypercatabolic state. It is extremely important for anesthesiologists to understand MH, but it is even more important to be able to accurately diagnose and effectively treat MH, should it arise. The earliest signs of an episode of MH following administration of succinylcholine are a rapid and unexplained tachycardia, a rise in $ETCO_2$ with increased minute ventilation, muscle rigidity, and masseter muscle contracture. Most people, due to the name malignant hyperthermia, believe that hyperthermia is a key early element; however, hyperthermia is usually a late sign of MH.

Other features of MH include acidosis, cyanosis, tachypnea, hypertension, hyperkalemia and cardiac dysrhythmias. The actual diagnosis of MH is based on clinical assessment. The best way to prevent a MH attack is through the avoidance of the known triggering factors, succinylcholine and all volatile anesthetics. The anesthesia circuit should be completely new, free from all volatile anesthetics with 100% oxygen flushed throughout the machine for 20–30 minutes. There are differing opinions and thoughts on prophylactic dantrolene prior to the start of the case. The newest theory is that dantrolene should not be given prophylactically if other steps are performed and no triggering agents are being used for the case.

If MH is suspected, rapid treatment is important. The current therapy is IV dantrolene, discontinuing any triggering agent being used and supportive therapy while monitoring for signs and symptoms of circularity collapse, acidosis and organ dysfunction

Immunologic disorders

The immunologic system is a very complex system with the primary function of protecting the body from infection. When this system is disrupted, it can lead to autoimmune disorders, allergic reactions/conditions, immunodeficiency syndromes and malignancies. There are a huge number of immunologic disorders and they are categorized in several different ways and broken down into two main groups. The first group is primary immunodeficiency diseases (PIDs) and the second is secondary or acquired immunodeficiency diseases. So far, according to the International Union of Immunological Societies, more than 150 PIDs and even more acquired diseases have been discovered and explored. These immune disorders are even further broken down and categorized by the component of the immune system affected and by whether the immune system is over or under active. The most well-known and most researched secondary immunodeficiency is human immunodeficiency virus infection/acquired immunodeficiency syndrome (HIV/AIDS). Below is a list of some of the major autoimmune disorders and PIDs:

Autoimmune disorders:

- Type 1 diabetes
- Celiac disease
- Juvenile dermatomyositis
- Juvenile idiopathic arthritis
- Scleroderma
- Lupus

PIDs:

- Severe combined immunodeficiency (SCID)
- DiGeorge syndrome
- Hyperimmunoglobulin E syndrome (Job's syndrome)
- Leukocyte adhesion deficiency (LAD)
- Wiskott–Aldrich syndrome
- Chronic granulomatous disease (CGD)
- Common variable immunodeficiency

- Autoimmune lymphoproliferative syndrome
- Selective IgA deficiency
- Ataxia telangiectasia

Preoperatively, it is important to do a full history and physical in pediatric patients with any known autoimmune disorders, PIDs or acquired immunodeficiency. There have been many airway complications associated with patients with these disorders, decreased cervical and temporomandibular mobility being the most common. Prior to proceeding to the operating room, all protective measures should be taken to ensure that the patient is protected from infectious agents.

Intraoperatively, it has been shown that the stress of surgery and anesthesia may result in lymphopenia and therefore further decrease the protective factors in these already immunocompromised patients. Children with these disorders undergo multiple procedures throughout their lifetime and kids with CNS involvement may have excessive and unwanted effects from the usual doses of opioids and sedatives.

Postoperatively, these patients may have rapid clinical deterioration following what may appear to be a minor procedure. Postoperative care should be tailored to each patient individually and must include the possibility of ventilation and other supportive measures in the recovery area.

Ataxia-telangiectasia syndrome	Telangiectases, cerebellar ataxia, peripheral nerve degeneration, immunodeficiency	Aseptic technique with invasive procedures; potential hyperkalemia with succinycholine; may have glucose intolerance

Chromosomal abnormalities

Chromosomal abnormalities reflect an abnormality of chromosome number or structure in one or more chromosomes. These abnormalities usually occur during meiosis or mitosis when there is an error in cell division. There are many types of these abnormalities, but they can be organized into two main groups: numerical disorders and structural disorders.

Numerical disorders, also known as aneuploidy, occur when an individual is missing either a chromosome from a pair (monosomy) or has more than two chromosomes of a pair (trisomy).

Monosomy:

- Turner syndrome – patient is born with only one X chromosome
- Trisomy 8
- Trisomy 9
- Trisomy 13
- Trisomy 18
- Trisomy 21

Structural abnormalities occur when the actual chromosome's structure is altered and can take several forms: deletions, duplications, translocations, inversions, insertions, rings and isochromosomes.

Deletions – portion of the chromosome is missing or deleted:

- Angelman's syndrome – 15q maternal deletion
- Cri du chat – 5p deletion
- DiGeorge syndrome – 22q11.2 deletion
- Prader–Willi syndrome – 15q paternal deletion

Duplications – portion of the chromosome is duplicated, resulting in extra genetic material:

- Fragile X syndrome – expansion of CGG trinucleotide repeat
- Klinefelter syndrome – 47, XXY
- Noonan syndrome – 12q24

Translocations – portion of one chromosome is transferred to another chromosome. There are two main types:

- Reciprocal – segments from two different chromosomes have been exchanged
- Robertsonian – entire chromosome has attached to another at the centromere
- Inversions – portion of chromosome has broken off, turned upside down and reattached
- Insertions – portion of one chromosome has been deleted and inserted into another chromosome

Rings – portion of a chromosome has broken off and formed a circle.

The preoperative assessment in patients with chromosomal abnormalities is extremely important as these patients can have a multitude of problems. The biggest concerns when confronted with a patient with chromosomal anomalies are the airway, cardiac status, respiratory status, renal function, coexisting craniofacial abnormalities, and behavioral difficulties.

Intraoperatively, many of these patients are on chronic seizure prophylaxis medications, which can interfere with certain anesthesia medications and agents. As stated before, patients with different chromosomal abnormalities are at risk for many intraoperative complications. The anesthesiologist should be aware of the preoperative assessment and be ready to treat any intraoperative complications that may arise.

The postoperative course of these patients can be somewhat difficult. Delayed extubation until the patient has full control of their airway is recommended in all patients with difficult airways. These patients have a high risk of developing rapid airway decline postsurgery and all ventilation and airway supplies should be readily available in the PACU in case of airway loss and the need for reintubation. The behavioral defects associated with these conditions can also be difficult to manage in the postoperative period.

Angelman syndrome	Severe mental retardation, "happy puppet syndrome"	Likely taking antiseizure medications
Cri du chat syndrome	Partial deletion of chromosome 5p, high-pitched cry	Difficult intubation described because of micrognathia and short neck; preoperative cardiac evaluation for congenital heart defects; risk of aspiration at baseline; airway obstruction secondary to hypotonia
DiGeorge syndrome (CATCH-22 syndrome)	Microdeletion on chromosome 22; cellular immunodeficiency	May be difficult intubation because of micrognathia; endobronchial intubation more likely with short trachea; preoperative cardiac evaluation for congenital heart defects; avoid nasal tubes with choanal atresia; monitor calcium; irradiate blood products
Down syndrome (trisomy 21 syndrome)	Trisomy 21	Airway obstruction; atlantoaxial instability; risk for subluxation may require preoperative neck films; smaller endotracheal tube by 1 mm; preoperative cardiac evaluation for congenital heart defects; bradycardia common after inhalation induction
Fragile X syndrome	Defect in X chromosome, mental retardation	Preoperative cardiac evaluation for mitral valve prolapse; may have behavioral difficulties, chronic antiseizure medication
Noonan syndrome	Sometimes referred to as male version of Turner syndrome	May be difficult intubation because of facial deformities and webbed neck; impaired blood clotting; preoperative cardiac evaluation for congenital heart defects; check preoperative renal function
Prader–Willi syndrome	Secondary to partial deletion of chromosome 15	Anesthetic concerns related to obesity; difficult mask ventilation; potential difficult airway; decreased functional residual capacity; perioperative respiratory complications; monitor perioperative glucose
Trisomy 8 syndrome	Mental retardation	May be difficult intubation; chronic anticonvulsant medication; preoperative cardiac evaluation
Trisomy 9 syndrome	Profound mental retardation	May be difficult intubation; chronic anticonvulsant medication; preoperative cardiac evaluation for congenital heart defects

Trisomy 13 syndrome (Patau syndrome)	Severe mental retardation, polydactyly; most die young	May be difficult intubation; preoperative cardiac evaluation; check preoperative renal function; placement of radial catheter may be difficult; chronic anticonvulsant medication
Trisomy 18 syndrome (Edwards syndrome)	Mental retardation and rocker bottom feet	May be difficult intubation; preoperative cardiac evaluation for congenital heart defects; malformations may pertain to the heart and kidneys
Turner syndrome	Caused by single X chromosome	May be difficult intubation because of micrognathia; preoperative cardiac evaluation for congenital heart defects; check preoperative renal function

Further reading

1. Baum VC, O'Flaherty JE. *Anesthesia for Genetic, Metabolic, and Dysmorphic Syndromes of Childhood.* Philadelphia PA: Lippincott Williams & Wilkins, 1999.
2. Davis PJ, Cladis FP, Motoyama EK. *Smith's Anesthesia for Infants and Children*, Eighth Edition. Appendix D, A22–A37. Philadelphia PA, Elsevier Mosby, 2011.
3. Fleisher LA. *Anesthesia and Uncommon Diseases*, Sixth Edition. Philadelphia, PA: Saunders (Elsevier), 2012.

Chapter 15

Neonatal: General considerations

Jennifer Aunspaugh

Introduction

Increasing advancements in perinatal care has greatly decreased the morbidity and mortality of critically ill neonates over the past 25 years, leading to less and less of them requiring exposure to anesthetic agents for surgery. However, many of the surviving neonates develop coexisting diseases that eventually require care by an anesthesiologist. This chapter will focus on anesthesia management for the neonate, taking in to consideration their developmental physiology, and some surgical disease states that may be encountered in the operating room.

General considerations

Infants are classified in two categories based on their postconceptual age at time of delivery. The term infant is defined as > 37 weeks gestation. Preterm infants are defined as those infants delivered at < 37 weeks gestation and can be categorized further as:

(1) Low birth weight = less than 2500 g
(2) Very low birth weight = less than 1500 g
(3) Extremely low birth weight = less than 1000 g

In the early 1950s, Virginia Apgar, an anesthesiologist at Columbia University, proposed a new method of evaluating the newborn infant's clinical status and whether the child needed prompt intervention to establish breathing. The Apgar score describes the condition of the newborn infant immediately after birth and, when properly applied, is a tool for standardized assessment (1–3). Five objective signs were identified as easy to determine and without interfering with the care of the newborn infant.

The Apgar comprises five components:

(1) Heart rate
(2) Respiratory effort
(3) Muscle tone
(4) Reflex irritability
(5) Color

Each sign is a score with a 0, 1, or 2 with the sum of the scores being the total score. These scores are determined at 1 min and 5 minutes following delivery of the infant with a score of 7 or higher suggesting the condition of the baby is good to excellent. The score was once inappropriately used alone to diagnose asphyxia. The National Resuscitation Program guidelines state that "Apgar scores should not be used to dictate appropriate resuscitation actions, nor should interventions for depressed infants be delayed until the 1 minute assessment" (1). This score has been widely used to evaluate term newborns, with limited use in preterm infants. However, Mujahid *et al.* found that in low birth weight infants, a low Apgar score correlates both with acidosis and mortality (4).

Organ system maturity

Cardiovascular system

It is important for anesthesiologists to consider developmental changes in heart rate, blood pressure, and cardiac output in the neonate. The development of the cardiovascular system is essentially complete by 8 weeks of gestation. Studies of isolated fetal muscle strips have shown that fetal myocardium cannot generate the same contractile force as adult myocardium throughout the entire range of the length–tension curve (5). Reduced numbers of underdeveloped mitochondria and maturational differences in various signaling pathways and related messenger systems are also characteristic of the neonatal myocardium.

The increased amount of noncontractile tissue in the neonate results in poor ventricular compliance and limited response to increased preload. Compliance of both ventricles progressively increases during fetal life

Essentials of Pediatric Anesthesiology, ed. Alan David Kaye, Charles James Fox and James H. Diaz. Published by Cambridge University Press. © Cambridge University Press 2015.

and the postnatal period so that maximal stroke volume occurs at a significantly reduced atrial pressure in the neonate compared with the fetus (6). The extraordinarily high metabolic rate of the neonate (oxygen consumption, 6 to 8 ml/kg/min, compared with 2 to 3 ml/kg/min in the adult) requires a proportional increase in cardiac output. The neonatal heart functions at close to maximal rate and stroke volume just to meet the basic demands for oxygen delivery (6). The cardiac output is commonly described as being primarily heart rate (HR) dependent due to a fixed stroke volume, but echocardiographic studies in human fetuses and neonates clearly demonstrate the capacity to increase stroke volume (6).

After birth, the neonatal heart has little ability to increase cardiac output through increases in preload and afterload; therefore, neonatal cardiac output is primarily heart rate dependent. The mechanism is unknown describing the heart rate dependent increase in immature myocardium therefore leading to increased cardiac output. Autonomic control of the heart in utero is mediated through the parasympathetic nervous system, predominantly. The sympathetic system reaches maturity by early infancy, whereas the parasympathetic system reaches maturity within a few days after birth (7). The relative imbalance of these two components of the autonomic nervous system at birth may account for the clinical observation that neonates are predisposed to exhibit marked vagal responses to a variety of stimuli. The mean heart rate in the first 24 hours of the life of the neonate is 120 beats per minute. Atropine and glycopyrrolate are drugs commonly used by anesthesiologists to increase the heart rate in neonates, and therefore increase cardiac output in times of hypotension during anesthesia.

Table 15.1 Heart rates related to age (6,8)

Age	*Heart rate, beats/min*
Premature	120–170
0–3 months	100–150
3–6 months	90–120
6–12 months	80–120
1–3 years	70–110
3–6 years	65–110
6–12 years	60–95
Adult	55–85

Understanding the differences in blood pressures of the neonate as compared to adults is important so that abnormal values can be further investigated. Accurate blood pressure measurement in children depends on the selection of an appropriate sized cuff. Neonates have a mean systolic of around 65 mmHg at birth that increases to 75 mmHg at 6 weeks. There is little change in the mean systolic blood pressure between the ages of 6 weeks and 1 year, followed by a gradual increase with age beyond 1 year (9). Normal blood pressure in newborns correlates with gestational age and birth weight.

There are significantly lower systolic and diastolic blood pressures in infants receiving ventilation and those born after birth asphyxia than in healthy infants (10).

Respiratory system

During the course of development, the infant upper airways undergo deep anatomic modifications (6). An infant's glottis is relatively small compared to the adult and epiglottis is proportionately larger (8). This difference is crucial in allowing the baby to suck, swallow, and breath simultaneously. Most newborn infants are obligate breathers. The glottis in infants is at the level of the C3–4 interspace; however, at around 2 years of age, the larynx begins to move to a lower position in the neck with the glottis being at the C4–5 interspace in adults. This lower position eliminates the ability to suck and breathe simultaneous, but this lowering is crucial for the development of complex speech and articulation (8).

The two main functions of the respiratory system are to supply sufficient oxygen and remove carbon dioxide. The development of the respiratory system begins during the fourth week of gestation. By 26 to 28 weeks of gestation, sufficient alveoli and surfactant are present to permit survival of some infants without exogenous surfactant. Before birth, the lungs are filled with fluid that must be replaced by air when making the transition to extrauterine life. With the first breath, the lungs are inflated with air and the fluid is removed via absorption through the pulmonary vascular and lymphatic system. The contact with the air containing oxygen results in vasodilatation and a large increase in pulmonary blood flow, at which time the pulmonary resistance acutely falls (6,8).

The noncompliant lungs of the infant may cause abnormal chest wall elasticity creating mild intercostal retractions. Additionally, neonates and infants are more dependent on the diaphragm for normal ventilatory function.

Table 15.2 Respiratory rates related to age (6,8)

Age	*Respiratory rate, breaths/min*
Premature	40–70
0–3 months	35–55
3–6 months	30–45
6–12 months	25–40
1–3 years	20–30
3–6 years	20–25
6–12 years	14–22
Adult	12–18

The respiratory rate is highest in the newborn period and gradually falls to adult values by adolescence. Young, especially premature, infants may normally show an irregular respiratory pattern. Term infants may normally display periodic breathing, seen during the first 24 hours and disappearing by 38 to 40 weeks of gestational age.

Renal system

The main purpose of the kidney is to maintain fluid and electrolyte homeostasis.

Urine production begins at approximately 12 weeks of gestation and continues throughout fetal life. The kidneys do not work until birth due to the placenta functioning as the primary organ of elimination of fetal metabolic waste. Although the kidneys are fully developed at 34 weeks gestation, postnatal functional changes occur in renal blood flow, glomerular filtration rate (GFR), and tubular function. GFR is one-third to one-fourth of those of the adult values in the neonatal period and increases within the first month of life (6).

After the 1st month of life, GFR increases progressively and reaches adult levels between 1 and 2 years of life (16). The serum creatinine concentration reflects the maternal level at birth and then declines during the first days of life (6,16).

In the newborn, the ability to concentrate urine is limited compared to the adult. For example, the maximum urine concentration of 600 mOsm/kg in newborns vs. 1200 mOsm/kg in adult counterparts (8).

Table 15.3 Factors leading to increased GFR afer birth

1. Systemic blood pressure
2. Hydrostatic pressure of glomeruli
3. Pore size of glomerular capillary wall
4. Plasma flow rate
5. Ultrafiltration coefficient

Hematopoietic and immunologic system

During the last 3 months of gestation, the bone marrow becomes the primary site of blood cell formation. The neonate generally has a higher hemoglobin and hematocrit compared to the older child and their hemoglobin (HgbF) also has a much higher affinity for oxygen than in the adult type (HgbA) (17). The preterm infant has a more exaggerated neonatal anemia due to low total body iron stores and a shorter lifespan of red cells (17). There is a physiologic drop in hemoglobin by 8–12 weeks that stimulates erythropoiesis. Hemoglobin produced postnatally is the adult type. This adult type hemoglobin displaces the HgbF by 4 months of age.

The white blood cell count is highest in the first days of life and drops steadily throughout childhood to finally reach adult values during adolescence. The production of platelets is regulated by thrombopoietin, which maintains a normal blood platelet count of 15–400 × 10^{a}/l with no age related differences (8).

After the first hours of life, the blood volume maintains a constant relationship to body weight throughout life. Average blood volume for a term infant is 85 ml/kg. The blood volume at approximately 6 months of age is 75 ml/kg, which is similar to older children and adults (18).

Digestive and endocrine systems

The gastrointestinal system is fully capable of taking over its functions at birth, as well as the endocrine and immunologic systems. The first bowel movement after birth, meconium, is normally discharged within the first 24 to 48 hours of life (8). Normal range of stool frequency varies greatly with breast fed infants usually having more stools than formula-fed infants. The frequency of bowel movements declines in the first few years of life and reaches adult habits by 4 years of age.

In neonates and younger infants, the lower esophageal sphincter tone is decreased and may lead to gastroesophageal reflux (8). Between 1:300 and 1:1000 infants have reflux significant enough to cause complications (19).

High rates of bilirubin production due to a shorter lifespan of red blood cells in the newborn cause a

Table 15.4 Relationship of motor milestones to age (6)

Motor milestone	Age
Supports head	3 months
Sits alone	6 months
Stands alone	12 months
Balances on one foot	3 years

Table 15.5 Relationship of fine motor/adaptive milestones to age (6)

Fine motor/adaptive milestones	Age
Grasps rattle	3 months
Passes cube hand to hand	6 months
Pincer grip	1 year
Imitates vertical line	2 years
Copies circle	3 years

Table 15.6 Relationship of language milestones to age (6)

Language milestones	Age
Squeals	1.5–3 months
Turns to voice	6 months
Combines two words	1.5 years
Composes short sentences	2 years
Gives entire name	3 years

Table 15.7 Relationship of personal–social milestones to age (6)

Personal–social milestones	Age
Smiles spontaneously	3 months
Feeds self crackers	6 months
Drinks from cup	1 year
Plays interactive games	2 years

common condition known as neonatal jaundice. Neonatal jaundice is a physiologic hyperbilirubinemia beginning during the second 24 hours of life, peaks around the 3rd day of life, and resolves itself by the end of the first week (20). This is generally a benign, self-limiting condition in the newborn, but should be monitored to prevent missing an indication for treatment (e.g., phototherapy) or a pathologic cause of jaundice.

In utero, glucose supply to the fetus is primarily from the mother. During the 3rd trimester, glycogen storage and capacity for degradation are developed. At birth, the maternal supply of glucose is abruptly interrupted and neonates then begin to meet their glucose needs by glucose intake, glycogenolysis or gluconeogenesis. Glycogenolysis allows a full term infant to maintain normal serum glucose concentrations during a 10–12 hour fast. Hepatic proglucose enzyme activity increases rapidly after birth. In the preoperative period, most newborns should receive an intravenous infusion containing 5% to 10% dextrose to prevent hypoglycemia. Normal glucose levels for the newborn are between 40 and 60 mg/dl.

Neurologic development in the neonate

The nervous system is anatomically complete at birth; functionally it remains immature with the continuation of myelination and synaptogenesis. An infant's normal mental development depends on the maturation of the central nervous system (6). This development may be affected by physical illness, inadequate psychosocial support, or poor nutrition conditions in preterm babies. The brain has two growth spurts, neuronal cell multiplication between 15 and 20 weeks of gestation, and glial cell multiplication commencing at 25 weeks and extending into the second year of life. Myelination continues into the third year. Malnutrition during this phase of neural development may have profound handicapping effects (6).

Cranial sutures are still open at birth and are easily palpable. The anterior fontanel is diamond shaped and soft at birth. It's size gradually decreases following birth and closes anywhere from 12 to 18 months of life. A bulging fontanel may indicate an increase in intracranial pressure. A sunken fontanel may be a sign of severe hypovolemia from various causes including dehydration (8). As myelination continues during the first two years of age, there is a rapid development of many motor and behavioral skills. Myelination is usually complete by 7 years of age.

Normal neonates show various primitive reflexes such as the grasp, rooting, sucking, Moro, and asymmetric tonic neck reflex. Milestones of development are useful indicators of mental development and possible deviations from normal. These milestones represent the *average*, and infants can vary in their rates of maturation of different body functions and still be within the normal range (6).

Cognitive development issues with anesthesia

Children can be delayed in many ways in both cognitive and motor development. In diagnosing a developmental abnormality, anesthesiologists must be aware of the difficulties to be faced: Infants born prematurely will be delayed and should be assessed in terms of their conceptional age. Infants with cerebral palsy or sensory deficits (auditory and visual) may have normal mental development, but the handicap may interfere with assessment of mental status. The effects of drugs should be considered (e.g., barbiturates for epilepsy) (6). In one recent study in infants $\leq$ 6 weeks having surgery for congenital heart disease, there was no evidence of an association between dose and duration of sedation/analgesia drugs during the operative and perioperative period and adverse neurodevelopmental outcomes (21). The FDA's National Center for Toxicological Research (NCTR) in animals has raised concerns about some anesthetic drugs that need to be investigated further to determine if there is a risk to infants and children younger than 4 years of age. However, this research is very limited and is not yet conclusive. Dangers to infants and children from anesthesia are unproven at this point. There is no direct evidence that anesthetics are unsafe for children (22).

Stress response in neonates

In newborn infants, metabolic activity is much more difficult to maintain because of a greater surface area, larger brain-to-body weight ratio, increased obligatory requirements for glucose, and smaller reserves for protein, carbohydrates, and fat. It is well known that surgical or nonsurgical injury triggers the release of "stress hormones," mainly catecholamines, corticosteroids, growth hormones, and glucagon, all of which stimulate a cascade of metabolic changes leading to substrate mobilization with the breakdown of protein, fat, and carbohydrate stores (23). Studies that investigated the cortisol response to surgical stress in children have shown that cortisol levels at least doubled during the surgery procedure and increased further during recovery (24). There are more extreme and prolonged stress responses in neonates during noncardiac surgery than in adult patients.

More recent studies are looking at the cortisol response in patients undergoing a nonstimulating procedure such as medical imaging. In these studies, while some children demonstrated a rise in their cortisol levels in response to anesthesia without surgery, the response was variable and often more pronounced during recovery (25). Recovery from anesthesia appears to be more physiologically stressful than anesthesia itself in patients undergoing medical imaging.

Neonatal resuscitation and transporting neonates

A team or persons trained in neonatal resuscitation should be promptly available to provide resuscitation for each of the more than 4 million infants born annually in the USA. The National Resuscitation Program, which was initiated in 1987 to identify infants at risk of requiring resuscitation, underwent major updates in 2006 and 2010 (26). Those physicians caring for neonates in an operating room or critical care setting should be PALS certified. Refer to the American Heart Association's PALS algorithms as well as the Neonatal Resuscitation Program for the most recent guidelines on neonatal resuscitation.

Special attention should be taken to assure the necessary equipment is available and functioning prior to transporting the neonate. Equipment necessary for transports includes a bassinet or transport cradle with a warming device installed in the transport bed, warming packs, or warm blankets available to maintain adequate temperature control during transport. Other equipment necessary for transport:

1. **Oxygen** with means of delivery based on airway stability of the neonate
2. **Emergency medications**
3. **Endotracheal tubes, LMAs, and laryngoscopes** of appropriate size for neonate
4. **Monitor** to include pulse oximetry, ECG, end-tidal carbon dioxide monitoring, and blood pressure measuring capabilities
5. **Suction**
6. **Support staff:** at least one person for unforeseen complications during transport

Medical states of the neonate

Apnea and bradycardia

During the first few days of life, premature infants encounter problems with the normal control of respiration. Resolution of apnea and establishment of a normal respiratory pattern is a major developmental milestone for many premature infants. The definition of "apnea of prematurity"(AOP) is a pause of breathing for more than 15–20 s, or accompanied by oxygen desaturation (SPO2 ≤80% for ≥ 4s) and bradycardia (heart rate < 2/3 of baseline for ≥ 4 s) in infants born less than 37 weeks of gestation (27). Severe apnea that lasts longer than 20 s is usually associated with bradycardia or desaturation 75% of the time.

The incidence of AOP is inversely correlated with gestational age and birth weight. Nearly all infants born at < 29 weeks gestation or < 1000 g exhibits AOP (27). The pathogenesis of AOP is poorly misunderstood, but is thought to be related to the "physiological" immature state of respiratory control in premature infants.

Factors that can be contributing to AOP (27):

- Intracranial hemorrhage
- Hypoxic ischemic encephalopathy
- Seizures
- Elevated body temperature
- Glucose of electrolyte imbalance
- Presence of patent ductus arteriosus with large shunt

Medications contributing to AOP (28):

- Narcotic analgesics
- Magnesium sulfate
- Anesthetic agents

Lastly, anemia can contribute to episodes of apnea because of lowered oxygen-carrying capacity of red blood cells leading to hypoxia, which results in respiratory depression (29).

AOP treatment options are fairly limited and include (27):

Prone positioning

Methylxanthine therapy (caffeine, theophylline, and aminophylline)

Nasal intermittent positive-pressure ventilation

Continuous positive airway pressure (4–6 cmH2O)

Sensory stimulation, CO2 inhalation and red blood cell tranfusions are not widely used and require further information.

Apnea is a very common symptom in premature infants. In the majority of infants, apnea is a time-limited problem, disappearing by term postconceptual age. The long-term consequences of severe, recurrent apnea-associated bradycadia and desaturation are not known. Many interventions and pharmacologic therapies remain unproven for long-term efficacy (27). Premature infants < 54 weeks should be monitored for at least 12 if not 24 hours postoperatively as they are at risk of apnea and bradycardia secondary to anesthesia exposure. Most centers have a policy monitoring anesthetic patients who are premature, with risk of apnea and bradycardia, undergoing an outpatient surgical procedure.

Anemia of prematurity

The development of anemia after birth in very premature, critically ill newborn infants is a well-described phenomenon (30). Erythropoietic activity from the bone marrow decreases immediately after birth in both full-term and preterm infants. In term infants, the hemoglobin concentration decreases during the 9th to 12th week to reach a nadir of 10 to 11 g/dl, and then increases. The decrease is due to a decrease in erythropoiesis and to some extent due to a shortened life span of the red blood cells. In preterm infants, the decrease in the hemoglobin level is greater and is directly related to the degree of prematurity. The nadir in premature infants is reached earlier (4 to 8 weeks) (31). This "anemia" is a normal physiologic adjustment to extrauterine life. Despite the reduction in hemoglobin, the oxygen delivery to the tissues may not be compromised because of a shift of the oxygen – hemoglobin dissociation curve (to the right), secondary to an increase of 2,3-diphosphoglycerate (32). Fetal hemoglobin is replaced by adult hemoglobin, which results in a shift in the same direction. In premature infants, reduced hemoglobin concentrations may be associated with apnea and bradycardia (33). Infants with anemia of prematurity have been found to have an inadequate production of erythropoietin. Some centers are now using recombinant human erythropoietin in VLBW infants to stimulate erythropoiesis and decrease the need for transfusions (34,35).

Iatrogenic phlebotomy loss remains a key contributor to neonatal anemia and the need for RBC transfusion. Estimates of NICU laboratory blood draws primarily in the first 6 weeks of life show that laboratory blood losses have been reported to range from 11 to 22 ml/kg per week. This is equivalent to 15–20% of the circulating blood volume (30).

Some nonpharmacological strategies for prevention and treatment of neonatal anemia (30):

- Increase initial blood volume (delaying cord clamping and cord "milking"
- Removing less blood with lab draws
- Increasing blood production

Hemoglobin values of full-term and preterm infants are comparable after the first year.

Bronchopulomonary dysplasia

Bronchopulmonary dysplasia (BP) is defined as a respiratory disease requiring supplemental oxygen for more than 28 days after birth. It is a form of chronic lung disease associated with prolonged mechanical ventilation and oxygen toxicity in preterm neonates (36). In a cohort study of premature infants in Denmark, BPD was a serious complication to prematurity and was diagnosed in 18.5% of the surviving infants (37). These babies exhibit bronchospasm more frequently and as many as 50% will require a hospital admission within the first year of life (38). Premature infants with BPD and severe pulmonary hypertension are at high risk of death, particularly during the first six months after diagnosis of pulmonary hypertension (37). Under anesthesia, the ex-BPD patient may not respond in quite the same positive therapeutic way as asthmatics do when given a beta 2-agonist bronchodilator or steroidal anti-inflammatory inhalational therapy. Preoperative preparation should focus on optimizing oxygenation, reducing airway hyperactivity, and correcting electrode abnormalities caused by chronic diuretic therapy. Adequate expiratory time to avoid excessive positive-pressure ventilation is important, and the potential for subglottic stenosis may necessitate using a smaller than expected tracheal tube (36). In view of increased airway reactivity, it would be prudent to plan an anesthetic without having to instrument the patient's airway in those infants with history of BPD but otherwise stable from a respiratory standpoint. In some centers, it is common practice to try and avoid general anesthesia for these children and consider regional anesthesia techniques as an alternative (38).

Intraventricular hemorrhage

Intraventricular hemorrhage (IVH) occurs in as many as one-third of micropremie infants (39). The severity of IVH, as defined by head ultrasound is graded as follows:

- Grade 1: hemorrhage limited to the germinal matrix
- Grade 2: hemorrhage extending into the ventricular system
- Grade 3: hemorrhage into the ventricular system and with ventricular dilatation
- Grade 4: hemorrhage extending into brain parenchyma

Risks factors for early onset: (during first day of life) (39)

- Fetal distress
- Vaginal delivery
- Reduced Apgar score
- Metabolic acidosis
- Severe hypercapnia
- Need for mechanical ventilation

Risk factors for late onset (weeks to months after birth) (39):

- Respiratory distress syndrome
- Seizures
- Pneumothoraces
- Hypoxemia
- Acidosis
- Severe hypocarbia
- Use of vasopressor infusions

Rapid fluctuations in cerebral blood flow; cerebral blood volume, and cerebral venous pressure appear to play a role in the development of IVH (40). Infants with grade 3 or 4 IVH are more likely to exhibit severe long-term neurocognitive sequelae. Antenatal glucocorticoids, or indomethacin may decrease the incidence and severity of IVH in patients with the confirmed diagnosis.

Kernicterus

In the extremely low birth weight (ELBW) infant, liver conjugation and bilirubin elimination is immature, bowel motility immaturity is present, faster red blood cell turnover occurs; as a result, these infants are at greater risk for kernicterus than neonates born at term. Kernicterus involves unconjugated bilirubin deposition in the pons, cerebellum, and basal ganglia (38). This can lead to serious neurological complications, including brain damage and hearing loss. Bilirubin levels are usually greater than 20–25 mg/dl. Some NICUs begin phototherapy in ELBW infants at birth; others wait for bilirubin to increase by 50% of the level at birth. Exchange transfusions are recommended for ELBW infants with bilirubins approaching 10 mg/dl./kg (38). Highly protein-bound agents such as furosemide, sulfonamides, ceftriaxone, and benzyl alcohol may displace bilirubin and increase the possibility of kernicterus (41).

Persistent pulmonary hypertension

Persistent pulmonary hypertension (PPHN) is a disease that is found usually secondary to hypoxic respiratory failure that was induced by significant lung pathology soon after birth (38). The PPHN can be caused by meconium aspiration, pneumonia, BPD, and infant respiratory distress syndrome. Intrauterine maternal factors causing PPHN are premature rupture of membranes, oligohydramnios, and sepsis. Inhaled nitric oxide (iNO) is a potent pulmonary vasodilator that has been shown to improve PPHN in near-term infants; however, the same benefit is not seen with ELBW or premature infants. High-frequency oscillatory ventilation of the ELBW infant is sometimes necessary to prevent lung injury via conventional mechanical ventilation (38).

Retinopathy of prematurity

Retinopathy of prematurity (ROP) is the leading cause of childhood blindness in industrialized countries and is the fifth leading cause of bilateral childhood blindness worldwide (42). The incidence and severity are closely correlated to lower birth weight and earlier postconceptional age. Caucasian and Hispanic children develop a more aggressive ROP that is more likely to lead to retinal detachment. The condition of ROP is a bilateral disease and 85% of children will develop bilateral retinal detachment even though one eye may precede the other (39).

The underlying development of ROP is incomplete vascularization of the retina. High levels of oxygen lead to regression of retinal capillaries. Wide fluctuations in SpO_2 levels have been shown to affect the development and progression of ROP (39). However, the actual acceptable range of oxygen requirement and exposure is not known. Clinical studies suggest that screening examinations be initiated at 31 weeks of postmenstrual age or at 4 weeks of chronologic age for infants born before 27 weeks postmenstrual age and be continued until 45 weeks of postmenstrual age or progression of retinal vascularization (38).

Laser and cryotherapy are common treatments for this condition. Because of the complexity and exact accuracy of the procedure, infants are usually intubated and paralyzed. Extubation of the infant may be possible after the procedure, but most of the time due to the prematurity or comorbidities of the infant, a small period of mechanical ventilation is required postoperatively.

Surgical disease states specific to neonates

Congenital cystic adenomatoid malformation

Congenital cystic adenomatoid malformation (CCAM) of the lung consists of cystic masses of pulmonary tissue and bronchial structures, neither of which participate in gas exchange (43). These cystic masses are categorized into macrocytic and microcytic and can compress surrounding lung tissue and impair normal lung development. It is most frequently associated with hypdrops fetalis due to the inability of the fetus's ability to swallowing, thus leading to amniotic fluid imbalance. Most of these cystic masses can be detected by ultrasound antenatally. If the congenital anomaly is found when the fetus is ≤ 32 weeks and there are signs of amniotic fluid imbalance, then the fetus will undergo a thoracotomy in utero with resection. Cystic lung anomalies diagnosed after 32 week in an asymptomatic fetus will undergo a thoracotomy with resection of the cystic lesion after delivery.

Part of the preanesthetic evaluation should include the results of the ultrasound of the mass. Note the size, and if it is compressing any major structures in the chest such as great vessels, lungs, or the heart. In CCAM anomalies can also be associated with diaphragmatic hernias or a cardiac lesion so it is important to rule out other congenital anomalies prior to undergoing thoracotomy for resection.

Perioperative anesthetic management will be discussed from the standpoint of an ex utero thoracotomy and resection, although if the CCAM is severe enough to create amniotic fluid imbalance or decreased lung development, the fetus will undergo a thoracotomy in utero to remove the CCAM.

Induction of anesthesia can be via inhalation or intravenous if the patient has a peripheral IV in situ. If the surgeon requires lung isolation in order to resect the CCAM, then a bronchial blocker may be considered or simply perform a mainstem intubation, particularly if the CCAM is left sided. Depending on the extent of the resection, an arterial line and second intravenous line or central line should be considered. A thoracic epidural should be considered for postoperative pain control. Most patients are extubated at the end of the procedure and admitted for postoperative care.

Hernia

Approximately one-third of preterm neonates will have an inguinal hernia and approximately 1% of term neonates. With incarceration or strangulation of bowel or gonads, emeregency correction is indicated (44).

Often, the children with inguinal hernias that were premature will have many comorbidities to consider prior to providing anesthesia for this procedure. Those who required mechanical ventilation for a significant period of time just after delivery may have a chronic lung disease or bronchopulmonary dysplasia. Spinal anesthesia may be appropriate for these patients to avoid postoperative mechanical ventilation requirement or worsening of lung disease.

In otherwise healthy children, general anesthesia with a regional block may be safely performed with 1 ml/kg of 0.25% bupivacaine with epinephrine (1:200 000) for a caudal block or ultrasound guided ilioinguinal and iliohypogastric nerve block for postoperative pain control. These children often receive an oral premedication prior to relieve any anxiety they may have about leaving their families in a strange environment. These patients can be induced with inhaled sevoflurane or intravenous propofol +/- an opioid to blunt instrumentation of the airway. The regional block is placed after the patient is under general anesthesia.

Overnight admission postoperatively with pulse oximetry and apnea monitoring may be indicated for those at risk.

Myelomeningocele

Myelomeningocele (MMC) affects 0.5 to 1 per 1000 live births annually (45). This is despite folic acid fortification. At least 75% of affected individuals reach early adulthood; most deaths occur during infancy and the preschool years due to respiratory and neurologic complications. Spina bifida is the most common of congenital anomalies of the central nervous system that are compatible with life. Myelomeningocele is the most common form of spina bifida and is defined as incomplete closure of the neural tube resulting in an extrusion of the spinal cord into a sac filled with cerebrospinal fluid (CSF). There is usually life-long neurological impairment of the lower extremities, urinary and fecal incontinence, the Arnold–Chiari malformation, and hydrocephalus requiring ventriculoperitoneal shunting (46). To prevent ongoing injury to the spinal cord, early repair is usually indicated. If it is an in utero repair, the ideal time is prior to 20 weeks, otherwise it should occur within the first few days after birth.

The special issue with these patients is how to position for intubation in order to not put pressure on the MMC and cause further damage.

Preanesthetic preparations include ruling out other comorbidities leading to increased anesthetic risks. Having adequate lab values and ensuring there is blood available in case of emergency or unforeseen complications. The patient should be on an antibiotic regimen prior to surgery for prophylaxis and the MMC should be covered with wet sponges to preserve the spinal cord. These patients often develop a latex allergy so making sure that the OR is prepared with latex-free products is of utmost importance in these patients.

Due to the young age of these infants, there is no need for an anxiolytic premedication. Using routine monitoring, the patient is positioned on the OR table in the lateral position for induction and intubation or can be positioned supine as long as there are support pads underneath the infant to avoid pressure damage of the nervous system structures making up the MMC. Patients can be induced with atropine and propofol IV. A neuromuscular blocking agent may be necessary for intubation.

Once the patient is successfully intubated, they will be positioned prone for the surgery. Maintenance anesthetic usually consist of an opioid-volatile agent combination with neuromuscular blocking agent if necessary. Most patients will be extubated at the end of the procedure and returned to an ICU setting.

Congenital lobar emphysema

Congenital Lobar Emphysema (CLE) is a developmental anomaly of the lower respiratory tract, characterized by hyperinflation of one or more of the pulmonary lobes (47). It has a prevalence of 1 in 20 000 to 1 in 30 000 patients and is associated with several factors.

In 50% of cases, there is associated decreased bronchial cartilage, vascular abnormalities that produce compression, bronchial stenosis, bronchogenic cysts, or congenital cytomegaloviral infection (47). If not diagnosed by ultrasound in utero, the age of onset can be from a few days after birth to 6 months and they commonly present with tachypnea, severe respiratory distress, tachycardia with hypotension, and cyanosis. It is often found accidentally on chest radiograph or due to a lateral shift of the cardiac sounds (48).

Airway management in patients with CLE is challenging. It is necessary to avoid further inflation and gas trapping in the diseased lung since this may compromise the normal lung. With further inflation of the diseased lung, the increased intrathoracic pressure can reduce the cardiac output. It is preferable to avoid positive-pressure ventilation until thoracotomy is performed and the diseased lung is isolated (47).

Preoperative assessment should consist of obtaining a chest radiograph and echocardiogram to assess any compression of normal structures. Routine labs, ABG, type, and cross of at least one unit of blood and one unit of plasma is necessary prior to inducing anesthesia.

Routine monitoring mandatory includes an arterial line for obtaining blood gases and hematocrit during the surgery. No anxiolytic premedication is necessary for infants, but IV atropine or glycopyrrolate should be considered with preoxygenation. If there is no IV, inhalation induction may be performed making sure to maintain spontaneous ventilation to limit the enlargement of the lobar emphysema. For an IV induction, one might consider using ketamine to maintain spontaneous respirations and prevent hemodynamic instability.

After the patient is intubated, one-lung ventilation is often necessary and can be obtained with either a selective main stem intubation or using a bronchial blocker. Maintenance of anesthesia depends on the severity of the lesion; total intravenous anesthesia or an inhalational agent are acceptable. These patients may require inotropic support. Re-expand the lungs prior to thoracic closure to prevent atelectasis. Extubation can be attempted if hemodynamically stable and meeting criteria. Spontaneous breathing reduces the strain on the bronchial stump and decreases the risk for significant air leak or development of a bronchopleural fistula.

Regional anesthetic techniques are very helpful, but IV opioids can be utilized for pain control, alternatively (48).

Sacrococcygeal teratoma

The incidence of sacrococcygeal teratoma (SCT) is 1–2 per 35–40 000 newborns. The prevalence is 0.25–0.5: 10 000 live births for any fetal teratoma, with sacrococcygeal accounting for over 50%, cranial 40%, and cervical 5.5%. Sacrococcygeal teratoma is more common in female than in male fetuses (1:4) (49).

Most SCTs are external with both solid and cystic components. A variety of tissues from the three primary germ layers are found in these teratomas. With smaller tumors, complete surgical resection usually occurs after delivery under elective, controlled conditions. The tumor can cause fetal congestive heart failure and even fetal demise if no treatment is performed. Massive hemorrhage into the tumor with fetal exsanguination may occur spontaneously in utero or be precipitated by labor and delivery (50). Predictors of poor outcome include diagnosis before 20 weeks gestation, delivery before 30 weeks, development of hydrops, low birth weight, Apgar score of less than 7, malignant histotypes, polyhydramnios, and placentomegaly (51).

These patients can have tumor lysis syndrome; therefore, it is imperative that electrolytes be closely followed prior to surgery. An echocardiogram and chest radiograph should be obtained to rule out other congenital anomalies or evidence of congestive heart failure. Depending on the severity of the mass and projected difficulty of resection, it may be appropriate for all members of the surgical team to meet to communicate concerns about the case. Blood products should be available prior to the start of the case and possibly considering activating a massive transfusion protocol if your institution has this in place.

Most infants will come to the operating room with an IV in situ, allowing for an IV induction with ketamine preferably for its hemodynamic stability properties. Once the patient is intubated, a central line and arterial line should be placed with sterile techniques. If the patient had significant respiratory distress at birth, the infant may already be intubated and sedated on arrival to the operating room. Maintenance is anesthesia can be achieved with a volatile agent and opioid mixture with neuromuscular blocking agent if necessary. If the patient is not on any kind of inotropic agent prior to surgery, it is important to have it available in the operating room.

Dopamine is a good agent to start with to treat hypotension and boost cardiac output during this massively bloody procedure with many fluid shifts. Postoperatively, the patient should be kept intubated, sedated, and transported to an ICU setting with standard monitoring for transport.

Vein of Galen malformation

Vein of Galen malformations (VGAMs) are rare congenital abnormalities (less than 1/25 000 deliveries), which can cause severe morbidity and mortality, particularly in neonates but also in infants and older children (52). The VGAM can be diagnosed in association with CHF (high output failure) in neonates, hydrocephalus in infants, or developmental delay that mostly manifests in childhood but may also occur at any age (53). In the past decade, endovascular treatment has emerged as the treatment of choice for VGAM presenting in infancy with heart failure. To date, however, endovascular treatment has been generally used on a selective basis in infants with VGAM, and in many series, neonates less than 1 month of age have not been treated because of perceived poor outcome (52). Unless the excess flow through the AVM is reduced by early neurointervention and aggressive management of cardiac failure, severe cerebral injury occurs (52). Pulmonary hypertension (PH) may also be associated with this disease; therefore, inhaled nitric oxide may be used to reduce PH during the initial emergency transcatheter embolization.

A chest radiograph and echocardiogram are definitely necessary preoperatively to assess the extent of cardiac failure and/or pulmonary hypertension. Routine labs should be assessed and blood products made immediately available to the neurointerventional suite.

If the neonate is not already intubated and sedated, then a slow, controlled induction may be successful with the use of hemodynamically stable IV agents such as ketamine or an inhalational induction with 70% Give oxygen, 30% nitrous oxide, and incremental amounts of sevoflurane until the patient is adequately anesthetized for IV placement and intubation. Anesthesia should be conservatively managed with oxygen/air mixture, choice of volatile agent; in addition, agents such as dopamine and diuretics for management of heart failure should be immediately on hand. Inhaled nitric oxide should be considered if the patient develops any signs of pulmonary hypertension. These patients should be kept intubated, sedated, and monitored in an ICU setting.

Most patients will require multiple embolizations within the first few weeks of life as part of a staged embolization to decrease cardiac failure and pulmonary hypertension.

References

1. Fei Li, Ting Wu, Xiaoping Lei, *et al.* The Apgar Score and infant mortality. *PLOS ONE* 2013; **8** (7): 1–8.
2. Apgar Virginia. A proposal for a new method of evaluation of the newborn infant. *Current Researches in Anesthesia and Analgesia* 1953; July-August: 260–7.
3. American Academy of Pediatrics. The Apgar Score. *Pediatrics* 2006; **117**: 1444.
4. Anwar Mujahid, Carbone Tracy, Hegyi Thomas, *et al.* The Apgar Score and its components in the preterm infant. *Pediatrics* 1998; **101**: 77.
5. De Swiet Michael, Fayers Peter, Shinebourne Elliot Anthony. Systolic blood pressure in a population of infants in the first year of life: The Brompton study. *Pediatrics* 1980; **65** (5): 1028.
6. Marciniak B. Growth and development. In Coté Charles J, Lerman Jerrold, Anderson Brian J, eds., *A Practice of Anesthesia for Infants and Children, 4th edn.* Phildelphia PA, Elsevier, 2013, pp.7–21.
7. Southall DP, Johnston F, Shinebourne EA, *et al*: 24-hour electrocardiographic study of heart rate and rhythm patterns in population of healthy children. *Br Heart J* 1981; **45**: 281–91.
8. Bissonnette B, Anderson Brian J, Bosenberg A, *et al.* General growth and tissue development throughout childhood. In *Pediatric Anesthesia Basic Principles – State of the Art – Future.* Shelton, CT: People's Medical Publishing House, 2011, pp. 20–42.
9. Hegyi Thomas, Anwar Mujahid, Carbone Mary Terese, *et al.* Blood pressure ranges in premature infants: II. The first week of life. *Pediatrics* 1996; **97** (3): 336–42.
10. Rigatto H, Brady JP, De La Torre Verduzco R. Chemoreceptor reflexes in preterm infants: I. The effect of gestational and postnatal age on the ventilatory response to inhalation of 100% and 15% oxygen. *Pediatrics* 1975; **55**: 604–13.
11. Coté CJ, Zaslavsky A, Downes JJ, *et al*: Postoperative apnea in former preterm infants after inguinal herniorrhaphy: a

combined analysis. *Anesthesiology* 1995; **82**: 809–22.

12. Liu LM, Coté CJ, Goudsouzian NG, *et al*: Life-threatening apnea in infants recovering from anesthesia. *Anesthesiology* 1983; **59**: 506–10.
13. Kurth CD, Spitzer AR, Broennle AM, *et al*: Postoperative apnea in preterm infants. *Anesthesiology* 1987; **66**: 483–8.
14. Southall DP, Richards JM, Johnstone PGB, *et al*: Study of cardiac rhythm in healthy newborn infants. *Br Heart J* 1980 **43**: 14–20.
15. Smith R, Cable B. Laryngeal disorders. In *Oski's Pediatrics: Principles and Practice*, ed. McMillan J, Feigin R, De Angelis C, *et al.* Philadelphia PA, Lippincott Williams & Wilkins, 2006, pp.1411–21.
16. Hoseini R, Otukesh H, Rahimzadeh N, Hoseini S. Glomerular function in neonates. *Iran J Kidney Dis* 2012; **6**: 166–72.
17. O'Brien RT, Pearson HA. Physiologic anemia of the newborn infant. *J Pediatr* 1971; **79**: 132–8.
18. Dallman P, Shannon K, Pearson HA. Developmental changes in red blood cell production and function. In *Rudolph's Pediatrics*, ed. Rudolph C, Rudolph A, Hostetter M, *et al.* New York: McGraw-Hill, 2002, 1519–23.
19. Orenstein S, Peters J, Kahn S, *et al.* Gastroesophgeal reflux. In *Nelson Textbook of Pediatrics*, ed. Kliegman R, Behrman R, Jenson H, *et al.* Philadelphia: Saunders, 2007, 1547–9.
20. Stevenson D, Madan A. Jaundice in the Newborn. In *Rudolph's Pediatrics*, ed. Rudolph C, Rudolph A, Hostetter M, *et al.* New York: McGraw-Hill, 2002, 164–9.
21. Guerra GG, Robertson CM, Alton GY, *et al.*; Western Canadian Complex Pediatric Therapies Follow-up Group. Neurodevelopmental outcome following exposure to sedative and analgesic drugs for complex cardiac surgery in infancy. *Pediatr Anesth* 2011; **21**: 932–41.
22. International Anesthesia Research Society. Smart Tots (Internet) 2013. http://www.smartots.org/research.
23. Anand KJS., Neonatal stress response to anesthesia and surgery. *Clin Perinatol* 1990; **17**: 207–14.
24. Anand KJS, Sippell WG, Schofield NM, *et al.* Does halothane anesthesia decrease the metabolic and endocrine stress response of newborn infants undergoing operation? *Br Med J* 1988; **296**: 668–72.
25. Rains PC, Rampersad N, DeLima J, *et al.* Cortisol response to general anesthesia for medical imaging in children. *Clin Endocrinol* 2009; **71**: 834–9.
26. Raghuveer TS, Cox AJ. Neonatal resuscitation: an update. *Am Fam Physician* Website 2011; **83** (8).
27. Zhao J, Gonzalez F, Mu D. Apnea of prematurity: from cause to treatement. *Eur J Pediatr* 2011; **170**: 1097–105.
28. Stokowski LA. A primer on apnea of prematurity. *Adv Neonatal Care* 2005; **5**: 155–70.
29. Bishara N, Ohls RK. Current controversies in the management of the anemia of prematurity. *Semin Perinatol* 2009; **33**: 29–34.
30. Carroll PD, Widness JA. Nonpharmacological, blood conservation techniques for preventing neonatal anemia: effective and promising strategies for reducing transfusion. *Semin Perinatol* 2012; **4**: 232–43.
31. O'Brien RT, Pearson HA. Physiologic anemia of the newborn infant. *J Pediatr* 1971; **79**: 132–8.
32. Delavoria-Papadolpulos M, Roncevic N, Oski FA. Postnatal changes in oxygen transport of term, premature and sick infants: the role of red cell, 2,3-diphosphoglycerate and adult hemoglobin. *Pediatr Res* 1971; **5**: 235–45.
33. Ross MP, Christensen RD, Rothstein G, *et al.* A randomized trial to develop criteria for administering erythrocyte transfusions to anemic preterm infants 1 to 3 months of age. *J Perinatol* 1989; **9**: 246–53.
34. Shannon KM, Keith JF, Mentzer WC, *et al.* Recombinant human erythropoietin stimulates erythropoiesis and reduces erythrocyte transfusions in very low birth weight preterm infants. *Pediatrics* 1995; **95**: 1–8.
35. Aher S, Malwatkar, Kadam S. Neonatal anemia. *Semin Fetal Neonatal Med* 2008; **13**: 239–47.
36. Ghazal EA, Mason LJ, Coté CJ. Preoperative evaluation, premedication, and induction of anesthesia. In Coté and Lerman's *A Practice of Anesthesia for Infants and Children.* Philadelphia: Elsevier Saunders, 2013, 31–63.
37. Ali Z, Schmidt P, Dodd J, Jeppesen DL. Predictors of bronchopulmonary dysplasia and pulmonary hypertension in newborn children. *Dan Med J* 2013; **60** (8): A4688.
38. Ing RJ, Ross KA. Specific problems and anesthesia management of extremely low birthweight infants. In Bissonnette B, Anderson BJ, Bosenberg A, Engelhardt T, *et al. Pediatric Anesthesia: Basic Principles – State of the Art – Future.* People's Medical Publishing House, USA, 2011; 1392–405.
39. Spaeth JP, Kurth CD. The extremely premature infant (micropremie). In Coté and Lerman's *A Practice of Anesthesia for Infants and Children.* Philadelphia: Elsevier Saunders, 2013, 733–45.

40. Mullaart RA, Hopman JC, Rotteveel JJ, *et al*: Cerebral blood flow fluctuation in neonatal respiratory distress and periventricular haemorrhage. *Early Hum Dev* 1994; **37**: 179–85.

41. Lovejoy FHJ. Fatal benzyl alcohol poisoning in neonatal intensive care units: a new concern for pediatricians. *Am J Dis Child* 1982; **136**: 974–5.

42. Lermann VL, Fortes Filho JB, Procianoy RS. The prevelance of retinopathy of prematurity in very low birth weight infants. *J Pediatr (Rio J)* 2006; **82**: 27–32.

43. Miller RK, Sieber WK, Yunis EJ. Congenital cystic adenomatoid malformation of the lung: a report of 17 cases and review of the literature. *Pathol Annu* 1980; **15**: 387–402.

44. Bachiller PR, Chou JH, Romanelli TM, Roberts JD. Neonatal emergencies. In Coté and Lerman's *A Practice of Anesthesia for Infants and Children.* Philadelphia: Elsevier Saunders, 2013, 746–65.

45. Hirose S, Meuli-Simmen C, Meuli M. Fetal surgery for myelomeningocele: panacea or peril? *World J Surg* 2003; **27**: 87–94.

46. Farmer D, von Koch C, Peacock W, *et al.* In utero repair of myelomeningocele: experimental pathophysiology, initial clinical experience, and outcomes. *Arch Surg* 2003; **138**: 872–8.

47. Ulku R, Onat S, Ozcelik C. Congenial lobar emphysema: differential diagnosis and therapeutic approach. *Pediatr Int* 2008; **50**: 658–61.

48. Lonnqvist PA. Management of the neonate: anesthetic considerations. In Bissonnette B, Anderson BJ, Bosenberg A, Engelhardt T, *et al. Pediatric Anesthesia: Basic Principles – State of the Art – Future.* People's Medical Publishing House, USA, 2011; 1437–75

49. Markovic I, Stamenovic S, Radovanovic Z, *et al.* Ultrasound and magnetic resonance imaging in prenatal diagnosis of sacroccygeal teratoma: case report. *Med Pregl* 2013; **66**: 254–7.

50. Brusseau R. Fetal intervention and the EXIT procedure. In Coté and Lerman's *A Practice of Anesthesia for Infants and Children.* Philadelphia: Elsevier Saunders, 2013, 766–88.

51. Abraham E, Parray T, Ghafoor A. Complications with massive sacrococcygeal tumor resection on a premature neonate. *J Anesth* 2010; **24**: 951–4.

52. Frawley GP, Dargaville PA, Mitchell PJ, Tress BM, Loughnan P. Clinical course and medical management of neonates with severe cardiac failure related to vein of Galen malformation. *Arch Dis Child Fetal Neonatal Ed* 2002; **87**: F144–9.

53. Li AH, Armstrong D, Terbrugge KG. Endovascular treatment of vein of Galen aneurysmal malformation: management strategy and 21-year experience in Toronto. *J Neurosurg Pediatr* 2011; **7**: 3–10.

Chapter 16

Neonatal surgical emergencies

Christina M. Pabelick, Shannon M. Peters, and Kim M. Strupp

Introduction

Although medicine in general and more specifically surgical and anesthetic techniques have advanced over the last 10 years, the number of neonatal surgical emergencies remains stable. In fact, due to the neonatal differences in regard to their anatomy, pharmacology, and physiology, neonatal mortality has been on a much slower decline during the last two decades in comparison to other age groups.[1] However, advances in perinatology have made it possible that critically ill newborns show improved survival.

The most common neonatal surgical emergencies affect the gastrointestinal system. This review will focus on the anesthetic management of neonatal surgical emergencies of the abdomen.

Pyloric stenosis

Pyloric stenosis is the most common gastrointestinal abnormality arising in neonates. It is more common in first-born, male infants and characterized by non-bilious, projectile vomiting. These infants tend to range from two to six weeks in age. The incidence is approximately 1 in 300 to 500 live births. The mechanism of pyloric stenosis is unknown but may be associated with exposure to systemic erythromycin and abnormal innervation of the pylorus.[2–5] Children with pyloric stenosis may have cleft palate and gastroesophageal reflux.[6] Clinically, one may be able to appreciate peristalsis along the anterior abdominal wall and palpate an olive-sized mass in the right upper quadrant of the abdomen. Radiographic confirmation is likely to occur and consists of ultrasonographic examination or rarely a barium swallow study.[2,4–7]

Pyloric stenosis is characterized by thickening of the musculature of the pylorus resulting in gastric outlet obstruction. Through extensive vomiting these children lose gastric juices, rich in hydrogen and chloride ions, resulting in the characteristic presentation of hypochloremic, hypokalemic metabolic alkalosis.[2,4–7]

Pyloric stenosis is not a surgical emergency; however, it may be considered a medical emergency due to severe dehydration, acid–base imbalances and electrolyte derangements. Pyloromyotomy is considered curative and may be performed open or laparoscopically. The laparoscopic route has become more common and allows these infants to resume their oral intake sooner and be dismissed from the hospital more quickly.[2,4–7]

Major anesthetic concerns include the degree of dehydration, and the extent of acid–base and electrolyte disturbances. It is imperative that these infants are well hydrated prior to undergoing surgical repair. These infants are at risk for aspiration and thorough gastric decompression is essential prior to induction of anesthesia. Gastric decompression may be achieved via the naso- or orogastric route. Prior to gastric decompression, it is common to administer atropine to blunt any vagal responses brought on by suctioning. Traditionally, these children were intubated awake. The current practice includes rapid sequence induction, modified rapid sequence, and even mask induction. Following induction and intubation, an oro- or nasogastric tube is placed to further decompress the stomach and also to insufflate air at the end of the operation. If air is detected within the abdomen, a full-thickness disruption of the pylorus requiring surgical repair may have occurred.[3,6–7] During the operative procedure and immediately postoperatively, opioids may be used to manage pain. However, there is a concern that alkalosis of the cerebrospinal fluid may predispose to respiratory depression and the administration of opioid analgesics may risk

Essentials of Pediatric Anesthesiology, ed. Alan David Kaye, Charles James Fox and James H. Diaz. Published by Cambridge University Press. © Cambridge University Press 2015.

postoperative respiratory depression and apnea.[3] These infants may be quickly transitioned to nonopioid analgesics, such as acetaminophen and ibuprofen. Once they have resumed oral intake without further emesis, these infants may be dismissed from the hospital.[3,5–6]

Key points

- Pyloric stenosis is a medical, not a surgical emergency
- It commonly presents in male infants at two to six weeks of life with nonbilious, projectile vomiting
- Hypochloremic, hypokalemic metabolic alkalosis is the key laboratory finding
- These children are at high risk of aspiration during induction of anesthesia
- Judicious gastric decompression is paramount and a (modified) rapid sequence induction is commonly performed
- Postoperatively, these children may be transitioned quickly to nonopioid analgesics and be dismissed home

Congenital diaphragmatic hernia

Congenital diaphragmatic hernia (CDH) involves herniation of the intra-abdominal contents (typically the midgut but may also include the stomach, portions of the colon, kidney, and liver) into the thoracic cavity. It is seen in 1 in 2500 to 4000 live births. It is most commonly (~ 90%) seen in the posterolateral position ("Bochdalek" hernia) and on the left; less commonly (~ 10%) it is anteromedial and referred to as a hernia of "Morgagni." CDH may be an isolated occurrence or seen with chromosomal abnormalities (e.g., chromosomal trisomies) as well as a part of a syndrome (e.g., CHARGE, Beckwith–Wiedemann, and pentalogy of Cantrell).[8–14]

Classically, CDH is defined by the presence of cyanosis, dyspnea, and apparent dextrocardia. On physical exam, a scaphoid abdomen and diminished or absent breath sounds over the thorax are appreciated. Occasionally, bowel sounds may be heard over the affected hemithorax.[6–7,14–15]

These infants present with a number of physiologic issues related to the degree of lung hypoplasia, pulmonary hypertension, and the effects of associated syndromes. The severity of lung hypoplasia depends on the degree of intestinal herniation. Mediastinal shift may occur in severe cases contributing to hypoplasia of the contralateral ("good") lung. In an infant with CDH, there are fewer alveoli to contribute to gas exchange, the alveoli have thicker walls, and there is decreased vasculature to the affected lung. The vasculature that is present tends to have thicker walls than normal contributing to the pulmonary hypertension.[6,9,15]

Embryologically, airway development occurs during the fourth and fifth week of gestation. Lung formation begins as the ventral bud in the foregut. Diaphragmatic closure occurs around the ninth week of gestation. If this does not proceed normally, the abdominal viscera may herniate into the pleural cavity. Research into the exact mechanism of CDH is ongoing; vitamin A and prenatal exposure to teratogens may play a role in the pathophysiology of CDH.[8,10–11,14]

Previously referred to as a surgical emergency, neonates with CDH are now medically optimized prior to entering the operating room, if possible. Since these infants are known to have pulmonary hypoplasia, there is no need for aggressive ventilation. On the contrary, survival has dramatically improved with the implementation of lung-protective ventilation strategies, which include low tidal volume ventilation, permissive hypercapnia, titrated F_iO_2 to maintain preductal saturations greater than or equal to 90%, and reduced peak airway and end-expiratory pressures. Use of high-frequency oscillatory ventilation (HFOV), implementation of inhaled nitric oxide (iNO), surfactant therapy, and early use of extracorporeal membrane oxygenation (ECMO) have further improved outcomes. Correction of acid/base disturbances is done in concert with lung protective ventilation strategies, thereby contributing to a reduction in shunting and improved pulmonary perfusion.[7–9,11,14]

Prenatal ultrasound may be diagnostic and shows displacement of the heart with bowel contents seen within the thorax. Radiologically, CDH may appear similar to congenital lobar emphysema, congenital cystic adenomatoid malformation, and extralobular sequestration. Once diagnosed, these neonates should be delivered at institutions in which pediatric surgeons, a neonatal intensive care unit, HFOV, iNO, and ECMO are available.[7–9,11,14]

When these infants arrive in the operating room, ventilatory goals remain the same as preoperative goals with lung-protective ventilation strategies. Careful attention should be given to hemodynamic and respiratory variables with decisive interventions to correct perturbations. If called to the delivery room of a suspected and undiagnosed CDH, aggressive positive-pressure ventilation should be avoided as this may cause gastric distention and may worsen pulmonary mechanics, causing additional respiratory distress. In addition, aggressive ventilation may contribute to contralateral pneumothorax, a feared complication. Gastric decompression should take place as the child enters the operating room and prior to commencing the surgical procedure. Nitrous oxide (N_2O) should be avoided as it may lead to visceral distension. The surgical procedure may occur via an open or minimally invasive approach. Reduction of intestinal contents may prove difficult and require a staged reduction with a chimney or silastic pouch. Postoperatively, these children typically return to the intensive care unit intubated and mechanically ventilated. Although reduction of the herniated viscera from the thoracic cavity is the goal of surgery, it does not solve the biggest physiologic conundrum for the patient – the degree of lung hypoplasia with resultant pulmonary hypertension.[6,9,11,15]

Outcomes in these children depend on the degree of pulmonary hypoplasia and severity of pulmonary hypertension. These children are also at risk for neurodevelopmental disability, difficulties with nutrition and orthopedic issues (e.g., pectus excavatum). Fetal surgical techniques are investigational and include tracheal occlusion. The occlusion of the trachea leads to an increase in fetal lung water, potentially leading to accelerated lung development.[6,8,11,14]

Key points

- CDH is classically defined by the presence of cyanosis, dyspnea, and apparent dextrocardia.
- A scaphoid abdomen with absent breath sounds and presence of bowel sounds over the thorax is commonly appreciated on physical examination
- The degree of pulmonary hypoplasia and pulmonary hypertension correlate with morbidity and mortality; intrathoracic position of the liver portends a worse prognosis
- Prenatal diagnosis of CDH should prompt referral to an institution capable of utilizing advanced therapies including HFOV, iNO, and ECMO to provide medical optimization prior to surgical intervention
- No longer considered a surgical emergency, medical optimization is key with implementation of lung-protective ventilation strategies, correction of acid/base disturbances, reducing shunting, and improving pulmonary perfusion
- The goals of optimizing pulmonary function include strategies to minimize pulmonary vasoconstriction, correction of acid–base disturbances, surfactant, iNO, proper sedation, and in some cases, muscle relaxation

Tracheoesophageal fistula and esophageal atresia

Tracheoesophageal fistula (TEF) and esophageal atresia (EA) are seen in 1 in 3000 to 4000 births. There are several different configurations of these lesions, which are depicted in Figure 16.1. Up to 25% of these children have additional congenital defects, whose incidence varies with the type of lesion present. TEF/EA is often seen in children with VATER or VACTERL association – vertebral, anal, cardiac, tracheoesophageal, renal, and limb anomalies. It may also be seen in children with CHARGE and DiGeorge syndrome as well as in various chromosomal trisomies (13, 18 and 21).[4,6–7]

Approximately 90% of all anomalies consist of a blind proximal esophageal pouch and a distal TEF. The second most common subtype consists of EA without a fistula (radiographically, there is no air bubble in the stomach). The third most common type is called the "H" type defect in which there is no EA but there is the presence of a TEF. These children often have recurrent respiratory infections that lead to a later diagnosis.[4,6–7,15]

The embryology of TEF/EA is incompletely understood. The trachea and esophagus arise from the foregut during weeks four and five of gestation. At some point, separation of the trachea from the esophagus needs to occur and the exact mechanism of this process is unknown. Although the exact mechanism of TEF/EA formation is unknown, abnormal molecular signaling along sonic hedgehog pathways, genetic defects in retinoic acid receptors, and defects in other genes and transcription factors are thought to play a role in this process.[4,6,16]

Prenatal diagnosis occurs in about 50% of cases. Clinical findings include maternal polyhydramnios (due to esophageal obstruction preventing the fetus

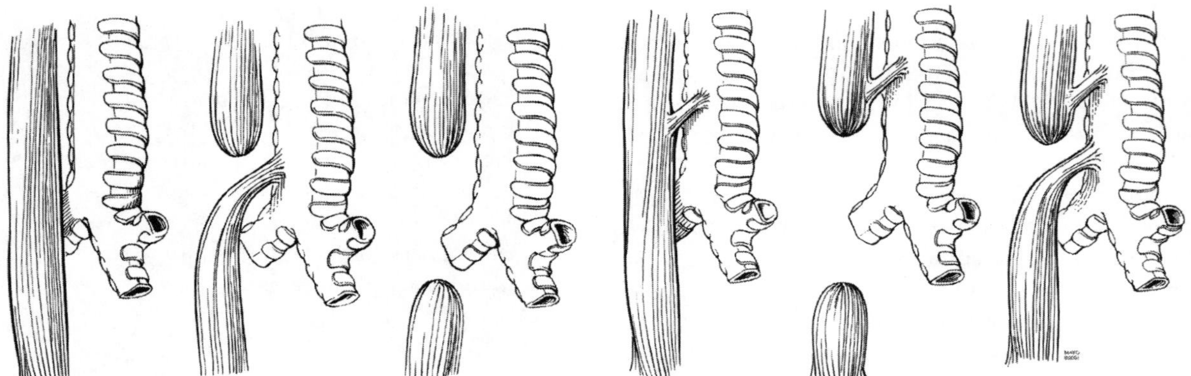

Figure 16.1 Schematic of the different types of tracheoesophageal fistula. By permission of Mayo Foundation for Medical Education and Research. All rights reserved.

from swallowing amniotic fluid) and a small or absent fetal gastric bubble. Preterm delivery is also common. Postnatally, these children present with excessive salivation and drooling, coughing, cyanosis, and difficulty swallowing. A suction catheter is unable to be passed into the stomach.[6,15–16]

Surgical correction of this anomaly is considered urgent and not emergent. Preoperatively, these infants should be NPO and positioned in the upright position to avoid aspiration of saliva. Frequent or continuous suctioning of the esophageal pouch is important. Preoperative work-up should exclude additional anomalies, such as those seen in VACTERL association. Cardiorespiratory status should be optimized and critical cardiac lesions ruled out by echocardiography. Children with low birth weight and cardiac anomalies have the highest mortality.[4,6–7,15]

The safest approach to airway management is to intubate these infants awake. However, an inhalation induction with spontaneous respiration and avoidance of muscle relaxants prior to securing the airway is a feasible and safe alternative. Avoidance of positive-pressure ventilation (PPV) is critical. Increased airway pressures will lead to gastric distension thereby worsening pulmonary mechanics. In some cases, bronchoscopy will be performed prior to definitive airway management to delineate the anatomy of the fistula tract. Alternatively, some advocate intentional mainstem intubation with an endotracheal tube (ETT) without a Murphy eye and removal of the ETT slowly until bilateral breath sounds are appreciated. If possible, the bevel of the ETT should be placed anteriorly within the airway to avoid ventilating the fistula tract. In the majority of cases of TEF/EA, the fistula tract is just proximal to the carina and placement of the ETT may fortuitously "plug" the tract. Continuous suctioning of the esophageal pouch is important. Invasive monitoring, such as arterial line placement, may be necessary in sicker children. Postoperatively, pain management may include opioids or regional anesthetic techniques including placement of a caudal epidural threaded to the thoracic region.[6–7,15]

The surgical procedure may be done thoracoscopically or with an open technique and may be primary or staged. Single-lung ventilation may need to be considered for video-assisted thoracoscopy. Surgical compression of the large airways provides ample opportunity for oxygenation and ventilation issues to arise intraoperatively. The procedure is usually performed through a right-sided approach unless there is a right-sided aortic arch. Blood from the surgical site may enter the trachea and cause plugging of the ETT. Therefore, strict vigilance is necessary to prevent catastrophic complications. In a primary repair, the surgical goal is to ligate the fistula and provide primary anastomosis of the proximal and distal esophageal segments, provided there is enough length to these segments. In situations in which this anastomosis is not possible, the operation may be delayed and several strategies employed: interventions to "stretch" the esophageal components may be performed, the child may be allowed to grow and there is no need for instrumented stretching techniques for later anastomosis, or an interposition graft may be placed (e.g., by utilizing a segment of bowel to bridge the gap). In critically ill children, a gastrostomy tube may be placed prior to undergoing definitive repair to allow for decompression of the stomach, prevention of reflux into the lungs, and as a conduit to feed the child in case surgery will be significantly delayed.[4,6–7,16]

Early postoperative complications include anastomotic breakdown and leaks. Later in life, these children have poor esophageal motility, which is thought to be related to poorly formed innervation of the esophagus. Long-term issues include gastroesophageal reflux and esophageal stenosis requiring frequent dilations. In addition, these children may have a degree of tracheomalacia. There is a risk these children may develop a tracheal diverticulum at the site of the TEF which may be unintentionally intubated later in life providing ventilation and oxygenation issues during future surgical encounters.[4,7,16]

Key points

- There are several anatomic variations of TEF/EA, but the most common lesion is a proximal, blind esophageal pouch with a distal tracheoesophageal fistula
- TEF/EA are associated with a number of other anomalies; one in particular is the VACTERL association
- Birth weight and cardiac anomalies correlate with mortality risk, meaning those with low birth weight and the presence of cardiac abnormalities have the highest mortality risk
- While the safest approach to airway management in these children is an awake intubation, inhalation induction with spontaneous ventilation and avoidance of muscle relaxation until the airway is secured avoids use of PPV and potentially gastric distension
- Intraoperatively, there is a high risk of ETT dislodgement and inadvertent ventilation of the fistula tract; significant signs include increased airway pressures, difficult ventilation, and stomach distension
- Postoperative outcomes depend on the type of repair, critical illness of the child, and comorbidities
- Anastomotic breakdown and leak are the most common postoperative complications

Abdominal wall defects: gastroschisis and omphalocele

Gastroschisis is an abdominal wall defect seen lateral to the umbilicus (commonly to the right). It is seen in 1 in 10 000 births. The defect typically contains only bowel and no sac covers the eviscerated contents, which exposes the bowel to the damaging effects of amniotic fluid. The umbilical cord remains separated from the defect.[6–7,17–18]

Omphalocele, on the other hand, is a midline defect of the umbilical ring. There is an intact umbilical sac and the umbilical cord is within the sac. Omphaloceles are seen in 1 in 4000 to 7000 births. The fascial defect seen is greater than 4 cm. If it is less than 4 cm, it is considered an umbilical hernia. The sac may contain stomach, bowel, and sometimes the liver. Embryologically, during gestational weeks seven to 12, the midgut herniates into the umbilical cord. By week 12, the gut should return to the abdominal cavity. The exact mechanism of an omphalocele is incompletely understood.[6–7,17–18]

Gastroschisis typically occurs earlier in gestation than omphalocele. The defect is thought to be due to abnormal development of the right omphalomesenteric artery or right umbilical vein leading to ischemia of the right abdominal wall. While the mechanism is not completely understood, there is likely an abnormal relationship between cell proliferation and apoptosis in the region of the defect.[7,15,17–18]

Gastroschisis is normally an isolated event for the neonate and may be related to a maternal exposure. Intestinal atresias may be seen in these children. In contrast, omphaloceles are commonly seen in association with other lesions and chromosomal abnormalities. Omphaloceles are associated with syndromes of midline defects including Beckwith–Wiedemann, Rieger's, prune belly syndromes, and trisomies 13, 15, 18, and 21. Two more specific associations include pentalogy of Cantrell and OEIS complex. Pentalogy of Cantrell is associated with omphalocele, diaphragmatic hernia, abnormalities of the sternum, ectopic and anomalous heart, and genetic abnormalities at Xq25 to Xq26.1. The OEIS complex is associated with omphalocele, bladder/cloacal exstrophy, imperforate anus, colonic atresia, sacrovertebral abnormalities, and meningomyelocele.[7,15,17–18]

Gastroschisis and omphaloceles may be identified by prenatal ultrasound. The presence of an abdominal wall defect should prompt additional evaluation for associated anomalies. Delivery of children with gastroschisis and nongiant omphaloceles is typically via the vaginal route.[15,17–18]

Preoperatively, attention should be given to fluid resuscitation, minimizing heat loss, treating associated infections, and avoiding trauma to the eviscerated bowel. If possible, formal work-up should evaluate for additional anomalies prior to operative intervention.[7,15,17–18]

The infant will present to the operating room with the eviscerated bowel in a sterile bowel bag to protect the bowel and to prevent heat and fluid loss. A nasogastric (NG) tube, if not already present, should be placed to decompress the bowel. Attention should be given to aggressive intravenous hydration and monitoring of electrolyte and acid–base disturbances. These infants may undergo an intravenous or inhalation induction; some anesthesiologists prefer to perform an RSI. An arterial line and central venous catheter are helpful. Monitoring the central venous pressure (CVP) to assess for changes in blood volume may be of particular assistance as the bowel is being reduced, since CVP may be utilized as a surrogate measure of intraabdominal pressure (IAP). Another method of monitoring changes in IAP as the viscera are being reduced is to measure postductal arterial saturations at two sites, typically the left upper extremity and a lower extremity. If the saturation drops or the waveform deteriorates in the lower extremity, compromised blood flow to the lower extremities may prompt surgical re-evaluation of the reduction. Neuromuscular blockade is helpful to facilitate reduction of the bowel. Nitrous oxide (N_2O) should be avoided as it may lead to distension of the bowel, impacting the ability of the surgeon to reduce it. Drastic increases in IAP may lead to impaired ventilation, hypotension, and ischemia of the bowel and intraabdominal organs (e.g., liver and kidneys).[6–7,15]

Repair of an abdominal wall defect may be primary or staged depending on the size of the defect. If the lesion is large or the infant is small, a staged repair is accomplished utilizing a "silo" chimney. The silo is sutured to the fascia and over the course of days to weeks, the eviscerated contents are slowly introduced into the abdomen. If the reduction occurs too quickly, diaphragmatic excursion and respiratory mechanics can be compromised and abdominal compartment syndrome may result. Signs of abdominal compartment syndrome include cyanotic legs due to inferior vena cava (IVC) compression and bowel ischemia.[6–7,17–18]

Postoperatively, these infants are commonly mechanically ventilated as respiratory compliance improves over the course of several days. These infants require parenteral nutrition as the resulting ileus is typically prolonged. Mortality and long-term complications are associated with the severity of coexisting anomalies, presence of postoperative complications (e.g., anastomotic leaks and breakdown), and complications secondary to parenteral nutrition. Small bowel obstructions are common as these children get older.[6–7,17–18]

Key points

Table 16.1 Important differences between gastroschisis and omphalocele

	Gastroschisis	Omphalocele
Incidence	1 in 10 000	1 in 4000 to 7000
Associated anomalies	Uncommon; intestinal atresias may be seen	Common; associated with pentalogy of Cantrell, OEIS complex, Beckwith–Wiedemann
Defect	To the right of the umbilical cord; *no sac* covers the defect	Defect of the umbilical ring; umbilical cord associated with the defect, which is covered with a sac
Embryology	Likely due to vascular compromise	Incompletely understood; failure of the gut to return to the abdomen during week 12 of development

Necrotizing enterocolitis

Necrotizing enterocolitis (NEC) is the most common gastrointestinal surgical emergency in neonates and the most common cause of death among neonates requiring gastrointestinal surgery. It primarily affects very low birth weight (VLBW) and low birth weight (LBW) neonates. Over 90% of infants with NEC are born prematurely.[19]

Utilizing the 2000 kids' inpatient database, Holman *et al.* used hospital discharge records to estimate hospital rates and mortality associated with NEC in the USA. The rate of hospitalization was 1.1 per

1000 live births (4464 hospital admissions). The median length of stay was 49 days, with an in-hospital mortality of 15.2%. Sixty six percent of infants were < 1500 g and 27% were 1500–2499 g. Those neonates who underwent surgical intervention were more likely to have a longer hospitalization and more likely to die than those treated medically. Nonhispanic Black neonates had the highest rate of NEC.[20] It rarely affects full term neonates; however, in this demographic it is often associated with an underlying condition such as perinatal asphyxia, polycythemia, respiratory distress, or congenital anomalies (myelomeningocele or congenital heart disease).[19]

The pathophysiology of NEC is poorly understood. It is characterized by a variable degree of intestinal necrosis and accompanying sepsis. Potential contributing factors include immature intestinal motility and digestion, immature intestinal circulatory regulation, immature intestinal barrier function, abnormal bacterial colonization, and immature intestinal innate immunity.[19] It is characterized by mucosal edema, coagulation necrosis, and hemorrhage. Several inflammatory mediators have been implicated including platelet activating factor, tumor necrosis factor alpha, and interleukins.[21]

The clinical presentation of NEC includes both gastrointestinal and systemic signs. Early signs of NEC are nonspecific and have considerable similarity to sepsis. These signs include feeding intolerance, delayed gastric emptying, abdominal distension, abdominal tenderness, bloody or mucoid stools, lethargy, apnea, respiratory distress, and hemodynamic instability.[19,22] Intestinal perforation, peritonitis and shock may occur. Radiographs and laboratory studies facilitate diagnosis and management. Early radiographs may reveal ileus with edematous bowel or an asymmetric bowel gas pattern. Pneumatosis intestinalis, pneumoperitoneum or portal venous air may confirm the diagnosis. Common laboratory abnormalities in NEC include hyperglycemia, thrombocytopenia, coagulopathy, anemia, leukocytosis or leucopenia, metabolic acidosis, and acute kidney injury.[15]

Medical treatment of NEC includes bowel rest with discontinuation of enteral feedings, abdominal decompression, fluid and electrolyte resuscitation, initiation of total parenteral nutrition (TPN), and broad-spectrum antibiotic therapy with anaerobic coverage. Hemodynamic support with volume and pressors as well as ventilatory support may be necessary. Hematologic abnormalities (anemia, thrombocytopenia, coagulopathy) should be corrected.[15,19,23–24]

Indications for operative intervention include intestinal perforation with free air, clinical deterioration despite maximal medical treatment, an abdominal mass with persistent intestinal obstruction or sepsis or development of an intestinal stricture.[22–24] Peritoneal drainage provides temporary decompression, drainage, and stabilization. However, 50% of patients require laparotomy 12 to 24 hours later. This technique is primarily utilized in infants < 1000 g who are expected to tolerate laparotomy poorly.[15,22–24]

The goal of laparotomy is to control sepsis and remove the gangrenous bowel while preserving as much bowel length as possible. Surgical techniques include resection with enterostomy and resection with primary anastomosis, depending on the viability of the distal segments of bowel. Panintestinal disease carries a higher complication rate and treatment may include either proximal diverting jejunostomy or the "clip and drop" technique.[22–23] The "clip and drop" technique involves resecting all segments of nonviable bowel, irrigation, clipping the ends of the bowel, and dropping the segments back into the abdomen. This procedure is followed by a second look 48–72 hours later.[25]

Preoperative evaluation includes assessment and correction of the respiratory, circulatory, hematologic, and metabolic disorders described previously. These patients will have increased crystalloid and colloid requirements due to massive third-space losses, bleeding, and disseminated intravascular coagulation (DIC). Potential adverse events associated with transport of these patients to the operating room include hypothermia, deterioration of oxygenation parameters, deterioration of ventilation parameters, and deterioration in platelet count. Limitations of operating in the neonatal intensive care unit (NICU) include inadequate lighting, inadequate surgical access, limited or no access to volatile anesthetics, reduced sterility, and limited or no ability to control room temperature. The decision whether to transport to the operating room should be made between the anesthesiologist, pediatric surgeon, and neonatologist.[15,26]

Intraoperative management is complicated by prematurity, hemodynamic instability, acidosis, respiratory failure, sepsis, coagulopathy, and electrolyte disturbances. Functional residual capacity (FRC) is reduced from abdominal distension. If the infant is not already intubated, expect rapid and profound desaturation with induction of anesthesia. Consideration should be given to a modified rapid sequence intubation (RSI) or awake intubation. Given the risk for retinopathy of prematurity, the FiO_2 should be titrated appropriately. If the patient is already intubated and ventilated in the NICU, attention should be given to the preoperative ventilator settings. If these settings cannot be achieved with the operating room ventilator, the NICU ventilator or oscillator should be brought to the operating room with appropriate personnel (e.g., respiratory therapist).[24] Volatile anesthetics may cause severe hemodynamic instability. An opioid-based technique with muscle relaxation will have less hemodynamic instability and provide adequate surgical conditions. Low-dose volatile anesthetic may be added depending on patient tolerance. Ketamine may also be used in the hemodynamically unstable neonate. N_2O should be avoided, especially in the presence of free air.[15,27]

Reliable intravenous access is imperative. Central venous access will facilitate administration of inotrope infusions. Peripheral or central venous access may be utilized for fluid and blood product administration, anesthetic administration, and correction of coagulopathy. Blood products including red blood cells, fresh frozen plasma, and platelets should be readily available. Ideally, the red blood cells should be fresh (minimize storage), leukocyte-reduced and potassium- and glucose-reduced. These neonates have massive volume requirements from evaporative losses, third-space losses and bleeding. Fluid and blood product requirements may total several blood volumes. Arterial access allows for close hemodynamic monitoring and arterial blood gas sampling, but may be challenging to obtain in this population. As in all surgical interventions in neonates, temperature regulation is important. Hypothermia is common due to the large fluid requirements. The operating room and intravenous fluids should be warmed. Close monitoring of glucose, hemoglobin, and electrolytes is recommended. Venous or arterial blood gas sampling should be utilized as well. Inotropic support with dopamine, epinephrine, and calcium may be necessary to maintain appropriate hemodynamics.[15,24,27] Typically these patients require postoperative mechanical ventilation and cardiovascular support. Long hospitalizations with prolonged TPN are common.[15]

Complications following surgical intervention include short bowel syndrome, wound dehiscence, intra-abdominal abscess, and intestinal strictures.[19,23] Patients with short bowel syndrome require long-term TPN, controversial bowel lengthening procedures or small bowel transplant. Long-term neurodevelopmental problems have been associated with VLBW survivors, especially those with surgical NEC.[15]

Key points

- NEC primarily affects premature infants of low birth weight or very low birth weight
- Medical management includes bowel rest, abdominal decompression, fluid and electrolyte resuscitation, initiation of TPN, broad-spectrum antibiotics, and correction of coagulopathy
- Hemodynamics and ventilation should be supported as necessary
- Central venous access is imperative; arterial access is helpful but may be challenging to obtain in this population
- Expect massive intraoperative volume requirements due to third-space losses, bleeding, and DIC

Imperforate anus

Anorectal malformations occur in approximately 1:5000 live births with a slight male predominance. They result from faulty separation of the rectum and urogenital system or failure of the anal membrane to rupture.[28] The diagnosis of imperforate anus encompasses a wide spectrum of malformations. These abnormalities range from mild stenosis of the anus or rectum to complex syndromes associated with other congenital anomalies. Imperforate anus is associated with trisomies 13, 18, and 21. It is part of the VACTERL Association: vertebral anomalies, imperforate anus, congenital cardiac anomalies, tracheoesophageal fistula, renal anomalies, and limb defects.[29] There is an association between anorectal malformations and maternal exposure to tobacco smoke and caffeine.[30]

Anorectal malformations are classified according to the presence or absence and location of a fistula. This classification determines the appropriate surgical correction. Surgical intervention may involve primary repair or protective colostomy followed by delayed repair.[31] The laparoscopic-assisted pull-through technique allows for primary repair without a colostomy.[32]

Preoperative evaluation should aim to identify the nature of the bowel obstruction and whether bowel perforation is present. These patients are at risk for aspiration, dehydration, electrolyte disturbances, and sepsis. Abdominal distension will impair ventilation. Induction of anesthesia should proceed with an awake intubation, rapid sequence intubation (RSI) or modified RSI. A difficult airway may be suspected in infants with associated congenital anomalies, such as tracheoesophageal fistula.[15] In addition, it is important to identify any associated defects. Preoperative evaluation with echocardiogram, renal and bladder ultrasound, spinal ultrasound, voiding cystourethrogram, and plain radiographs of the abdomen and lower spine is warranted.[29]

These infants may be anesthetized with volatile anesthetics or an opioid-based technique. Neuromuscular blocking agents may facilitate surgical exposure. However, when nerve stimulation is utilized to identify the anal sphincter, muscle relaxation should be avoided. Nitrous oxide (N_2O) is avoided due to the risk of increasing bowel distension.[15] Tobias presented a case report of an infant with palliated congenital heart disease who successfully underwent anorectoplasty under combined general and spinal anesthesia.[33] When considering neuraxial anesthesia or analgesia, the possible association with lumbosacral abnormalities and tethered cord should be considered.

Intraoperative management requires careful monitoring of fluid status and replacement of fluids, electrolytes, and blood products as necessary. Peripheral access is typically adequate for these surgical procedures, except in cases of marked cardiorespiratory instability.

Postoperative mechanical ventilation and hemodynamic support may be required. In addition, many infants require TPN.[15] Long-term complications include fecal incontinence, constipation, urinary incontinence, and sexual inadequacy.[31]

Key points

- Associated syndromes (VACTERL associations and trisomy 21) should be considered in preoperative evaluation and planning
- Preoperative evaluation with echocardiogram, renal and bladder ultrasound, spinal ultrasound, voiding cystourethrogram, and plain radiographs of the abdomen and lower spine is warranted
- Consider aspiration risk with induction of anesthesia
- Consider potential need for nerve stimulation to assist in identification of the anal sphincter prior to administration of a muscle relaxant

Intestinal obstruction

Obstructive lesions in neonates may be divided into three categories: congenital, mechanical, and functional. They occur anywhere along the gastrointestinal tract from the esophagus to the anus. Congenital obstructive lesions include atresias, stenosis or webs of the esophagus, pylorus, duodenum, jejunum, ileum, or colon. Mechanical causes include malrotation, intussusceptions, incarceration, perforation, and volvulus. Functional causes include meconium ileus and Hirschprung's disease.[24]

Clinically, patients with intestinal obstruction present with vomiting, abdominal distension, and failure to pass stool. Maternal polyhydramnios may be a sign of intestinal obstruction. Gas-filled loops of bowel may be seen on radiographs. Loss of gastric, biliary, and pancreatic secretions leads to dehydration, electrolyte abnormalities, and hypovolemia. These abnormalities should be monitored and corrected appropriately.[24] Failure to recognize and treat an intestinal obstruction may result in intestinal perforation, bowel necrosis, or sepsis.[15]

Duodenal atresia or stenosis is the most common intestinal atresia, occurring in 1:5000 to 1:10 000 live births. It is commonly associated with other anomalies including Down syndrome, cystic fibrosis, renal anomalies, congenital cardiac anomalies, intestinal malrotation, esophageal atresia, imperforate anus, intraluminal diaphragm, membranous web, and annular pancreas.[29,34] Prenatal ultrasound in the late second or third trimester may be diagnostic. Infants present with bilious emesis and a scaphoid abdomen. The "double-bubble" sign on an abdominal radiograph is created by a dilated stomach and a dilated proximal duodenum. Failure to provide treatment with resuscitation and gastric decompression may lead to dehydration, weight loss, and hypochloremic alkalosis.[15,29] Prior to operative intervention, evaluation for associated skeletal, spinal, and cardiac anomalies should be completed. Postoperative complications include delayed gastric emptying, a slow return to feeding, gastroesophageal reflux, gastritis or peptic ulcer, megaduodenum, blind-loop syndrome, adhesions causing obstruction and rarely, late stenosis.[29]

Jejunolileal atresias are associated with prematurity, polyhydramnios, and cystic fibrosis. The proposed etiology involves intrauterine vascular accidents. The risk of jejunoileal atresia is increased by maternal vasoconstrictive medications and maternal cigarette smoking during the first trimester. Extra-intestinal anomalies are uncommon (except in patients with cystic fibrosis).[15,29] Clinical presentation depends on the location of the atresia and the severity of disease. Proximal obstructions present with bilious emesis and a scaphoid abdomen whereas distal obstructions present with significant abdominal distension. Volvulus and perforation may occur pre- or postnatally. Flat and decubitus radiographs aid in the diagnosis showing dilated loops of bowel with air-fluid levels and a paucity of gas distal to the obstruction. A contrast enema will show a small unused colon. Treatment includes gastric decompression, fluid resuscitation, and broad-spectrum antibiotics. Operative repair most commonly includes excision of dilated and atretic bowel followed by primary end-to-end anastomosis; TPN is required postoperatively until return of bowel function.[29]

Malrotations occur in 1:6000 live births. They result from abnormalities in rotation of the bowel, which occurs during the 10th–12th week of gestation. The bowel does not develop appropriately. Instead areas of ischemia, atresia, and volvulus develop. Without adequate fixation, the small bowel may rotate around its mesentery. These abnormalities lead to strangulation of bowel, bloody stools, abdominal distension, peritonitis, and hypovolemic shock.[15,35] Patients often present within the first 1 to 2 months of life, but may not present until much later (including adulthood). Associations have been identified with cardiac (heterotaxia), esophageal, urinary, and anal anomalies. All patients with gastroschisis, omphalocele, and congenital diaphragmatic hernia have some degree of intestinal malrotation or nonrotation.[15,29]

Missing the diagnosis of malrotation has catastrophic consequences. Initially infants present with irritability, bilious emesis, and a scaphoid abdomen. This presentation progresses to abdominal distension, tenderness, abdominal wall erythema, and hematemesis or melena. Peritonitis, sepsis, shock, and death result from compromise of the mesentery. Treatment involves aggressive fluid resuscitation, gastric decompression, and broad-spectrum antibiotics. Immediate operative intervention is warranted in the presence of volvulus.[29]

Surgical repair of a malrotation may be performed open or laparoscopically and involves Ladd's procedure. First the bowel is eviscerated and the intestines are untwisted in a counterclockwise direction. Ladd's peritoneal band is lysed and an appendectomy is performed. The bowel is observed for recovery of vascular perfusion to the involved intestine. Necrotic bowel is excised and the bowel is reconnected with a primary anastomosis or proximal and distal stomas are formed. Complications include short bowel syndrome and the need for chronic total parenteral nutrition (TPN).[15,29,35]

All patients with intestinal obstructions are at significant risk of aspiration on induction of anesthesia. Rapid sequence intubation (RSI), modified RSI or awake intubation should be considered. Preoperative gastric decompression should be considered.[24] Ventilation is compromised by abdominal distension due to the high, fixed position of the diaphragm.[15]

Key points

- Intestinal obstruction presents with maternal polyhydramnios, bilious emesis, failure to pass stool, and abdominal distension
- Treatment involves fluid resuscitation, correction of electrolyte disorders, and gastric decompression prior to operative intervention
- There is a significant risk for aspiration on induction of anesthesia

Summary and conclusions

Neonates presenting for a surgical emergency may present overall healthy but may also be critically ill. Although abdominal, neonatal surgical emergencies encompass a variety of defects and diseases, their anesthetic management has a lot in common. Due to the fact that these are neonates, differences in anatomy, pharmacology, physiology, and temperature regulation must be taken into account. This is particularly important in cases where the risk of aspiration upon induction of anesthesia is very high and/or the neonate has comorbidities. In general, proper preoperative evaluation, planning, and meticulous attention to detail are important for optimal postoperative outcomes.[1]

References

1. D. J. Mellor and J. Lerman. Anesthesia for neonatal surgical emergencies. *Semin Perinatol* 1998; **22**: 363–79.
2. G. Aspelund and J. C. Langer. Current management of hypertrophic pyloric stenosis. *Semin Pediatr Surg* 2007; **16**(1): 27–33.
3. G. Hammer, S. Hall, and P. J. Davis. Anesthesia for general abdominal, thoracic, urologic, and bariatric surgery. In P. J. Davis, F. P. Cladis and E. K. Motoyama. *Smith's Anesthesia for Infants and Children,* Eighth Edition. Philadelphia PA, Elsevier, 2011; pp.745–85.
4. B. Naik-Mathuria and O. O. Olutoye. Foregut abnormalities. *Surg Clin N Am* 2006; **86**(2): 261–84.
5. S. Pandya and K. Heiss. Pyloric stenosis in pediatric surgery. *Surg Clin N Am* 2012; **92**(3): 527–39.
6. J. D. Roberts Jr., T. M. Romanelli, and I. D. Todres. Neonatal emergencies. In C. J. Cote, J. Lerman and I. D. Todres. *A Practice of Anesthesia for Infants and Children.* Philadelphia PA, Elsevier, 2009; pp. 746–65.
7. J. Lerman, C. J. Cote, and D. Steward. General and thoracoabdominal surgery. In J. Lerman, C. J. Cote and D. Steward. *Manual of Pediatric Anesthesia.* Philadelphia PA, Elsevier, 2009; pp. 336–97.
8. R. Brown and A. Bosenberg. Evolving management of congenital diaphragmatic hernia. *Paediatr Anaesth* 2007; **17**: 713–19.
9. A. Garcia and C. Stolar. Congenital diaphragmatic hernia and protective ventilation strategies in pediatric surgery. *Surg Clin N Am* 2012; **92**(3): 659–68.
10. A. M. Holder, M. Klaassens, D. Tibboel, *et al.* Genetic factors in congenital diaphragmatic hernia. *Am J Hum Genet* 2007; **80**: 825–45.
11. D. W. Kays. Congenital diaphragmatic hernia and neonatal lung lesions. *Surg Clin N Am* 2006; **86**(2): 329–52.
12. V. Moyer, F. Moya, R. Tibboel, *et al.* Late versus early surgical correction for congenital diaphragmatic hernia in newborn infants. *Cochrane Database Syst Rev* 2010.
13. M. Mugford, D. Elbourne, and D. Field. Extracorporeal membrane oxygenation for severe respiratory failure in newborn infants. *Cochrane Database Syst Rev* 2008.
14. P. D. Robinson and D. A. Fitzgerald. Congenital diaphragmatic hernia. *Paediatr Respir Rev* 2007; **8**(4): 323–35.
15. C. Brett and P. J. Davis. Anesthesia for general surgery in the neonate. In P. J. Davis, F. P. Cladis, and E. K. Motoyama. *Smith's Anesthesia for Infants and Children, Eighth Edition.* Philadelphia PA, Elsevier Mosby, 2011; pp. 554–88.
16. A. Goyal, M. O. Jones, J. M. Couriel, and P. D. Losty. Oesophageal atresia and tracheo-oesophageal fistula. *Arch Dis Child-Fetal* 2006; **91**: F381–4.
17. D. J. Ledbetter, S. Dauger, E. Gordon, *et al.* Gastroschisis and omphalocele. *Surg Clin N Am* 2006; **86**(2): 249–60.
18. D. J. Ledbetter. Congenital abdominal wall defects and reconstruction in pediatric surgery: Gastroschisis and omphalocele. *Surg Clin N Am* 2012; **92**(3): 713–27.
19. P. W. Lin and B. J. Stoll. Necrotizing enterocolitis. *Lancet* 2006; **368**: 1271–83.
20. R. C. Holman, B. J. Stoll, A. T. Curns, *et al.* Necrotizing enterocolitis hospitalisations among neonates in the USA. *Paediatr Perinat Ep* 2006; **20**: 498–506.
21. T. P. Fox and C. Godavitarne. What really causes necrotising enterocolitis? *ISRN Gastroenterol* 2012; 2012:628317.
22. Y. S. Guner, N. Chokshi, M. Petrosyan, *et al.* Necrotizing enterocolitis – bench to bedside: novel and emerging strategies. *Semin Pediatr Surg* 2008; **17**: 255–65.
23. A. Pierro. The surgical management of necrotising enterocolitis. *Early Hum Dev* 2005; **81**: 79–85.
24. R. Brusseau and M. E. McCann. Anaesthesia for urgent and emergency surgery. *Early Hum Dev* 2010; **86**: 703–14.
25. W. G. Vaughan, J. L. Grosfeld, K. West, *et al.* Avoidance of stomas and delayed anastamosis for bowel necrosis: the "clip and drop" technique. *J Pediatr Surg* 1996; **31**: 542–5.
26. G. Frawley, G. Bayley, and P. Chondros. Laparotomy for necrotizing enterocolitis: Intensive care nursery compared with operating theatre. *J Paediatr Child H* 1999; **35**: 291–5.
27. S. C. Hillier, G. Krishna, and E. Brasoveanu. Neonatal anesthesia. *Semin Pediatr Surg* 2004; **13**(3): 142–51.
28. R. Stevenson. Rectum and anus. In R. Stevenson, J. Hall, and R. Goodman. *Human Malformations and Related Anomalies.* New York, Oxford University Press, 1993; pp. 493–9.
29. D. Juang and C. L. Snyder. Neonatal bowel obstruction. *Surg Clin N Am* 2012; **92**: 685–711.
30. E. A. Miller, S. E. Manning, S. A. Rasmussen, *et al.* Maternal exposure to tobacco smoke, alcohol and caffeine, and risk of anorectal atresia: National Birth Defects Prevention Study 1997–2003. *Paediatr Perinat Epidemiol* 2008; **23**: 9–17.

31. A. Pena and A. Hong. Advances in the management of anorectal malformations. *Am J Surg* 2000; **180**: 370–6.

32. K. E. Georgeson, T. H. Inge, and C. T. Albanese. Laparoscopically assisted anorectal pull-through for high imperforate anus – A new technique. *J Pediatr Surg* 2000; **35**(6): 927–31.

33. J. D. Tobias. Combined general and spinal anesthesia in an infant with single-ventricle physiology undergoing anorectoplasty for an imperforate anus. *J Cardiothorac Vasc Anesth* 2007; **21**(6): 873–5.

34. A. R. Mustafawi and M. E. Hassan. Congenital duodenal obstruction in children: A decade's experience. *Eur J Pediatr Surg* 2008; **18**: 93–7.

35. A. J. Millar, H. Rode, and S. Cywes. Malrotation and volvulus in infancy and childhood. *Semin Pediatr Surg* 2003; **12**(4): 229–36.

Chapter 17

Pathophysiology of pain

Lisgelia Santana

Introduction

The initial reception of noxious inputs perceived to be painful is by the specialized endings of primary afferent neurons known as nociceptors. Reception of noxious input occurs in functionally specialized free nerve endings of the skin, muscle, joints, blood vessels, fascia, viscera, and dura. Nociceptor subtypes respond best to either mechanical, thermal, or chemical stimuli (1,2). Common types of cutaneous nociceptors are A-delta mechanoreceptors and C polymodal nociceptors that relay the transduced information about potentially harmful input via A-delta and C-fibers, respectively (3,4).

The axons that relay information about noxious input from the skin and other tissues to the central nervous system fall characteristically into the range of small, unmyelinated fibers with conduction velocities less than 2.5 m/sec for C-fiber nociceptors, and small fibers wrapped in a thin layer of myelin produced by Schwann cells with a conduction velocity of 4 to 30 m/sec in the case of the A-delta fibers. Primary afferent C-fibers are more numerous than myelinated primary afferents in peripheral nerves. They bring sensory information into the CNS through the dorsal root. The sensory afferent fibers have their cell bodies in the dorsal root ganglia (or cranial nerve ganglia) located outside the spinal cord or brainstem. Noxious mechanical, temperature, and chemical (nociceptive) information are first relayed across a synapse located in the spinal cord before transmission to the brainstem sites (including ventral posterolateral thalamus).

As many central neuronal circuits, glutamate is the primary neurotransmitter substance in the primary afferent nociceptors and its action is modulated by neuropeptides coreleased at their terminal endings, such as calcitonin gene-related peptide (CGRP), substance P, neurokinin A, adenosine triphosphate, adenosine, galanin, and somatostatin (5). All of these substances have been identified in the dorsal root ganglia; however, they are produced and transported quickly to terminal endings in the spinal cord and thus may not necessarily be evident in the dorsal root ganglia without further manipulations.

In general, large myelinated primary afferent fibers carrying sensory discriminative information (tactile, pressure, vibratory sense) enter via the dorsal horn of the spinal cord (Lissauer's tract), and turn to ascend uncrossed input into the dorsal horn. The smaller myelinated and unmyelinated fibers carry information about temperature and nociceptive input perceived as pain in humans. The fibers enter the Lissauer's tract, then innervate the gray matter core of the spinal cord where neuronal cell bodies and dendrites receive their arborized synaptic endings.

The gray matter at the core of the spinal cord is a matrix of synaptic terminations and cells forming the first tier of processing and integration of sensory information. The gray matter of the spinal cord has been decribed topographically as ten laminae by Rexed (6) based on the histologic appearance; these include laminae I to VI. Laminae VII to IX and lamina X are involved in somatic and autonomic motor function, respectively. Somatic C nociceptor afferent endings are distributed mainly to laminae I and II in the same and adjacent segments, whereas visceral C afferents can extend for more than five segments before they terminate. Somatic C nociceptors end rather focally in the spinal cord gray matter, whereas visceral C nociceptors are widely distributed in laminae I, II, V, X ipsilaterally as well as in laminae III and X contralaterally (7,8). Cutaneous A-delta mechanical nociceptors terminate in the ipsilateral laminae I and V.

Essentials of Pediatric Anesthesiology, ed. Alan David Kaye, Charles James Fox and James H. Diaz. Published by Cambridge University Press. © Cambridge University Press 2015.

There are two parallel pain system ascending pathways bringing nociceptive information to higher brain centers. The spinothalamic tract brings primarily cutaneous nociceptive information and sends its axons across the midline in the spinal cord before ascending to the thalamus. The postsynaptic dorsal column pathway brings primarily visceral nociceptive information. Uncrossed axons are sent up the dorsal column to synapse in the dorsal column nuclei, in the dorsal medulla midline. A crossed axonal projection from the dorsal column nuclei ascends as the medial lemniscus, bringing information about visceral pain to the thalamus. The ventral posterolateral nucleus of the thalamus is the principal sensory relay nucleus providing discriminative site-specific information about pain to the somatosensory cortex, SI and SII. Other thalamic nuclei receive nociceptive information provided to frontal, insular, and anterior cingulated cortices for affective responses to pain, including nuclei of the medial and intralaminar thalamus. Finally, descending modulatory systems impact nociceptive processing through complex brainstem circuitry (9).

Pain assessment in infants and children

Pain is both a sensory and emotional personal experience, making assesement complex (10). It is now well accepted by neuroscientists and pain specialists that the nervous system is sufficiently developed to process nociception before birth, and consequently, children must be assumed to experience pain from birth onward (11).

Due to a more robust inflammatory response and the lack of central inhibitory influence, infants and young children actually may experience a greater neural response, i.e., more pain sensation and pain-related distress, following noxious stimulus than do adults. The impact of a painful experience on the young nervous system is so significant that long-term effects can occur, including a lowered pain tolerance for months after the event that produced the pain (12).

The assessment of children's pain is problematic as younger children or some with develpmental delays often can not express or describe their pain. Accurate assessment of children's pain is needed to diagnose conditions and guide a treatment. Over the past 20 years, significant research attention has been devoted to developing instruments to quantify children's pain. In 2007, the Pediatric Initiative on Methods, Measurement, and Pain Assessment in Clinical Trials (Ped-Immpact) commissioned a review to identify measures to use in pediatric pain clinical research trials. It included one self report (13) and one observational study (14).

In the adult world there is a recommendation to assess pain intensity by asking patients to rate their pain on numerical rating scales, with 0 indicating no pain and 10 indicating the worst pain posible (15). As children are more limited in understanding the number concepts, a variety of other rating scales have been developed in which children provide a graphic representation of pain intensity by marking a point on a line (VAS), pointing to or coloring a certain level on a pain "thermometer," selecting from a series of faces depicting different levels of pain, or counting different numbers of simple, tangible objects such as poker chips. The VAS system consists of a 100 mm horizontal line with anchors indicating "no pain" at the left endpoint and "worst pain possible" at the right endpoint. The child makes a vertical line to indicate how much pain he/she feels. Extensive evidence supports VAS pain ratings as valid indicators of children's pain. Children's VAS scores have been shown to correlate significantly with parent ratings of children's pain (16) and with medical personnel ratings (17). The VAS score correlates positively with postoperative recovery (18). The VAS score has been shown to be sensitive to changes in pain following analgesic medications (19). Advantages of VAS include ease of administration, low cost, and the fact that the scale yields ratio data. It is recommended as most appropriate for children over 8 years of age (20).

Faces scales consist of a set of line drawings or photographs of faces that depict pain states (21). Faces scales have been shown to correlate highly with other self-report indices (22), ratings by parents and nurses (21), and to be sensitive to analgesic and non-pharmacological interventions (23). A popular faces scale, The Oucher, provides different photographs for Caucasian, Hispanic, and black children, and can be used from 3–12 years old (24). The Wong–Baker Faces Scales has no ethnicity distinctions. It is well accepted in children over 6 years of age (25).

The poker chip tool or pieces of hurt tool (26) is a very simple pain intensity measure, consisting of four red chips that represent "pieces of hurt" (with one chip indicating a little hurt and all four chips indicating the most hurt). This straightforward, concete measure has been used in 3- to 8-year-olds from a variety of cultures for acute procedure-related and postoperative pain (27).

The FLACC (Face, Leg, Activity, Cry and Consolability) Scale is a behavioral scale that had been validated for assessment of postoperative pain in children between the ages of 2 months and 7 years (28). For less than two months of age, CRIES has been used as a behavioral modality scale. The CRIES scale: Assesses Crying, Oxygen requirement, Increased vital signs, facial Expression, Sleep. An observer provides a score of 0 to 2 for each parameter based on changes from baseline. The scale is useful for neonatal postoperative pain.

Postoperative pain

Providing analgesia in the setting of moderate to severe pain, especially in the setting of surgery or trauma, is an important ethical responsibility of the medical profession, especially for anesthesiologists. The pain of surgery is not confined to the duration of the procedure itself but persists for some time afterward. Typically, after minor surgery, not only is there persisting pain for hours, days, or weeks depending on the location and severity of injury but changes in sensitivity at the operation site itself and the surrounding area. The trauma, manipulation, and damage at the wound site after surgery result in local inflammation. Inflammation is characterized by an altered perception (hypersensitivity) of pain that includes an enhanced pain sensation to a noxious stimulus (hyperalgesia) and an abnormal sensation of pain to previously nonnoxious stimuli (allodynia). In addition, there may be spontaneous or ongoing pain. The hyperalgesia that follows tissue injury can be divided into primary and secondary hyperalgesia. Primary hyperalgesia develops at the site of an injury and appears to arise largely from peripheral nociceptor sensitization. Surrounding this is a zone of secondary mechanical hyperalgesia, which is proposed to arise from central plastic changes in spinal cord connectivity modifying CNS responsiveness to future stimuli.

The pain arising from the surgical wound differs from the pain of a needle because it activates a number of new mechanisms within the nervous system. Local consequences of inflammation include the release of allogenic substances from damaged cells, recruitment of inflammatory cells, and release of further mediators from cells in the vicinity. This include H+ and K^+, serotonin, histamine, bradykinin, prostaglandins, nitric oxide, cytokines, and growth factors (29). These may directly activate peripheral nociceptors to cause pain, but more often they act indirectly to sensitize nociceptors and alter their response properties to subsequent stimuli (30).

Post-traumatic pain

Trauma is a major source of morbidity and mortality in the USA, as well as throughout the world. Pediatric unintentional physical injuries continue to be the leading cause of morbidity and mortality in children aged ≥ 1 year in the USA. According to the National Center for Health Statistics (2006), 34.3% of all deaths for children aged 1–4 years and 39.0% of all deaths for children aged 5–14 years resulted from unintentional injury in 2004.

Until recently, the prevailing dogma was that children did not perceive or remember painful occurrences as intensely or as unpleasantly as did adults. There also was fear, often unfounded, that treating traumatic pain would mask the symptoms of progressive injury. Such assumptions are false, and it is no longer appropriate simply to restrain children or to withhold analgesia. Although emergency medicine has made major strides in the treatment of pediatric trauma pain, multiple erroneous reasons have been offered not to treat pain in children. The most prevalent assumption is that children, especially infants, do not feel pain. Because the very young child is unable to verbalize and, thus, report pain, physicians simply may deny its existence. In fact, nociceptive neural pathways are in place by 23 to 24 weeks' gestation. Term and preterm newborns have fully developed pain transmission pathways, but lack fully developed pain inhibitory systems. Thus, they may feel even more pain than older children in similar situations.

Children's perceptions of pain are influenced by many factors including: Gender, age, cognitive level, family learning, past pain experience, culture, emotion, expectation, parental response, perception of control, relevance, coping style, etc. Children's expectations of pain come from their own memory of previous painful experiences and those learned from family or culture (31).

Analgesia for head trauma

Acute pain management of head trauma patients presents several unique considerations. First, it is difficult to assess the level of pain in patients with an altered mental status. Patients who are unable to voice their pain may be mistakenly believed to not have pain. There are also concerns that the sedating effects of opioid could interfere with adequate neurological assessment. As a result, trauma patients with head injuries are less likely to receive opioids than patients with comparable injuries who have not sustained head trauma (32). Analgesic treatments include the use of non-sedating analgesic agents and opioid-reducing strategies wherever possible, to minimize the sedating effects of opioids. Acetaminophen is a good choice for mild to moderate pain. Use of NSAIDs such as ibuprofen and ketorolac are best avoided in any patient at risk for intracranial bleeding due to platelet-inibitory effects. For moderate to severe pain, shorter acting opioids such as fentanyl, or remifentanil as an infusion can be used. In head injury patients with chest trauma, chest analgesia (thoracic epidural or intercostals nerve block) reduces pulmonary morbidity and decreases hypoventilation due to poor respiratory mechanics, splinting, and resultant atelectasis. Hypoventilation and resultant hypercarbia can lead to increased intracranial pressure in patients with traumatic brain injury.

Analgesia in the setting of burn injury

Burn injury in children continues to be a major epidemiologic problem around the globe. Nearly a fourth of all burn injuries occur in children under the age of 16, of whom the majority are under the age of five. Burn injuries often cause very severe pain associated with the injury itself, as well as with the multiple interventions that follow. Pain management is a critical piece in the overall care of the burned child. Severe pain is a major consequence of burn injury, and it has been demonstrated that it is often inadequately treated (33). Anxiety and depression are confounding components in a major burn and can further decrease the pain threshold. The different types of pain must be taken into account (acute, procedure-related pain versus background, or baseline pain) in the development of an effective pain regimen. High-dose opioids are commonly used to manage acute breakthrough pain and pain associated with burn procedures, and morphine is currently the most widely used drug at burn centers in North America (34). As alterations in morphine clearance do not seem to be an effect of burn injury and most burned patients will develop tolerance to its effects, titration to the appropriate level of pain control and frequent reassessment are important. In addition, the combination of opioids and benzodiazepines (with appropriate monitoring) can be used successfully for procedural sedation, as daily wound care and dressing changes are commonplace and can be associated with significant pain.

Due to the concerns of tolerance, withdrawal, and opioid-induced hyperalgesia (35), the use of a multimodal pain management regimen has been advocated. For background analgesia, analgesics such as acetaminophen can be used for their opioid-sparing effect. Ketamine, an N-methyl-D-aspartic acid (NMDA) antagonist has been used with increased frequency for procedural sedation. Advantages for its use include preserved muscle tone and protective airway reflexes, reduced risk of respiratory depression, and reduced hemodynamic effects (36). Regional anesthetic techniques may also serve as a useful opioid-sparing adjunct for burn injuries limited to an extremity. Lastly, a variety of other techniques including music therapy, hypnotherapy, massage, behavioral techniques, and even virtual reality techniques have been successfully used to reduce pain during wound care (37).

Pain in the neonate

Scientific research in recent years has continued to confirm that neonates, especially when preterm, are more sensitive to nociceptive stimuli than older children. Neonates are capable of mounting robust physiological, behavioral, hormonal, and metabolic responses to such stimuli, responses that can have adverse short- and long-term effects (38,39). Several lines of evidence suggest that early and repeated exposure to painful stimuli during a period fundamental to nervous system development leads to persistent behavioral changes and a smaller volume of the sensory areas of the brain in ex-preterm infants (40,41).

In 2006, the American Academy of Pediatrics and the Canadian Pediatric Society published new guidelines (42) recommending that each health care facility that treats neonates establish a neonatal pain control program. The responsibilities of this program include:

- Providing routine assessments to detect neonatal pain
- Reducing the number of painful procedures
- Preventing or treating acute pain from bedside invasive procedures
- Anticipating and treating postoperative pain following surgery
- Avoiding prolonged or repetitive pain and stress during neonatal intensive care

Despite these recommendations, acute neonatal pain results from 8.5 million untreated painful procedures annually in neonatal intensive care units in Europe (43), which extrapolates to 120 million painful procedures performed annually in newborns worldwide.

Nonpharmacological approaches for procedural pain and postoperative pain

Prevention

Acute procedural pain can be minimized by using indwelling catheters for blood sampling, by planning procedures with an analgesic approach (44). Procedures must be limited to those absolutely necessary for the diagnostic or therapeutic management of neonates (45). Touch in preterm infants at 32 weeks through gentle massage appeared to have analgesic effects (46).

Non-nutritive sucking

The pacifying effects of non-nutritive sucking were clearly shown in multiple studies that reported decreased crying, lower heart rates, and increased oxygenation in term and preterm neonates during painful procedures like heel sticks and venipuncture (47,48).

Sweet solutions

The analgesic effect of sucrose was first reported by Blass *et al.* in 1991 (49). A systematic Cochrane review in 2010 including 44 studies and 3496 infants concluded that sucrose is safe and effective for reducing procedural pain in neonates (50). In another meta-analysis, doses of 0.24 g sucrose given 2 minutes before painful stimuli were effective for term neonates (50), providing analgesia for 5–7 minutes. Repeated doses may be required if the procedure exceeds this duration. For painful procedures that involve breaking the skin, 24% sucrose can be placed directly on the infant's tongue, using the following doses:

- 24–26 weeks gestation: 0.1 ml
- 27–31 weeks gestation: 0.25 ml
- 32–36 weeks gestation: 0.5 ml
- > 37 weeks gestation: 1 ml

Administration of a sweet solution with a pacifier was synergistic (51,52), providing stronger analgesic effects than either intervention alone.

Skin-to-skin contact (kangaroo care)

Gray *et al.* found that 10–15 minutes of kangaroo care between mothers and their term newborns reduced crying, grimacing, and heart rate during heel-stick procedures (53). Johnston *et al.* showed that kangaroo care significantly reduced the acute pain responses of preterm neonates at 32–36 weeks and 28–32 weeks gestation (54,55).

Breastfeeding analgesia

Breastfeeding maintained throughout a procedure relieved heel-stick pain in term neonates more effectively than swaddling (56). In another study, Carbajal *et al.* found that breastfeeding effectively reduced venipuncture-associated pain in term neonates (57).

Local anesthesia

Several topical anesthetics, including lidocaine–prilocaine cream, 4% tetracaine gel, liposomal lidocaine, and lidocaine/tetracaine gel, are now available (58). Efficacy data suggest that lidocaine–prilocaine cream and tetracaine gel are ineffective for heel sticks, but decrease pain during venipunctures. Lidocaine–prilocaine cream decreases circumcision pain; tetracaine gel is safe but ineffective for venous catheterization in neonates. When applied to intact skin, lidocaine–prilocaine cream requires 60 minutes and tetracaine gel requires 30–45 minutes to produce local anesthesia (58,59). Both preparations are safe for single use in preterm and term neonates.

Surgical pain in neonates

Pain is an inevitable consequence of surgery at every age. Pain is of particular importance in the neonate because of the evidence of improved clinical outcomes, including decreased mortality, when adequate pain control is achieved (60,61). Tissue injury, which occurs during all forms of surgery, elicits profound physiologic responses. The more marked these responses to surgery, the greater the morbidities and mortality (62). Improving pain management and improving outcomes in the neonate require a coordinated strategy of pain reduction, which must be multidimensional, requires a team approach, and should be a first priority in perioperative management. Despite fears that analgesics (particularly with opioids) may lead to respiratory depression and an increase in postoperative complications, such effects have never been shown in randomized, controlled trials. Indeed, postoperative respiratory compromise associated with the pain of a thoracotomy can be relieved by adequate analgesia (63,64).

Because of the physiologic and metabolic immaturity of the neonate, doses of medications that are effective for the reduction of pain may be close to the doses that cause toxicity. Therefore, the concept of a "balanced analgesia" has arisen, whereby several approaches to pain reduction can be used simultaneously to decrease the dosage required of each medication and, thereby, reduce toxicity. Early and effective pain treatment is associated with a lower total dose of medications, although therapy should be guided by ongoing pain assessment.

As far as possible, stress and preoperative pain should be relieved before surgical interventions. An infant who is stressed and disturbed, unclothed, hypothermic, overstimulated by noise and light, and already experiencing pain will have elevated basal concentrations of adrenal cortical and medullary hormones and will be susceptible to further stress and complications postoperatively.

Postoperatively, opioids can be given by continuous infusion or by regular bolus. Randomized trials do not show any substantial benefit of continuous infusion of opioids over intermittent dosing, probably because of the long half-life of many of these agents in the neonate (65). In neonates aged 1–7 days, the clearance of morphine is one-third that of older infants and elimination half-life approximately 1.7 times longer (66,67). In appropriately selected cases, the s.c. route of administration is a useful alternative to the IV route (68,69). The s.c. route is contraindicated when the child is hypovolemic or has significant ongoing fluid compartment shifts (70).

Fentanyl, sufentanil, alfentanil, and remifentanil may have a role after major surgery and in intensive care practice. Remifentanil is very titratable and has a context-insensitive half-time with extremely rapid recovery because of esterase clearance, but transition to the postoperative phase is difficult to manage and may be complicated by acute tolerance.

Postoperative ketorolac use in infants and neonates has been described (71,72). However, the risk of renal failure or insufficiency is not known. A comparison of ibuprofen and indomethacin for closure of patent ductus arteriosus indicated oliguria as an adverse effect, occurring more in the indomethacin group (73). Renal blood flow depends on prostaglandins, especially during stressful periods (as in neonates in the postoperative course). Studies in premature neonates have shown that the glomerular filtration rate decreases in neonates with use of ibuprofen (74). With the evidence currently available, ketorolac and other NSAID use is associated with risk of renal compromise in the neonatal period.

Acetaminophen is rapidly absorbed from the small bowel, and oral formulations in syrup, tablet, or dispersible forms are widely available and used in pediatric practice. Suppository formulations vary somewhat in their composition and bioavailability, with lipophilic formulations having higher bioavailability. Absorption from the rectum is slow and incomplete, except in neonates; IV acetaminophen is currently not approved for children less than 2 years of age in the USA (75). There are limited neonatal IV acetaminophen pharmacokinetic data available for comparison with the prodrug pharmacokinetics in neonates, attributable in part to its off-label use in children weighing <10 kg in other countries.

Chronic pain states

We will briefly discuss the diagnosis and management of some common chronic pain syndromes diagnosed in pediatric patients who are referred to the chronic pain

Table 17.1 Acetaminophen for postoperative analgesia in infants

Age	Oral loading dose	Oral maintenace dose	Rectal loading dose	Rectal maintenance dose	Maximum daily dose oral or rectal	Duration at maximum dose
Preterm 28–32 weeks	20 mg/kg	15 mg/kg up to 12 hourly	20 mg/kg	15 ml/kg up to 12 hourly	35 mg/kg/day	48 hours
Preterm 32–38 weeks	20 mg/kg	20 mg/kg up to 12 hourly	30 mg/kg	20 mg/kg up to 12 hourly	60 /kg/day	48 hours
0–3 months	20 mg/kg	20 mg/kg up to 8 hourly	30 mg/kg	20 mg/kg up to 12 hourly	60 mg/kg/day	48 hours

clinic for management. Chronic pain (defined as persistent and recurrent pain for more than 3 months by the International Association for the Study of Pain) is a significant problem in the pediatric population, conservatively estimated to affect 20% to 35% of children and adolescents around the world (76,77). Some of the most common complaints include headaches, abdominal pain, chest pain, neuropathic pain, back pain, pelvic pain, cancer-related pain, and pain due to chronic illnesses such as sickle cell, cystic fibrosis, and collagen vascular diseases (e.g., juvenile idiopathic arthritis, systemic lupus erythematosus, scleroderma). Because prevalence rates vary considerably across studies, it is difficult to make general conclusions regarding the pervasiveness of different pains in children and adolescents.

Chronic pain in children is the result of a dynamic integration of biological processes, psychological factors, and sociocultural factors considered within a developmental trajectory. Children may experience physical and psychological sequelae and their families may experience emotional and social consequences as a result of pain and associated disability. Childhood pain brings significant direct and indirect costs from healthcare utilization and lost wages due to taking time off work to care for the child (78). Other studies provide convincing evidence to suggest that childhood chronic pain predisposes both for the continuation of pain and the development of new forms of chronic pain in adulthood (79).

Chronic pain in children and teenagers is a dramatically growing problem, with hospital admissions for youngsters with the condition rising nine-fold between 2004 and 2010, a new study suggests. The most common type of chronic pain among kids in the study was abdominal pain, which was reported in 23 percent of cases, according to the study. For the study, researchers gathered information on 3752 children admitted to 43 pediatric hospitals throughout the USA. The typical chronic pain patients were white and female, with an average age of 14. The average hospital stay was 7.32 days, according to the study. The vast majority of the patients in the study received additional diagnoses while in the hospital, with an average of ten diagnoses per child. Children were diagnosed with conditions such as abdominal pain, mood disorders, constipation, and nausea. Altogether, 65 percent of patients received a gastrointestinal diagnosis, and 44 percent received a psychiatric diagnosis. The mean length of stay was 7.32 days; 12.5% were readmitted at least once within 1 year (80).

A multidisciplinary initial evaluation should include a complete medical and pain history, including onset, intensity, quality, location, duration, variability, predictability, exacerbating, and alleviating factors, history of previous medications or treatments and side effects. Psychosocial assessment of the child and family focuses on an assessment of the child's emotional functioning, coping skills, and impact of pain on daily life including sleeping, eating, school, social and physical activities, and family and peer interactions. A complete physical and neurological examination should be performed with the focus on but not limited to the affected area. Basic vital signs and growth parameters, pertinent laboratories and radiological studies should also be obtained. Also, previous evaluation and communication with other pediatric specialist groups should be available. A basic multidisciplinary pediatric pain clinic should consist of a pain management physician, physical medicine, and rehabilitation staff and behavioral therapy professionals.

Complex regional pain syndrome

Previously known as reflex sympathetic dystrophy, CRPS type 1 has been well described in the pediatric population and it does not involve a nerve damage, and the most common precipitating event is trauma. The mechanisms that generate neuropathic pain are varied and complex. Patients often report a burning spontaneous pain felt in the distal part of the affected extremity. Charasteristically, the pain is disproportionate in intensity to the inciting event, they have mechanical or thermal allodynia and/or hyperalgesia. Autonomic abnormalities include swelling and changes in sweating and skin blood flow. There are trophic changes in nails and hair, changes in color and temperature.

Formerly referred to as causalgia, **CRPS type 2** is less common, has evidence of obvious nerve damage, and there are few reports in the literature. Injuries to peripheral nerves may involve crush, transection, compression, demyelination, axonal degeneration, inflammation, or ischemia.

Predominantly CRPS occurs in one extremity. A series of 70 patients evaluated at the Children's Hospital Boston, Boston, MA, during a 41-month period showed a high female-to-male ratio (approximately 6:1) and that occurrences were more common in the lower extremities than upper extremities (81). A 54% history of trauma was founded in another study among 46 patients (82).

Given the relative lack of data on the causes of CRPS, it is not surprising that approaches to treatment have varied. Several case reports described successful treatment with single therapies of transcutaneous electronic nerve stimulation (TENS), Bier blocks, lumbar sympathetics block, thermal biofeedback, medications such as gabapentin, intravenous ketorolac, ketamine, and lidocaine, intrathecal ziconotide, pamidronate, and others. Wilder *et al.* showed 57% of patients improved with conservative treatment alone, consisting of physical therapy, TENS, cognitive behavioral therapy, and tricyclic antidepressants, whereas 28 of 37 patients benefited from interventional sympathetic blocks (81). Subsequent studies have shown the value of aggressive physical therapy without use of pharmacological agents or interventional nerve blocks. One of the first studies was an extended clinical series by Sherry *et al.* that focused on 103 patients treated in a "reflex neurovascular clinic" during a nearly 13-year period. Exercise therapy that focused on aerobic exercise weight-bearing, functional activities, and hydrotherapy was at the core of intervention, administered 5 to 6 hours daily, in addition to evening and weekend regimens that ranged from 45 minutes to 3 hours. Complete resolution of pain and full function were restored in 92% of patients, and long-term data for 49 patients indicated lasting benefit for most patients. Recurrent episodes occurred 31% of the time but generally resolved with reinitiation of rehabilitative strategies (83). Meier *et al.* showed that aggressive physical therapy and cognitive behavioral interventions were effective in treating 20 children and adolescents for both pain and regional and systemic autonomic responses (84). Low *et al.* described outcomes among 20 children diagnosed as having CRPS during a 4-year period. Treatment consisted of intensive physiotherapy and psychological therapy, although 70% received adjuvant medications (amitriptyline and/or gabapentin) for analgesia and to facilitate participation in physiotherapy. Although most children had complete resolution of symptoms with this treatment regimen, 40% required treatment as inpatients, and 20% had a relapse episode (85). In 2005, continuous peripheral nerve blocks provided at home were used in 13 children between 9 and 16 years of age who had intractable CRPS with substantial short-term benefit. A double-blind, placebo-controlled crossover trial was conducted with 23 patients 10 to 18 years of age who had unilateral lower limb CRPS. A catheter was placed along the lumbar sympathetic chain, and patients received intravenous lidocaine and lumbar sympathetic saline or lumbar sympathetic lidocaine and intravenous saline. Immediate short-term differences were noted as mean pain intensity of allodynia to brush, and pinprick temporal summation was reduced in the latter group, as well as reduction in pain intensity from pretreatment for allodynia to brush, pinprick, pin-prick temporal summation, and verbal pain scores. Findings led the authors to assert that a component of pain in CRPS may be mediated by abnormal sympathetic activity (86).

After reviewing the available literature on treatments of CRPS in children and adolescents, Wilder concluded that, although an array of treatments may have some benefit, the mainstay of treatment appears to be physical therapy involving desensitization, strengthening, and functional improvement (87).

Headaches

Headache is a common reason why pediatric patients seek medical care. Headaches can result from any of a number of causes, such as genetic predisposition, trauma, an intracranial mass, a metabolic or vascular disease, or sinusitis, to name a few. Headaches have a significant impact on the lives of children and adolescents, resulting in school absence, decreased extracurricular activities, and poor academic achievement.

The most common primary headaches in pediatrics are migraine and tension-type headaches, representing the ends of a spectrum of manifestations of similar pain mechanisms. These two types of headache can be episodic, or they can exist in a chronic, daily form. Migraine headaches account for most primary childhood headaches. Migraine can be divided into two groups: migraine with aura, and migraine without aura. Pediatric migraines are often bilateral, and clear localization of the pain can be difficult to obtain from children. Migraines in children are often of shorter duration than they are in adults. Migraine is identified by at least five attacks fulfilling the following criteria:

- Duration between 1 and 48 hours
- At least two of the following: (1) unilateral or bilateral, (2) pulsating, (3) moderate to severe in intensity, (4) aggravation by, or causing avoidance of, routine physical activity
- During the headache, at least one of the following must be present: (1) nausea or vomiting, (2) photophobia or phonophobia

- Typical aura with migraine consists of the presence of visual, sensory, or speech symptoms or any combination of the three. In addition, development is gradual and the aura lasts no more than 60 minutes

Tension-type headaches are benign. They manifest as a bandlike sensation around the head, and they may be associated with neck and/or shoulder pain. These headaches often become worse as the day progresses and can last for days. They may be associated with stressful events at home or school, and they may be temporarily relieved by sleep.

Other types of headaches are benign intracranial hypertension, post-traumatic, sinus headaches, infection, tumors, etc.

Long-term prognostic studies of pediatric headache are scarce, but Brna *et al.* reported that at 20-year follow-up, 73% of pediatric headache patients in their study continued to suffer from headache. In a follow-up study of 200 patients from a headache clinic over 6 years, 48% of initial migraineurs remained migraine sufferers; 26% became tension-type headache sufferers; and 26% became headache-free (88).

Management

Treatment of pediatric headache is of three basic types:

- Symptomatic
- Abortive
- Preventive

Drugs used in symptomatic treatment are chosen according to the following:

- Headache type and frequency
- Type of symptoms present
- Adverse-effect profile
- Comorbidities present

Nonpharmacologic treatment of migraine and tension-type headaches includes the following:

- Elimination of identified precipitants
- Lifestyle changes
- Stress relief

Abortive therapy for migraine and tension-type headaches may include the following:

- Triptans (sumatriptan, almotriptan, rizatriptan, and others)
- Isometheptene and ergotamines
- Analgesics

Prophylactic therapy for migraine and tension-type headaches may include the following:

- Beta blockers
- Tricyclic agents and cyproheptadine
- Anticonvulsants
- Calcium channel blockers

Treatment of chronic daily headache (CDH) may include the following:

- Combination of therapies used for tension and migraine headache
- Discontinuance of over-the-counter analgesics and all narcotics
- Tricyclic antidepressants (TCAs)
- Psychological, behavioral, and relaxation interventions (sometimes with TCAs)
- Hypnosis
- Abortive therapy, if the CDH pattern includes well-defined migraine attacks

Abdominal pain

Recurrent abdominal pain (RAP) is a common problem among school-aged children. The pain must occur at least once per month for three consecutive months, be accompanied by pain-free periods, and be severe enough to interfere with normal activities. Some studies report that as many as 25% of school-aged children will experience recurrent abdominal pain, with the highest prevalence in young girls. Children with RAP frequently describe diffuse periumbilical pain that is poorly localized. Pain is often worse at night but rarely awakens the child from sleep. Many children will experience other symptoms such as headaches, nausea, and dizziness (89).

Organic pathology has been associated with "red flags" such as weight loss, pain awakening the child at night, fevers, pain far from umbilicus, dysuria, guaiac positive stool, anemia, elevated sed rate. Despite considerable controversy concerning the underlying cause of RAP, almost all studies have found that only 10% of children seem to have a recognizable organic disease. The lack of a readily identifiable cause for RAP does not imply psychogenic causes. A subgroup of patients will have lactose intolerance, constipation, ureteropelvic junction obstruction, inflammatory bowel disease, or endometriosis (90–93). Some studies have suggested that RAP may be a precursor to irritable bowel syndrome in adults (94,95). The diagnosis is based on history, physical exam, family history, and review of symptoms. A psychosocial history is essential to learn how the child and family cope with pain and to identify school avoidance and reinforcers of pain. A significant component of treatment is education and reassurance that no serious organic illness appears likely. It should be emphasized that the child's pain is real. Treatment is based on improving function and reducing maladaptive pain behaviors through emphasis on cognitive behavioral therapies, as well as to treat underlying anxiety and depression. Participation in normal family and social activities and return to school is essential. Medication trials with neuropathic medications and antispasmodics are sometimes used, but there is limited data (96–98).

Sickle cell pain

Sickle cell pain ranges from acute vaso-occlusive episodes to chronic, daily pain. Acute painful episodes are characterized by an abrupt and usually unpredictable onset of severe ischemic pain. Vaso-occlusive episodes typically produce pain in extremities, chest, lower back, and abdomen, and may be caused by variety of factors such as infection, dehydration, hypoxia, and acidosis. Acute episodes account for most of the ED and hospital visits. Chronic pain may develop as painful episodes become more frequent and severe. Bone infarction or necrosis may result in debilitating chronic pain conditions such as aseptic necrosis of the hip, vertebral compression fractures, and chronic low back pain.

Hospitalization is necessary for patients who are unable to tolerate oral opioids because of vomiting, or if the patient has severe escalating pain requiring intravenous analgesics. Patient-controlled analgesia offers patients the ability to rapidly titrate opioids according to wide fluctuations in pain intensity in vaso-occlusive episodes.

Medications for chronic pain

Acetaminophen

Beware of hepatic failure associated with toxic dosing. Avoid PR route in patients receiving antineoplastic agents. No antiplatelet effect. The suggested dosing regimen is:

10–15 mg/kg PO q4h
20–30 mg/kg PR q4h
Max daily dose
90 mg/kg/day (children)
60 mg/kg/day (infants)
30 mg/kg/day (neonates)

Ibuprofen

Anti-inflammatory effects. Gastric, platelet, and kidney effects. The suggested dosing regimen is:

4–10 mg/kg PO q 6h
Max daily dose
40 mg/kg/day (children)

Naproxen

Anti-inflammatory effects. Gastric, platelets and kidney effects. The suggested dosing regimen is:

5–7 mg/kg PO q 8–12h
Max daily dose
40 mg/kg/day (children)

Ketorolac

Anti-inflammatory effects. Gastric, platelet, and kidney effects. Useful for patients unable to tolerate oral dosing.

0.25–0.5 mg/kg IV q 6h up to a maximum of 5 days

Nortriptyline and amitriptyline

Useful for neuropathic pain, screen for for rhythm disturbances, check levels. Side effects include dry mouth, constipation, orthostatic hypotension, palpitations.

Starting dose 0.1–0.2 mg/kg at bedtime; titrate as clinically indicated up to 1.5 mg/kg/day. Some patient need divided dosing.

Gabapentin

Useful for neuropathic pain, reduce dose for renal impairment, monitor for hematologic and hepatic toxicity. The suggested dosing regimen is:

5 mg/kg/day PO divided TID; titrate maximum 50 mg/kg/day

Carbamazepine

Monitor for hematologic and hepatic toxicity. Side effects include dizziness, tinnitus, diplopia, urinary retention, Stevens–Johnson syndrome.

Start at 10 mg/kg/day divided BID; titrate to a maximum of 20 mg/kg/day

Propanolol

Use with caution in patients with bronchospastic disease. Screen for rhythm disturbances.

1 mg/kg POBID

Venlafaxine

An SSRI chemically similar to opioid tramadol. Useful for neuropathic pain and chronic pain with depression. The dosing regimen is:

1–2 mg/kg dose divided BID or TID; caution if used with TCAs or other SSRI because of reported arrhythmias

Lidocaine

Membrane stabilizer. For neuropathic pain, headaches, refractory visceral pain. Measure plasma levers every 8–12

Start 150 mcg/kg/h

Valproate

Neuropathic pain, migraine prophylaxis, mood stability. Blood dyscrasias, hepatotoxicity, dose divided TID, monitor plasma level, periodic CBC and LFTs. The dosing regimen is:

10–60 mg/kg

Tramadol

Absence of respiratory depression, weak opioid, inhibitory effect on central neuronal norepinephrine and serotonin reuptake systems. More recently, noted actions include a local anesthetic, anti-inflammatory effects in rats (99). The dosing regimen is:

1 mg/kg PO every 6h

Complementary and alternative pain management

A descriptive definition of complementary and alternative medicine devised by the US National Center for Complementary and Alternative Medicine: "a group of diverse medical and health care systems, practices, and products that are not generally considered part of conventional medicine."

In the Complementary and Alternative Medicine (CAM) Research Methodology Conference, April 1995, CAM was defined as "a broad domain of healing resources that encompasses all health systems, modalities, and practices and their accompanying theories and beliefs, other than those intrinsic to the politically dominant health system of a particular society or culture in a given historical period. CAM includes all such practices and ideas self-defined by their users as preventing or treating illness or promoting health or well-being."

The lack of consensus in the definition of CAM makes comparison across pediatric studies complicated. What we know now is that those with chronic unresponsiveness to conventional treatment in pediatric patients are using more CAM. Rates of CAM use among pediatric patients with chronic conditions such as cancer, rheumatoid arthritis, and cystic fibrosis range from 30 to 70% (100,101). The increased interest in CAM approaches for pain symptoms in the pediatric and general populations has focused attention on questions of safety and efficacy. There are only case reports available and controlled studies are needed to determine whether CAM approaches can be safe and effective for pain in children.

Both Dr. Zesler and Dr. Tsao published a report to evaluate the empirical evidence for the efficacy of CAM approaches for pediatric pain problems (102). Unfortunately for procedural and acute postoperative pain they did not find any efficacious treatment, only promising and possibly efficacious treament.

For a treatment to be considered 'efficacious,' there must be a minimum of two between-group experiments conducted by at least two independent research groups showing that the intervention is superior to a no-treatment control, an alternative treatment or a placebo; or that the intervention is equivalent to a previously established treatment (103). For a designation of 'possibly efficacious' only one between-group study that meets these criteria is sufficient.

Hypnosis or guided imagery has been used in at least two published studies on postoperative pain in children (104,105). In one study, 52 children (aged 7–19 years) were randomly assigned to a single session of hypnosis which included suggestions for favorable postoperative outcomes 1 week prior to surgery or standard care (105). The hypnosis group evidenced significantly lower postoperative pain ratings and shorter length of hospital stays compared with controls, although the groups did not differ on anxiety or the amount of pain medication received. Huth and colleagues (104) randomly assigned 73 children (aged 7–2 years) to: (i) a treatment condition involving the viewing of a videotape on the use of imagery and then listening to a 30-minute audiotape of imagery 1 week prior to surgery (T1); or (ii) an attention control group. The treatment group also listened to the audiotape 1–4 h after surgery (T2) and 22–27 h after discharge at home (T3). The control group received standard care, including an equal amount of preoperative attention as the experimental group. The imagery group reported less pain and anxiety at T2 than controls; there were no group differences in pain or anxiety at T3 group. Hypnosis also had been shown to be efficacious in procedural pain in pediatric oncology such as bone marrow aspiration and lumbar puncture. Wild and Espie (44) discuss nine studies conducted on the effects of hypnosis on painful procedures. Following guidelines published by the Canadian Task Force on the Periodic Health Examination (106), Wild and Espie rated each study on a scale ranging from 1(e.g., randomized controlled trials with very low risk of bias) to 4 (expert opinion). All of the studies except for three fell in the 2 category (i.e., case–control or cohort studies with a high risk of confounding or bias and a significant risk that the relationship is not causal). The three highest rated studies were ranked in the 2 category (i.e., well-conducted case–control or cohort studies with a low risk of confounding or bias and a moderate possibility that the relationship is causal).

One study found no effects of hypnosis compared with cognitive–behavioral coping skills in alleviating pain and distress during BMA in 30 patients (age 5–15 years) (107), whereas another study found that hypnosis was significantly more effective than distraction in reducing distress, pain, and anxiety during venipuncture, BMA, and LP in highly hypnotizable children (age 3–8 years) (108). The third study found a small effect for hypnotic imaginative involvement BMAs in younger (3–6 years) but not in older children (7–10 years) (109).

Most of the studies with strong evidence about CAM in pediatrics are on chronic pain management. For example it is well known that acupuncture, hypnosis, and thermal biofeedback are efficacious for pediatric migraines. There has only been one randomized, controlled study on acupuncture in children with chronic pain. In this study by Pintov and colleagues, 22 patients aged 7–15 years with migraine headaches received either true acupuncture or placebo acupuncture (superficial needling) (110). The true acupuncture group (n=12) was treated according to the principles of traditional Chinese medicine with needles inserted subdermally. Children, as well as their parents and the nurses who administered the pain measures, were all unaware of study group assignment. Both groups received ten weekly treatment sessions and no children received prophylactic medications. The results showed that the true acupuncture group had clear reductions in migraine frequency and severity. In addition, B-endorphin levels rose significantly in the true acupuncture group. No such changes, however, were observed in the placebo group.

Several studies published since the 1980s have examined the effects of biofeedback (BFB) on pain in children, with the majority focused on pediatric migraine and a few on tension headache. The most frequently studied forms of BFB for head pain in children are skin temperature or thermal biofeedback. Thermal biofeedback (TBF) typically involves monitoring visual and /or auditory feedback from a thermistor placed on the fingers. Electromyographic (EMG) biofeedback involves monitoring visual and/ or auditory feedback from electric impulses generated from the frontalis muscle. One study (111) has compared TBF (HWB; handwarming) with an attention placebo (HCB; handcooling) and waiting list in 36 children (mean age 12.8 years) with pediatric migraine. The results indicated that a significantly greater proportion of the HWB group (53.8%) achieved clinically significant improvement (i.e., 50% reduction in symptoms) compared with the HCB group (10%) at post-treatment, and 3, and 6 month follow-ups.

Only one published study has specifically examined the impact of massage on chronic pain in children (112). In this study, 20 children with juvenile rheumatoid arthritis (JRA) aged 5–14 years received either a daily 15 minute massage by their parents or a daily 15 minute relaxation session with their parents. At the conclusion of the 30-day trial, the massage group experienced less pain according to both child and parent report compared with controls. A physician who was unaware of group assignment also rated the massage group as having less pain and less morning stiffness.

The only other controlled study of massage for children's pain examined distress during dressing changes in pediatric burn patients (113). Prior to dressing changes, 24 children (mean age 2.5 years) were randomly assigned to receive either massage therapy or attention control (i.e,. casual chat with the therapist). Children in the massage group received a 15 minute massage from a trained therapist conducted according to a standardized protocol, applied to areas of the body that were not burned. Independent raters unaware of group assignment rated children's distress before and during the procedure. Massage patients evidenced minimal distress behaviors (aside from an increase in torso movements), whereas the control group showed increased facial grimacing, crying, torso movement, leg movement, and reaching out. These results support the beneficial effects of massage for procedural pain in pediatric burn patients.

There has been a single randomized control trial investigating the effects of peppermint oil compared with placebo for pain and related symptoms in 50 children (ages 8–12 years) with irritable bowel syndrome (114). By the end of the 2 weeks' trial, a significantly greater proportion of the treatment group (71%) reported improvements in severity of symptoms compared with controls (43%).

Conclusion

A multidisciplinary approach to pediatric chronic pain integrates pharmacology therapy, physical therapy and rehabilitation and cognitive behavioral techniques to provide effective pain control, maintenance of normal functioning, and optimal quality of life, sleep, and school work.

References

1. Belmonte C, Cervero F. *Neurobiology of Nociceptors.* Oxford, Oxford University Press, 1996.
2. Kumazawa T, Kruger L, Mizumura K. *The Polymodal Receptor: A Gateway to Pathological Pain.* Progress in Brain Research, vol. **113**. Amsterdam, Elsevier, 1996.
3. Willis WD, Cogeshall RE. *Sensory Mechanisms of the Spinal Cord,* 2nd edn. New York, Plenum Press, 1991.
4. Willis WD, Coggeshall RE. *Sensory Mechanisms of the Spinal Cord,* 2nd edn. New York, Plenum Press, 2004.
5. Chung K, Briner RP, Carlton SM, *et al.* Immunohistochemical localization of seven different peptides in the human spinal cord. *J Comp Neurol* 1989; **280**: 158–70.
6. Rexed B. The cytoarchitectonic organization of the spinal cord in the cat. *J Comp Neurol* 1952; **96**: 415–66.
7. Morgan MM, Fields HL. Pronounced changes in the activity of nociceptive modulatory neurons in the rostral ventromedial medulla in response to prolonged thermal noxious stimuli. *J Neurophysiol* 1994; **72**: 1161–70.
8. Sugiura Y. *Spinal Organization of C-fiber Afferents Related with Nociception or Non-nociception.* Progress in Brain Research, vol. **113**. New York, Elsevier, 1996, pp. 319–39.
9. Besson JM, Chaouch A. Peripheral and spinal mechanism of nociception. *Physiol Rev* 1987; **67**: 67–186.
10. Melzack R., Wall PD. Pain mechanisms: A new theory. *Science* 1965; **150**: 971–9.
11. Andrews K, Fitsgerald M. Cutaneous flexion reflex in human neonates: a quantitative study of threshold and stimulus-response characteristics after single and repeated sitmuli. *Dev Med Child Neurol* 1999; **41**: 696–703.
12. Taddio A, Katz J, Ilersich AL, Koren G. Effect of neonatal circumcision on pain response during subsequent routine vaccination. *Lancet* 1997; **349**: 599–603.
13. Stinson J., Kavanagh T. Yaamda J, Gill N, Stevens B. Systemic review of the psychometric properties, interpretability and feasibility of self-report pain intensity measures for use in clinical trials in children and adolescents. *Pain* 2006: **125**; 143–7.
14. von Baeyer C., Spagrud L. Systematic review of observational measures of pain for children and adolescents aged 3 to 18 years. *Pain* 2007; **1227**: 140–50.
15. Dworkin R, Turk D, Farrar J, *et al.* Core outcome measures for chronic pain clinical trials: IMMPACT recommendations. *Pain* 2005; **113**: 9–19.
16. Luffy R, Grove F. Examining the validity, reliability, and preference of three pediatric pain measurement tools in African-American children. *Pediatr Nurs* 2003; **29**: 54–9.
17. Gragg R, Rapoff M, Danosky M, *et al.* Assessing chronic musculoskeletal pain associated with rheumatic disease: Further validation of the pediatric pain questionnaire. *J Pediatr Psychol* 1996; **21**: 237–50.
18. Beyer J, Aradine C. Patterns of pediatric pain intensity: A methodological investigation of a self-report scale. *Clin J Pain* 1987; **3**: 130–41.
19. Romsing J, Moller-Sonnergaard J, Hertel S, Rasmussen, M. Postoperative pain in children. Comparison between ratings of children and nurses. *J Pain Symptom Manage* 1996; **11**(1): 42–6.
20. Stinson J, Kavanagh T, Yamada J, Gill N, Stevens F. Systematic review of the psychometric properties, interpretability and feasibility of self-report pain intensity measures for use in clinical trials in children and adolescents. *Pain* 2006; **125**: 143–57.

21. Chambers C, Giesbrecht K, Craig K, Bennett S, Huntsman E. A comparison of faces scales for the measurement of pediatric pain: Children's and parents' ratings. *Pain* 1999: **83**: 25–35.

22. Spafford P, von Baeyer CL, Hicks CL. Expected and reported pain in children undergoing ear piercing: A randomized trial of preparation by parents. 2002. *Behav Res Ther* 2002; **40**: 253–66.

23. Gold J, Hyeon Kim S, Kant A, Joseph M, Rizzo A. Effectiveness of virtual reality for pediatric pain distraction during IV placement. *Cyber Psychol Behav* 2006; **9**(2): 207–12.

24. Beyer J. Judging the effectiveness of analgesia for children and adolescents during vaso-occlusive events of sickle cell disease. *J Pain Symptom Manage* 2000; **19**: 63–72.

25. Wong D, Baker C. Pain in children: Comparison of assessment scales. *Pediatr Nurs* 1988; **14**: 9–17.

26. Hester N, Foster R, Kristensen K. Measurement of pain in children: Generalizability and validity of the pain ladder and the poker chip tool. *Adv Pain Res Ther*, 1990; **15**: 79–84.

27. Stinson J, Petroz G, Tait G, *et al.* E-Ouch: usability testing of an electronic chronic pain diary for adolescents with arthritis. *Clin J Pain* 2006; **22**: 295–305.

28. Merkle SI, Shayevitz JR, Voepel-Lewis T, Malviya S. The FLACC: A behavioral scale for scoring postperative pain in young children. *Pediatr Nurs* 1997; **23**: 292–7.

29. Woolf CJ, Costigan M. Transcriptional and posttranslational plasticity and the generation of inflammatory pain. *Proc Natl Acad Sci USA* 1999; **96**: 7723–30.

30. Yaksh TL. Spinal systems and pain processing: development of novel analgesic drugs with mechanistically defined models. *Trends Pharmacol Sci* 1999; **20**: 329–37.

31. Joseph M, Brill J, Zeltzer L. Pediatric pain relief in trauma. *Pediatr Rev* 1999; **20** (3): 75–83.

32. Neighbor ML, Honner S, Kohn MA. Factors affecting emergency department opioid administration to severely injured patients. *Acad Emerg Med* 2004; **11**: 1290–6.

33. Singer AJ, Thode HC., Jr. National analgesia prescribing patterns in emergency department patients with burns. *J Burn Care Rehabil* 2002; **23**: 361–5.

34. Martin-Herz SP, Patterson DR, Honari S, *et al.* Pediatric pain control practices of North American Burn Centers. *J Burn Care Rehabil* 2003; **24**: 26–36.

35. Cuignet O, Pirson J, Soudon O, Zizi M. Effects of gabapentin on morphine consumption and pain in severely burned patients. *Burns* 2007; **33**: 81–6.

36. 53. Gregoretti C, Decaroli D, Piacevoli Q, *et al.* Analgo-sedation of patients with burns outside the operating room. *Drugs* 2008; **68**: 2427–43.

37. Stoddard FJ, Sheridan RL, Saxe GN, *et al.* Treatment of pain in acutely burned children. *J Burn Care Rehabil* 2002; **23**: 135–56.

38. Anand KJS, Scalzo FM. Can adverse neonatal experience alter brain development and subsequent behavior? *Biol Neonate* 2000; **77**: 69–82.

39. Fitzgerald M. Development of pain pathways and mechanisms. In Anand JKS, Stevens BJ, McGrath PJ, eds. *Pain in Neonates*, 2nd edn. Amsterdam, Elsevier, 2000, pp. 9–21.

40. Grunau RVE. Long-term consequences of pain in human neonates. In Anand JKS, Stevens BJ, McGrath PJ, eds. *Pain in Neonates*, 3rd edn. Amsterdam, Elsevier, 2007, pp. 55–76.

41. Peterson BS, Vohr B, Staib LH, *et al.* Regional brain volume abnormalities and long-term cognitive outcome in preterm infants. *JAMA* 2000; **284**: 1939–47.

42. Batton DG, Barrington KJ, Wallman C. Prevention and management of pain in the neonate: an update. *Pediatrics* 2006; **118**: 2231–41.

43. Carbajal R, Rousset A, Danan C, *et al.* Epidemiology and treatment of painful procedures in neonates in intensive care units. *JAMA* 2008; **300**: 60–70.

44. McIntosh N, van Veen L, Brameyer H. Alleviation of the pain of heel prick in preterm infants. *Arch Dis Child Fetal Neonatal Ed* 1994; **70**: F177–81.

45. Anand KJS, Johnston CC, Oberlander TF, *et al.* Analgesia and local anesthesia during invasive procedures in the neonate. *Clin Ther* 2005; **27**: 844–76.

46. Jain S, Kumar P, McMillan DD. Prior leg massage decreases pain responses to heel stick in preterm babies. *J Paediatr Child Health* 2006; **42**: 505–8.

47. Golianu B, Krane E, Seybold J, Almgren C, Anand KJS. Non-pharmacological techniques for pain management in neonates. *Semin Perinatol* 2007; **31**: 318–22.

48. Corbo MG, Mansi G, Stagni A, *et al.* Nonnutritive sucking during heelstick procedures decreases behavioral distress in the newborn infant. *Biol Neonate* 2000; **77**: 162–7.

49. Blass EM, Hoffmeyer LB. Sucrose as an analgesic for newborn infants. *Pediatrics* 1991; **87**: 215–18.

50. Stevens B, Yamada J, Ohlsson A. Sucrose for analgesia in newborn infants undergoing painful procedures. *Cochrane Database Syst Rev* 2010; **1**: CD001069.

51. Blass EM, Watt LB. Suckling- and sucrose-induced analgesia in human newborns. *Pain* 1999; **83**: 611–23.

52. Carbajal R, Chauvet X, Couderc S, Olivier-Martin M. Randomised trial of analgesic effects of sucrose, glucose, and pacifiers in term neonates. *BMJ* 1999; **319**: 1393–7.

53. Gray L, Watt L, Blass EM. Skin-to-skin contact is analgesic in healthy newborns. *Pediatrics* 2000; **105**: e14.

54. Johnston CC, Stevens B, Pinelli J, *et al.* Kangaroo care is effective in diminishing pain response in preterm neonates. *Arch Pediatr Adolesc Med* 2003; **157**: 1084–8.

55. Johnston CC, Filion F, Campbell-Yeo M, *et al.* Kangaroo mother care diminishes pain from heel lance in very preterm neonates: a crossover trial. *BMC Pediatr* 2008; **8**: 13.

56. Gray L, Miller LW, Philipp BL, Blass EM. Breastfeeding is analgesic in healthy newborns. *Pediatrics* 2002; **109**: 590–3.

57. Carbajal R, Veerapen S, Couderc S, Jugie M, Ville Y. Analgesic effect of breast feeding in term neonates: randomised controlled trial. *BMJ* 2003; **326**: 13.

58. Taddio A, Ohlsson A, Einarson TR, Stevens B, Koren G. A systematic review of lidocaine–prilocaine cream (EMLA) in the treatment of acute pain in neonates. *Pediatrics* 1998; **101**(2): E1.

59. Taddio A, Gurguis MG, Koren G. Lidocaine–prilocaine cream versus tetracaine gel for procedural pain in children. *Ann Pharmacother* 2002; **36**: 687–92.

60. Anand KJ. Consensus statement for the prevention and management of pain in the newborn. *Arch Pediatr Adolesc Med* 2001; **155**: 173–80.

61. Anand KJ, Sippell WG, Aynsley-Green A. Randomised trial of fentanyl anaesthesia in preterm babies undergoing surgery: effects on the stress response. *Lancet* 1987; **1**(8526): 234.

62. Saarenmaa E, Neuvonen PJ, Fellman V. Gestational age and birth weight effects on plasma clearance of fentanyl in newborn infants. *J Pediatr* 2000; **136**: 767–70.

63. Soto RG, Fu ES. Acute pain management for patients undergoing thoracotomy. *Ann Thorac Surg* 2003; **75**: 1349–57.

64. Cass LJ, Howard RF. Respiratory complications due to inadequate analgesia following thoracotomy in a neonate. *Anaesthesia* 1994; **49**: 879–80.

65. Bouwmeester NJ, Anand KJ, van Dijk M, *et al.* Hormonal and metabolic stress responses after major surgery in children aged 0–3 years: a double-blind, randomized trial comparing the effects of continuous versus intermittent morphine. *Br J Anaesth* 2001; **87**: 390–9.

66. Anderson BJ, Meakin GH. Scaling for size: some implications for paediatric anaesthesia dosing. *Paediatr Anaesth* 2002; **12**: 205–19.

67. Buttner W, Finke W. Analysis of behavioural and physiological parameters for the assessment of postoperative analgesic demand in newborns, infants and young children: a comprehensive report on seven consecutive studies. *Paediatr Anaesth* 2000; **10**: 303–18.

68. McNicol LR. Post-operative analgesia in children using continuous subcutaneous morphine. *Br J Anaesth* 1993; **71**: 752–6.

69. Taddio A, Goldbach M, Ipp M, *et al.* Effect of neonatal circumcision on pain responses during vaccination in boys. *Lancet* 1994; **344**: 291.

70. Wolf AR, Lawson RA, Fisher S. Ventilatory arrest after a fluid challenge in a neonate receiving sc morphine. *Br J Anaesth* 1995; **75**: 787–9.

71. Moffett BS, Wann TI, Carberry KE, Mott AR. Safety of ketorolac in neonates and infants after cardiac surgery. *Paediatr Anaesth* 2006; **16**: 424–8.

72. Burd RS, Tobias JD. Ketorolac for pain management after abdominal surgical procedures in infants. *South Med J* 2002; **95**: 331–3.

73. Van Overmeire B, Smets K, Lecoutere D, *et al.* A comparison of ibuprofen and indomethacin for closure of patent ductus arteriosus. *N Engl J Med* 2000; **343**: 674–81.

74. Allegaert K, Cossey V, Debeer A, *et al.* The impact of ibuprofen on renal clearance in preterm infants is independent of gestational age. *Pediatr Nephrol* 2005; **20**: 740–3.

75. Arana A, Morton NS, Hansen TG. Treatment with paracetamol in infants. *Acta Anaesthesiol Scand* 2001; **45**: 20–9.

76. King S, Chambers CT, Huguet A., *et al.* The epidemiology of chronic pain in children and adolescents revisited: A systematic review. *Pain* 2011; **152**: 2729–38.

77. Stanford EA, Chambers CT, Biesanz, JC, Chen E. The frequency, trajectories and predictors of adolescent recurrent pain: A population-based approach. *Pain* 2008; **138**(1): 11–21.

78. Ho IK, Goldschneider KR, Kashikar-Zuck S, *et al.* Healthcare utilization and indirect burden among families of pediatric patients with chronic pain. *J Musculoskelet Pain* 2008; **16**(3); 155–64.

79. Walker LS, Dengler-Crish CM, Rippel S, Bruehl S. Functional abdominal pain in childhood and adolescence increases risk for chronic pain in adulthood. *Pain* 2010; **150**(3); 568–72.

80. Coffelt T, Bauer B, Carroll A. Inpatient characteristics of the child admitted with chronic pain. *Pediatrics* 2013; **132**(2): e422–9.

81. Wilder RT, Berde CB, Wolohan M, *et al.* Reflex sympathetic dystrophy in children. Clinical characteristics and follow-up of seventy patients. *J Bone Joint Surg Am* 1992; **74**(6): 910–19.

82. Murray CS, Cohen A, Perkins T, Davidson JE, Sills JA. Morbidity in reflex sympathetic dystrophy. *J. Arch Dis Child* 2000; **82**(3): 231–3.

83. Sherry DD, Wallace CA, Kelley C, Kidder M, Sapp L. Short- and long-term outcomes of children with complex regional pain syndrome type I treated with exercise therapy. *Clin J Pain* 1999; **15**(3): 218–23.

84. Meier PM, Alexander ME, Sethna NF, *et al.* Complex regional pain syndromes in children and adolescents: regional and systemic signs and symptoms and hemodynamic response to tilt table testing. *Clin J Pain* 2006; **22**: 399–406.

85. Low AK, Ward K, Wines AP. Pediatric complex regional pain syndrome. *J Pediatr Orthop* 2007; **27**(5): 567–72.

86. Meier PM, Zurakowski D, Berde CB, Sethna NF. Lumbar sympathetic blockade in children with complex regional pain syndromes: a double blind placebo-controlled crossover trial. *Anesthesiology* 2009; **111**(2): 372–80.

87. Wilder RT. Management of pediatric patients with complex regional pain syndrome. *Clin J Pain* 2006; **22**(5): 443–8.

88. Brna P, Dooley J, Gordon K, Dewan T. The prognosis of childhood headache: a 20-year follow-up. *Arch Pediatr Adolesc Med* 2005; **159**(12): 1157–60.

89. Apley J, Naish N. Recurrent abdominal pains: a field survey of 1,000 school children. *Arch Dis Child* 1958; **33**: 165.

90. Feldman W, McGrath P, Hodgson C, *et al.* The use of dietary fiber in the management of simple, childhood, idiopathic recurrent abdominal pain. Results in a prospective, double-blind, randomized, controlled trial. *Am J Dis Child* 1985; **139**: 1216.

91. Wewer V, Andersen LP, Paerregard A, *et al.* The prevalence and related symptomatology of *H. pylori* in children with recurrent abdominal pain. *Acta Paediatr* 1998; **87**: 830.

92. Khetan N, Torkington J, Watkin A, *et al.* Endometriosis: presentation to general surgeons. *Ann Roy Coll Surg Engl* 1999; **81** (4): 255–9.

93. Irish MS, Pearl RH, Caty MG, *et al.* The approach to common abdominal diagnosis in infants and children. *Pediatr Clin North Am* 1998; **45**(4): 729.

94. Hyams JS, Hyman PE, Rasquin-Weber A. Childhood recurrent abdominal pain: resemblance to irritable bowel syndrome. *J Dev Behav Pediatr* 1999; **20**(5): 318.

95. Walker LS, Guite JW, Duke M, *et al.* Recurrent abdominal pain: potential precursor of irritable bowel syndrome in adolescents and young adults. *J Pediatr* 1998; **132**(6): 1010–15.

96. Gold N, Issenman R, Roberts J, *et al.* Well-adjusted children: an alternate view of children with inflammatory bowel disease and functional gastrointestinal complaints. *Inflamm Bowel Dis* 2000; **6**(1): 1–7.

97. Compas BE, ThomThromsen AH. Coping and responses to stress among children with recurrent abdominal pain. *J Dev Behav Pediatr* 1999; **20**: 323.

98. Sanders M, Shepherd RW, Cleghorn G, *et al.* The treatment of recurrent abdominal pain in children: A controlled comparison of cognitive–behavioral family interventions and standard pediatric care. *J Consult Clin Psychol* 1994; **62**(2): 306–14.

99. Benzon H. *Raj's Practical Management of Pain*, 4th edn. Philadelphia, Elsevier, 2008.

100. Grootenhuis MA, Last BF, de Graaf-Nijkerk JH, van der Wel M. Use of alternative treatment in pediatric oncology. *Cancer Nurs* 1998; **21**: 282–8.

101. Stern RC, Canda ER, Doershuk CF. Use of nonmedical treatment by cystic fibrosis patients. *J Adolesc Health* 1992; **13**: 612–15.

102. Tsao JCI, Zeltzer L. Complementary and alternative medicine approaches for pediatric pain: A review of the state of the science. *eCAM* 2005; **2**: 149–59.

103. Chambless DL, Hollon SD. Defining empirically supported therapies. *J Consult Clin Psychol* 1998; **66**: 7–18.

104. Huth MM, Broome ME, Good M. Imagery reduces children's post-operative pain. *Pain* 2004; **110**: 439–48.

105. Lambert SA. The effects of hypnosis/guided imagery on the postoperative course of children. *J Dev Behav Pediatr* 1996; **17**: 307–10.

106. Wild MR, Espie CA. The efficacy of hypnosis in the reduction of procedural pain and distress in pediatric oncology: a systematic review. *J Dev Behav Pediatr* 2004; **25**: 207–13.

107. Liossi C, Hatira P. Clinical hypnosis versus cognitive behavioral training for pain management with pediatric cancer patients undergoing bone marrow aspirations. *Int J Clin Exp Hypn* 1999; **47**: 104–16.

108. Smith JT, Barabasz A, Barabasz M. Comparison of hypnosis and distraction in severely ill children undergoing painful medical

procedures. *J Counseling Psychol* 1996; **43**: 187–95.

109. Kuttner L, Bowman M, Teasdale M. Psychological treatment of distress, pain, and anxiety for young children with cancer. *J Dev Behav Pediatr* 1988; **9**: 374–81.

110. Pintov S, Lahat E, Alstein M, Vogel Z, Barg J. Acupuncture and the opioid system: implications in management of migraine. *Pediatr Neurol* 1997; **17**: 129–33.

111. Scharff L, Marcus DA, Masek BJ. A controlled study of minimal-contact thermal biofeedback treatment in children with migraine. *J Pediatr Psychol* 2002; **27**: 109–19.

112. Field T, Hernandez-Reif M, Seligman S, *et al.* Juvenile rheumatoid arthritis: benefits from massage therapy. *J Pediatr Psychol* 1997; **22**: 607–17.

113. Hernandez-Reif M, Field T, Largie S, *et al.* Childrens' distress during burn treatment is reduced by massage therapy. *J Burn Care Rehabil* 2001; **22**: 191–5.

114. Kline RM, Kline JJ, Di Palma J, Barbero GJ. Enteric-coated, pH-dependent peppermint oil capsules for the treatment of irritable bowel syndrome in children. *J Pediatr* 2001; **138**: 125–8.

Chapter

18 Otolaryngology

Sungeun Lee and Dua M. Anderson

Providing anesthesia for otolaryngology procedures can present a variety of challenges and considerations. The wide range of procedures continues to expand as surgical equipment and techniques evolve. Many of these procedures involve the airway in some capacity, and thus require the anesthesia provider to have a clear understanding of each facet of the surgical plan, as well as maintain constant communication with the surgeon to safely share the airway. This section will outline some of the considerations for commonly performed surgeries of the ear, nose, and throat in children.

Airway procedures

Anatomy and physiology

It is imperative to have a thorough understanding of pediatric airway anatomy and physiology in order to provide safe anesthetic care during airway procedures. Distinctions in pediatric airway anatomy include, but are not limited to: a large tongue, long and narrow epiglottis, and a high larynx. In addition, the narrowest part of the airway in pediatric patients is the cricoid ring, as opposed to the glottic inlet in adults. The cricothyroid membrane is comparatively short, making emergent urgent needle cricothyroidotomy more challenging.

Even healthy infants are predisposed to hypoxia due to two main factors. First, functional residual capacity is less than closing capacity, partially due to the decreased recoil from chest wall elasticity. Also, young infants have a higher metabolic requirement than older children and adults. Infants also encounter respiratory fatigue earlier. This is due to the fact that the diaphragm plays a more significant part in ventilation in young infants. Since tidal volumes vary less in smaller patients, any increase in minute ventilation occurs predominantly via an increased respiratory rate. This requires increased work for the diaphragm, leading to fatigue (1).

Bronchoscopic procedures

Indications

Indications for bronchoscopy can be classified as diagnostic or therapeutic. Evaluation for airway obstruction, with or without intervention via dilation, and foreign body extraction are the more common indications.

Preoperative considerations and premedication

Coexisting diseases need the usual consideration and evaluation. In addition, the indication for bronchoscopy dictates the anesthetic plan. If the patient has undergone airway evaluation in the past, thorough chart review should be done to determine certain specifics: grade of direct laryngoscopy view, ability to mask ventilate when necessary, significant airway obstruction with induction of anesthesia, size of endotracheal tube that fit in the airway, and any post-procedure edema or stridor.

In young infants, premedication for anxiolysis is not indicated and sedation prior to proper monitoring and equipment availability could lead to unnecessary complications. An anticholinergic should be considered for both its antisialagogue and vagolytic effects.

Induction and intubation

General anesthesia is induced while maintaining spontaneous ventilation whenever possible. Lidocaine (2–4% with dose max of 5 mg/kg) is then sprayed in the airway to minimize airway reactivity. This adds to the depth of anesthesia for a very stimulating procedure. At this point, the airway can be secured with an

Essentials of Pediatric Anesthesiology, ed. Alan David Kaye, Charles James Fox and James H. Diaz. Published by Cambridge University Press. © Cambridge University Press 2015.

endotracheal tube (in order to size the airway), or the bronchoscope can be directly inserted. However, if part of the evaluation involves assessment of airway dynamics such as vocal cord mobility or tracheal wall collapse, placing an ETT will restrict this part of the evaluation. A dose of dexamethasone (0.5 mg/kg) in anticipation of airway swelling should be considered soon after induction.

If the evaluation will be via flexible bronchoscopy, introduction of the scope via a laryngeal mask airway and an attachment with a sealed port allows inhaled anesthetic to continue via LMA.

Maintenance and emergence

Maintenance of anesthesia can occur via inhalational or intravenous agents. A ventilating bronchoscope includes a side port allowing connection to a breathing circuit or supplemental oxygen. The patient can be spontaneously ventilating or assisted with positive pressure. In reality, during rigid bronchoscopy, there will be numerous occasions when the bronchoscope or ETT is placed and removed from the trachea. A TIVA (total intravenous anesthetic) technique allows maintenance of a consistent level of anesthesia during these times. Propofol, remifentanil, ketamine, and dexmedetomidine (as infusions and/or boluses) have all been used with success (1–4).

Analgesia with IV acetaminophen should suffice for this procedure. Post-procedure opioids, if necessary, can be administered in the recovery area. Awake extubation, or observation of patient's airway until stable, in the operating room is recommended after airway intervention has occurred.

Complications and postoperative course

Hypoxia during the procedure can occur for a variety of reasons. Bronchospasm can occur due to manipulation of the airway during insufficient anesthetic depth.

Hypercarbia can result due to insufficient ventilation via the bronchoscope. This is more likely to occur in smaller patients, due to the small-diameter, higher-resistance bronchoscope. Incomplete exhalation through the narrow passage can lead to air trapping. An appropriately sized bronchoscope should have a leak to allow for passive airflow to occur around the apparatus.

Complications can include injury from the rigid instruments. Airway edema is common after bronchoscopic procedures, even if no intervention was made. Racemic epinephrine may improve postoperative stridor.

Tonsillectomy, adenoidectomy, and abscess drainage

Patient population

Tonsillectomy is one of the most commonly performed pediatric otolaryngology procedures. In 2006, an estimated 530 000 tonsillectomies, with or without adenoidectomy, and 132 000 adenoidectomies, with or without tonsillectomies, were performed in patients less than 15 years of age (5).

Indications and associated pathologies

Indications for this common surgery can be broadly categorized as infectious versus obstructive. Epidemiological trends have shifted: surgical indications have shifted from infection toward upper airway obstruction (6).

Obstructive sleep apnea (OSA) or sleep disordered breathing is a common indication for pediatric adenotonsillectomy. The incidence of pediatric OSA has been estimated to be anywhere between 0–5% (7). In extreme cases, OSA can result in alveolar hypoventilation, pulmonary hypertension, and cor pulmonale. Neurological sequelae such as impaired growth, behavioral issues, or cognitive impairment are possible. These secondary effects may have yet to be identified in the child's work-up.

If the surgical indication is peritonsillar abscess, the patient may present with profound dehydration due to impaired oral intake. With a peritonsillar abscess, considerable airway distortion and edema can be present, making direct laryngoscopy (or even mask ventilation) difficult. Preoperative nebulized racemic epinephrine can be considered. Additional equipment and personnel assistance should be arranged for a difficult airway if needed. Drainage of an abscess may or may not include tonsillectomy. Significant airway edema may worsen with the procedure, possibly requiring prolonged intubation to allow time for reduction in swelling.

Preoperative considerations and premedication

Medical evaluation should include assessment for risk factors for increased perioperative complications. Of particular note are: OSA (especially with severe apnea on sleep study), obesity, age less than 3 years old, and craniofacial anomalies (8). History of unusual bleeding or bruising is a risk factor given the innate risk of postoperative bleeding with this procedure, and any underlying coagulopathy needs to be evaluated and addressed.

Since a major indication for adenotonsillectomy is chronic infection of the upper airway (URI), many children presenting for tonsillectomy have concurrent or recent URIs. The usual risk to benefit ratio needs to be considered. However, it may not be practical to wait for a window when the child does not have a concurrent or recent URI.

Premedication with oral midazolam is appropriate in most cases. Careful consideration should be given to patients with severe airway obstruction, with noisy breathing at baseline while awake. Sedation in these patients can cause more clinically significant airway obstruction and therefore should be done in the setting of close monitoring and observation in the preoperative area. Arrangements for awake or sedated IV should be made at this time if mask induction is not appropriate for a patient due to multiple airway and cardiac risk factors.

Adjuncts to the premedication can be considered such as acetaminophen (15 mg/kg) or ibuprofen (10 mg/kg) (see Postoperative course, below).

Induction and intubation

Induction can proceed via standard inhalation induction, or an intravenous induction may be elected if the patient's comorbidities dictate that having intravenous access prior to induction is the safer plan. Intubation can proceed with or without muscle relaxation. As a typical adenotonsillectomy is a short procedure, thought should be given to the duration of muscle relaxation required, and dosed accordingly. Alternatively, a dose of remifentanil (3–4 mcg/kg) can be administered to facilitate tracheal intubation, avoiding medium- to long-acting muscle relaxant (9). Either laryngeal mask airways or endotracheal tubes (ETT) are used, depending on provider, institution, and surgeon preference. If an ETT is chosen, a preformed tube such as the Oral RAE® can be useful in allowing the surgeon to position the mouth gag and suspension apparatus.

As always, consideration must be given to the indication for adenotonsillectomy and associated airway abnormalities. Advanced laryngoscopic devices or techniques such as video laryngoscopy or fiberoptic laryngoscopy may be advisable in the case of gross adenotonsillar hypertrophy or other dysmorphism.

Maintenance and intraoperative medications

Maintenance with volatile or intravenous anesthetic is appropriate. Typically dexamethasone (0.5 mg/kg) is given to reduce airway edema and helps prevent postoperative nausea and vomiting (PONV) (10). Similarly, prophylaxis with ondansetron (0.1 mg/kg with max of 6 mg) or a similar agent is indicated due to the high incidence of PONV in tonsillectomy patients.

Intraoperative administration of opioids should be done judiciously given this high-risk population. Opioid-sparing agents should be utilized whenever possible. If oral acetaminophen was not administered as part of a premedication, a rectal (30 mg/kg) or IV (15 mg/kg, depending on age of the child) dose should be given intraoperatively.

Emergence, extubation, and recovery

Either deep or awake extubation is acceptable (11). However, appropriate considerations should be made: severe airway obstruction, difficult mask ventilation, or difficult direct laryngoscopy should dictate an awake extubation. Deep extubation can be associated with less coughing (coughing can dislodge the tonsillar bed clot and result in hemorrhage). Lateral decubitus positioning with head down (i.e., recovery position) is recommended (12). Emergence agitation or delirium should be managed to help prevent hypertension affecting the integrity of the surgical site clot.

Apnea monitoring: If the child has OSA or sleep disordered breathing, longer postanesthesia observation is indicated, though the data are not yet clear for how long. Many centers have opted for 6 hours or overnight observation with continuous oximetry monitoring rather than day surgery for this population.

Postoperative course: pain, PONV, hemorrhage

Postoperative pain control can be achieved with opioid-based therapy, but opioid-sparing agents are recommended whenever possible. Scheduled acetaminophen and nonsteroidal anti-inflammatory agents (NSAIDs) in an alternating dosing schedule can reduce the opioid requirement significantly. Many providers have been hesitant to use NSAIDs after tonsillectomy due to the risk of postoperative hemorrhage, but emerging data in children and adults show no increased risk of bleeding (13). Codeine-based analgesia has been linked with postoperative deaths in children and, in February of 2013, the FDA issued a Black Boxed Warning, which is the FDA's strongest warning, to all codeine containing products. Codeine is contraindicated for use after tonsillectomy and/or adenoidectomy (14). Patients who rapidly metabolize codeine to morphine can develop respiratory depression from high circulating levels of morphine, and the pediatric population with chronic airway obstruction (OSA) is at particular risk for respiratory depression (15,16). However, the FDA warning does not distinguish particular higher-risk patients because it is too difficult to determine or predict which patients are ultra-fast metabolizers of codeine.

The incidence of postoperative nausea and vomiting (PONV) after adenotonsillectomy may be as high as 8% (17). Significant reduction in incidence (by 50%) and severity of PONV has been shown with intraoperative IV dexamethasone (18).

Primary hemorrhage in the immediate postoperative period is more common in older children, patients with chronic tonsillitis, intraoperative bleeding, or postoperative hypertension. The overall incidence for secondary hemorrhage is 3%, and usually occurs 7–10 days postoperatively (19). Tonsillar hemorrhage is a true emergency, and presents several challenges. Acute blood loss can be massive, but may not be reflected in a measured hematocrit. Patients may present with hemorrhagic shock or with ongoing vomiting. Any patient with post-adenotonsillectomy hemorrhage should be treated as having a full stomach, and a rapid sequence induction is indicated.

Multiple well-functioning suction devices need to be ready, as well as surgical personnel on standby for possible airway intervention.

Tracheostomy

Considerations for pediatric tracheostomy are largely influenced by whether the procedure is elective or emergent.

Elective indications

Usual indications for elective tracheostomy in the pediatric population are prolonged ventilator dependence or airway stenosis (20). In most cases, the patient will already be intubated and the procedure is performed in this state until an incision is made in the trachea and the tracheotomy tube is ready to be inserted.

Preoperative and induction considerations

Regardless of the indication for tracheostomy, comorbidities should be assessed prior to the anesthetic. Appropriate backup airway equipment should be available. Induction can be achieved via inhalational induction through the in situ endotracheal tube. If the patient is a known difficult airway, maintaining spontaneous ventilation should be considered given the possibility of losing the airway during the surgical procedure.

Maintenance and emergence considerations

Maintenance is via a balanced anesthetic technique. Patients will often require ventilator support at the conclusion of the case given the likely pre-existing need. Consider sedation for the immediate postop period, especially if transport from operating room to intensive care unit is involved.

Emergent

There are several unique situations to consider for an emergent tracheostomy.

If attempts at securing an airway have been unsuccessful, surgeons should proceed to surgical airway while mask ventilation is maintained as well as possible. Inserting a laryngeal mask airway to assist in ventilation while the surgical airway is being secured is also a valid option (21).

Another technique is ventilating via a rigid bronchoscope while the surgical airway is being obtained. This is only feasible in certain infants and neonates. An appropriately sized rigid bronchoscope in a small infant or neonate's airway is sufficient to ventilate without using extremely high positive pressures. This is applicable in situations where the glottic opening is normal to visualize but subglottic stenosis prevents proper ventilation. A rigid bronchoscope can stent past the stenosis to provide ventilation while a tracheostomy is being performed in an emergent situation.

Choanal atresia repair

Choanal atresia is obstruction of the posterior nasal airway. It can be partial or complete, membranous or bony, unilateral or bilateral. It occurs as a result of abnormal persistence of the oronasal membrane. The incidence is 1 in 7000 live births. It is more common in females (2:1), more bony (9:1), and more unilateral (2:1) (22).

Associations

Half of all cases are associated with congenital anomalies, most notably the CHARGE association (coloboma, heart disease, atresia-choanal, retarded growth, genital abnormalities, ear deformity). Other associations include Apert's syndrome (craniosynostosis, syndactylism, difficult airway) and Fraser's syndrome (laryngeal/tracheal stenosis, congenital heart disease, GU anomalies, renal agensis/hypoplasia).

Presentation

Bilateral choanal atresia can present more emergently given that neonates are obligate nose breathers. Respiratory distress, which is typically relieved by crying and worsened with feeding, is the most common presentation for bilateral atresia. Unilateral atresia does not present acutely unless the patent side becomes obstructed. Presentation is usually later in infancy due to chronic nasal discharge.

Surgical repair

For bilateral choanal atresia, surgical repair is necessary in early infancy. Unilateral defects can be repaired later in childhood.

Preop considerations

Due to the high rate of association with other congenital anomalies, a thorough medical evaluation needs to be completed prior to the patient undergoing surgical repair. There may be underlying cardiac issues, as well as appropriate planning in preparation for a difficult airway.

Intraop considerations

Standard inhalational or intravenous induction and intubation is appropriate for this procedure. A preformed ETT such as the oral RAE® tube may be preferred to facilitate access to the surgical area. A balanced maintenance technique should be considered to facilitate an awake extubation. A dose of intravenous dexamethasone (dose: 0.5 mg/kg) at the start of the case should be considered if airway edema is anticipated.

Emergence, extubation, and recovery considerations

Bloody secretions from the surgery may be in the patient's stomach at the conclusion of the case. Prior to emergence, suctioning of the stomach with an orogastric tube should be considered. Airway edema may be a factor at the conclusion of the case, especially if the operative time was prolonged. Patients may require intubation until the airway edema resolves.

Recovery and postop considerations include age appropriate monitoring. Neonates undergoing surgical repair should remain on continuous pulse oximetry and apnea monitoring overnight.

Adequate pain management is important. In addition to patient comfort, it is important that the nasal stents that are placed at the end of surgery remain in place to ensure patency of the nasal passages.

Laryngeal reconstruction for subglottic stenosis

Laryngeal tracheal reconstruction (LTR) is the definitive treatment for significant subglottic stenosis.

Patient population, indications, and associated pathologies

Subglottic stenosis can be congenital or acquired. Acquired lesions are due to injury that leads to tissue inflammation, scarring, and narrowing. Congenital malformations range from thin tracheal webs to tracheal stenosis, which involves cartilaginous rings. Associations include trisomy 21, pulmonary hypoplasia, and tracheoesophageal fistulas. Tracheomalacia, caused by weakening of the support structures of the trachea, can be primary or secondary (acquired). Secondary tracheomalacia is caused by a variety of external sources of weakening, such as vascular rings, compression from the innominate artery, or aberrant vessels (23).

Not all patients who have tracheal stenosis require reconstruction. Other surgical interventions can be made such as endoscopic dilations, laser treatment of scars, or injection of scar tissue with steroids or other agents.

Preoperative considerations and premedication

It is important to have a detailed understanding of the surgical plan since the airway will be shared with the surgical team. Reconstruction can be categorized as a single or double-staged repair. The single-staged LTR involves a cartilage graft to widen the airway, with no tracheostomy left behind. The patient is orally intubated with an ETT to allow for healing prior to extubation. The double stage LTR differs in that a tracheostomy is left in place during the healing time and a stent is left in the grafted area. The second step occurs several weeks later when a microdirect laryngoscopy is performed, the stent is removed, and the airway is assessed for decannulation.

All relevant comorbidities should be considered preoperatively. Patients may have history of prematurity with associated chronic lung disease. Reactive airway disease and recurrent pulmonary infections are common, and these issues should be optimized prior to major airway surgery (24).

Standard premedication is appropriate.

Induction, maintenance

Patients presenting for LTR have tracheostomies in place. Inhalational induction via *in situ* tracheostomy or standard intravenous induction can occur. Once a deep level of anesthesia is obtained via combination of narcotic, inhaled anesthetic and topical lidocaine, airway manipulation can commence. A cuffed tracheostomy tube or a cuffed endotracheal tube should be placed to minimize debris and blood entering the lower airway worsening bronchospasm and ventilation.

Maintenance is via inhaled anesthetic or propofol infusion. Postoperative plans should be made for continued sedation and ventilation if necessary in the intensive care setting.

Laser procedures

Uses for the laser in the trachea and larynx include treatment of hemangiomas, vocal cord lesions, laryngomalacia, papillomas, stenosis, and postsurgical changes leading to granuloma formation. The vast majority of laser procedures in otolaryngology will involve some type of direct or microdirect laryngoscopy, so the principles for bronchoscopic procedures (above) will also apply.

The additional risks inherent to laser use in the airway primarily revolve around injury and fire risk. Literature suggests the incidence of airway fires may be as high as 1.5% in otolaryngoscopic anesthesia (25). Use of the laser provides the third part of the "fire triad" as the ignition source, with fuel (tissue or ETT plastic) and oxidizer (oxygen or nitrous oxide) already present. Tracheal intubation is often not required, and may even be undesirable depending on the surgical indication and patient factors. If an ETT is required, a laser tube (typically metallic coated) and saline-filled balloon are recommended. Inspired oxygen concentration should be $< 30\%$, and *exhaled* oxygen concentration should also be monitored, ideally until $< 30\%$ (26). Special care should also be given to protect the patient's eyes. Further attention to all personnel in the operating room should include appropriate eyewear and evacuation of the laser-induced smoke plume (19).

Otologic procedures

Myringotomy and tubes

If general anesthesia is required for myringotomy, with or without ear tube placement, intubation is typically not required. Analgesic plan should include oral, IV, or rectal acetaminophen or a nonsteroidal anti-inflammatory, with or without opioids. Standard inhalational induction is common given the young population. Anesthesia can be maintained via mask airway or placement of a laryngeal mask airway.

Cochlear implant, tympanoplasty, and mastoidectomy

One of the most salient anesthetic considerations for invasive otologic surgery is the need for nerve monitoring. Facial nerve monitoring is accomplished with continuous electromyographic (EMG) input from percutaneous needle electrodes in the orbicularis oris and oculi muscles (19). The effects of non-depolarizing muscle relaxants on the neuromuscular junction can impair the sensitivity of EMG monitoring, and should be avoided. Caution should be used with nitrous oxide as an adjunct, as middle ear space expansion is a risk, and PONV risk is high in middle ear surgery.

When cochlear nerve activity is monitored, the auditory brain response (ABR) is often used. The ABR has varying sensitivity to different anesthetic agents, minimal with fentanyl and nitrous oxide, but much more with volatile anesthetics (27). Propofol-based TIVA can be useful, as this can lower blood pressure (helping to provide a bloodless operative field) and provide sedation or general anesthesia in a dose-dependent manner (19). An adjunct infusion such as remifentanil, alfentanil, or ketamine can blunt noxious stimuli while minimizing interference with ABR (28,29). These adjuncts can thereby lower the required propofol dose, further minimizing its effects on ABR.

Emergence and postoperative considerations

As with any head and neck procedure, hypertension and coughing should be avoided with emergence. Postoperative nausea and vomiting (PONV) is common with middle and inner ear surgeries, so two agents such as an HT3 blocker (e.g., ondansetron) and a steroid (e.g., dexamethasone) should be used. A greater auricular nerve block could be appropriate as this can also provide analgesia and reduce PONV (30).

References

1. Hu S, Dong HL, Sun YY, *et al.* Anesthesia with sevoflurane and remifentanil under spontaneous respiration assisted with high-frequency jet ventilation for tracheobronchial foreign body removal in 586 children. *Paediatric Anaesthesia*. 2012. doi: 10.1111/j.1460-9592.2012.03874.x (Epub ahead of print).
2. Shen X, Hu CB, Ye M, Chen YZ. Propofol–remifentanil intravenous anesthesia and spontaneous ventilation for airway foreign body removal in children with preoperative respiratory impairment. *Paediatric Anaesthesia*. 2012; **22**(12): 1166–70.
3. Malherbe S, Whyte S, Singh P, *et al.* Total intravenous anesthesia and spontaneous respiration for airway endoscopy in children– a prospective evaluation. *Paediatric Anaesthesia*. 2010; **20**(5): 434–8.
4. Cai Y, Li W, Chen K. Efficacy and safety of spontaneous ventilation technique using dexmedetomidine for rigid bronchoscopic airway foreign body removal in children. *Paediatric Anaesthesia*. 2013; **23** (11): 1048–53.
5. Cullen KA, Hall MJ, Golosinskiy A. Ambulatory surgery in the USA, 2006. *National Health Statistics Reports*. 2009: **28**(11): 1–25.
6. Erickson BK, Larson DR, St Sauver JL, Meverden RA, Orvidas LJ. Changes in incidence and indications of tonsillectomy and adenotonsillectomy, 1970–2005. *Otolaryngology – Head and Neck Surgery*. 2009; **140**(6): 894–901.
7. Marcus CL, Brooks LJ, Draper KA, *et al.* Diagnosis and management of childhood obstructive sleep apnea syndrome. *Pediatrics*. 2012; **130** (3): e714–55.
8. Johnson LB, Elluru RG, Myer CM, 3rd. Complications of adenotonsillectomy. *Laryngoscope*. 2002; **112**(8 Pt 2 Suppl 100): 35–6.
9. Bouvet L, Stoian A, Rimmele T, *et al.* Optimal remifentanil dosage for providing excellent intubating conditions when co-administered with a single standard dose of propofol. *Anaesthesia*. 2009; **64**(7): 719–26.
10. Karaman M, Ilhan AE, Dereci G, Tek A. Determination of optimum dosage of intraoperative single dose dexamethasone in pediatric tonsillectomy and adenotonsillectomy. *International Journal of Pediatric Otorhinolaryngology*. 2009; **73** (11): 1513–15.
11. von Ungern-Sternberg BS, Davies K, Hegarty M, Erb TO, Habre W. The effect of deep vs. awake extubation on respiratory complications in high-risk children undergoing adenotonsillectomy: A randomised controlled trial. *European Journal of Anaesthesiology*. 2013; **30**(9): 529–36.
12. Ravi R, Howell T. Anaesthesia for paediatric ear, nose, and throat surgery. *Continuing Education in Anaesthesia, Critical Care & Pain*. 2007; **7**(2): 33–7.
13. Riggin L, Ramakrishna J, Sommer DD, Koren G. A 2013 updated systematic review & meta-analysis of 36 randomized controlled trials; no apparent effects of non steroidal anti-inflammatory agents on the risk of bleeding after tonsillectomy. *Clinical Otolaryngology*. 2013; **38**(2): 115–29.
14. FDA Drug Safety Communication. Safety review update of codeine use in children; new Boxed Warning and Contraindication on use after tonsillectomy and/or adenoidectomy. 2013. http://www.fda.gov/Drugs/DrugSafety/ucm339112.htm. (Accessed September 1, 2013). Epub 02/20/2013.
15. Kelly LE, Rieder M, van den Anker J, *et al.* More codeine fatalities after tonsillectomy in North American children. *Pediatrics*. 2012; **129**(5): e1343–7.
16. Voelker R. Children's deaths linked with postsurgical codeine. *JAMA*. 2012; **308**(10): 963.
17. He XY, Cao JP, Shi XY, Zhang H. Dexmedetomidine versus morphine or fentanyl in the management of children after tonsillectomy and adenoidectomy: a meta-analysis of randomized controlled trials. *Annals of Otology, Rhinology, and Laryngology*. 2013; **122**(2): 114–20.
18. Steward DL, Grisel J, Meinzen-Derr J. Steroids for improving recovery following tonsillectomy in children. *Cochrane Database of Systematic Reviews*. 2011 (8): CD003997.
19. Bissonnette B. *Pediatric Anesthesia: Basic Principles, State of the Art, Future*. Shelton, CT: People's Medical Publishing House, 2011.

20. Deutsch ES. Tracheostomy: pediatric considerations. *Respiratory Care*. 2010; **55**(8): 1082–90.
21. Wrightson F, Soma M, Smith JH. Anesthetic experience of 100 pediatric tracheostomies. *Paediatric Anaesthesia*. 2009; **19**(7): 659–66.
22. Menasse-Palmer L, Bogdanow A, Marion RW. Choanal atresia. *Pediatrics in Review/American Academy of Pediatrics*. 1995; **16**(12): 475–6.
23. Tatekawa Y, Muraji T. Surgical strategy for acquired tracheomalacia due to innominate artery compression of the trachea. *European Journal of Cardio-thoracic Surgery*. 2011; **39**(3): 412–13.
24. Rowe RW, Betts J, Free E. Perioperative management for laryngotracheal reconstruction. *Anesthesia and Analgesia*. 1991; **73**(4): 483–6.
25. Heine P, Axhausen M. Anesthesia and laser surgery of the laryngo-nasal-ear region. *Der Anaesthesist*. 1988; **37**(1): 10–18.
26. Remz M, Luria I, Gravenstein M, *et al*. Prevention of airway fires: do not overlook the expired oxygen concentration. *Anesthesia and Analgesia*. 2014; **58**(2): 87–8.
27. Kileny PR, Niparko JK, Shepard NT, Kemink JL. Neurophysiologic intraoperative monitoring: I. Auditory function. *American Journal of Otology*. 1988; **9**: Suppl: 17–24.
28. Tooley MA, Stapleton CL, Greenslade GL, Prys-Roberts C. Mid-latency auditory evoked response during propofol and alfentanil anaesthesia. *British Journal of Anaesthesia*. 2004; **92**(1): 25–32.
29. Akin A, Esmaoglu A, Tosun Z, *et al*. Comparison of propofol with propofol–ketamine combination in pediatric patients undergoing auditory brainstem response testing. *International Journal of Pediatric Otorhinolaryngology*. 2005; **69**(11): 1541–5.
30. Suresh S, Barcelona SL, Young NM, *et al*. Postoperative pain relief in children undergoing tympanomastoid surgery: is a regional block better than opioids? *Anesthesia and Analgesia*. 2002; **94**(4): 859–62.

Chapter

19 Plastic and cleft–craniofacial surgery

Brenda C. McClain, Alexander Y. Lin, and Naila A. Ahmad

General principles of pediatric plastic surgery

Pediatric plastic surgery improves the unique human qualities required for social interaction: appearance, speech, and hands (1). Each of these elements allows communication, which is essential for a child's psychosocial development (2–4). As many procedures involve the external structures of the mouth and nose such as the lips, tongue, palate, and nasal bones, cartilage and septum, good communication is critical, as the plastic surgery team and the anesthesia team must both take responsibility for this shared area. Many reconstructions require complex osteotomies that increase the surface area of bleeding bone edges, which could be catastrophic in smaller patients, requiring vigilance by all members in the operating room.

Plastic surgery is derived from the Greek word *plastikos* meaning "to shape." However, shaping the body is limited by blood supply, as each incision and movement of tissues causes devascularization. The two main tools to move tissue while maintaining blood supply are: grafts versus flaps (5–9). Grafts do not have a blood supply, and are placed in a recipient site that must be highly vascularized in order for the grafted tissue to survive on diffusion alone, until neovascularization occurs at about 48 hours. This delay in neovascularization limits the amount of tissue that can be grafted. If the recipient site lacks surface vascularity, such as exposed bone, or requires significant tissue coverage to protect vasculature or viscera, a flap is required. Flaps have a known blood supply, and as long as the blood supply is preserved, significant amounts of tissue can be transferred, including skin, fat, fascia, muscle, and bone. Local and regional flaps can move neighboring tissue based on neighboring blood supply. In areas of limited local tissue, free flaps may be required, which require detaching a flap at its known artery and vein, and then performing microvascular anastomosis at the recipient artery and vein.

Plastic surgeons have also developed direct molding technologies. Tissue expansion increases the volume of local flaps that are usually of better color or hair-bearing match than more distant tissues. This is a staged procedure, which entails a preliminary step of placing a silicone expander with a subcutaneous port that can be injected with saline weekly. When enough tissue has been expanded, a second procedure will be needed to remove the tissue expander and utilize the expanded local flaps (10). Distraction osteogenesis is a process that can be used to grow significant amounts of bone, rather than being limited by smaller bone grafts (11). This staged procedure starts with osteotomies in the bone to expand, placement of distraction hardware that can be lengthened by the parents daily to widen the osteotomy a small amount each day. After a consolidation period, osteogenesis replaces the bone gap, and a second procedure is needed to remove the distraction hardware.

The final principle of pediatric plastic surgery that differs from adults is the rapid wound healing and growth of the child. Different regions of the body grow at different rates, and the development of bones, teeth, sinuses, affects the overlying soft tissue structures, and these timelines must be respected, as surgery can interfere with growth centers (12,13). Even when surgery is appropriate, the rapid changes of the child need to be taken into account, and overcorrection is often necessary to match the rapid growth. The timing of surgery may be more urgent, as wounds or fractures may quickly heal or fuse inappropriately (14–16).

Essentials of Pediatric Anesthesiology, ed. Alan David Kaye, Charles James Fox and James H. Diaz. Published by Cambridge University Press. © Cambridge University Press 2015.

General principles of anesthesia in pediatric plastic surgery

Although a majority of infants and children who undergo anesthesia for plastic surgery procedures are ASA 1 and 2 patients, a thorough history of the patient is required to investigate for coexisting disease, syndromes, or inherited compounding factors. Evaluation for sleep disordered breathing or obstructive sleep apnea (OSA) is mandatory since OSA occurs in 37.5% of children with cleft palate, and up to 82% of children with syndromic craniofacial anomalies (17).

The preservation of spontaneous respirations at the induction of anesthesia is best accomplished by an inhalational induction technique. Appropriate airway equipment must be readily available within reach. The use of oral airways, stylets, and nasal trumpets may be needed soon after induction. Direct laryngoscopy may be challenging due to a small mouth opening compounded by a large tongue. The presence of a cleft palate can make maneuvering the laryngoscope blade difficult as it can lodge within the cleft. Hand-held video laryngoscopes improve visualization, but guiding the endotracheal tube through the glottic opening can be challenging even in a normal airway. With fiberscopes (e.g., Bonfils, flexible fiberoptic scope) the endotracheal tube is threaded on to the scope prior to insertion of the unit into the mouth enabling continuous visualization (10). The use of fiberscopes requires an appreciable amount of experience and should be a technique in the armamentarium of the pediatric anesthesiologist whose interests lie in the management of this patient population.

The position of the endotracheal tube depends on the working surgical field required, and can range from oral intubation with oral RAE to nasal intubation. For the patient with a tracheostomy and a mature stoma, the tracheostomy tube can be removed before or after induction, and replaced with a cuffed endotracheal tube for ventilation. The outer diameter of the endotracheal tube must be sized relative to the tracheostomy tube. Regardless of the type of intubation, the endotracheal tube must be secured firmly without causing pressure necrosis. The bed may be turned 180° for better access to the head by the plastic surgery team. The circuit must be detached prior to turning the bed, to avoid inadvertent extubation. Shoulder rolls and head rests are frequently employed to gain better oral access. Reassessment of breath sounds, once in the final position, is key since the depth of the endotracheal tube is position-dependent. Because of field avoidance with the 180° position, paralysis is utilized to prevent patient movement and possible dislodgement of the endotracheal tube. If alcohol-based preps are used, oxygen tension may need to be lowered initially to avoid operating room fires. A throat pack may be used, and its removal must be documented at the end of the case. Local anesthetic with epinephrine must be monitored for dosage toxicity. Bone bleeding may be reduced with permissive hypotension.

In all head and neck procedures where extubation is planned, it is imperative that the patient demonstrate adequate respiratory function and a degree of alertness that allows ready assessment of motor and sensory function. Extubation should be performed in an awake, yet calm patient who demonstrates self-supported ventilation. For oral procedures, the plastic surgery team must communicate with the anesthesia team to identify the regions of repair that are at risk and cannot afford to sustain trauma from oro-gastric suctioning, bite blocks, mouth guards, oral or nasal trumpets, or compression from face masks. The classical method of airway management via snug mask fit for bag mask ventilation must be avoided, as this could disrupt the repair. Elbow splints may be placed after surgery to prevent children from putting their hands in their mouths.

Facial reconstruction

The primary drivers of facial growth can be thought of as arising from the craniofacial skeleton, with the overlying soft tissue responding to this bony growth. Most facial reconstruction utilizes local flaps that contain similar tissues. Ear reconstruction and nasal reconstruction have more specific anesthesia concerns.

Ear microtia reconstruction

Microtia is the congenital absence of a normal external ear. This usually requires three to four staged plastic surgery procedures, with several months between stages to allow vascular growth (18). Microtia may be associated with inner ear anomalies, which require evaluation and treatment by the pediatric otolaryngologist. For the external ear reconstruction, the first stage is the most complex, as a large block of cartilage at the synchondrosis of the 6th, 7th, and 8th ribs is harvested and carved into the shape of an ear, to place under a very thin skin flap under the microtia remnant. This is usually performed at approximately

6–12 years of age, or older. The main anesthetic issue is the risk of pleural injury during the rib harvest, and therefore a Valsalva is performed at the end of the rib harvest to assess for pleural injury that may require needle aspiration of free air or insertion of a temporary chest catheter.

Rhinoplasty and septoplasty

Rhinoplasty and septoplasty reshapes the cartilage, bone, and soft tissue of the nose and septum to improve appearance and nasal airflow (19,20). Oral intubation with the bed turned gives full access to the plastic surgeon. Local anesthetic with epinephrine is essential given the high vascularity of this area. Often, cartilage is required and harvested from the septum, ear, or rib. Osteotomies of the nasal pyramid may be needed, with postoperative internal and external splints. One of the anesthesia risks postoperatively, especially in a strong male teenager, is that the postnasal bleeding may lead to laryngospasm or airway obstruction while the patient is waking up and taking a deep breath against a closed airway, leading to negative pressure pulmonary edema (NPPE) (20); NPPE presents as acute pulmonary edema, which may require reintubation and prolonged convalescence. Its postoperative incidence can be reduced with postnasal suctioning, local anesthetic, and a slower emergence (21).

Hand surgery

Hand surgery can be congenital or trauma. Similar principles of soft tissue management are used, with the specialized management for bones, tendon, nerves, and vessels. The airway may potentially be secured with LMA, or even sedation and local anesthetic. Tourniquet control is standard, and perioperative antibiotics need to be given prior to the tourniquet going up. Local anesthetic toxicity needs to be monitored if a Bier block is used. Fluoroscopy is usually necessary, and requiring shielding of the patient and caregivers. Children are nonadherent, and frequently need a cast after surgery to avoid disruption of the repair.

Hand trauma

In hand trauma, fractures may be fixated via reduction only, percutaneous pinning, or open reduction and internal fixation with hardware (22,23). Tendon repairs usually require additional incisions to expose the length of the tendon. Nerve repairs require wound exploration and operating room microscope, as well as potential sural nerve harvest for nerve grafts (24,25). Vessel repair requires microvascular anastomosis, and avoidance of vasoconstrictors (26,27).

Congenital hand anomalies

There are multiple congenital hand anomalies, which can be categorized as formation problems, differentiation problems, duplication, overgrowth, undergrowth, amniotic band sequence, and skeletal anomalies (28,29). The most common hand anomalies include syndactyly, or fusions of adjacent figures that may involve bone, and polydactyly, or additional digits usually on the radial or ulnar aspect (thumb or small finger). Syndactyly requires separation with flaps and grafts to reconstruct the inner surfaces. Polydactyly requires excision with reconstruction of remaining bone, tendon, and collateral ligaments. A final example of congenital hand anomaly is thumb hypoplasia, which in milder forms requires tendon balancing, first webspace deepening, collateral ligament reconstruction, but in more advanced cases, treatment is thumb amputation followed by pollicization. Pollicization entails dissecting out the structures of the index ray and transferring it as a complex flap to the position of the thumb, to create functional four-fingered hands. Most hand surgery is done around 1 year of life, to allow for neuroplasticity in learning to use the reconstructed hand.

Cleft lip–nose–palate

Cleft lip–nose–palate are the most common birth defects in the USA, occurring in 1 in 590 live births (23–25). From an epidemiologic standpoint, these are frequently separated into cleft lip–nose with or without palate (CLNP), or isolated cleft palate only (CPO), which both exhibit different degrees of severity (Figure 19.1). Syndromic association occurs in CLNP in about 15%–30% of cases, whereas in CPO about 50%. The most common syndrome associated with CPO is velocardiofacial syndrome (VCF), or chromosome 22q11 deletion. Incidence of CLNP is approximately 1 in 700 for Caucasians, twice as common in Asian descent, half as common for African descent; in CPO it is about 1 in 1500 among all ethnicities (30). There are some variations in the cleft care protocol among different centers, but the plastic surgery and anesthesia principles are similar. Cleft lip–nose repair is usually performed at 3 to 6 months of age, cleft palate at 9 to 12 months, alveolar bone grafting at 7 to 10 years, potential orthognathic surgery at 16 to 18 years, with possible

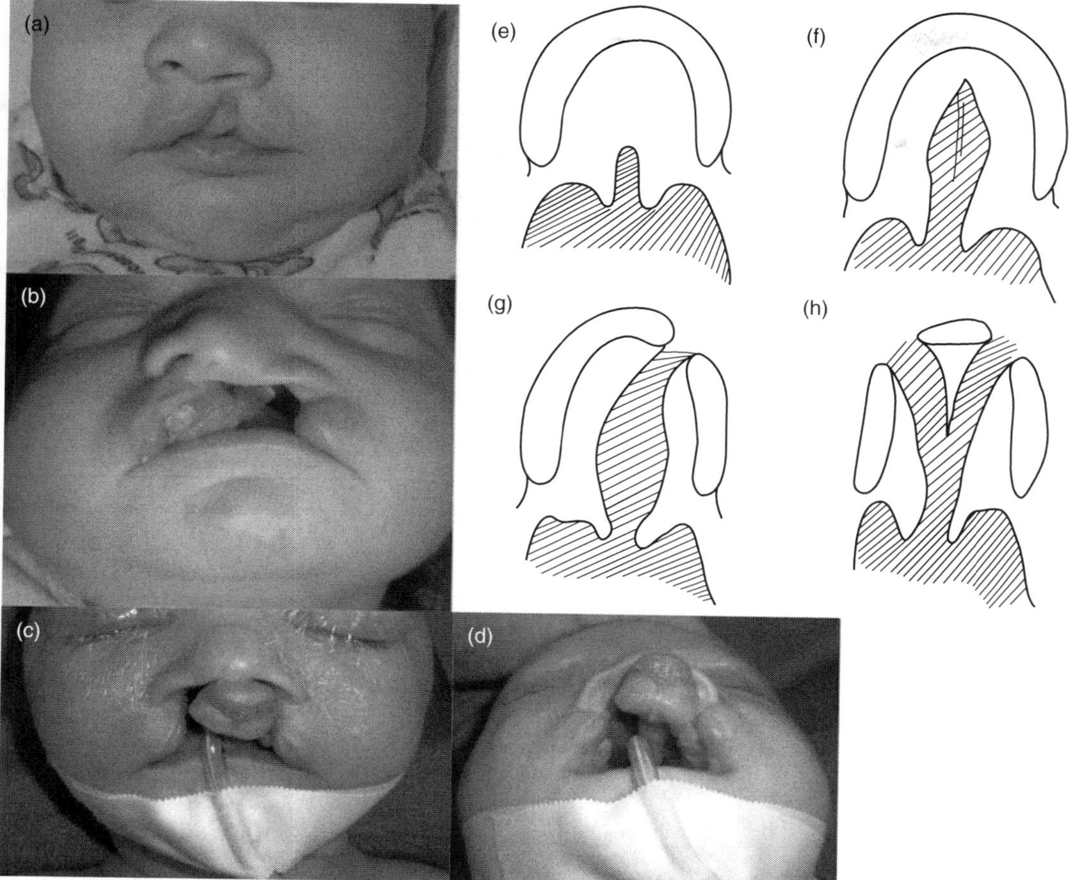

Figure 19.1 Continuum of cleft lip–nose (from top to bottom): **(a)** left unilateral cleft lip–nose, incomplete; **(b)** left unilateral cleft lip–nose–palate, complete; **(c)**, **(d)** two views of intubated bilateral cleft lip–nose–palate, complete. Diagram of Veau classification of cleft palates: **(e)** Veau I – soft palate only; **(f)** Veau II – soft and posterior hard palate; **(g)** Veau III – the common complete unilateral cleft lip–nose–palate; **(h)** Veau IV – complete bilateral cleft lip–nose–palate.

revisions of the lip or nose or palate throughout childhood (25). Given the possibility of significant scarring or pharyngeal tissue obstruction from previous speech surgery, it is critical to know the plastic surgery history of these patients prior to intubation.

Cleft lip repair and infant cleft rhinoplasty

Cleft lip–nose repair is performed under general anesthesia with the bed turned. An oral RAE tube is preferred, centered over the lower lip, to keep the tube away from the nose and the upper lip. Precise markings are made that may delay incision time, so it is important to discuss the timing of the perioperative antibiotics. Injection with local anesthetic with epinephrine is performed for hemostasis and pain control. The lip is opened at the markings to expose the mucosa and orbicularis oris muscles, and then a buccal sulcus incision is used to elevate and advance the cleft side as a cheek-ala-lip advancement flap. Oral mucosa is balanced, and the clefted orbicularis oris muscle is reconstructed. A rhinoplasty is performed via dissection of the nasal cartilages, and reshaping with sutures and nasal stents. Finally the skin is closed geometrically to recreate a more normal lip. On extubation, it is important to avoid trauma to the freshly reconstructed lip and nose. These patients can usually go home the next day.

Cleft palate repair and secondary speech surgery

Cleft palate primary repair, as well as secondary speech surgery, has a much higher airway risk, given the retropharyngeal location of surgery and swelling.

The function of the palate is to allow normal human speech via velopharyngeal competence, or when the velum (Latin for soft palate) apposes the posterior pharynx to prevent loss of spoken air through the nasopharynx. The normal velum contains the transversely paired levator veli palatini muscles, and the hard palate anatomically consists of a primary and a secondary portion that are respectively anterior and posterior to the incisive foramen. Velopharyngeal insufficiency (VPI) results in hypernasal speech that is difficult to understand and inhibits communication (31). Primary cleft palate repair is usually done around 9 to 12 months of age, before there is full speech development. Patients are monitored annually for hypernasality by the cleft team's speech language pathologist for possible revision speech surgery such as palate lengthening, sphincter pharyngoplasty (SP), or posterior pharyngeal flap (PPF) (26).

The sequences of repair for primary cleft palate surgery and secondary speech surgery are similar. A turned bed, shoulder roll, and oral RAE tube well-taped in the midline will accommodate a Dingman mouth retractor for full intraoral access. The mouth retractor puts pressure on the tongue, and therefore is released for several minutes each hour to avoid tongue ischemia or reperfusion injury and subsequent edema which could result in airway obstruction. Temporary tongue sutures are placed to allow postoperative tongue retraction if needed. Local anesthetic with epinephrine is used. In palate repair, flaps are designed to be elevated off the hard palate, which may lead to bone bleeding. The malpositioned levator veli palatine muscles are reconstructed for velopharyngeal competence. The palatal flaps are brought midline to close the cleft, frequently leaving raw lateral edges with bone bleeding that may benefit from more epinephrine injection or permissive hypotension. In SP, the posterior tonsillar pillars are elevated as flaps and inset transversely at the junction of the adenoids and the posterior pharynx, to dynamically augment the posterior aspect of the velopharyngeal complex. In PPF, a rectangular flap of pharyngeal tissue is elevated and sewn to the soft palate, which creates a static near-obstruction of the nasopharyngeal outlet, with two lateral ports that allow air passage. Patients with VCF may have anomalous carotid branches in the posterior pharyngeal wall that are at risk during PPF procedure (27).

As all of these operations add tissue to the nasopharyngeal airway; they all have risks of postoperative swelling and airway obstruction. Bone edges may be bleeding that require gastric or retropharyngeal suctioning. However, it is vital to avoid injuring the tenuous palatal flaps in oral suctioning, or the SP or PPF in nasal suctioning. It is advisable to use a soft suction and aim laterally and inferiorly into the buccal area to avoid injuring these fresh flaps. The plastic surgeon may intraoperatively position a nasal trumpet or airway to bypass the surgical site. Steroids intraoperatively and postoperatively may be used to further reduce airway swelling.

Alveolar bone grafting

The most common form of cleft lip–nose-palate is the complete form, which results in the cleft going from the palate, through the alveolus-maxilla, through the lip–nose. This cleft of the alveolus is not repaired until ages 7 through 10 before eruption of the cleft tooth, via bone grafting (32). Intubation is via oral RAE taped down the center with the bed turned. The plastic surgeon typically harvests bone from the iliac crest via a hip incision. The cleft of the alveolus and maxilla is exposed, and the nasal fistula and palatal fistula are closed to create a vascularized area for the bone graft. Both the hip donor site and the oral flaps are closed. The bone is harvested and placed into the alveolar-maxillary gap, and the mucosal flaps are closed. Typically, there is more pain in the hip donor site than the oral portion, and therefore local anesthetic or even anesthetic pump may be considered. Other donor site morbidities include hematoma, and the risk of injury to the lateral femoral cutaneous nerve that could result in meralgia paresthetica.

Cleft orthognathic surgery and adult cleft rhinoplasty

Approximately 25% of children with clefts will have significant maxillary hypoplasia that places them in a severe underbite (also called class III malocclusion, or negative overjet) that affects eating, speech, and appearance. These children may need a Le Fort I maxillary advancement, but scar tissue from multiple previous operations, or tethering from a posterior pharyngeal flap, can lead to a high relapse rate (33). Additionally, a large advancement may have greater risk of loss of blood supply to the maxilla. Distraction osteogenesis can solve these problems, by advancing the osteotomized maxilla 1 mm per day, thereby stretching the scar and soft tissues (34). Hardware can be internal, or external with a halo connected to the scalp with screws, and connected to the maxilla with a dental splint and vertical bar. The halo makes postoperative airway access more difficult, and full communication with the plastic surgery team will reveal whether the vertical bar can be removed prior to intubation, or only mild sedation is needed. In general, maxillary advancement surgery is deferred until skeletal maturity (16 to 18 years of age), otherwise the mandible can continue to grow past the advanced maxilla, leading again to an apparent underbite relationship.

Finally, as the child grows, nasal or septal asymmetry that may have once been minor, can become magnified with airway obstruction. Many patients will require a finishing adult cleft septorhinoplasty that may require additional cartilage from the septum, ears, or ribs, to counteract the scarred tissue. If the patient requires maxillary repositioning, it is best to defer rhinoplasty until after Le Fort I, as maxillary movement changes position of the nose.

Craniofacial, maxillary, and mandibular disorders

Etiology of craniofacial malformations

Craniofacial anomalies result from dysregulation of hindbrain rhombomeres, resulting in one or more perturbations of the first three branchial arches. Rhombomeric dysregulation is likely from mutations in gene expression of neural crest cells that perturb normal fetal development (39). As a result, many craniofacial disorders have characteristic visceral and skeletal anomalies associated that are pathognomonic for a given syndrome. Other theories suggest that premature suture closure is a result rather than a cause of craniofacial anomalies, with the perturbation originating in the cranial base (40). Due to the multiple mechanisms of craniofacial growth (direct osteogenesis, conversion of cartilage, sutural deposition, and periosteal remodeling), complete correction often requires multiple surgeries that must be staged at appropriate times during growth, from infancy to adulthood.

Calvarial physiology

The skull of the fetus is composed of five bones united by fibrous sutures. Between the two frontal bones is the metopic suture, which undergoes normal closure at about 7 to 8 months of age. The sagittal suture overlies the midline between the paired parietal bones. The coronal sutures lay transversely between the frontal bones and parietal bones. The lambdoid sutures form a lambda-shape between the occipital bone and the parietal bones. The sutures maintain malleability during passage through the birth canal and allow for rapid brain expansion during the first year of life (41). Fontanelles are gaps that lie at the suture junctions: the anterior fontanelle joins the metopic, coronal, and sagittal sutures, whereas the posterior fontanelle joins the lambdoid and sagittal sutures. The posterior fontanelle closes by age 6 months while the anterior fontanelle closes by age 18 months. Craniosynostosis is the premature, usually congenital, pathologic fusion of one or more sutures. The rapidly expanding brain cannot separate the fused suture, forcing brain growth at the other sutures, resulting in abnormal compensatory growth parallel to the fused suture (42). The frequency of the various single suture synostoses is: sagittal > metopic > coronal >> lambdoidal. Sagittal craniosynostosis leads to an anterior–posterior long head shape or scaphocephaly (43). Metopic craniosynostosis leads to trigonocephaly or a triangular-shaped forehead and supraorbital rim, that retrudes the eyelids laterally, resulting in pseudohypotelorism and difficulty closing the eyes. Unilateral coronal or lambdoidal synostosis results in asymmetric plagiocephaly (44). Closure of both coronal sutures leads to brachycephaly, or a short anterior–posterior distance, which is frequently syndromic. While the majority of cases are nonsyndromic, craniosynostosis can be found as part of over 100 syndromes, with multiple coexisting diseases that require an interdisciplinary approach and careful timing of interventions (45).

Facial clefts

Facial clefts is a comprehensive term used to describe various types of gaps in facial structures, including the common cleft lip–nose–palate. These anomalies are clefts through the facial bones, leading to derangement of the overlying soft tissues. The most frequently used classification was described by plastic surgeon Paul Tessier, who described 15 clefts numbered 0 to 14 dividing the face like a clock, with the orbits as the centers. Not including common cleft lip–nose–palate, facial clefts occur at a rate of 1.4 to 4.8 per 100 000 live births, and are frequently associated with syndromes such as hemifacial microsomia, frontonasal dysplasia, or holoprosencephaly (46).

Co-existing disease in craniofacial anomalies

Thorough awareness of the spectrum of craniofacial disorders and associated anomalies is essential to surgical and anesthetic management of this patient population. A full review of systems is required for optimal anesthetic management.

Airway compromise

Thorough awareness of the spectrum of craniofacial disorders and associated anomalies is essential to surgical and anesthetic management of this patient population. A full review of systems is required for optimal anesthetic management. Airway management is a leading concern due maxillary or mandibular deformities that impact airway mechanics leading to airway compromise and pulmonary dysfunction. Obstructive sleep apnea is a frequent finding in children with cleft and craniofacial disorders, and should remain in the forefront when considering methods of postoperative pain management (47). Perioperative airway compromise can occur from edema, bleeding, intra- or perioral mechanical devices, opioid-induced sedation, or inability to handle secretions.

Cardiac

Coexisting cardiac anomalies may require additional surgeries, such as in velocardiofacial syndrome (also known as Shprintzen–Goldberg syndrome), Williams syndrome, Wolf–Hirschorn, or van der Woude syndrome (48). Approximately 28% of patients with cleft lip have some type of cardiac anomaly.

Neurological

Raised intracranial pressure (ICP) can occur in both nonsyndromic and syndromic craniosynostosis. Elevated ICP is often subclinical and can be found even in children with less severe phenotypic features. Only 25 percent of children with raised intracranial pressure have papilledema on fundoscopic exam. Radiographic evidence such as a copper-beaten appearance of the skull may be nonspecific. Thus, measurement of ICP is recommended if the risk–benefit of surgical correction is unclear (49,50).

Hearing loss

Thirty percent of genetic hearing loss is associated with craniofacial abnormalities (51). The hearing loss can be sensorineural, conductive, or mixed. Embryogenic aberration in the first and second branchial arches results in malformations of the craniofacial skeleton and the ossicles of the middle ear. Hemifacial microsomia, Goldenhar, Stickler, Treacher Collins, Crouzon, Pfeiffer, and Shprintzen syndromes and Pierre Robin sequence are a few of the craniofacial malformations with hearing loss (51).

Ophthalmalogical

Syndromic craniosynotosis results in restricted growth of the orbital bones that lack enough volume to house the globes, resulting in exotropia, proptosis, and occasionally hypertelorism. The retruded supraorbital rim sets back the upper eyelid, preventing normal eyelid closure, which risks conjunctivitis, keratopathy, and even blindness. Fronto-orbital advancement (FOA), described later, advances the supraorbital rim to restore upper eyelid function. If timing of FOA needs to be deferred, a tarsorraphy can also protect the globe. Poor vision is found in about 50% of these patients (52). Colobomas, glaucoma, and cataracts are less frequent causes of decreased vision. Fundoscopic exams are notable for papilledema in over 50% of patients with syndromic craniosynostosis (53). Asymmetric craniofacial anomalies, such as nonsyndromic unicoronal craniosynostosis, have increased risk of strabismus (54).

The craniosynostoses

Nonsyndromic craniosynostosis

Nonsyndromic craniosynostosis (NSC) is a clinically and genetically heterogeneous condition that has the characteristics of a multifactorial trait with possible gene–gene or gene–environment interactions (55). Craniosynostosis is a common malformation occurring in 3–5 per 10 000 live births. Nonsyndromic craniosynostosis usually involves only one suture, although occasionally more than one suture may be involved. Between the two frontal bones is the metopic suture, which undergoes normal closure at about 7 to 8 months of age. The sagittal suture overlies the midline between the paired parietal bones. The coronal sutures lay transversely between the frontal bones and parietal bones. The lambdoid sutures form a lambda-shape between the occipital bone and the parietal bones. Sagittal craniosynostosis leads to an anterior–posterior long head shape or scaphocephaly (56). Metopic craniosynostosis leads to trigonocephaly or a triangular-shaped forehead and supraorbital rim, that retrudes the eyelids laterally resulting in pseudohypotelorism and difficulty closing

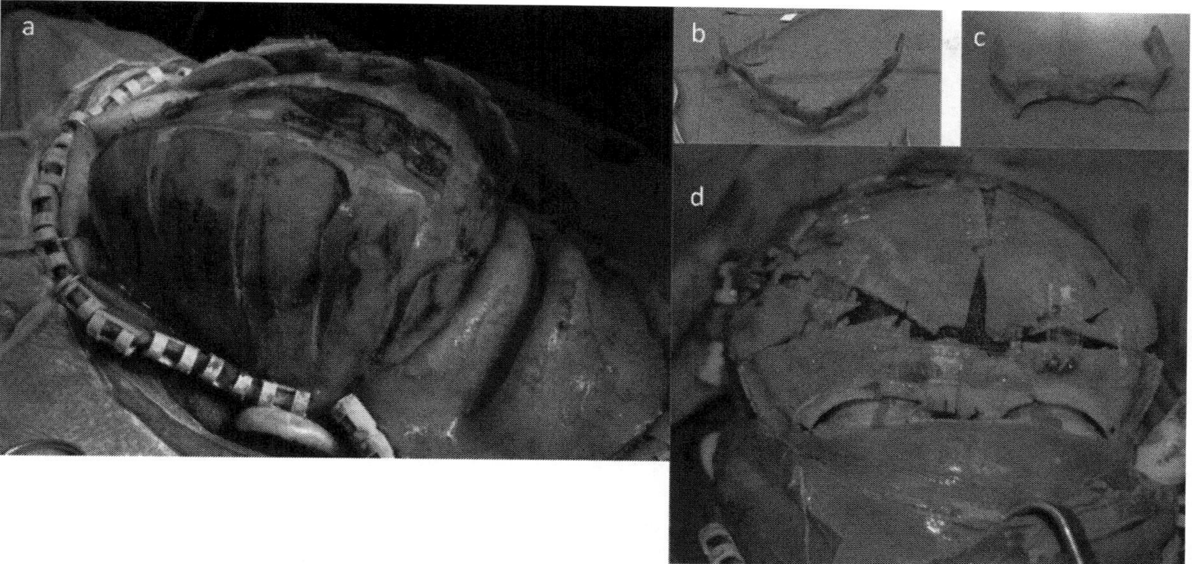

Figure 19.2 Nonsyndromic craniosynostosis intraoperative: **(a)** sagittal craniosynostosis undergoing lateral barrel stave osteotomies to widen the calvarium, **(b)** metopic craniosynostosis triangular fronto-orbital bandeau before, and **(c)** after reshaping, with **(d)** final anterior view showing bandeau and forehead reconstruction with resorbable sutures and plates. Note the increased surface area of bone edges that are at risk for bleeding; increasing surface area is necessary to solve the problem of increasing calvarial volume.

the eyes. Unicoronal craniosynostosis leads to asymmetric anterior craniosynostotic plagiocephaly with ipsilateral raised orbital rim and contralateral frontal bossing and nasal chin deviation contralaterally (57). Bicoronal craniosynostosis is seen more often in association with a syndrome and leads to retrusion of the supraorbital rim bilaterally, with a AP-short head shape, or craniosynostosis brachycephaly. Finally, unilambdoid craniosynostosis is very rare and leads to asymmetric craniosynostotic plagiocephaly with ipsilateral mastoid bossing and contralateral parietal bossing with facial changes.

In sagittal craniosynostosis, cranial vault remodeling is performed in the supine or prone position with the bed turned 180 degrees. The sphinx position is less common, given the increased risk for air embolism. Hair is shaved and prepped. Local epinephrine is frequently used for improving hemostasis, as well as Raney clips along the scalp edges. When the bone is exposed, the neurosurgery team can perform craniotomies. The plastic surgery team performs reconstruction via bone reshaping, bone grafts, and fixation with sutures and resorbable plates and screws (Figure 19.2). In patients with craniosynostosis that involves the supraorbital rims (metopic or coronal craniosynsotosis), the supraorbital rims require fronto-orbital advancement (FOA), in addition to the cranial vault remodeling. For FOA, the plastic surgery team must additionally perform osteotomies to elevate the supraorbital rim as a fronto-orbital bandeau, taking care to minimize pressure on the globes or dura. The fronto-orbital bandeau is reshaped and advanced to create a more normal brow that allows normal eyelid function and globe protection (Figure 19.2). At the end of the case, a scalp drain is placed and the galea and scalp are closed. The patient is usually extubated before transfer to the ICU for monitoring.

Syndromic craniosynostosis

The most well known of these syndromes are the acrocephalosyndactyly syndromes, which consist of multisutural craniosynostosis involving at least the coronal sutures, midface hypoplasia with obstructive sleep apnea, and hand and foot anomalies. Most of these anomalies are related to mutations in the fibroblast growth factor receptor (FGFR) family. This protein's function includes signaling of immature cells to become bone cells during embryonic development. The three most recognized are Apert, Crouzon, and Pfeiffer syndromes. Typically, the bicoronal craniosynostosis causes supraorbital rim retrusion, and the midface hypoplasia causes infraorbital rim deficiency,

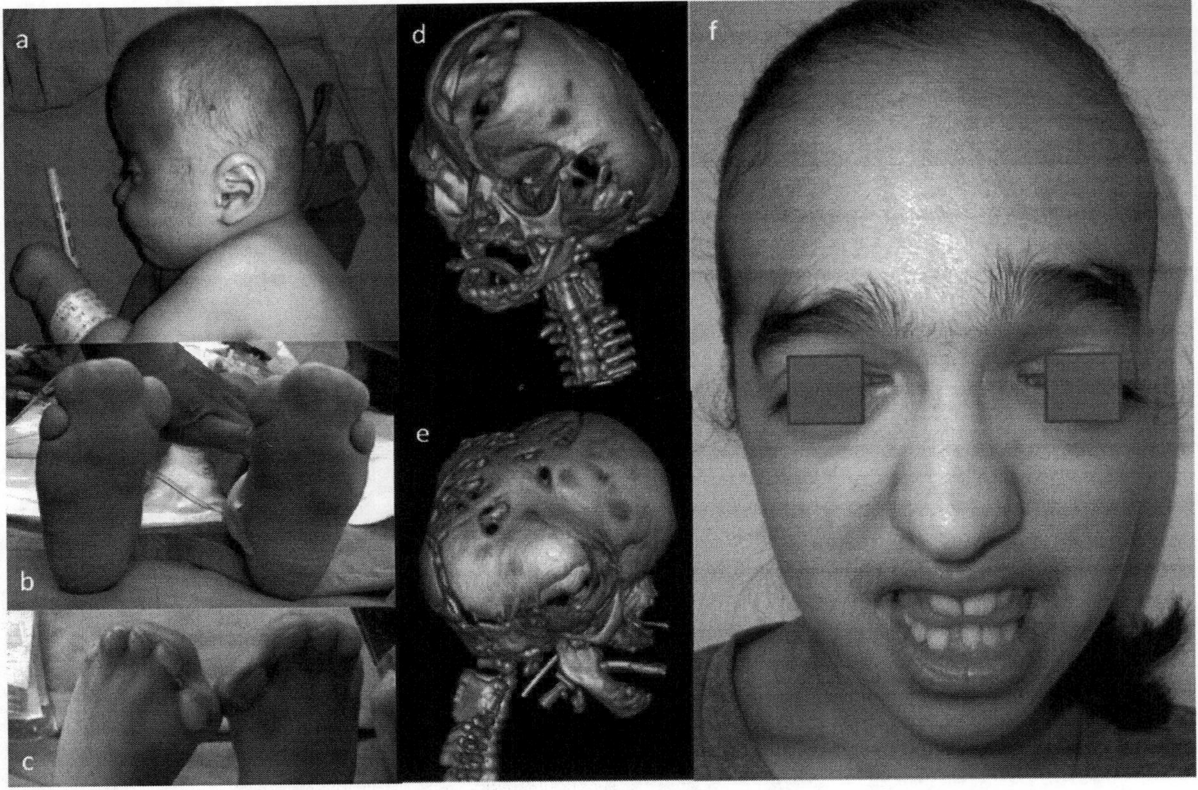

Figure 19.3 Syndromic craniosynostoses: Apert syndrome infant with **(a)** bicoronal craniosynostosis with fronto-orbital retrusion and brachycephaly with mitten syndactyly, and note the **(b)** plantar and **(c)** dorsal aspects of the bilateral complex syndactyly of the toes; **(d)** oblique and **(e)** sagittal views of Pfeifer syndrome infant 3-D CT reconstruction with kleeblattschadel cloverleaf multisutural craniosynostosis and hypoplastic midface and shallow orbits; **(e)** teenager with Crouzon status post infant fronto-orbital advancement and midface advancement, now with persistent hypoplastic maxilla relative to mandible as she grows, as well palpebral fissures with negative canthal tilt.

thus leading to insufficient orbital housing and exorbitism, or globe exposure. The sequence of repairs for these children is complex, as experience has shown that early cranial vault reconstruction leads to relapse, and revision is difficult with the scarred, relapsed bone. The current management is to defer the fronto-orbital advancement until they are at least 9 to 12 months of age, or even older to await adequate bony stock that is less susceptible to relapse (58). If elevated ICP requires earlier release, a combination of craniectomies, posterior vault expansion or distraction, and ventriculoperitoneal shunting may be necessary preliminary procedures until the bone is ready for FOA.

Apert syndrome

Apert syndrome is an autosomal dominant disorder from mutation of FGFR2 (59). This gene produces a protein called fibroblast growth factor receptor 2 whose functions include the signaling of immature cells to become bone cells during embryonic development. The phenotype includes midface hypoplasia especially at the nasal bridge, maxillary deformity with high-arched palate and dentoalveolar distortion, shallow orbits with exophthalmos and hypertelorism. Deformities of the ossicles result in ear disease and hearing loss. Children with Apert syndrome have complex bilateral syndactyly of the hands and feet, involving at least three digits or toes, and sometimes all five (mitten syndactyly) (Figure 19.3a, b, c). Some degree of fusion of the cervical vertebra occurs in approximately 70% of patients, of which C5–C6 fusion is the most common (59). Intracranial hypertension results in delayed mentation. Hyperhidrosis and acne are seen in nearly all patients. Apert syndrome is a more severe clinical entity than Crouzon syndrome, because Apert has worse airway compromise and cervical limitations (60).

Crouzon syndrome

Crouzon syndrome is also a syndromic bicoronal craniosynostosis due to autosomal dominant mutations in FGFR2, but children have normal hands and feet, and often normal intelligence. The syndrome was first described in 1912 by Louis Edouard Octave Crouzon (61). Other features include a parrot-beaked nose, short upper lip, hypoplastic maxilla, and relative mandibular prognathism. Its incidence is 1:25 000 to 1:60 000 live births (59). More than 30 mutations of FGFR2 have been identified that can cause Crouzon syndrome. The hypoplastic orbits lead to proptosis and a predilection for optic nerve impingement. Poor visual acuity and even blindness have been reported (62). The cervical spine has been noted to undergo progressive fusion where the posterior elements fuse first, followed by fusion of the vertebral bodies. The C2–C3 fusion and C5–C6 fusion occur with equal frequency. The occurrence of butterfly vertebrae is prevalent in association with Crouzon syndrome (63).

Pfeiffer syndrome

Pfeiffer syndrome is caused by autosomal dominant mutation of FGFR1 or FGFR2, resulting in bicoronal craniosynostosis, exorbitism, midface hypoplasia, with the unique phenotype of broad thumbs and great toes, and more severe forms include cloverleaf-shaped multisutural synostosis (Kleeblattschadel), hydrocephalus, and cervical anomalies (Figure 19.3d, e).

Pfeiffer syndrome (PS) is divided into three subtypes based on physical findings. Children with type I, also known as classic Pfeiffer syndrome, usually have normal intelligence and a normal life span. Types II and III are more severe forms of Pfeiffer syndrome that often involve problems with the nervous system such as megalencephaly, midline disorders, malformations of the amygdala, and hippocampus, and ventricular wall alterations. Kleeblattschadel is seen in type II, but not type III. The brain anomalies in PS result from the combination of mechanical deformations and intrinsic developmental disorders due to FGFR2 hyperactivity (64). Skeletal anomalies include elbow ankylosis and sacrococcygeal defects.

Craniofacial anomalies with mandibular hypoplasia

Craniofacial (hemifacial) microsomia and Goldenhar syndrome

Craniofacial microsomia (CFM), sometimes called hemifacial microsomia, is the second most common facial anomaly. It is thought to be due to hypoplasia of the first and second branchial arches leading to variable hypoplasia of the mandible, orbit, ear (both external ear microtia and internal ear hearing loss), facial nerve, and soft tissue. When associated with vertebral anomalies and epibulbar dermoids, it is known as oculo-auriculo-vertebral (OAV) or Goldenhar syndrome, where incidence ranges from 1:3500–1:5600 with a male: female ratio of 3:2. This syndrome has a wide spectrum of severity, including unilateral or bilateral presentation, heterogeneous anomalies of various organ systems, ocular anomalies including colobomas or microphthalmos, auricular anomalies including microtia and ear appendices, and lateral facial clefts (Tessier #7), cleft palate, dental malformations, and mental retardation (65). Plastic surgery options include jaw surgery such as mandible distraction osteogenesis, and staged microtia reconstruction.

Treacher Collins syndrome

Treacher Collins syndrome (TCS) is an autosomal dominant condition of variable phenotypic expression, caused by mutations in the TCOF1 gene. The incidence ranges from 1 in 25 000 to 1 in 50 000 live births (66). The primary issue is hypoplasia of the zygomatico-maxillary complex including the lateral orbits, resulting in a downward sloping lateral canthi with coloboma or hypoplasia. Additionally, there is bilateral symmetric otomanidbular hypoplastic anomalies, resulting in different degrees of microtia, temporomandibular joint dysfunction, and micrognathia that can lead to glossoptosis and airway obstruction that requires mandible distraction osteogenesis. The combination of midface and mandibular hypoplasia leads to a unique craniofacial phenotype that has been described as a bird-like face.

Pierre Robin sequence

Pierre Robin sequence, or Robin sequence (RS), is classified as a sequence, as only approximately 25% of patients are syndromic. The RS is defined by the triad of mandibular micrognathia, glossoptosis, and airway obstruction. Frequently, there is also an associated wide u-shaped cleft palate only of the secondary palate (Veau II with intact alveolus). The sequence is thought to originate with the hypoplastic mandible, leading to posterior displacement of the tongue and glossoptosis, resulting in obstruction of the airway by the base of the tongue (67). It is critical to have a wide armamentarium of anesthetic approaches for intubation of these children, as these are some of the most difficult airways to secure. For patients with prolonged intubation, extubation should be in the ICU or OR setting with adequate personnel, in case the airway needs to be resecured urgently.

Nearly half of these patients can be initially treated nonsurgically by placing the patient in a nonsupine position during sleeping and eating to avoid supine-dependent glossoptosis. A nasal trumpet may be used to provide air passage past the root of the tongue. Many of these nonsurgical patients will have eventual mandibular catch-up growth around 6 to 9 months of age (68). The primary symptoms that are indications for surgery are: airway obstruction that cannot be maintained at room air, inability to feed given the airway obstruction, or lack of weight gain likely due to wasting calories during severe obstructive sleep apnea. The surgical treatment involves ensuring that the surgical disease is due to tongue-base collapse, and not due to any etiology other than the tongue: neurologic diseases that are associated with loss of tone, or primary airway diseases such as laryngomalacia or tracheomalacia. These diagnoses require a multidisciplinary approach with services such as neurology, sleep medicine, otolaryngology, and pulmonary medicine. Although nontongue etiologies are uncommon, it is critical to diagnosis these as treatment would then be tracheostomy with its concomitant morbidities, including social costs of home care. Much more commonly, the primary issue is tongue-base collapse, and the plastic surgery team can perform surgery on the tongue or mandible to move the tongue forward to restore the airway and normal development of the child (69).

Craniofacial surgery of midface and jaws

Midface advancement procedures

Midface hypoplasia can be corrected with midface advancement procedures, usually performed with distraction osteogenesis to reliably achieve significant anterior advancement. These procedures carry with them risks of blood loss requiring transfusions from the multiple osteotomy sites, risks of airway swelling requiring prolonged postoperative intubation, injury to the globes, and in intracranial approaches there are risks to the dura. A Le Fort III advancement is subcranial, with frontozygomatic osteotomies at the lateral orbital rim extending across the entire orbital floor and frontonasal junction, across the zygomatic arches, and down through the pterygomaxillary junction to section off the entire maxilla and zygoma and infraorbital rims as a single unit (70). The monobloc advancement can be thought of as a Le Fort III segment joined to a fronto-orbital bandeau as a single unit, and therefore requires neurosurgical craniotomies for exposure (71). A bipartition procedure can be thought of as a monobloc divided down the center with removal of midline bone to additionally correct hypertelorism (58). These midface advancement procedures require bicoronal scalp incision to expose the orbits and zygoma. For the Le Fort III, the osteotomies can be performed through this incision. In monobloc procedure, neurosurgical frontal craniotomies expose the supraorbital rim from above, allowing the plastic surgeon to create the monobloc osteotomies. Pressure on the globes may cause oculocardiac reflex with increased vagal tone, and must be communicated with the anesthesia team. An upper buccal sulcus intraoral incision may be used to finish the maxillary osteotomies. Once the osteotomies are confirmed, internal hardware distractors are placed, or the incisions are first closed and external halo distractor is placed. There may be significant swelling that may necessitate maintaining intubation and mechanical ventilation postoperatively.

Skull reconstruction

Skull defects may result from trauma, infection, or previous surgery. The gold standard for reconstruction is autologous bone grafts from the calvarium, ribs, or iliac crest (15,16). The anesthesia risks are similar to craniosynostosis reconstruction discussed above. After exposure of the skull, bone graft is harvested. Small pieces of bone graft can be harvested via split-thickness calvarial osteotomies. For larger pieces of bone graft, neurosurgical craniectomies may be needed for full-thickness bone. Particulate bone graft between resorbable plates can also reconstruct bony calvarial defects. Regardless of technique used, the risks of blood transfusion, injury to dura, and air embolism need to be monitored.

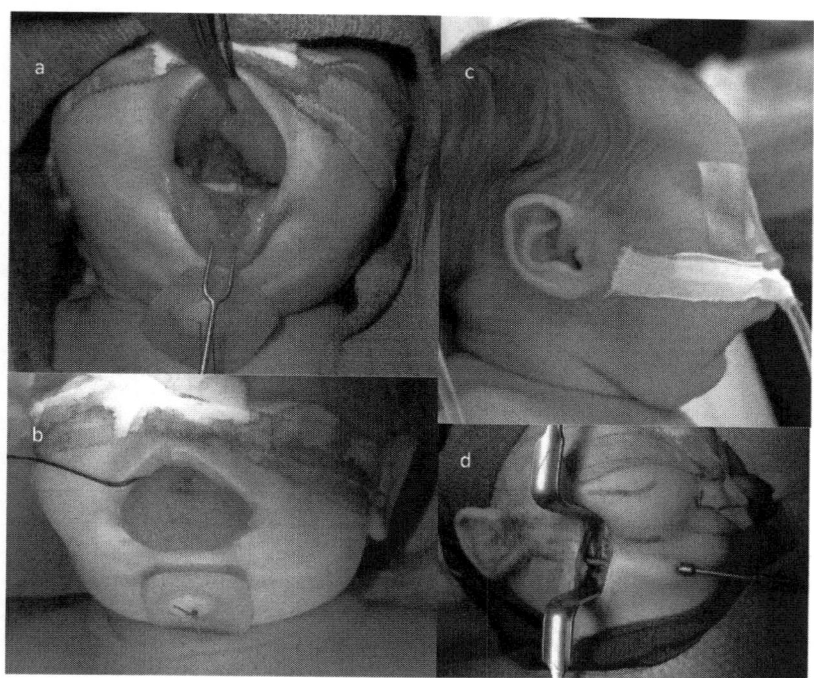

Figure 19.4 Pierre Robin sequence, nonsyndromic: **(a)** intraoperative tongue–lip adhesion: **(a)** exposed tongue and lower lip musculature with pull through button in place, and **(b)** at the end of procedure; **(c)** shows mandibular micrognathia, **(d)** shows intraoperative view of mandible distractor hardware being tested after placement; note anteriorly directed activating rods for distraction osteogenesis.

Tongue-lip adhesion (TLA)

This procedure attaches the anterior tongue to the lower lip to reduce glossoptosis (69). It is usually performed with nasotracheal intubation to allow complete access to the tongue without risk of extubation. The bed may remain unturned, to allow the anesthesia team close access to the airway. The plastic surgeon raises flaps on the ventral surface of the tongue and the inside of the lower lip, to secure the intrinsic tongue musculature to the orbicularis oris muscle of the lip. Given the risk of dehiscence from the strength of the tongue, this muscular adhesion is usually reinforced with a button at the base of the tongue sewn to the mandible or a second button below the chin (Figure 19.4a, b). Most protocols keep the patient intubated postoperatively for several days to reduce the risk of dehiscence, and therefore a nasogastric feeding tube is usually placed intraoperatively. After extubation, the button may be left in place longer to allow further healing. The patients usually breathe and feed better after TLA, which buys time for the mandible to catch up in growth.

Mandible distraction osteogenesis (MDO)

Some Robin sequence patients do not exhibit catch-up mandibular growth, or have such severe glossoptosis or micrognathia that they need early mandibular distraction osteogenesis (MDO) (72). In addition, MDO can be used in symptomatic Treacher Collins or craniofacial microsomia. This procedure advances the mandible forward, which also brings the tongue anteriorly, and can rapidly solve the pathoanatomy of RS. The MDO is performed with nasotracheal intubation. The bed may remain unturned to allow the anesthesia team close access to the airway. The MDO can be with external hardware (via intraoral incisions), or with internal hardware placement (via extraoral submandibular skin incisions). The submandibular incision approach requires nerve monitoring for the marginal mandibular nerve, and therefore paralytics should be avoided. Depending on the severity of the preoperative symptoms, the patients may remain intubated postoperatively, until enough distraction has proceeded, before they are extubated (Figure 19.4b).

Craniomaxillofacial trauma

Craniomaxillofacial trauma has slightly decreased in incidence with the advent of improved automobile safety with seatbelts and airbags. Facial trauma is still common, and, as in all trauma, securing the airway is of paramount priority. More commonly, the airway is secured for decreased sensorium. Less frequently is direct airway obstruction from panfacial fractures, foreign bodies, swelling, or massive hemorrhage, all of which may need emergent surgical airway. Rarely there is severe enough bleeding in the parapharyngeal spaces that require nasal packing, balloon catheter tamponade, or interventional radiology embolization. Brain and cervical spine injury must be ruled out before focusing on the treatment of the fractures and soft tissue (16).

Craniomaxillofacial fractures can be roughly categorized to the following bony structures: frontal sinus, orbital walls, orbital floor and zygomaticomaxillary complex, naso-orbito-ethmoid (NOE) region, maxilla and palate, mandible and dentoalveolus. The key access incisions for these fractures are bicoronal scalp incisions, periorbital incisions, facial incisions, and intraoral incisions (16). Soft tissue reconstruction is discussed in later sections.

The principal differences between children and adults is that children have more pliable bone with potential growth, lack frontal and maxillary sinuses, and their jaws are filled with teeth. This latter principle impedes the liberal use of plates and screws for fracture fixation, as the hardware may damage the unerupted adult tooth buds. Depending on the age of the child, wire fixation may be appropriate, or resorbable plates and screws (73). A brief period of maxillomandibular fixation (MMF), where the jaws are wired shut with wires or elastics, is commonly used to reduce hardware burden, and therefore nasotracheal intubation is usually necessary for fractures involving the jaws.

Once the airway is secured, the bed is usually turned to allow full access to the plastic surgery team. Frontal sinus and NOE fractures frequently require bicoronal incision for exposure. Orbital reconstruction requires eyebrow or eyelid incisions to expose the orbital walls and floor, with risks of globe pressure that may trigger the oculocardiac reflex. Jaw fractures can usually be accessed through intraoral buccal sulcus incisions or external facial incisions. The fractures are reduced and fixated, and MMF may be necessary. Except in the worst panfacial fractures, most patients are extubated, even with MMF.

Orthognathic surgery

Orthognathic surgery is the alignment of the lower two-thirds of the face involving the maxilla, mandible, and chin (74). The maxilla can be moved forward or backward with Le Fort I osteotomies. The mandible can be advanced with bilateral sagittal split osteotomies (BSSO), or reduced with BSSO or vertical reduction osteotomies. Genioplasty can be performed to reduce or advance the chin for normal facial harmony. Restoring occlusion is a key principle, and therefore intraoperative or postoperative MMF via nasotracheal intubation is necessary. Positioning requires shoulder roll and the bed turned. Maxillary and mandibular osteotomies can have significant bone bleeding that may benefit from arterial line placement and blood loss monitoring or permissive hypotension, although actual transfusions are uncommon as patients are usually larger teenagers. An MMF is sometimes required postoperatively, and patients can usually be extubated at the end.

Anesthetic principles in craniofacial reconstruction

Craniosynostosis reconstruction involves reconstruction of the skull and orbits. Ideally, this operation is usually performed in early childhood before 12 months of age to prevent growth restriction of the rapidly growing brain, and to take advantage of the rapid calvarial bone regeneration in this age group. Given the nadir in hemoglobin production that occurs in this age group, cranial reconstruction places the patient at significant risk of the complications associated with major blood loss. Due to the high vascularity of the scalp and bone, blood loss can be rapid and insidious. Constant communication between the anesthesia team and surgical team is absolutely essential, especially with regards to periods of anticipated blood loss.

Adequate vascular access is critical. The patients require at least two large-bore peripheral catheters for fluid resuscitation. An arterial catheter is needed for blood pressure monitoring and as a sampling line for blood work (74). During the neurosurgical craniotomies, there is risk of dural tear and venous air embolism. Air embolism can occur if the head is elevated above the level of the heart as occurs with the seal or sphinx position because the cut surfaces of the cranium and exposed sinuses can entrain air. Monitoring for air embolism is essential. A precordial Doppler positioned over the right atrium is used for detection of large volumes of air that present as muffled heart sounds or the classic mill-wheel murmur. Maintenance of a stable air–oxygen mixture is required since end-tidal CO_2 is monitored for declines in values and is a sensitive indicator of the presence of an air embolus. Paralytics are necessary to reduce the chance of Valsalva or unplanned movement. If an air embolus is suspected, then the surgical field must be flooded and covered, the patient placed in Trendelenburg position with the right side up (i.e., left lateral decubitus position). This may be helpful in displacing the air bubble to allow flow into the ventricle. Air aspiration from a central line has been described but this practice is of limited success (75). The use of central venous pressure monitoring in managing hypotension has been suggested as a standard of care; however, the utility of this practice is questioned since studies show that the presence of a CVP catheter did not prevent or shorten the duration of hypotensive events (74). A Foley catheter is needed to assess renal perfusion via quantity and quality of urine output.

Hemorrhage can occur in an occult fashion at several sites including scalp, open bone edges, and hidden, unsuspected pooling of blood in the drapes. In addition, cranial vault expansion usually requires extensive osteotomies to increase skull volume, and therefore contains more surface area of bleeding bone edges than most other neurosurgical or otolaryngologic procedures. Stricker *et al.* found the mean blood loss to be 1.4 blood volumes in 36 subjects studied (74). Hence, cross-matched blood has to be available and ready in the room prior to major reconstruction procedures for potential transfusion, especially prior to craniotomies.

Upon reinfusion, stored red blood cells (RBCs) need to function properly in delivering oxygen to the tissues. The loss of 2,3-disphosphoglycerate (2,3-DPG) during storage results in an increase in oxygen affinity that may compromise the ability of the stored erythrocytes to deliver oxygen to the tissues. After reinfusion the RBC 2,3-DPG level returns to half-normal in 4 hours, and to normal in 24 hours. Our institutional policy is to use banked PRBCs that have been stored less than 7 days because the (1) oxygenating capacity will be better, and (2) the potential for hyperkalemia is lessened since massive transfusion may be necessary. Potassium levels have been documented to reach 50 meq/l in stored blood by Day 30 (76). Avoidance of acidosis, hypotension, and hypoxia are essential since any of these three states can trigger fibrinolysis and coagulopathy.

Trauma guidelines for massive transfusion have suggested from 1:1 to 1:2.4 volumes of fresh frozen plasma to packed red blood cells and $>$ 1:2 platelets to PRBCs in an attempt to limit the occurrence of a dilutional coagulopathy. These blood replacement schema are usually instituted once losses equal or exceed 0.5 total blood volumes. Permissive hypotension or hypotensive resuscitation is a technique where fewer fluids or blood is used in the early period of hemorrhage, although enough crystalloid is given to maintain mean pressures within the autoregulatory curve. Additionally, the use of albumin may cause temporary derangement of laboratory values. Transfusion rates may be potentially decreased by utilizing permissive hypotension, a cell saver, preoperative administration of erythropoietin, or intraoperative antifibrinolytics such as tranexamic acid or epsilon-aminocaproic acid (77). Each of the aforementioned techniques or products has its unique risks and benefits.

Summary

Plastic and cleft–craniofacial surgery move tissues while maintaining blood supply to treat anomalies that affect human interaction: appearance, speech, and hands. Many of the oral and maxillomandibular facial procedures place the patient at risk of airway compromise. Reconstruction procedures require extensive osteotomies with potential blood loss and swift changes in hemodynamic stability, and therefore constant communication between the anesthesia team and plastic surgery team is essential. This is especially critical in the pediatric patient, as their airway and blood volume are more limited.

References

1. Lin AY, Losee JE. Pediatric plastic surgery. In Zitelli BJ, McIntire S, Nowalk AJ, editors. *Zitelli and Davis' Atlas of Pediatric Physical Diagnosis*. 6th edn. Philadelphia, PA: Saunders/Elsevier; 2012, pp. 889–919.
2. Habal MB. Improving the quality of life of patients through pediatric plastic and craniofacial surgery. *J Craniofac Surg* 2013; **24**(1): 21–7.
3. Wong KW, Forest CR, Goodacre TE, Klassen AF. Measuring outcomes in craniofacial and pediatric plastic surgery. *Clin Plastic Surg* 2013; **40**(2): 305–12.
4. Klassen AF, Stotland MA, Skarsgard ED, Pusic AL. Clinical research in pediatric plastic surgery and systematic review of quality-of-life questionnaires. *Clin Plastic Surg* 2008; **35**(2): 251–67.

5. Jacob G, Robison JG, Otteson TD. Increased prevalence of obstructive sleep apnea in patients with cleft palate. *Arch Otolaryngol Head Neck Surg* 2011; **137**(3): 269–74.
6. Hallock GG, Morris SF. Skin grafts and local flaps. *Plastic Reconstr Surg* 2011; **127**(1): 5e–22e.
7. Sadove AM, Eppley BL. Major craniomaxillofacial reconstruction aided by microsurgical tissue transfer. *J Craniofac Surg* 1990; **1**(2): 77–87.
8. Mathes SJ, Nahai F. *Reconstructive Surgery: Principles, Anatomy & Technique*. New York, St Louis: Churchill Livingstone, Quality Medical Publishing; 1997.
9. Glotzbach JP, Levi B, Wong VW, Longaker MT, Gurtner GC. The basic science of vascular biology: implications for the practicing surgeon. *Plastic Reconstr Surg* 2010; **126**(5): 1528–38.
10. Kaufman J, Laschat M, Hellmich M, Wappler F. A randomized controlled comparison of the BonfilsÂ fiberscope and the GlideScope Cobalt AVL video laryngoscope for visualization of the larynx and intubation of the trachea in infants and small children with normal airways. *Pediatr Anesth* 2013; **23**: 913–19.
11. Christophel JJ, Gross CW. Pediatric septoplasty. *Otolaryngol Clin North Am* 2009; **42**(2): 287–94, ix.
12. van der Heijden P, Korsten-Meijer AG, van der Laan BF, Wit HP, Goorhuis-Brouwer SM. Nasal growth and maturation age in adolescents: a systematic review. *Arch Otolaryngol Head Neck Surg* 2008; **134**(12): 1288–93.
13. Smartt JM, Low DW, Bartlett SP. The pediatric mandible: I. A primer on growth and development. *Plastic Reconstr Surg* 2005; **116**(1): 14e–23e.
14. Gorlin RJ. Fibroblast growth factors, their receptors and receptor disorders. *J Cranio-maxillo-facial Surg* 1997; **25**(2): 69–79.
15. Losee JE, Afifi A, Jiang S, Smith D, *et al.* Pediatric orbital fractures: Classification, management and early follow-up. *Plastic Reconstr Surg* 2008; **122**(3): 886–97.
16. Losee JE, Jiang S. Craniofacial fractures. In Bentz M, Bauer B, Zuker R, editors. *Principles and Practice of Pediatric Plastic Surgery*. 2nd edn. St. Louis, MO: Quality Medical Publishing; 2008, pp. 1047–72.
17. Gasparini G, Di Rocco C, Saponaro G, *et al.* Evaluation of obstructive sleep apnea in pediatric patients with facio-craniostenosis: A brief communication. *Child's Nervous System [Internet]*. 201210.1007/s00381-012-1821-x. [cited 2013 Oct 31] Available from: http://link.springer.com.ezp.slu.edi/article/10.1007%2Fs00381-012-1821-x/fulltext.html.
18. Brent B. Microtia repair with rib cartilage grafts: a review of personal experience with 1000 cases. *Clin Plastic Surg* 2002; **29**(2): 257–71, vii.
19. Christophel JJ, Gross CW. Pediatric septoplasty. *Otolaryngol Clin North Am* 2009; **42**(2): 287–94, ix.
20. Lawrence R. Pediatric septoplasty: a review of the literature. *Int J Pediatr Otolaryngol* 2012; **76**(8): 1078–81.
21. Westreich R, Sampson I, Shari CM, Lawson W. Negative-pressure pulmonary edema after routine septorhinoplasty: discussion of pathophysiology, treatment, and prevention. *Arch Facial Plast Surg* 2006; **8**(1): 8–15.
22. Campbell RM, Jr. Operative treatment of fractures and dislocations of the hand and wrist region in children. *Orthop Clin North Am* 1990; **21**(2): 217–43.
23. Corley FG, Jr., Schenck RC, Jr. Fractures of the hand. *Clin Plast Surg* 1996; **23**(3): 447–62.
24. Strauch B, Goldberg N, Herman CK. Sural nerve harvest: anatomy and technique. *J Reconstr Microsurg* 2005; **21**(2): 133–6.
25. Kaufman Y, Cole P, Hollier L. Peripheral nerve injuries of the pediatric hand: issues in diagnosis and management. *J Craniofac Surg* 2009; **20**(4): 1011–15.
26. Chapman KL, Hardin-Jones MA, Goldsten JA, *et al.* Timing of palatal surgery and speech outcome. *Cleft Palate Craniofac J* 2008; **45**(3): 297–308.
27. Sloan GM. Posterior pharyngeal flap and sphincter pharyngoplasty: the state of the art. *Cleft Palate Craniofac J* 2000; **37**(2): 112–22.
28. Swanson AB. A classification for congenital limb malformations. *J Hand Surg* 1976; **1**: 8–22.
29. Netscher DT, Baumholtz MA. Treatment of congenital upper extremity problems. *Plast Reconstr Surg* 2007 **199**(5): 101e–129e.
30. Unal C, Ozdemir J, Hasdemir M. Clinical application of distal ulnar artery perforator flap in hand trauma. *J Reconstr Microsurg* 2011; **27**(9): 559–65.
31. Marsh JL. Management of velopharyngeal dysfunction: differential diagnosis for differential management. *J Craniofac Surg* 2003; **14**(5): 621–8.
32. Daw JL, Jr., Patel PK. Management of alveolar clefts. *Clin Plastic Surg* 2004; **31**(2): 303–13.
33. Dowling PA, Espeland L, Sandvik L, Mobarak KA, Hogevold HE. LeFort 1 maxillary advancement: 3-year stability and risk factors for relapse. *Am J Orthod Dentofacial Orthop* 2005; **128**(5): 560–7; quiz 669.
34. Baek SH, Â Lee JK, Lee JH, Kim MJ, Kim JR. Comparison of treatment outcome and stability between distraction osteogenesis

and LeFort I osteotomy in cleft patients with maxillary hypoplasia. *J Craniofac Surg* 2007; **18**(5): 1209–15.

35. Campbell RM, Jr. Operative treatment of fractures and dislocations of the hand and wrist region in children. *Orthop Clin North Am* 1990; **21**(2): 217–43.

36. Corley FG, Jr., Schenck RC, Jr. Fractures of the hand. *Clin Plastic Surg* 1996; **23**(3): 447–62.

37. Gold NB, Westgate MN, Holmes LB. Anatomic and etiological classification of congenital limb deficiencies. *Am J Med Genet* 2011; Part A. **155A**(6): 1225–35.

38. Netscher DT, Baumholtz MA. Treatment of congenital upper extremity problems. *Plast Reconstr Surg* 2007; **199**(5): 101e–129e.

39. Limme M. [Physiology of craniofacial development]. [Article in French] *Acta Otorhinolaryngol Belg* 1993; **47**(2): 93–101.

40. Boutros S, Shetye PD, Ghali S, *et al.* Morphology and growth of the mandible in Crouzon, Apert, and Pfeiffer syndromes. *J Craniofac Surg* 2007; **18** (1): 146–50.

41. NIH. NIDCR Source: The Centers for Diseases Control and Prevention (CDC) National Birth Defects Prevention Network (NBDPN). 2004 to 2006 cleft lip and palate data collected from 14 states. This page last updated: July 18, 2013.

42. Okada H, Gosain AK. Current approaches to management of nonsyndromic craniosynostosis. *Curr Opin Otolaryngol Head Neck Surg* 2012; **20**: 310–17.

43. Ocampo RV, Jr., Persing JA. Sagittal synostosis. *Clin Plastic Surg* 1994; **21**(4): 563–74.

44. Posnick JC. Unilateral coronal synostosis (anterior plagiocephaly): current clinical perspectives. *Ann Plastic Surg* 1996; **36**(4): 430–47.

45. Boyadjiev SA. Genetic analysis of non-syndromic craniosynostosis. International Craniosynostosis Consortium. *Orthod Craniofac Res* 2007; **10**(3): 129–37.

46. Fearon JA. Rare craniofacial clefts: A surgical classification. *J Craniofac Surg* 2008; **19**(1): 110–12.

47. Caprioglio A, Zucconi M, Calori G, Troiani V. Habitual snoring, OSA and craniofacial modification. Orthodontic clinical and diagnostic aspects in a case control study. *Minerva Stomatol* 1999; **48**(4): 125–37.

48. Venkatesh R. Syndromes and anomalies associated with cleft. *Indian J Plast Surg* 2009 October; **42**(Suppl): S51–S55.

49. Okada H, Gosain AK. Current approaches to management of nonsyndromic craniosynostosis. *Curr Opin Otolaryngol Head Neck Surg* 2012; **20**: 310–17.

50. Eley KA, Johnson D, Wilkie AOM, *et al.* Raised intracranial pressure is frequent in untreated nonsyndromic unicoronal synostosis and does not correlate with severity of phenotypic features. *Plast Reconstr Surg* 2009; **130**(5): 690e–697e.

51. Lunardi S, Forli F, Michelucci A, *et al.* Genetic hearing loss associated with craniofacial abnormalities. Sadaf Naz (ed.) *InTech*, Available from: http://www.intechopen.com/books/hearing-loss/genetic-loss-associated-with-craniofacial-abnormalities. Published online March 28, 2012.

52. Kreiborg S, Cohen MM. Ocular manifestations of Apert and Crouzon syndromes: Qualitative and quantitative findings. *J Craniofac Surg* 2010; **21**(5): 1354–7.

53. Bannik N, JoostenÂ KF, van Veelen NLC, *et al.* Papilledema in patients with Apert, Crouzon and Pfeiffer syndrome: Prevelance, efficacy of treatment, and risk factors. *J Craniofac Surg* 2008; **19** (1): 121–7.

54. Ricci D, Vasco G, Baranello G, Salerni A, *et al.* Visual function in infants with non-syndromic craniosynostosis. *Dev Med Child Neurol* 2007; **49**: 574–6.

55. Boyadjiev SA. Genetic analysis of non-syndromic craniosynostosis. International Craniosynostosis Consortium. *Orthod Craniofac Res* 2007; **10**(3): 129–37.

56. Ocampo RV, Jr., Persing JA. Sagittal synostosis. *Clin Plastic Surg* 1994; **21**(4): 563–74.

57. Posnick JC. Unilateral coronal synostosis (anterior plagiocephaly): current clinical perspectives. *Ann Plastic Surg* 1996; **36**(4): 430–47.

58. Greig AV, Britto JA, Abela C, *et al.* Correcting the typical Apert face: combining bipartition with monobloc distraction. *Plastic Reconstr Surg* 2013; **131**(2): 219e–230e.

59. Carinci F, Pezzetti F, Locci P, *et al.* Apert and Crouzon syndromes: Clinical findings, genes and extracellular matrix. *J Craniofac Surg* 2005; **16**(3): 361–8.

60. Stavropoulos D, Tarnow P, Mohlin B, Kahnberg KE, Hagberg C. Comparing patients with Apert and Crouzon syndromes – clinical features and cranio-maxillofacial surgical reconstruction. *Swed Dent J* 2012; **36**(1): 25–34.

61. Tanwar R, Iyengar AR, Nagesh KS, Subhash BV. Crouzon syndrome: A case report with review of literature. *J Indian Soc Pedod Prev Dent* 2013; **31**(2): 118–20.

62. Wilkie AO, Slaney SF, Oldridge M, *et al.* Apert syndrome results from localized mutations of FGFR2 and is allelic with Crouzon syndrome. *Nat Genet* 1995; **9**: 165–72.

63. Anderson PJ, Evans RD, Harkness WJ, Hayward RD, Jones BM. The cervical spine in

Crouzon syndrome. *Spine* 1997; **22**: 402–5.

64. *Am J Med Genet A*. 2012 Nov;158A(11):2797–806. doi: 10.1002/ajmg.a.35598. Epub 2012 Sep 17. Central nervous system malformations and deformations in FGFR2-related craniosynostosis.
65. Vinay C, Reddy RS, Uloopi KS, Madhuri V, Sekhar RC. Craniofacial features in Goldenhar syndrome. *J Indian Soc Pedod Prev Dent* 2009; **27**(2): 121–4.
66. Posner JC, Ruiz RL. Treacher Collins syndrome: Current evaluation, treatment, and future directions. *Cleft Palate Craniofac J* 2000; **37**(5): 483.
67. Schaefer RB, Gosain AK. Airway management in patients with isolated Pierre Robin sequence during the first year of life. *J Craniofac Surg* 2003; **14**(4): 462–7.
68. Schaefer RB, Stadler JA, 3rd, Gosain AK. To distract or not to distract: an algorithm for airway management in isolated Pierre Robin sequence. *Plast Reconstr Surg* 2004; **113**(4): 1113–25.
69. Argamaso RV. Glossopexy for upper airway obstruction in Robin sequence. *Cleft Palate Craniofac J* 1992; **29**(3): 232–8.
70. Nout E, Cesteleyn LL, van der Wal KG, *et al.* Advancement of the midface, from conventional Le Fort III osteotomy to Le Fort III distraction: review of the literature. *Int J Oral Maxillofac Surg* 2008; **37**(9): 781–9.
71. Bradley JP, Gabbay JS, Taub PJ, *et al.* Monobloc advancement by distraction osteogenesis decreases morbidity and relapse. *Plast Reconstr Surg* 2006; **118**(7): 1585–97.
72. Polley JW, Figueroa AA. Distraction osteogenesis: its application in severe mandibular deformities in hemifacial microsomia. *J Craniofac Surg* 1997; **8**(5): 422–30.
73. Smith DM, Bykowski MR, Cray JJ, *et al.* 215 mandible fractures in 120 children: demographics, treatment, outcomes and early growth data. *Plast Reconstr Surg* 2013; **131**(6): 1348–58.
74. Stricker PA, Lin EA, Fiadjoe JE, *et al.* Evaluation of central venous pressure monitoring in children undergoing craniofacial reconstruction surgery. *Anesth Analg* 2013; **116**(2): 411–19.
75. Emby DJ, Ho K. Air embolus revisited – a diagnostic and interventional radiological perspective (bubble trouble and the dynamic Mercedes Benz sign). *SA J Radiol* 2006; **10**: 3–7.
76. Adias TC, Moore-Igwe B, Jeremiah ZA. Storage-related haematological and biochemical changes of CPDA-1 whole blood in a resource-limited setting. *J Blood Disord Transf* 2012; **3**: 124.
77. Stricker PA, Zuppa AF, Fiadjoe JE, *et al.* Population pharmacokinetics of epsilon-aminocaproic acid in infants undergoing craniofacial reconstruction surgery. *BJA* 2013; **110**(5): 788–99.

Chapter

20 Pediatric ophthalmology

Amit Prabhakar, Adam J. Broussard, Charles James Fox, Ofer N. Eytan, and Alan David Kaye

Introduction

Ophthalmology pertains to the study of the anatomy, physiology, pathology, and treatment of the eye. Vision is an integral mammalian sense that has allowed for evolutionary survival and progression. The eyes are used to aggregate a large amount of information from our environment and process that information for the brain and body to use. The eye relies on numerous complex physiologic processes and intricate anatomic supporting structures that work synergistically for optimal performance. However, this complexity also yields the eye and its supporting structures to be vulnerable to a wide array of pathology. Pathology of the eye can be narrowed down and categorized as chronological diseases that are more predominant in certain age groups. As such, the pediatric population is subject to a unique set of disorders distinct from adult ophthalmologic pathology. This chapter will review the anatomy, physiology, pharmacology, and pathology pertinent to the pediatric population.

General considerations

Anatomy and physiology

The eye is an embryological extension of the central nervous system originating from various aspects of the ectoderm, neural crest cells, and mesoderm (1). The developed eye can be divided into three distinct anatomical compartments known as the anterior, posterior, and vitreous chambers. Each chamber uses complex physiologic mechanisms to maintain its own unique microenvironment essential for proper functionality.

Anterior chamber

The anterior chamber includes the space between the cornea and iris diaphragm. The primary purpose of the structures in the anterior eye are to form an image that the posterior eye can understand and process. The cornea is the transparent, avascular outer layer of the eye. It is composed of five distinct layers of cells and fibrous tissue (2). The stroma is made up of evenly spaced collagen fibrils and accounts for up to 90% of the total cornea (3). The stroma is then lined with epithelial and basement membranes anteriorly and posteriorly respectively. These membranes are essential to maintain a hydration balance that also plays a role in corneal transparency (3). Transparency of the cornea is lost at the limbus, which is the junction between the cornea and the opaque sclera (2).

The iris is visible through the cornea and is responsible for eye color. Its main functions are to control pupillary size and limit excess light from reaching the lens (4). Pupillary constriction and dilation are controlled by two key muscles, the iris sphincter and dilator pupillae muscles respectively. The iris sphincter is controlled by the parasympathetic nervous system. The dilator pupillae muscles are controlled by the sympathetic nervous system (4). The ciliary body is attached to the iris anteriorly. The ciliary muscle is a smooth muscle with both longitudinal and circular fibers which contribute to altering the shape of the lens via nonelastic microfibrils, also known as zonules (2).

The lens is composed of 65% water and 35% protein (2). Similar to the cornea, it is both avascular and transparent. Transparency of the lens is maintained by a network of regularly arranged cell fibers which continue to grow throughout life. The lens is surrounded and anchored by an elastic extracellular matrix known as the capsule. As mentioned previously, the lens has the ability to change shape via the zonules of the ciliary body. This ability allows for adjustments in refractory power.

Essentials of Pediatric Anesthesiology, ed. Alan David Kaye, Charles James Fox and James H. Diaz. Published by Cambridge University Press. © Cambridge University Press 2015.

The anterior chamber is bathed by a fluid called the aqueous humour. This fluid is a clear solution of electrolytes formed by active secretion and ultrafiltration from the ciliary body in the posterior chambers (2). It serves two primary purposes. First, it is used to provide the cornea with nutrients. Secondly, it serves a key role in the optical pathway by providing refraction.

Vitreous chamber

The vitreous chamber consists of the space between the anterior eye and the retina. It is composed of a three-dimensional network of collagen fibrils and hyaluronic acid molecules that form a gel-like substance (5). These molecules of hyaluronic acid are capable of holding large quantities of water. This chamber primarily serves to ensure proper propagation of light and protect the retina.

Posterior chamber

The posterior chamber includes the space between the iris anteriorly, the lens and zonule posteriorly, and the ciliary body. This chamber is also known as the neurosensory layer because it is comprised of the photoreceptors responsible for transduction, or the conversion of light into electrical energy (2,5). The retina is a complex structure of ten layers of photoreceptors and supporting structures. The outermost layer is the retinal pigment epithelium (RPE). This layer is made of opaque cells which help to reduce light scattering. The RPE also provides metabolic support for the photoreceptors via the regeneration and recycling of photopigments. This process helps the eye to adjust to varying levels of light and darkness. The two main types of photoreceptors found in the retina are the rods and cones. Cones are primarily located in the fovea centralis and are responsible for fine details and color perception. Rods are more prevalent peripherally and are responsible for peripheral vision and vision in low light (6).

Accommodation

The eye is able to adjust rapidly to objects at different distances via the process of accommodation. This process is accomplished by alterations in the refractory power of the lens, which is controlled by ciliary muscle contraction and relaxation. Ciliary muscle contraction relaxes the zonule fibers resulting in a more globular shape of the lens and a increase in refractory power. Ciliary muscle relaxation results in taut zonule fibers, flattening of the lens, and a decrease in refractory power (2).

Blood supply

The blood supply of the eye originates from the ophthalmic artery, a direct branch of the internal carotid artery. The ophthalmic artery then gives off three branches: the central retinal artery, the anterior ciliary arteries, and the posterior ciliary arteries. These vessels then branch off into smaller vessels to provide essential nourishment.

Lacrimal gland

The lacrimal apparatus is primarily responsible for production of the tear film. The major lacrimal gland occupies the superior temporal anterior portion of the eye (2). Lacrimal gland ducts open into the palpebral conjunctiva at the upper eyelid. The tear film consists of the mucoid, aqueous, and oily layers. The mucoid layer is produced by goblet cells in the conjunctival epithelium and serves to improve the wetting properties of the tears (5). This layer rests directly on the eye. The aqueous layer is made from the lacrimal gland and has both nutritional and immunologic functions. It is composed of proteins, glucose, electrolytes, immunoglobulins, oxygen, and lysozymes. The oily layer is produced by the meibomian glands and is the most superficial. This layer helps to prevent excess evaporation. Normally, tears drain into the lacrimal sac via puncta and cannaliculi. The lacrimal sac then drains into the nasolacrimal duct which opens into the inferior meatus of the nose (5).

Extraocular muscles

Movement of the eye is facilitated by six muscles: the superior, inferior, lateral, and medial recti, and the superior and inferior oblique muscles. Contraction of the inferior, superior, medial, and lateral recti results in eye movement corresponding to their name. The superior oblique is responsible for intorsion, depression, and abduction. The inferior oblique is responsible for extorsion, elevation, and abduction. The lateral rectus is innervated by the sixth cranial nerve. The superior oblique is supplied by cranial nerve four. Cranial nerve three is responsible for innervation of the remaining muscles. With the exception of the inferior oblique, these muscles all originate from a fibrous ring called the annulus of Zinn at the orbital apex.

Basic pharmacology of the eye

The physiology and function of the eye is dictated primarily by the actions of cholinergic and adrenergic receptors. These receptors have various broad actions that are not completely understood and are still actively being investigated. Researchers have studied these targets extensively and have developed numerous pharmacological agents for the treatment of diseases. The majority of these drugs are applied topically with differing levels of absorption dependent on drug solubility.

Adrenergic receptors

Adrenergic receptors are found throughout the eye. Both alpha and beta receptors are found predominantly in the smooth muscle cells of the iris, blood vessels in the conjunctiva, ciliary processes, and aqueous outflow tract. Alpha-1 receptors in the iris mediate the contraction of the dilator pupillae muscle resulting in mydriasis (7). Administration of alpha-2 agonists also result in mydriasis. Alpha-1 stimulation has also been found to inhibit outflow of aqueous humour resulting in an increase in intraocular pressure. Alpha-2 agonists vasoconstrict the ciliary body and prevent excess production of aqueous thus reducing intraocular pressure (8). Beta-2 receptors in the ciliary body produce aqueous humour when stimulated (9). Topical beta blockers prevent the ciliary body from releasing aqueous and thus are widely used to decrease intraocular pressure (9).

Cholinergic receptors

Muscarinic receptors can also be found throughout the eye. Stimulation of cholinergic receptors act on the smooth muscle of the iris and result in miosi (10). Conversely, antagonism of these receptors results in mydriasis via action of the dilator pupillae muscles. Ciliary muscle contraction seen with muscarinic agonists has also been found to decrease intraocular pressure by opening up the trabecular meshwork and increasing outflow of the aqueous humour (10).

Oculocardiac reflex

The oculocardiac reflex (OCR) is a result of pressure or torsion of the extraocular muscles. The afferent limb is transmitted by the ophthalmic division of CN5. The efferent limb is transmitted by the vagus nerve. The reflex results in bradycardia, ectopy, or even cardiac arrest. Prophylaxis with atropine can be given to avoid or mitigate OCR.

Pathology

Enucleation

Enucleation may be required for trauma, malignancy, infection, or blind painful eye. Like other ophthalmologic procedures, special attention should be given to OCR and PONV. Blood loss can be significant but rarely requires transfusion. Postoperative pain can be significant.

Retinopathy of prematurity

Retinopathy of prematurity (ROP) is a multifactorial vasoproliferative retinopathy of preterm newborns. Risk increases with greater prematurity and lower birth weights. Hyperoxia is a major risk factor for ROP but does not cause ROP alone. Retinal vasculogenesis typically completes at 44 weeks postconception. In ROP, normal vasculogenesis stops and disordered reactive vasculogensesis and fibrous tissue formation take place in the retina and vitreous humor. This vasoproliferation can lead to scarring and retinal detachment. Retinal detachment results in visual impairment and blindness experienced by ROP patients. To prevent blindness, laser or cryotherapy is used to prevent the progression of vasculogenesis and lessen the risk of retinal detachment. Since these patients are premature neonates, all typical neonate precautions should be taken. Special attention should be given to the airway and respiratory system when preparing these patients for surgery. Since ROP is related to hyperoxia, it is likely that these patients received oxygen for a pulmonary condition. This pulmonary history must be elicited. The child may have been intubated and have airway stenosis. The delicate and precise nature of this procedure necessitates intubation and paralysis. Intraoperative oxygen saturation should be maintained between 90–95%. Neonates, especially following this procedure, are at risk of postoperative apnea and bradycardia. Close monitoring and possible prolonged intubation may be required.

Penetrating trauma

Penetrating ocular trauma can be particularly difficult cases to balance the various risks and safety of the patient. These cases are typically booked emergently.

The patients should be treated as if they have a full stomach. The patient will likely have IV access as intravenous antibiotic therapy is indicated emergently to prevent endophthalmitis. Any increase in intraocular pressure can cause prolapse of intraocular contents, worsening the injury and decreasing the chance of restoring vision. This includes crying, coughing, and straining. While premedication can help calm the patient, the risk of aspiration must be weighed. Aspiration prophylaxis can be given preoperatively. Induction must result in ideal conditions for intubation to prevent bucking, coughing, or sympathetic response to intubation. The patient must be adequately deep prior to attempting intubation. Since these children will likely have preoperative IVs, an IV induction is possible. The risk of using succinylcholine versus a nondepolarizing neuromuscular blocker must be weighed. Although succinycholine will raise IOP, it is less than the increase with bucking. Maintenance of anesthesia interoperatively can be provided with inhalational agents or propofol infusion. If deemed to be a low aspiration risk, deep extubation will decrease the rise in IOP postop. Otherwise, IV lidocaine can be given to decrease coughing and the child should be extubated awake.

Tear duct probing (dacryocystorhinostomy)

Otherwise healthy infants typically present for nasolacrimal duct probing on an outpatient basis. The surgery is normally brief and minimally stimulating. This should be taken into account prior to premedicating the child. The case can usually be performed with general mask or LMA anesthesia. The patency of the duct is confirmed by touching a second probe inserted in the nostril or by injecting fluorescein dye in the lacrimal duct and seeing it on a pipe cleaner placed in the nostril. Blood, dye, or secretions may accumulate in the oropharnyx. The patient can be placed in Trendelenburg or on a shoulder roll to prevent laryngospasms. Any secretions should be suctioned prior to lightening anesthesia.

Strabismus repair

Strabismus repair is a very common pediatric ophthalmologic procedure. Strabismus can be associated with malignant hyperthermia and myopathies, so increased attentiveness should be paid to possible signs. Although these serious conditions may be present, the majority of patients are healthy. No special testing is needed unless otherwise warranted. Minimal sedation should be use as these cases can be quite short and the surgeon may want to examine the child shortly after surgery. An IV or inhalational induction is typical. Sux should be avoided because of the association with MH and myopathies and it may interfere with forced duction during the surgery. Atropine can be given at induction or be drawn up and easily accessible in case of occulocardic reflex. As with all eye surgeries, PONV is especially increased following strabismus repair. Pharmacological pretreatment should be given intraoperatively to prevent PONV. Local anesthetic injection or eye drops and NSAID PO/PR/IV can be use to decrease opiate use. This will also decrease PONV. In addition, early PO intake and ambulation should not be forced upon the child as this will also increase nausea.

References and further reading

1. Cook CS, Sulik KK, Wright KW. Embryology. In Wright KW, Speigel PH, Thompson LS, eds. *Handbook of Pediatric Eye and Systemic Disease*. 1st edn. New York: Springer, 2006, pp. 1–61.
2. Galloway NR, Amoaku WMK, Galloway PH, Browning AC. Basic anatomy and physiology of the eye. In *Common Eye Diseases and their management*. 1st edn. London: Springer, 2006, pp. 7–15.
3. Jones LW, Jones DA. Non-inflammatory corneal complications of contact lens wear. *Contact Lens and Anterior Eye* 2001; **24**(2): 73–9.
4. Nicolas CM, Robman LD *et al.* Iris colour, ethnic origin, and progression of age-related macular degeneration. *Clinical and Experimental Ophthalmology* 2003; **31**(6): 465–9.
5. Kaufman PL, Alm A. *Adler's Physiology of the Eye*. 10th edn. St. Louis, MO: Mosby, 2003.
6. Ang LP, Ang LP. Current understanding of the treatment and outcome of acute primary angle-closure glaucoma: An Asian perspective. *Annals, Academy of Medicine, Singapore* 2008; **37**(3): 210–15.
7. Curtin DM, Buckley C. Review of alpha adrenoceptor function in the eye. *Eye* 1989; **3**: 472–6.
8. Matsuo T, Cynader MS. Localization of alpha-2 adrenergic receptors in the human eye. *Ophthalmic Research* 1992; **24**: 213–19.
9. Wax MB, Molinoff PB, Alvarado J, Polansky J. Characterization

of beta-adrenergic receptors in cultured human trabecular cells and in human trabecular meshwork. *Investigative Ophthamology and Visual Science* 1989; **30**: 51–7.

10. Nietgen GW, Schmidt J, Hesse L *et al.* Muscarinic receptor functioning and distribution in the eye: molecular basis and implications for clinical diagnosis and therapy. *Eye* 1999; **13**: 285–300.
11. Weaver RG, Tobin JR. Ophthalmology. In Cote CJ, Lerman J, Todres ID, eds. *A Practice of Anesthesia for Infants and Children*. 4th edn. Philadelphia, PA: Saunders Elsevier, 2009.
12. Lee C, Luginbuehl I, Bissonnette B, Mason LJ. Pediatric diseases. In Hines RL, Marschall KE, eds. *Stoeling's Anesthesia and Co-existing Diseases*. 5th edn. Philadelphia, PA: Churchill Livingstone, 2008.
13. Ophthalmology. In Lerman J, Cote CJ, Stewart DJ, eds. *Manual of Pediatric Anesthesia*. 6th edn. Philadelphia: Churchill Livingstone, 2010.
14. Kovatsis PG. Open globe injury repair. In Litman RS, ed. *Pediatric Anesthesia Practice*. 2nd edn. New York: Cambridge University Press, 2007.
15. Kovatsis PG. Lacrimal duct probing and irrigation. In Litman RS, ed. *Pediatric Anesthesia Practice*. 2nd edn. New York: Cambridge University Press, 2007.
16. Vanzillotta PP, Litman RS. Stabismus repair. In Litman RS, ed. *Pediatric Anesthesia Practice*. 2nd edn. New York: Cambridge University Press, 2007.

Chapter

21 Orthopedic surgery

Carl Lo, Deepa Kattail, and Dolores B. Njoku

Anesthesia for orthopedic surgery can offer distinct challenges for the pediatric anesthesiologist. In addition to the potential for life-threatening surgical blood loss or even management of tourniquet pain, the pediatric anesthesiologist may be faced with significant coexisting diseases which include but are not limited to cardiopulmonary, oncologic, or other systemic diseases.

Coexisting diseases

Cardiopulmonary disease

Managing the patient with significant cardiac disease presents a unique comorbidity when delivering anesthesia for pediatric orthopedic surgery. For example, 25% of patients with idiopathic scoliosis can also have mitral valve prolapse. Where cardiac disease usually comes into play with orthopedic surgery is when pulmonary dysfunction from restrictive lung disease promotes pulmonary hypertension. In this section we will present some of the more common patient conditions with cardiopulmonary disease that may be encountered when delivering anesthesia to pediatric patients for orthopedic surgery.

Marfan syndrome is a variable, autosomal dominant connective tissue disorder. It involves mutation in the fibrillin 1 gene on chromosome 15. Marfan syndrome patients usually present in orthopedic surgery with spine pathology such as kyphoscoliosis, spondylolisthesis, and atlantoaxial subluxation (1). Other surgical presentations include neonatal hip dislocation, protrusio acetabulae, pes planus, hand/wrist instability, and shoulder/knee instability (2). The currently accepted diagnostic tool are the Ghent criteria, which include skeletal, ocular, cardiovascular, pulmonary, and integumentary organ systems (3). A diagnosis of Marfan syndrome requires at least two major criteria in two systems and involvement of a third. Major criteria include dilation of ascending aorta, dissection of ascending aorta, lens dislocation, dural ectasia, proven mutation, family history, and > four skeletal findings (which include pectus carinatum, pectus excavatum requiring surgery, wrist and thumb signs, scoliosis > 20 degrees or spondylolisthesis, reduced elbow extension, pes plenus, and protrusion acetabulae).

Evaluation of the airway is critical in caring for patients with Marfan syndrome who require orthopedic surgery. Compared to the general population, radiographic analysis of Marfan syndrome patients shows increased atlantoaxial translation, larger odontoid height, and basilar impression. Thus the cervical bony and ligament abnormalities in these patients may place them at increased risk for atlantoaxial rotatory instability (4). Hence in clinical practice we suggest that intubation should be attempted without dramatic cervical movement to avoid injury to the spinal cord.

Evaluation of the respiratory system should include chest wall deformities as well as questioning for history of pneumothorax. A number of patients with Marfan syndrome can develop recurrent spontaneous pneumothorax that may be missed if a focused past medical history is not obtained. Additionally, while it is well known that scoliosis may also cause restrictive lung disease in these patients, scoliosis progression is much faster in Marfan syndrome patients than in the general population.

Progressive enlargement of the aorta and aortic dissection is a major cause of morbidity and potential mortality in Marfan syndrome patients. Careful preoperative evaluation must include an echocardiogram to rule out severe ascending aortic dilation, pulmonary artery dilation, aortic valve, and mitral valve

Essentials of Pediatric Anesthesiology, ed. Alan David Kaye, Charles James Fox and James H. Diaz. Published by Cambridge University Press. © Cambridge University Press 2015.

regurgitation. The risk for aortic rupture increases substantially when the diameter at sinus Valsalva exceeds 5.5 cm. Thus it is recommended that these children receive serial transthoracic echocardiography at age 6 years old, with 2 month intervals and subsequent intervals depending on aortic diameter and rate of progression. Prophylactic aortic root surgery is then recommended when the diameter of sinus Valsalva exceeds 5.5 cm in adult or 5.0 cm in children (5). Traditionally, beta-blockers are used for these patients to reduce the systolic ejection impulse and aortic dilation in order to decrease the risk of aortic dissection. Beta-blockers are shown to lower cardiac mortality, decrease need for preventive aortic surgery, and decrease the rate of aortic dissection. Thus a beta-blocker is generally continued in perioperative settings (6). Recently, the use of angiotensin II blockade therapy in Marfan syndrome has been shown to significantly slow the rate of aortic root dilation (7). However, angiotensin II blockade is not usually given on the day of surgery because of severe hypotension following induction of anesthesia seen with this class of drugs. Anesthetic evaluation should ensure beta-blocker is not discontinued preoperatively. Sudden myocardial contractility or blood pressure increase should be avoided to minimize the risk of aortic dissection. It is recommended to monitor blood pressure and heart rate stability with an arterial line, especially if the patient has pre-existing aortic root enlargement.

Increased aggressive medical and prophylactic surgical intervention has successfully reduced the morbidity and mortality associated with aortic dilation and aortic dissection. Thus, the life expectancy has increased significantly for Marfan Syndrome patients (8), making these patients likely candidates for orthopedic surgery

Congenital malformations

Many patients with congenital malformations require orthopedic surgery. Patients with cerebral palsy and Down syndrome are included in this area in addition to patients with osteogenesis imperfecta (OI) and spina bifida. In this section we will focus on OI since other syndromes will be covered in other areas.

Osteogenesis imperfecta (OI) is a genetic disorder of connective tissue that involves abnormal collagen synthesis. It inherits in an autosomal dominant pattern with sporadic mosaics, and also rarely with recessive forms. There is a wide spectrum of severity of disease. Type I patients are asymptomatic individuals with occasional fractures and normal stature. Type II involves perinatal lethality, small for gestational age, respiratory distress, limb deformities with multiple fractures. Type III is the most severe phenotype in children with short stature, multiple fractures, progressive deformities, and hearing loss (9). Other features relevant to anesthesia include restricted neck and jaw mobility, severe chest wall deformity and kyphoscoliosis that may restrict pulmonary function, cleft palate, premature atherosclerosis, and valvular heart disease. These patients often present to orthopedic surgeries for recurrent fractures or deformity that impairs function (10).

Anesthetic evaluation includes assessing risk of fractures of mandible, maxillary surface, and cervical spine during airway manipulation. Excessive extension of cervical spine may cause atlantoaxial subluxation and dislocation. Fiberoptic intubation may offer a safe method in establishing the airway in experienced hands. Appropriate use of a laryngeal mask airway may offer an alternative to endotracheal tube placement or extensive pressure applied by face mask ventilation.

Thorough cardiac evaluation is recommended, as these patients are predisposed to pulmonary insufficiency and restrictive lung disease (from kyphoscoliosis) that may lead to pulmonary hypertension and cor pulmonale. Preoperative spirometric tests and blood analysis may be helpful to demonstrate baseline pulmonary function. Platelet abnormalities may be present and patients may be on desmopressin (DDAVP) to reverse the platelet dysfunction.

Patients with OI under general anesthesia have additional unique challenges. Because of extreme bone fragility, positioning and transporting require special precautions. Meticulous padding is recommended to avoid further fractures. Frequent blood pressure cuff cycling may cause humeral fractures, therefore arterial line placement is recommended in all but extremely short surgical cases. Because venous access may be difficult in these patients, central venous access should be considered early. Succinylcholine should be avoided for two reasons: (1) lethal hyperkalemic response may occur due to up-regulation of acetylcholine receptors from denervated or immobilized body parts, (2) the potential of muscle contraction-induced fractures. Nerve stimulation can also lead to contraction-induced fractures. Lastly, OI patients may demonstrate a hypermetabolic state demonstrated by excessive diaphoresis, hyperthermia, tachycardia, and tachypnea, therefore atropine and glycopyrrolate should be used judiciously due to excessively increased body temperature (11). The routine pediatric anesthesia practice of using a warming blanket, heating the surgical room temperature, and humidified gases should be adjusted according to the patient's core temperature. However this hyperpyrexia reaction is not associated with malignant hyperthermia (12–15).

Myopathic disease

Myopathic disease is another broad category that includes but is not limited to muscular dystrophy. We will focus on muscular dystrophy since understanding of the anesthetic implications of this disease covers issues encountered by a large portion of these patients.

Muscular dystrophy: Duchenne muscular dystrophy and Becker muscular dystrophy are the most common type of muscular dystrophies. Duchenne muscular dystrophy is a rapidly progressive, X-linked recessive disease with an incidence of 1 in 3500 live male births (16). Becker muscular dystrophy is much rarer X-linked disease and demonstrates much slower progression, variable severity of symptoms, and approximate incidence is 1 in 18 000 live male births. Both diseases are caused by defects in the production of dystrophin; however, in Duchenne muscular dystrophy the dystrophin is nonfunctional while in Becker's some function of dystrophin is retained. The lack of dystrophin prevents integration of the glycoprotein complex into muscle cell membrane leading to cellular and membrane instability, with eventual increase in creatine phosphokinase (CPK). Definite diagnosis can be achieved through muscle biopsy. Clinical symptoms include muscle weakness, frequent falls, muscle contractures of Achilles tendons, pseudohypertrophy (enlargement) of tongue and calf. Most patients suffer from progressive degeneration of skeletal, cardiac, and smooth muscles. Patients develop symmetric proximal muscles weakness, gait disturbance, and in the case of Duchenne's many patients are wheelchair bound by age 12. Death may occur from recurrent pulmonary infections and cardiomyopathy.

Patients often present for orthopedic surgeries because of lower extremities joints contractures, metatarsus adductus, and rigid forefoot equinocavovarus impeding ambulation. Therefore, properly timed surgery and bracing have helped some patients to extend their ability to ambulate (17). Patients may also present for spine fusion because of progressive scoliosis. These patients are particularly challenging and should be approached in a multidisciplinary and collaborative fashion.

Anesthetic concerns include perioperative respiratory and cardiac complications. Respiratory muscle degeneration may present as retention of airway secretions due to ineffective cough. Patients with kyphoscoliosis can present with severe restrictive lung disease with pulmonary hypertension. Preoperative cardiac evaluation by pediatric cardiology is important because many of these patients have cardiac muscle involvement resulting in dilated or hypertrophic cardiomyopathy.

Succinylcholine is contraindicated for routine use due to a severe hyperkalemia response. An association with malignant hyperthermia has been suggested because of case reports of intraoperative deaths from unexplained cardiac arrests and cardiac failure. However, recent studies suggest that patients with muscular dystrophy do not have an increased risk of malignant hyperthermia (MH) compared with the general population (18). Although muscular dystrophy patients are unlikely to develop MH, exposure to volatile anesthetics may be associated with life-threatening rhabdomyolysis. Therefore, it is recommended to treat these patients like MH-susceptible patients because of possible "anesthesia induced rhabdomyolysis." The use of "trigger-free" anesthetics such as TIVA technique and "clean" anesthesia machines have emerged as popular anesthetics for muscular dystrophy patients.

Anesthesia-induced rhabdomyolysis that may develop in these patients following exposure to halogenated volatile anesthetics in itself is not without challenges. If anesthetic-induced rhabdomyolysis is suspected, serial serum potassium levels should be measured and immediately treated. Treatments include IV sodium bicarbonate, insulin with 10% dextrose, hyperventilation to shift potassium back to intracellular space, IV hydration and mannitol to prevent renal failure, and calcium chloride to antagonize the myocardial effects (19). Even so, it may be difficult to differentiate anesthesia-induced rhabdomyolysis and malignant hyperthermia. Anesthesia-induced rhabdomyolysis shows acute hyperkalemia cardiac arrest without any systemic signs of hypermetabolism such as rapid increase of end-tidal CO_2, metabolic acidosis, tachypnea, tachycardia, and fever.

Because of diminished muscle strength and weak laryngeal reflexes, these patients are also sensitive to nondepolarizing muscle relaxants. They also may be sensitive to sedative effects of pharmacologic agents utilized to induce and maintain general anesthesia. Hence, there should be a low threshold for ventilation in the postoperative period.

Neuromuscular disease

Even though neuromuscular diseases are rare, they present great challenges to anesthesiologists for diagnostic studies or surgery. With a diminished neuromuscular system, there is increased sensitivity to neuromuscular blockers that can result in postoperative respiratory failure, poor ambulation resulting in delayed recovery, and pulmonary aspiration.

Neuromuscular diseases include abnormality of any major component of the motor unit from motor neuron, neuromuscular junction, peripheral nerve, and muscle. Defects in any of the above components can result in autonomic, sensory, and motor defects. In this group we find myasthenia gravis, Lambert–Eaton myasthenic syndrome, and cerebral palsy.

Myasthenia gravis and Lambert–Eaton myasthenic syndrome are two major disorders of neuromuscular disorders. Myasthenia gravis is an autoimmune disease where IgG antibodies destroy the nicotinic acetylcholine receptor in postsynaptic neuromuscular junctions. Clinical presentation includes easy fatigability of skeletal muscle, especially after repeated use. Other symptoms range from ocular muscle weakness such as ptosis and diplopia, limb muscles weakness, bulbar symptoms with laryngeal and pharyngeal muscle weakness, and respiratory muscle weakness requiring ventilation support. The treatment of choice is pyridostigmine that indirectly increases the total amount of acetylcholine to exert its neuromuscular effect. However, with excessive amount of pyridostigmine, a cholinergic crisis may occur from excessive amounts of acetylcholine. Symptoms of cholinergic crisis include salivation, lacrimation, urination, defecation, GI dysfunction, emesis, bradycardia, and bronchoconstriction. An edrophonium (tensilon) test can differentiate between the two: if symptoms improve with edrophonium, then the most likely cause of weakness is myasthenia gravis, but if symptoms are worse, then a cholinergic crisis is the more likely culprit. Medical treatment includes anticholinesterase in mild disease. Moderate to severe disease requires a combination of anticholinesterase with corticosteroids, azathioprine, cyclosporine, and intravenous immunoglobulin (IVIG). Plasmapheresis is reserved for patients with severe respiratory compromise (20). For younger patients, including the pediatric population, clinical improvement can follow immediately after thymectomy (21).

Anesthetic concerns involve mostly respiratory status. Pulmonary aspiration risk is increased in these patients, therefore premedication with H2 blockers, metoclopramide, and sodium bicitrate is sometimes recommended. Nondepolarizing neuromuscular blockers are often avoided, as these patients are extremely sensitive. Risk factors for postoperative ventilation after surgery include disease longer than 6 years, peak inspiratory pressure of greater magnitude than -25 cm H_2O, vital capacity less than 4 ml/kg, and pyridostigmine dose greater than 750 mg/day. Infants of myasthenia gravis mothers may present with neuromuscular weakness symptoms for up to 1 month, until the effects of antiacetylcholine receptor antibodies from the mother diminish.

The Lambert–Eaton myasthenic syndrome is a paraneoplastic syndrome characterized by proximal muscles weakness that improves with repeated effort. Its pathophysiology involves antibodies against presynaptic voltage-gated calcium channels, reducing the amount of acetylcholine released to motor end plates. It typically involves malignancy, or rarely idiopathic autoimmune disease. Treatment includes corticosteroid, guanidine hydrochloride and 3,4-diaminopyridine, and plasmapheresis. Anesthetic concerns also involve increased risk of pulmonary aspiration and pulmonary insufficiency. These patients are exquisitely sensitive to both depolarizing and nondepolarizing muscular blockers (22).

Oncologic disease

Oncologic disease in children is mostly a multiorgan system diseae. In these conditions, children often present for orthopedic surgery for tumor excisions – most commonly primary bone sarcomas such as osteosarcoma, Ewing sarcoma, and chondrosarcoma (23). Careful preoperative evaluation is imperative as many of these patients are on chemotherapeutic agents that have profound anesthetic implications. Many chemotherapeutic agents have myelosuppression properties, thus anemia and thrombocytopenia can be significant. Availability of packed red blood cells and platelets is recommended. Similarly, patients can be leukopenic with white blood cell dysfunction and are at high risk for infection. Hand hygiene and a strict protocol for central line placement should be enforced to minimize procedure-related infection. Conversely, some malignancies predispose patients to polycythemia, leukocytosis, and thrombocytosis. These patients will have an increased chance for thrombus formation, emboli, hypertension, and stroke. Other side effects of chemotherapeutic agents may include cardiomyopathy by doxorubicin, pulmonary fibrosis by bleomycin, hepatotoxixity by idarubicin and methotrexate, neurotoxicity by vincristine, and nephrotoxicity by cisplatin. Patients undergoing radiation therapy may present with pericardial effusion, pericarditis, and more seriously, cardiac tamponade. Suspicion of cardiomyopathy warrants an extensive cardiac evaluation and consultation.

There is a large variability of complexity of orthopedic oncologic surgeries performed, ranging from a simple bone biopsy, to amputation, or radical hemipelvectomy requiring staging. Therefore it is important for anesthesiologists to have a good understanding of surgical involvement in order to perform proper perioperative management. Tumors are often vascular increasing the potential for large blood loss, especially if significant neovascularization has occurred. Location of metastasis is also a determination for hemorrhage. Pelvic metastases are often vascular in origin, thus preoperative embolization should be considered for a large tumor mass. Surgeries involving tumors of spine or pelvis increase the possibility of massive hemorrhage. Thorough preparation with ample blood products, adequate IV access, and arterial line monitor is essential prior to large tumor resection.

There are anesthetic techniques to minimize blood loss or blood transfusion; however, some may not be commonly used. The choice of technique to minimize blood loss and blood transfusion is patient-dependent. One technique, acute normovolemic hemodilution as an example, requires withdrawing the patient's own blood for storage and supplementing intravascular volume with crystalloid in a 3 to 1 ratio to achieve an acute normovolemic hemodilution stage. The blood withdrawn from patients is kept at room temperature, but must not be transfused back to patients longer than 8 hours after collection. Its advantage includes a reduction in the need for allogeneic transfusion, lower cost than cell saver, and minimal risk of ABO incompatibility. However this technique is inconvenient for anesthesiologists performing the procedure, and its use must be weighed against the possibility of acute anemia requiring vasopressors, as a result of hemodilution and decreased systemic vascular resistance. Another technique is preoperative autologous donation. This involves preoperative donation, up to three or more units before elective surgery. It requires the least equipment and decreases the need for allogeneic transfusion. However, anemia is usually the limiting factor, and patients can be given supplemental iron therapy between each donation. The use of cell saver has sometimes been suggested but it may be controversial in some oncologic diseases.

Some oncology patients have increased risk of hypercoagulation, thrombosis, and stroke; therefore the use of antifibrinolytics is debatable. One theory is that antifibrinolytics can cause increased thrombus formation, emboli, and stroke. Another theory suggests that the antifibrinolytics only stabilize the existing clots instead of forming new thrombosis. Multiple studies and the Cochrane database fail to demonstrate an increased incidence of postoperative thrombosis with the use of antifibrinolysis (24). Therefore, antifibrinolysis should not be withheld in cancer patients, especially if the surgery has a large potential for blood loss.

Perioperative pain management plays a significant role in patient satisfaction, early ambulation, decreased thrombosis formation, and lower stress response. Upper extremity tumor resection pain involves brachial plexus innervation. Interscalene, supraclavicular, infraclavicular, or axillary block may provide complete surgical anesthesia or postoperative analgesia. Lower extremity tumor resection is a big risk factor for postoperative DVT formation, therefore neuraxial anesthesia is not only an important postoperative analgesia modality, it also decreases the rate of deep vein thrombosis (DVT) and provides early ambulation. Spine and pelvic tumor resection may involve larger blood loss and hemodynamic changes. Spine surgery might require additional monitoring such as somatosensory evoked potentials (SSEPs), motor evoked potentials (MEPs), and electromyography (EMG). Neuraxial anesthesia for intraoperative and postoperative analgesia may be considered in spine and pelvic tumor resection.

Another important perioperative consideration that is rarely encountered is tumor lysis syndrome. This syndrome is usually associated with chemotherapy or even spontaneous occurrence, and it is possible to be triggered by anesthetics (25). Tumor lysis syndrome produces severe metabolic derangement from acute lysis of large numbers of tumor cells. It results in acidosis, hyperkalemia, hyperphosphatemia, increased uric acid, and lactic acidosis. Anesthesiologists must be prepared to treat electrolyte abnormalities, metabolic, and respiratory acidosis, and even consider dialysis if the patient's condition continues to deteriorate.

Systemic disease

Many systemic diseases can affect morbidity in patients requiring anesthesia for orthopedic surgery. Juvenile idiopathic arthritis (JIA) is the most common rheumatic disease of childhood (26). Juvenile idiopathic arthritis is defined as persistent arthritis for more than 6 weeks with an onset at younger than 16 years of age (27). It involves inflammation of the synovium of multiple joints, including spine, hip, and extremity joints. Systemic manifestation includes spiking fever, rash, uveitis, and other organ systems.

Preoperative evaluation should include medications, their possible adverse side effects, and thorough airway evaluation. Medical treatment includes nonsteroidal anti-inflammatory drugs (NSAIDs), corticosteroids, and other disease-modifying drugs such as methotrexate, sulfasalazine, leflunomide, cyclophosphamide, gold, and antitumor necrosis factor medications. Complications of NSAIDS include gastrointestinal bleed, CNS effect, and renal adverse effects such as papillary necrosis or tubular necrosis. Thrombocytopenia, leukopenia, and anemia might result from the use of methotrexate.

Preoperative evaluation of the airway is imperative because of the possibility of difficult or near-impossible intubation. First, the flexion deformity of the cervical spine may make neck flexion and extension impossible. Second, temporomandibular arthritis may limit the effective mouth opening (28). Finally, cricoarytenoid arthritis narrows the laryngeal opening making tracheal intubation difficult (29). Another danger for tracheal intubation is atlantoaxial subluxation. It is defined radiographically as distance from the anterior arch of the atlas to the odontoid process greater than 3 mm. This displaced odontoid process may compress the cervical cord, medulla, or vertebral arteries (30). Sudden neck movement by endotracheal intubation may cause displacement of the odontoid that results in paraplegia or sudden death. When radiographic evidence of atlantoaxial stability is lacking, direct laryngoscope should not be attempted. Fiberoptic intubation should be performed after the child has been adequately anesthetized while maintaining spontaneous ventilation. Neuromuscular junction blockers should only be administered after a definite airway has been established. Patients with JIA may also have systemic manifestations of pleural effusion, pneumonitis, and pleuritis. Myocarditis and conduction system delay are also possible.

Clinical science

Anterior, posterior, and combined spine fusion

Anterior spinal surgery

Anterior thoracic spinal surgeries may require video-assisted thoracoscopic surgery in specific deformities such as severe kyphosis and lordosis in cerebral palsy patients (31). This approach allows for anterior releases, diskectomies, and anterior instrumentation and fusion. This approach has the added advantage of less chest wall compromise than open thoracotomy using several small portal incisions. However, one-lung ventilation is rarely produced with a double-lumen endotracheal tube in children. More commonly, directed mainstem intubation or bronchial blockers are utilized (32) in the pediatric population (33). One-lung ventilation may be difficult in patients with restrictive lung disease, compromising oxygenation and ventilation. A CPAP may be added to nonventilated lung and PEEP to the ventilated. Complications of the anterior approach include arterial and venous puncture, hemothorax, pneumothorax, spinal cord injury, and paralysis.

Posterior spinal surgery

During posterior spine fusion, the vertebral laminae, facet joints, and the spinous processes are removed while bone for grafting is obtained from the iliac crest or ribs. Posterior fusion extends from one vertebra above the curve to the second vertebra below. Instrumentation techniques may include Harrington rod insertion (34), segmental spinal instrumentation that allows for three-dimensional correction, and the Cotrel–Dubousset segmental spinal instrumentation system that is complex with more potential blood loss (35).

Postoperative visual loss is a devastating complication of prone spinal surgery, and the most common type is ischemic optic neuropathy. The biggest risk factors include large blood loss and duration of prone position greater than 6 hours (36). Other complications of prone position surgeries may include loss of airway control such as ETT disconnect, kinking, upper airway edema, neck hyperflexion and hyperextension, corneal abraision, and brachial plexus neuropathy.

Combined spine fusion

Simultaneous combined anterior and posterior fusion were performed in years past on rare occasions for patients with severe disability and failed spinal operations (37). In these situations, the simultaneous combined fusion actually resulted in shorter surgical times, less blood loss, fewer days spent in the hospital, and better correction of the spinal deformity. Also, the complications were less frequent and less severe with the continuous procedure (38). However, recent experience suggests no clear advantage for the combined procedure in routine cases and the need should be determined on a case-to-case basis since patients requiring these procedures may have additional comorbidities.

Anesthesia management

Blood loss should always be anticipated in spine surgeries. Hence each patient should have PRBCs and fresh frozen plasma available. Risk factors for large blood loss include prolonged surgical time, number of vertebral levels fused, children with neuromuscular scoliosis, anesthetic technique that affects hemodynamic stability, and coagulopathy (39). Methods to decrease blood loss include controlled hypotension, intraoperative normovolemic hemodilution, and use of antifibrinolytics such as aminocaproic acid and tranexamic acid (40). Crystalloid or colloid may be used with success while transfusion of FFP and/or PRBCs is reserved for additional resuscitation.

Hypotension is a feared occurrence during spine surgery, and hypovolemia is usually the primary cause. Because cardiac resuscitation is difficult in the prone position, hemodynamic stability is essential. Adequate volume resuscitation may be difficult in pediatric patients, but following urine output is a convenient trend – with the goal of at least 0.5–1 ml/kg/h. Low urine output and metabolic acidosis upon blood gas analysis may indicate poor end-organ perfusion and spinal cord blood flow.

Postoperative paralysis and visual loss are the most feared neurologic complication of spine surgery, thus understanding spinal cord blood flow is essential in the management of these patients. The anterior two-thirds of spinal cord blood flow is supplied by one anterior spinal artery and, and the posterior one-third of the spinal cord is supplied by a pair of posterior spinal arteries. Each vertebral level also receives multiple segmental arteries, with the most important one being the artery of Adamkiewicz (arteria radicularis magna) that is usually derived from T9–12. Injury to this artery during surgery can cause *anterior spinal cord syndrome* which results in motor paralysis while preserving vibration and proprioception function.

In order to minimize intraoperative spinal cord injury, multiple monitoring techniques have emerged, including the intraoperative wake up test, somatosensory evoked potential (SSEP), motor evoked potential (MEP), and the electromyogram (EMG). The intraoperative wake up test is easily performed as long as the administered inhaled anesthetics are not above 0.5 MAC. The SSEP consists of posterior afferent sensory component of the spinal cord. Electrodes are usually placed at peripheral nerves, and receiving electrodes are placed at CNS. The MEP consists of anterior efferent motor component of the spinal cord. Electrodes are stimulated at CNS and received at peripheral nerves. These monitors have anesthetic implications. A high level of inhalation gas (greater than one MAC), hypotension, hypothermia, hypoxemia, severe anemia, and hypocarbia can increase latency and decrease amplitude of SSEP and MEP (41). Nitrous oxide decreases the amplitude, while etomidate increases both amplitude and latency. Neuromuscular blockers interferes with both MEP and EMG. Therefore by eliminating the above variables that can affect SSEP, MEP, and EMG, any acute changes in signals may suggest a spinal cord insult.

A multimodal approach is recommended for postoperative pain control. If remifentanyl is the sole agent used for analgesia, patients may acutely develop opioid tolerance during the surgery, and the postoperative pain will be difficult to treat (42). Therefore long-acting narcotics such as hydromorphone, fentanyl in a long-acting dosage format, methadone or morphine are necessary. Epidural catheters with local anesthetics and narcotics, or intrathecal morphine may produce reliable postoperative pain control (43). The use of nonsteroidal anti-inflammatory drugs (NSAIDs) can be controversial. The NSAIDs may decrease morphine consumption, decrease somnolence, pruritus, constipation, and enhance analgesia in comparison with patients who do not receive ketorolac (44). However, the use of NSAIDs may inhibit bone healing and increase postoperative bleeding from its antiplatelet effect, even though these side effects are debatable clinically (45).

Chest wall reconstruction

The most common chest wall reconstructions involve pectus chest deformities, which occur in 1 in every 300 to 400 white male births, and less commonly in females (46). Interestingly, these procedures are currently performed by general pediatric surgeons.

Pectus excavatum (sternal depression) is approximately six times more common than pectus carinatum (protrusion). Clinical presentation is less apparent until puberty when rapid linear growth occurs. Symptoms sometimes include dyspnea with mild exercise, chest pain, easy fatigue, palpitations, tachycardia, exercise-induced wheezing, and frequent upper respiratory infections. However, in some cases pectus excavatum is asymptomatic. An association with scoliosis is most common, and rarely it is associated with congenital heart disease, Marfan syndrome, and other connective tissue disease (47).

Surgical indications include rapid progression of deformity, paradoxical movement of the chest wall with inspiration, cardiac compression or displacement, pulmonary compression, mitral valve prolapse, and significant restriction disease on pulmonary function testing (48). Usually surgery is discouraged in children less than 5 years old due to risk of disruption of normal chest wall growth and future chest wall restriction. There are two surgical approaches, the classic open approach (Ravitch) and minimally invasive approach (Nuss procedure).

Anesthetic management includes a careful preoperative evaluation. Echocardiogram is useful because the depressed sternum may compress the right atrium and right ventricle, causing mild to severe diastolic function. Mitral valve prolapse is common and should be evaluated. Restrictive lung disease with decreased forced vital capacity and maximal ventilatory volumes is more common than obstructive airway disease. Because of possible cardiac compression, diastolic function and arrhythmia may be present. Both IV and mask induction are acceptable. With restrictive lung disease, there will be decreased FRC, and hypercarbia may exacerbate pulmonary hypertension. Tracheal intubation with controlled ventilation is necessary. Insertion of thoracic or lumbar epidural catheter with local anesthetics and narcotics is highly recommended for postoperative pain control. Otherwise a large amount of IV narcotics is needed, making postoperative extubation more difficult. Thoracic epidural catheter theoretically provides more analgesia than lumbar epidural catheter, but it is more difficult to insert, especially when inserted in pediatric patients under general anesthesia. Intraoperative deterioration characterized by increased ventilatory pressure, hypotension, and hypoxemia could indicate tension pneumothorax. Blood loss is usually minimal. Paradoxical chest wall movement may occur during spontaneous ventilation after surgery, suggesting hypoventilation, flail chest, and atelectasis. Since pneumothorax is very common, immediate postoperative chest X-ray is essential for possible chest tube placement (49–51).

Tourniquet management

Arterial tourniquets are utilized to create a bloodless surgical field for orthopedic extremity surgeries. Systemic effects are numerous, from both inflation and deflation of the tourniquet. Tourniquet inflation results in increase in circulating blood volume and systemic vascular resistance. Central venous pressure and systolic blood pressure can transiently increase (52). These hemodynamic changes are usually well tolerated in healthy children. Deflation of tourniquet reliably increases end-tidal CO_2. This phenomenon can be explained by returning of acidic and hypercapnic venous blood from the ischemic extremity back to central circulation. Increasing spontaneous ventilation can help compensate for the increased end-tidal CO_2. In patients with controlled ventilation, respiration rate needs to be increased to normalize end-tidal CO_2. The increased CO_2 results in increased cerebral blood flow, which can dangerously elevate intracranial pressure in patients with brain injury. Tissue ischemia after tourniquet inflammation promotes release of tissue plasminogen activator, causing systemic thrombolysis when the tourniquet is released (53).

Temperature effects from tourniquet management cannot be ignored. During general anesthesia, most of the initial temperature loss is from distribution of heat from central compartment to peripheral compartment. With tourniquet inflation there is reduced metabolic heat transfer, and it results in an increase in core body temperature. This hyperthermia effect is more significant in children (54). On the other hand, tourniquet deflation results in decrease in central temperature due to distribution of hypothermic ischemic extremity blood back to central circulation.

Tourniquets can also induce local effects. These include nerve injury, muscle injury, vascular injury, and skin injury. Peripheral nerve injuries from tourniquet inflation are well documented. These injuries range from sensory deficit, motor deficit, or both. Neuropathy occurs more often in the upper extremity than the lower extremity; the radial nerve is the most common upper extremity neuropathy and sciatic nerve is the most common lower extremity neuropathy (55). Therefore tourniquet inflation time should be limited as short as possible, usually 2 hours for healthy patients and shorter for trauma, or sickle cell disease patients.

Sickle cell disease is a unique condition when discussing utilization of tourniquets for orthopedic surgery. In sickle cell disease patients, hypoxia, acidosis, and circulatory status are avoided to prevent red blood cell sickling and thrombosis. There are two case reports of tourniquets initiating sickle cell crisis (56), but there are centers which routinely use tourniquets on sickle cell patients by maintaining hydration and avoid acidosis without any complications (57). Therefore the risk: benefit ratio of tourniquets on sickle cell patients should be evaluated and individualized. For surgery longer than 2 hours, tourniquets should be deflated every 2 hours to allow 10 minutes of reperfusion (58). An average adult would need an inflation pressure of 200 mmHg for the upper limb and 250 mmHg for the lower extremity. Children require less tourniquet pressure to achieve a bloodless field: 173 mmHg for upper limb and 176 mmHg for the lower extremity (59).

Tourniquet pain is a gradual onset and dull aching sensation at the site of the tourniquet extremity. In awake adult patients, this pain becomes unbearable in 45 to 60 minutes, despite an adequate regional block or neuroaxial anesthesia (60). This pain subsides quickly after the tourniquet is deflated. Its exact mechanism of action is unknown and is difficult to treat; an IV narcotic is often not helpful. In anesthetized children it is generally thought that tourniquet pain may be occurring when unexplained hypertension is seen.

Tourniquet-induced hypertension is defined as over 30% increase in either systolic or diastolic baseline blood pressure (61). This occurs more often in general anesthesia than in spinal anesthesia, and occurs more often in lower extremity surgery than in upper extremity surgery. Preoperative IV ketamine, 0.25 mg/kg or more, can significantly decrease tourniquet-induced systemic arterial pressure increase in patients under general anesthesia (62).

Finally, tourniquet use can affect the pharmacokinetics of anesthetics. Medication given prior to tourniquet inflation may be sequestered in the ischemic extremity, and then redistributed to the central compartment after tourniquet deflation. This may prolong the desired effect of anesthetics. Anesthetics given after tourniquet inflation may have enhanced effects due to lower volume of distribution. Therefore medications should be carefully titrated during tourniquet use, especially when more than one extremity is involved.

References

1. Demetracopoulos CA, Sponseller PD. Spinal deformities in Marfan syndrome. *Orthop Clin North Am* 2007; **38**: 563–72.
2. Joseph KN, Bowen JR *et al.* Orthopaedic aspects of the Marfan syndrome. *Clin Orthop* 1992; **277**: 251–60.
3. De Paepe A, Devereux RB, Dietz HC, *et al.* Revised diagnostic criteria for the Marfan syndrome. *Am J Med Genet* 1996; **62**: 417–26.
4. Herzka A, Sponseller PD, Pyeritz RE. Atlantoaxial rotatory subluxation in patients with Marfan syndrome. A report of three cases. *Spine* 2000; **25**: 524–6.
5. Dean, JC. Management of Marfan syndrome. *Heart* 2002; **88**: 97–103
6. Ladouceur M, Fermanian C, Lupoglazoff JM, *et al.* Effect of beta-blockade on ascending aortic dilatation in children with the Marfan syndrome. *Am J Cardiol* 2007; **99**: 406–9.
7. Brooke BS, Habashi JP, Judge DP, *et al.* Angiotensin II blockade and aortic-root dilation in Marfan syndrome. *N Engl J Med* 2008; **358**: 2787–95.
8. Sharkey AM. Cardiovascular management of Marfan syndrome in the young. *Curr Treat Options Cardiovasc Med* 2006; **8**: 396–402.
9. Basel D, Steiner RD. Osteogenesis imperfecta: recent findings shed new light on this once well-understood condition. *Genet Med* 2009; **11**: 375–85.
10. Kocher MS, Shapiro F. Osteogenesis imperfecta. *J Am Acad Orthop Surg* 1998; **6**: 225–36.

11. Ryan CA, Al-Ghamdi AS, Gayle M, Finer NN. Osteogenesis imperfecta and hyperthermia. *Anesth Analg* 1989; **68**: 811–14.
12. Hall RMO, Henning RD, Brown TCK: Anaesthesia for children with osteogenesis imperfecta. *Paediatr Anaesth* 1992; **2**: 115–19.
13. Porsborg P, Astrup G, Bendixen D, *et al.* Osteogenesis imperfecta and malignant hyperthermia: Is there a relationship? *Anesthesia* 1996; **51**: 863–5.
14. Cheung MS, Glorieux FH. Osteogenesis imperfecta: update on presentation and management. *Rev Endocr Metab Disord* 2008; **9**: 153–60.
15. Cunningham A, *et al.* Osteogenesis imperfecta: Anesthetic management of a patient for cesarean section: A case report. *Anesth Analg* 1984; **61**: 91–3.
16. Morris P. Duchenne muscular dystrophy: a challenge for the anaesthetist. *Paediatr Anaesth* 1997; **7**: 1–4.
17. Siegel IM. Maintenance of ambulation in Duchenne muscular dystrophy. The role of the orthopedic surgeon. *Clin Pediatr* 1980; **19**: 383–8.
18. Davis M. Malignant hyperthermia and muscular dystrophies. *Pediatric Anesthes* 2009; **109**: 1043–8.
19. Hayes J. Duchenne muscular dystrophy: an old anesthesia problem revisited. *Pediatr Anesth* 2008; **18**: 100–6.
20. Massey JM. Treatment of acquired myasthenia gravis. *Neurology* 1997; **48**: S46–S51.
21. d'Empaire G, Hoaglin DC, Perlo VP, *et al.* Effect of prethymectomy plasma exchange on postoperative respiratory function in myasthenia gravis. *J Thorac Cardiovasc Surg* 1985; **89**: 592.
22. Small S, Ali HH, Lennon VA, *et al.* Anesthesia for unsuspected Lambert–Eaton myasthenic syndrome with autoantibodies and occult small cell lung carcinoma. *Anesthesiology* 1992; **76**: 142.
23. Anderson R. Anesthesia for patients undergoing orthopedic oncologic surgeries. *J Clin Anesth* 2010; **22**: 565–72.
24. Hendry DA. Antifibrinolytic use for minimizing perioperative allogeneic blood transfusion. *Cochrane Database Syst Rev* 2007; **17**(4): CD001886.
25. Farley-Hills E, *et al.* Tumour lysis syndrome during anaesthesia. *Paediatr Anaesth* 2001; **11**: 233–6.
26. Helmick CG, Felson DT, Lawrence RC, *et al.* Estimates of the prevalence of arthritis and other rheumatic conditions in the USA. Part I. *Arthritis Rheum* 2008; **58**: 15–25
27. Hashkes PJ, Laxer RM. Medical treatment of juvenile idiopathic arthritis. *JAMA* 2005; **294**: 1671–84.
28. Pedersen TK, Jensen JJ, Melsen B, *et al.* Resorption of the temporomandibular condylar bone according to subtypes of juvenile chronic arthritis. *J Rheumatol* 2001; **28**: 2109–15.
29. Jacobs JC, Hui RM. Cricoarytenoid arthritis and airway obstruction in juvenile rheumatoid arthritis. *Pediatrics* 1977; **59**: 292–4.
30. Hodgkinson R. Anesthetic Management of a parturient with severe juvenile rheumatoid arthritis. *Anesth Analg* 1981; **60**: 611–12.
31. Sucato DJ. Thoracoscopic anterior instrumentation and fusion for idiopathic scoliosis. *J Am Acad Orthop Surg* 2003; **11**: 221–7.
32. Campos JH. An update on bronchial blockers during lung separation techniques in adults. *Anesth Analg* 2003; **97**: 1266–74.
33. Hammer GB, Harrison TK, Vricella LA, *et al.* Single lung ventilation in children using a new paediatric bronchial blocker. *Paediatr Anaesth* 2002; **12**: 69–72.
34. Harrington PR, Dickson JH. Spinal instrumentation in the treatment of severe progressive spondylolisthesis. *Clin Orthop* 1976; **117**: 157–63.
35. Richards BS, Johnston CE. Cotrel–Dubousset instrumentation for adolescent idiopathic scoliosis. *Orthopedics* 1987; **10**: 649–54.
36. Lee LA, Roth S, Posner KL, *et al.* The American Society of Anesthesiologists postoperative visual loss registry. *Anesthesiology* 2006; **105**: 652–9.
37. O'Brien JP, Dawson MH, Heard CW, *et al.* Simultaneous combined anterior and posterior fusion: a surgical solution for failed spinal surgery with a brief review of the first 150 patients. *Clin Orthop Relat Res* 1986; **203**: 191–5
38. Shufflebarger HL. Anterior and posterior spinal fusion staged versus same-day surgery. *Spine* 1991.
39. Nuttail GA, Horlocker TT, Santrach PJ, *et al.* Predictors of blood transfusions in spinal instrumentation and fusion surgery. *Spine* 2000; **25**: 596–601.
40. Urban MK, Beckman J, Gordon M. *et al.* The efficacy of antifibrinolytics in the reduction of blood loss during complex adult reconstructive spine surgery. *Spine* 2001; **26**: 1152–6.
41. Kumar A, Bhattachrya A, Makhija N. Evoked potential monitoring in anaesthesia and analgesia. *Anaesthesia* 2000; **55**: 225–41.
42. Crawford MW, Hickey C, Zaarour C, *et al.* Development of acute opioid tolerance during infusion of remifentanil for pediatric scoliosis surgery. *Anesth Analg* 2006; **102**: 1662–7.
43. Urban MK, Jules-Elysee K, Urquhart B. Reduction in postoperative pain after spinal fusion with instrumentation using

intrathecal morphine. *Spine* 2002; **27**: 535–7.

44. Reuben SS, Connelly NR, Steinberg R. Ketorolac as an adjunct to patient-controlled morphine in postoperative spine surgery patients. *Reg Anesth* 1997; **22**: 343–6.

45. Pradhan BB, Tatsumi RL, Gallina J, *et al.* Ketorolac and spinal fusion: does the perioperative use of ketorolac really inhibit spinal fusion? *Spine (Phila Pa)* 1976; **33**: 2079–82.

46. Jaroszewski D. Current management of pectus excavatum: a review and update of therapy and treatment recommendations. *JABFM* 2010; **10**: 2

47. Shaul D. Pectus carinatum guideline. *American Pediatric Surgical Association*; 2012.

48. Jaroszewski D. Current management of pectus excavatum: a review and update of therapy and treatment recommendations. *JABFM* 2010; **10**: 2.

49. Shamberger RC, Welch KJ. Surgical correction of pectus carinatum. *J Pediatr Surg* 1987; **22**: 48.

50. Malek M.H., Fonkalsrud E.W., Cooper C.B., *et al.*: Ventilatory and cardiovascular responses to exercise in patients with pectus excavatum. *Chest* 2003; **124**: 870–82.

51. Robicsek F. Surgical treatment of pectus excavatum. *Chest Surg Clin N Am* 2000; **10**: 277–96.

52. Valli H., Rosenberg PH, Kytta J, *et al.* Arterial hypertension associated with the use of a tourniquet with either general or regional anaesthesia. *Acta Anaesthesiol Scand* 1987; **31**: 279–83.

53. Kam PC, Kavanagh R, Yoong FF, *et al.*: The arterial tourniquet: pathophysiological consequences and anaesthetic implications. *Anaesthesia* 2001; **56**: 534–45.

54. Estebe JP, Le NA, Malledant Y, *et al.* Use of a pneumatic tourniquet induces changes in central temperature. *Br J Anaesth* 1996; **77**: 786–8.

55. Middleton RW, Varian JP. Tourniquet paralysis. *Aust NZ J Surg* 1974; **44**: 124–8

56. Kam PC, Kavanagh R, Yoong FF, *et al.* The arterial tourniquet: pathophysiological consequences and anaesthetic implications. *Anaesthesia* 2001; **56**: 534–45.

57. Adu-Gyamfi Y, Sankarankutty M, Marwa S. Use of a tourniquet in patients with sickle-cell disease. *Can J Anaesth* 1993; **40**: 24–7.

58. Kam PC, Kavanagh R, Yoong FF, *et al.* The arterial tourniquet: pathophysiological consequences and anaesthetic implications. *Anaesthesia* 2001; **56**: 534–45.

59. Lieberman JR, Staneli CT, Dales MC. Tourniquet pressures on pediatric patients: a clinical study. *Orthopedics* 1997; **20**: 1143–7.

60. Gielen MJ, Stienstra R. Tourniquet hypertension and its prevention: a review. *Reg Anesth* 1991; **16**: 191–4.

61. Kaufman RD, Walts LF. Tourniquet-induced hypertension. *Br J Anaesth* 1982; **54**: 333–6.

62. Satsumae T. Preoperative small-dose ketamine prevented tourniquet-induced arterial pressure increase in orthopedic patients under general anesthesia. *Anesth Analg* 2001; **92**: 1286–9.

Chapter 22

Trauma

James E. Hunt, Terry G. Fletcher, and Joe R. Jansen

Pediatric trauma

Pediatric trauma accounts for 25% of all trauma in the USA.[1] On an annual basis, trauma kills almost as many children in the USA as cancer, cerebrovascular disease, chronic respiratory disease, congenital anomalies and heart problems, influenza, pneumonia, and septicemia combined.[1]

Unintentional trauma occurs more often in lower socioeconomic levels, in males, and in African-Americans and Native Americans.[1] Pediatric trauma occurs more often in urban areas/population centers.[2] Nonaccidental trauma as a result of physical assault or abuse occurs in 10–15% of trauma cases.[3]

Pediatric trauma rates are bimodal in distribution across age ranges, with peaks occurring at 0–3 yrs and 15–19 yrs.[2] Pediatric trauma incidence, and trauma-related death, is more likely in males than females.[2] Brain trauma is responsible for up to 80% of all trauma deaths, and over 70% of deaths from trauma occur at time of injury.[1] Death from blunt trauma outnumbers death from penetrating trauma.[2] Case fatality rates in children < 3 y/o are twice that of children 8–10 y/o, and case fatality rates in children > 16 y/o are three to four times that of children 8–10 y/o.[2] Death resulting from intentional harm most often occurs in children < 4 y/o.[1]

Falls are the number one cause of pediatric trauma overall and the most common cause of nonfatal, unintentional trauma in children under 14 y/o.[1] Trauma related to motor vehicle accidents (MVAs) is the number one cause of fatal and nonfatal injuries overall in children > 14 y/o – primarily as a result of traumatic brain injury or cervical spine injury.[1] Nonfatal trauma related to motor vehicle traffic occurs more often in females; fatal trauma related to motor vehicle traffic occurs more often in males.[1]

Males are 1.5 times more likely to suffer traumatic brain injury (TBI) versus females; African Americans have the highest death rate from TBI.[1] A TBI is the most common reason for a child to require intensive care or develop a life-long disability.[1] Rates of TBI are higher among lower socioeconomic classes.[1] Penetrating brain injury is more likely in 15–19 y/o children secondary to increased use of firearms.[2] Trauma related to firearms causes the highest case fatality rate in children across all ages in the USA.

Maltreatment

Nonaccidental trauma is reported at much lower annual rates than actual occurrence in the USA: estimates of incidence and victim or parental self-reports differ by as much as ten-fold.[1] Maltreatment occurs in indirect proportion to age in children – adolescents are less likely to suffer abuse or recurrence of abuse versus infants.[1] Potential maltreatment is often addressed by pediatric anesthesiologists in trauma scenarios, and should be an integral part of comprehensive secondary and tertiary trauma evaluations.[1]

Neglect occurs at rates approximating five times rates of physical abuse. More than 75% of deaths attributed to abuse occur in children under 4 y/o.[1] Maltreatment – in the form of neglect, physical abuse and sexual abuse – occurs more than three times as often in disabled children versus nondisabled children.[1] Children with disabilities or special needs may be less likely to articulate or effectively communicate their anxiety or fear when asked about possible abuse secondary to communication or behavioral barriers (e.g., nonverbal communication, receptive or expressive language deficits, altered sensory responses).

Bruising over bony prominences (e.g., shins, knees, forehead, chin, forearms) on a 4 y/o child is

Essentials of Pediatric Anesthesiology, ed. Alan David Kaye, Charles James Fox and James H. Diaz. Published by Cambridge University Press. © Cambridge University Press 2015.

consistent with hazards of normal activity; bruising over bony prominences on a child ≤ 1 y/o is less consistent with hazards of increasing mobility or exploration, and more consistent with inflicted injury.[1] Injuries to padded and protected areas (e.g., abdomen, buttocks, cheek, ears, genitalia, or neck) are always suspicious.[1] Maltreatment can be associated with persistent inferior deviation of pupils ("sun-setting sign") or retinal hemorrhages in infants, as a result of brain injury (e.g., "shaken-baby").[1] Every patient should have genitalia/anus examined when abuse is suspected – as part of a comprehensive evaluation and documentation scenario.[1]

Initial management and resuscitation

Principles of initial management in the injured child are the same as principles of managing injured adults: pediatric trauma patients undergo the same primary and secondary surveys as adults, and the primary survey follows the same ABCDE format used in adult ATLS.[1]

Initial management of obstructive airway in a young child or infant should involve jaw thrust +/- suction – while keeping the cervical collar on.[1] However, in pediatric trauma, a modified GCS of ≤ 8 is always an indication for intubation.[4] Intubation of pediatric trauma victims in the prehospital setting is successful < 60% of the time; therefore, all pediatric trauma patients presenting to the ED intubated should have placement of the ETT verified by direct laryngoscopy or $ETCO_2$ measurement.[1]

Rapid-sequence induction may be used in pediatric trauma if no contraindications or difficult airway, but urgency of securing airway must take priority over risk of aspiration.[4] Conversely, preoxygenation or inhalation induction by forcefully holding a facemask on an awake child will contribute to worsening physiologic and psychologic stress – both during and after anesthesia – therefore appropriate anxiolysis or sedation should be considered prior to holding facemask on a fearful or agitated child.[4]

Venous access in pediatric trauma patients should be obtained where able, in order to accomplish initial, and possibly life-saving, resuscitation.[4] Attempts should initially focus on obtaining two large-bore (appropriate for age/size) peripheral IVs – or intraosseous (IO) access if peripheral IV access is not immediately available upon initiation of resuscitation.[4] If chest trauma exists, access may be needed in both upper and lower extremities to account for possible disruption of great vessels; if abdominal trauma exists, then access may be needed in upper extremities.[4] For a child who is critically ill, an arterial line may be necessary for continued management, but efforts to obtain arterial line access should not delay proceeding with life-saving surgery.[4] Congruently, establishment of central venous access may be highly important, but is not considered an initial or first-line procedure in management of hemodynamic instability.[4]

Cardiogenic shock is rare in pediatric trauma – although direct chest trauma can produce pneumothoraces, disruption of great vessels, cardiac tamponade, and direct myocardial injury.[4] Abdominal injuries are more common in children than thoracic injuries, and blunt trauma injuries are more common than penetrating trauma injuries.[4] High spinal cord injury produces loss of sympathetic tone in the arterial system with subsequent hypotension and spinal shock – which requires treatment with fluids and vasopressors.[5]

Initial resuscitation in the pediatric trauma patient with hypovolemia begins with isotonic crystalloid in 20 ml/kg IV/IO bolus.[1] Glucose-containing solutions should be avoided in young trauma victims – especially if traumatic brain injury is suspected.[4] Blood products (10 ml/kg) should be considered after repeated isotonic crystalloid boluses totaling 40–60 ml/kg have not produced stable blood pressure.[4] The need for transfusion of blood products during initial resuscitation is uncommon in pediatric trauma patients, and may signal need for surgical intervention.[1]

In pediatric trauma, shock is most associated with hypovolemia.[4] Young children will usually exhibit almost normal blood pressure until > 25% of circulating blood volume is lost.[1] Tachycardia is an earlier sign of impending shock than hypotension in pediatric trauma victims because of more robust physiologic efforts (higher sympathetic tone) expended to maintain blood pressure versus adults.[1] Mottling, delayed capillary refill, thready pulse, impaired consciousness, or cyanosis are all earlier indicators of shock in pediatric trauma versus hypotension.[1] Hypotension as a result of hypovolemia is an ominous sign of impending cardiovascular collapse in children.[1]

Children are equally likely to exhibit recall of trauma and anesthesia-related events as adults.[4] Acutely injured children will also commonly have pre-existing diagnoses and comorbidities (e.g., asthma, developmental delay, autism spectrum behaviors,

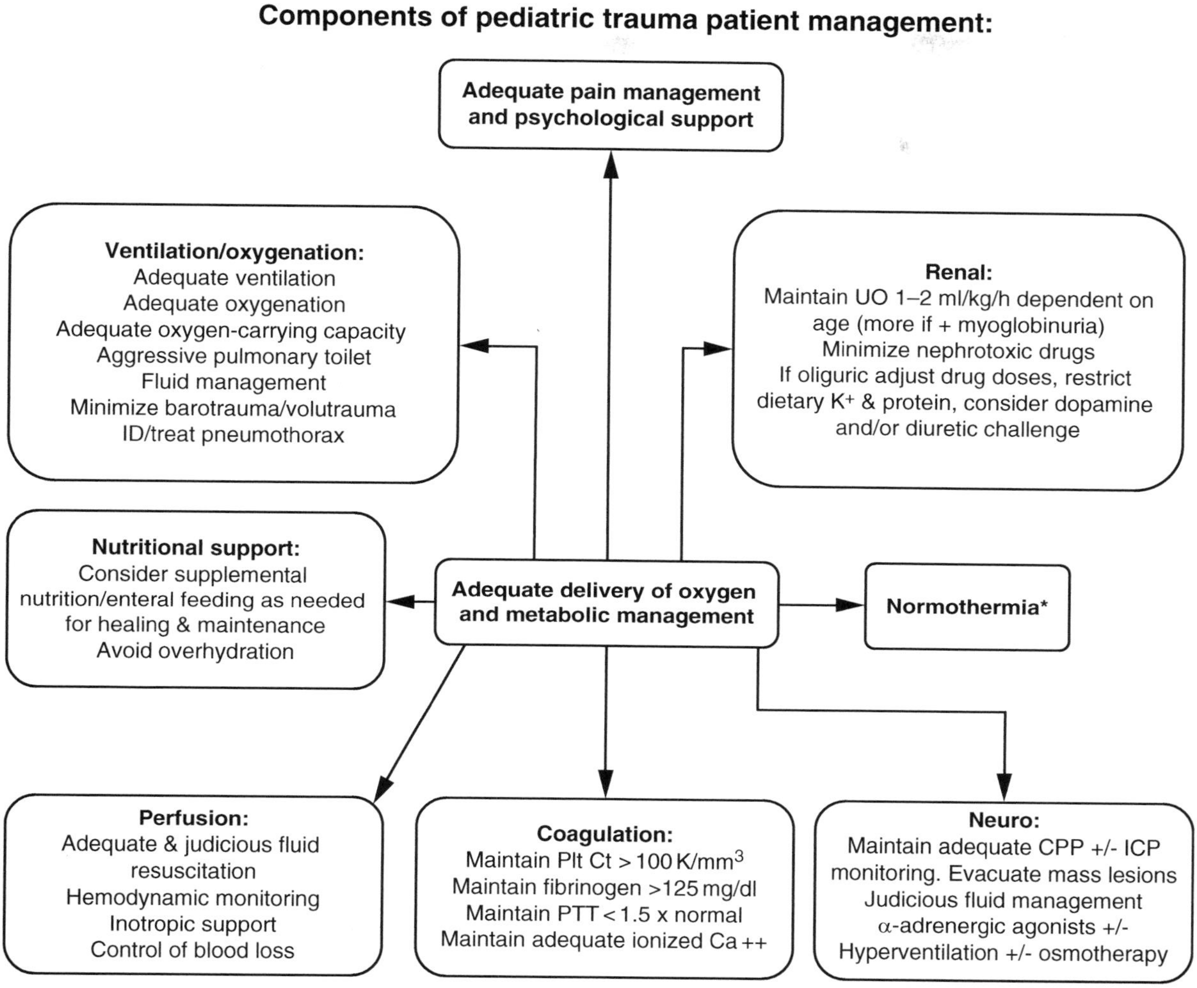

Components of pediatric trauma patient management:

Adequate pain management and psychological support

Ventilation/oxygenation:
Adequate ventilation
Adequate oxygenation
Adequate oxygen-carrying capacity
Aggressive pulmonary toilet
Fluid management
Minimize barotrauma/volutrauma
ID/treat pneumothorax

Renal:
Maintain UO 1–2 ml/kg/h dependent on age (more if + myoglobinuria)
Minimize nephrotoxic drugs
If oliguric adjust drug doses, restrict dietary K^+ & protein, consider dopamine and/or diuretic challenge

Nutritional support:
Consider supplemental nutrition/enteral feeding as needed for healing & maintenance
Avoid overhydration

Adequate delivery of oxygen and metabolic management

Normothermia*

Perfusion:
Adequate & judicious fluid resuscitation
Hemodynamic monitoring
Inotropic support
Control of blood loss

Coagulation:
Maintain Plt Ct > 100 K/mm^3
Maintain fibrinogen >125 mg/dl
Maintain PTT < 1.5 x normal
Maintain adequate ionized Ca ++

Neuro:
Maintain adequate CPP +/- ICP monitoring. Evacuate mass lesions
Judicious fluid management
α-adrenergic agonists +/-
Hyperventilation +/- osmotherapy

Modified from Coté's *A Practice of Anesthesia for Infants and Children*, 5th edn, 2013, Elsevier.
UO = urine output, CPP = cerebral perfusion pressure, ICP = intracranial pressure.
*Some centers may employ hypothermia protocols for neuroprotection.

Figure 22.1 Components of pediatric trauma patient management.

seizure disorder) that need to be considered in planning management.[4]

Airway and induction

The first step in relieving airway obstruction will often be initiating a jaw thrust +/- suction.[1] Pediatric trauma patients should all be considered to have cervical spine injury and a full stomach.[1] The cervical collar should not be taken off a sedated/anesthetized patient, and removal of the anterior portion of the collar should only be considered for access during invasive or surgical airway procedures (e.g., retrograde, tracheostomy).

Pediatric trauma patients with altered consciousness are equally as likely to require intubation as adults.[1] The angle of the pediatric nasopharynx is more acute versus adult anatomy, and makes nasotracheal intubation more difficult.[1] Rhinorrhea or ecchymoses around the eyes may be associated with facial fractures and basilar skull fractures.[1] The tongue of an infant or young child is relatively larger in size, the midface is relatively smaller in proportion,

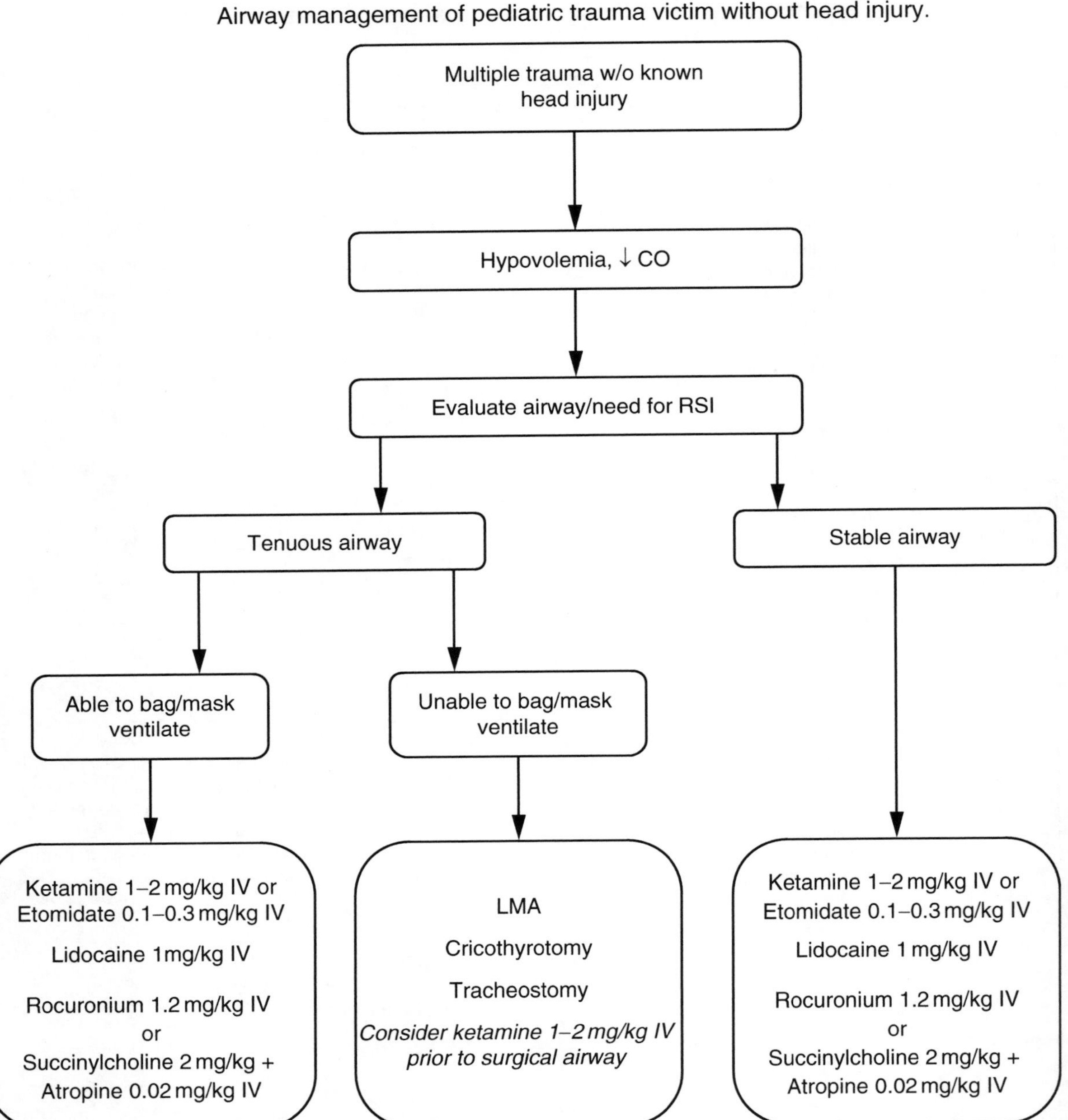

Modified from Coté's *A Practice of Anesthesia for Infants and Children*, 5th edn, 2013.
CO = cardiac output, RSI = rapid sequence induction, LMA = laryngeal mask airway, IV = intravenous.

Figure 22.2 Airway management of pediatric trauma victim without head injury.

Table 22.1 Common pediatric trauma patient induction medications

Medication	IV dosing (mg/kg)	Advantages	Disadvantages
Atropine	0.01–0.02	↓ Vagal response	↑ HR, flushing, hyperpyrexia, sedation, agitation
Glycopyrrolate	0.01	↓ Vagal response, antisialogue, no sedation or agitation	Longer acting versus atropine
Lidocaine	1–1.5	↓ Hemodynamic and intracranial responses to intubation	Cardiovascular toxicity in doses > 5 mg/kg
Fentanyl	0.001–0.003	↓ Hemodynamic and intracranial responses to intubation, analgesia	↓ HR, chest wall and glottic rigidity
Midazolam	0.05–0.2	Sedation, amnesia, anxiolysis	↓BP when used in combination with opioids in hypovolemic patients
Ketamine	1–2	Sympathomimetic, supports spontaneous respirations	↑ Salivation, may increase ICP
Propofol	1–3	Sedative–hypnotic	↓ BP
Etomidate	0.2–0.3	Hemodynamic stability, no cardiac depression	Possible adrenal suppression
Rocuronium	0.6–1.2	High dose = rapid onset and vagolytic properties	Intermediate–long duration depending on dose, cannot be quickly antagonized in absence of sugammadex
Succinylcholine	2	Rapid onset and ultra-short duration	May cause ↓ HR, may cause ↑ ICP and gastric pressures, hyperkalemia in patients with muscular dystrophy, crush injury, burns, sepsis, motor neuron lesions, prolonged immobilization

Source: Modified from Coté's *A Practice of Anesthesia for Infants and Children*, 5th edn, Elsevier 2013.

and the larynx and glottic opening are more anterior versus adults.[1] A child's airway is also relatively smaller in diameter, and shorter in length; small positional changes of the ETT are therefore more likely to result in extubation.[1]

There are no absolute standard induction agents for pediatric trauma patients – induction agents should be chosen based on needs of the individual patient.[1] Propofol should be reserved for patients who are hemodynamically stable.[1] Succinylcholine is contraindicated in crush injuries, long-bone fractures, and patients with susceptibility to malignant hyperthermia or significant hyperkalemia.[1] Fentanyl may cause hypotension (especially in hypovolemic patients), bradycardia, and chest wall and glottic rigidity.[4] Etomidate may decrease survival in septic patients because of the risk of adrenal suppression.[1] Ketamine may contribute to worsening increased ICP in children and adults with intracranial injury.[4] Rocuronium cannot be rapidly reversed without suggamadex.[4] Remifentanil may be useful during induction because it attenuates hemodynamic and intracranial responses to intubation while exhibiting rapid onset and offset similar to propofol or succinylcholine.[1]

Intraoperative management and massive transfusion

The most common reason for immediate operative treatment in pediatric trauma is evacuation of epidural or subdural hematoma; the next most common is laparotomy for abdominal trauma.[5] In children, simultaneous laparotomy and craniotomy are rare, as is penetrating chest wall trauma.[5] Most pediatric trauma patients do not require immediate anesthesia and surgery, but may report to OR after initial resuscitation and stabilization for secondary surgery, soft tissue injury, or treatment of fractures.[5]

As in adult trauma, life-threatening injuries may not allow time to fully cross-match blood prior to need for patient transfusion.[5] If time for full cross-match is insufficient, then type-specific uncross-matched blood is preferable; if type-specific blood cannot be readily available, then O-negative uncross-matched blood is used.[5] If massive transfusion with O-negative blood is commenced, then the anesthesiologist should continue with O-negative even after cross-match is available, secondary to risk of presence of anti-A and anti-B antibodies in the O-negative blood – and subsequent risk of hemolytic anemia.[5] Massive transfusion in a pediatric patient can be defined as transfusion of 50% of EBV in 3 hours or more than one whole blood volume in 24 hours.[5] Once again, a CVL is not necessary before massive transfusions/resuscitation, and delay for CVL establishment can be life-threatening: obtaining adequate IV or IO access must be a major priority.[5]

Calcium chloride may be necessary in pediatric and adult trauma scenarios requiring massive blood transfusion secondary to chelation of calcium by citrate in preserved blood products. Transfusion-related hypocalcemia is more likely with rapid administration of PRBCs.[1] Platelet transfusion of 0.1–0.2 units/kg is usually adequate to achieve surgical hemostasis after dilutional thrombocytopenia secondary to massive blood transfusions: platelet counts of 50 000 are adequate for surgical hemostasis.[1] An FFP/PRBC ratio of 1:1 to 1:1.5 are most common in pediatric massive transfusion protocols, as ratios greater than 1:2 are associated with lower 24-hour mortality rates.[1] Initial cryoprecipitate dose of 0.1 unit/kg is recommended for bleeding abnormalities after massive transfusion, DIC, and decreased fibrinogen levels.[1]

An unconscious patient with head trauma is not at risk for intraoperative recall; re-establishing hemodynamic stability must be the higher priority.[5] Treatment for prevention of recall can be initiated after hemodynamic stability is attained. Nitrous is not useful for induction or maintenance in pediatric trauma patients because of risk of expansion of encapsulated air in abdomen, chest, or cranium.[5] Scopolamine may be useful as an amnestic agent in unstable trauma patients.[5]

Traumatic brain injury and spinal cord injury

Traumatic brain injury (TBI) is the most common reason pediatric trauma victims develop life-long disability.[1] Pediatric traumatic brain injury (TBI) occurs 1.5 times as often in males versus females, and occurs more often in a bimodal distribution – in ages 0–4 y/o and 15–19 y/o.[1] Infants and toddlers are less prone to penetrating brain trauma, but are more prone to blunt injury from falls or falling objects (e.g., large TVs).[5] Diminished cognition and memory failure is often subtle and invisible during early trauma recovery and can be influenced by many factors such as drugs, anxiety, and hypoxia.[1]

Airway evaluation must occur early in trauma management, and before transport from ED trauma suite to CT imaging or OR suite.[1] Fundoscopic examination of the child with suspected TBI may reveal retinal hemorrhages indicative of shaken baby syndrome, and should be included in the evaluation of the trauma patient.[1]

Open fontanelles and cranial sutures may initially attenuate increased ICP in infants or neonates, but do not prevent its development or danger to brain tissue.[4] Trauma-related intracranial bleeding in infants and neonates can lead to hypovolemic shock because the head is a significantly larger fraction of the body, and open fontanelles and cranial sutures may provide greater potential space for accumulation of blood.[4] Intracranial hemorrhage often requires surgical intervention, and the pediatric anesthesiologist must be prepared for emergent transition to OR – as children are more susceptible to secondary brain injury (i.e., decreased CPP, hypoxia, hyperthermia, seizures).[4] Full fontanelles, split cranial sutures, or sun-setting sign are all associated with increased ICP or brain injury in infants.[5] Hypertension, bradycardia, and irregular respirations (Cushing's triad) are associated with impending brain herniation.[5]

The subarachnoid space is smaller in a child and thereby offers less buoyancy and protection from injury overall.[1] Monitoring ICP and CBF are essential in the pediatric TBI patient: ICP can be evaluated with intraventricular catheters, subarachnoid bolts, and epidural sensors; CBF can be evaluated by Doppler. Cerebral metabolic demands can be assessed via IJ bulb catheters or NIRS.[1]

Maintenance of cerebral blood flow and oxygen delivery is the major goal of managing head trauma.[5] Hyperthermia will increase oxygen demand in the brain of a pediatric trauma patient and can thereby contribute to tissue hypoxia and extension of infarction zones.[1] Cerebral perfusion pressure requirements will change across ages for pediatric patients: recent guidelines recommend maintenance of CPP of 40 mmHg in young children and 65 mmHg in teenagers (generally = MAP of 60 mmHg in young children and 85 mmHg in teenagers).[5] Hypertonic saline (3%) and mannitol may be used as osmotic agents to decrease cerebral edema and thereby decrease ICP.[1] Hyperventilation to $PaCO_2 < 35$ mmHg should only be used in the pediatric TBI patient with signs of impending brainstem herniation (e.g., decerebrate/decorticate posturing or unequal/unreactive pupils) despite efforts to control ICP, as hyperventilation to decrease ICP contributes to decreased cerebral blood flow, and is detrimental to brain tissue in watershed areas.[5] CSF drainage may be necessary in pediatric TBI management if ICP is unresponsive to less aggressive measures.[1]

Cervical spine injury is less associated with head injury in young children (despite proportionally larger head size/weight) because the spine is more mobile and less prone to fracture.[4] However, spinal cord injury without radiographic abnormality (SCIWORA) may occur in up to 50% of young children, and ATLS guidelines now allow for substitution of CT for cervical spine radiographs.[4] Cervical spine injuries are more likely to occur at C1–C4 in patients < 10 y/o, versus C5–C7 in patients > 10 y/o.[1]

Pseudosubluxation (anterior displacement of C2 over C3) usually occurs in children under 7 y/o.[1] Pseudosubluxation and increased distance between the Dens and arch of C1, of up to 4 mm, can be a normal variant in children under 7 y/o.[1] Both variants are difficult to discern versus spinal injury on plain radiographs.

In older children, an odontoid or open mouth view can be used to evaluate the superior cervical vertebrae, but younger children present more difficulty evaluating the upper cervical spine.[4] Physical examination of the awake/alert pediatric patient is reliable for evaluation of suspected spinal injury, but MRI should be considered for evaluation of cervical spinal cord in young trauma patients with uncertain radiographic results or inability to obtain clinical clearance (e.g., not alert, nonconversant, significant behavioral or intellectual disability, positive neurologic deficits, distracting pain, or cervical tenderness).[1]

Drowning

Drowning is consistently ranked high as a cause of accidental deaths for all age groups in the U.S.[6] Contrary to popular legend, drowning victims rarely exhibit efforts at gaining attention/help before loss of swimming ability.[6]

Most drowning victims may aspirate up to 22 ml/kg, but significant impairment of pulmonary gas exchange can occur after aspiration of as little as 1 to 3 ml/kg of fluid and 10–15% of drowning victims demonstrate no evidence of fluid aspiration on autopsy.[6] Victims may also swallow large amounts of fluid; gastric content aspiration is common in freshwater and seawater drowning.[6]

Drowning victims suffer shunting and hypoxia secondary to loss of sufficient surfactant and damage of the alveolar-capillary interface.[6] Cardiac dysrthymias are not the final common pathway of terminal drowning.[6] Comorbidities, circumstances of event, and duration of hypoxia will affect individual drowning victims and possible development of cardiac dysrthymias, but the final common pathologic event is tissue ischemia – and the brain is the critical end organ for drowning.[6] Irreversible brain damage occurs after 4–8 minutes of drowning-related hypoxia; recovery of normal brain function is unlikely after 8–10 minutes.[6]

Secondary brain edema is common in drowning events: hypoperfusion-related damage can continue after effective CPR has begun as posthypoxic cerebral edema formation continues and elevations in ICP will be encountered.[6] Routine measurement of ICP is not recommended for near-drowning victims, and may only introduce additional risk/morbidity; aggressive therapies to reduce ICP have not improved overall patient outcomes.[6]

Ventilation/perfusion mismatch occurs in both freshwater and seawater drownings, if by different physical manifestations.[6] Freshwater is hypotonic to plasma, while seawater is three times more concentrated than plasma.[6] Freshwater in the bronchoalveolar tree dilutes pulmonary surfactant and diminishes alveolar surface tension; reduction of alveolar surfactant promotes atelectasis and hypoxic ventilation/perfusion (V/Q) mismatch.[6] Seawater in the bronchoalveolar tree draws fluid from the capillary lumen into the alveolar sacs; hypoxic V/Q mismatch occurs secondary to continued perfusion of fluid-filled alveoli.[6]

Secondary electrolyte disturbances in drownings are rare; neither freshwater nor seawater contributes directly to primary renal injury.[6] Drowning can lead to renal hypoperfusion and hypoxia-related acute tubular necrosis, but glomerular filtration is typically preserved.[6] Hyperglycemia following near-drowning has been associated with poor outcomes in children.[6]

Immersion in water less than 25 °C can trigger ventricular fibrillation and asystole, but sinus bradycardia and atrial fibrillation are common under conditions of hypoxia and hypothermia.[6] Appearance of Osborn waves on ECG heralds dangerous proximity to critical ventricular fibrillation thresholds in the hypothermic patient.[6]

One in five near-drowning victims will have normal chest radiographs; it is common for initial films to demonstrate little or no pulmonary injury patterns.[6] Pulse oximetry can be an unreliable method for trending oxygenation in pediatric near-drowning victims secondary to peripheral vasoconstriction and hypothermia.[6] Frequent ABGs will be necessary.[6] Hyperbaric therapy is not the most effective method of reversing hypoxia postsubmersion injury: supplemental oxygen combined with positive-pressure ventilation has been described as the most effective treatment in reversing hypoxia postaspiration. Postaspiration pneumonia is not a common complication of near-drowning.[6] Patients with suspected drowning in grossly contaminated water should undergo bronchoscopy, with samples sent for gram stain and culture.[6] Prophylactic antibiotics are not routinely recommended for victims of near-drowning.[6]

Facial injury

The majority of facial injuries in young children is caused by falls, and occurs more often in males than females.[1] Facial trauma tends to be less severe in children under 5 years of age, and more often involves soft tissue injuries.[1] Compared to soft-tissue injuries, the incidence of dental injuries diminishes throughout childhood.[1] There is an increase in soft tissue injury of the face in adolescence – probably related to concurrent increase in aggressive and risky activities.[1] Facial fractures are the least common form of pediatric facial trauma, and nasal fractures make up approximately 50% of fracture injuries.[1]

In anticipated difficult airway related to facial injury, it may be necessary to transport the child to an OR suite – along with an anesthesiologist and otolaryngologist – prior to intubation.[1] Efforts should concentrate on establishing hemodynamic stability before transport to OR, so that inhalation/IV induction will be better tolerated.[1] In children, crepitus at the neck is associated with tracheal disruption and fiber optic intubation should be considered to avoid false passage of the ETT.[1] Zone I neck trauma (area between thoracic outlet and cricoid cartilage containing proximal common carotids, vertebral and subclavian arteries, esophagus, trachea, thoracic duct, and thymus) is associated with the worst morbidity and mortality prognosis in young children.[1]

All pediatric trauma patients should be considered as possible cervical spine injury and treated accordingly during initial airway management: inline stabilization is especially necessary in pediatric trauma victims who have suffered head injury or loss of consciousness.[1]

Flexible fiberoptic laryngoscopy remains the gold standard approach to nonemergent difficult airway in pediatric patients; patient cooperation may require planning for sedation or induction with maintenance of spontaneous respiration.[4] Use of rigid videolaryngoscopy, light wand, retrograde intubation, or other alternative techniques can be considered if equipment and expertise are immediately available, but placement of SGA (e.g., LMA, ILMA) through which blind or fiberoptic intubation can be accomplished is recommended as part of the ASA difficult airway algorithm in emergent airway scenarios.[4] Consideration for rapid transition to percutaneous or surgical airway must be part of any emergent pediatric airway management plan. Muscle relaxants are not usually necessary to accomplish use of fiberoptic laryngoscopy in pediatric trauma patients, and should be avoided until the airway is secured.[1]

Retractions and grunting without immediate hypoxia may be related to pain in young children but may also be related to chest or airway trauma; any increased work of breathing or signs of airway/

pulmonary distress should be evaluated and possible need for intubation considered – pain alone can lead to significant pulmonary compromise secondary to splinting.[5] Rapid-sequence induction involves considerable risk for children with hypovolemia or congenital cardiac disease; the anesthesiologist must consider alternatives and methods.[5]

Thoracic injuries

Trauma-related cardiac tamponade is rare in pediatric thoracic-injury victims – and will typically exhibit associated hypotension and pulsus paradoxus.[5] Myocardial enzyme studies are reliable for cardiac evaluation in young children, and should be considered if suspected myocardial injury is present.[5] Cardiac and great vessel trauma is less common in children, but nearly 90% of pediatric cardiac trauma patients will exhibit evidence of injury to other organ systems.[5]

Rib fractures and flail chest occur less often in children versus adults, as a result of having a more cartilaginous rib cage, but when a child suffers significant pulmonary injury, mortality increases tenfold.[1] Unilateral hemothorax can hold up to 40% of a young child's blood volume, and thereby produce dangerous hemodynamic instability.[1] A cartilaginous rib cage does not protect against transmission of forces to lung and mediastinal structures; transmission is more easily transferred secondary to decreased bony support.[1]

Abdominal injuries

Rapid deceleration or shearing injuries are most commonly associated with pediatric abdominal injuries.[1] Solid organs (kidneys, liver, and spleen) are more commonly injured, versus hollow visceral organs (3rd and 4th portions of duodenum, terminal ileum and sigmoid colon). Great vessel, GU tract, pancreas, and pelvis injuries are rare in pediatric trauma.[1] Death from abdominal injuries is usually secondary to hemorrhage.[1]

The extent of abdominal injury is often scored on a scale from 1 to 5 based on radiographic findings (higher number = more severe injury).[1] The decision to operate is based on clinical scenario (e.g., evidence of continued hemodynamic instability despite appropriate resuscitation); radiographic staging of abdominal organ injuries may influence the trauma team's decision, but does not determine need for operative intervention.[1] Success rates for nonoperative management of liver, spleen, and kidney trauma in pediatric patients exceed 90%.[1]

Gastric dilatation (as result of swallowing air) in children can inhibit vagally mediated tachycardic response to hypovolemia, as well as mimic peritonitis and limit diaphragmatic excursion.[1] Lap-belt injury complex is composed of soft-tissue injury, intra-abdominal injuries, and orthopedic injuries: bruising/ecchymosis or degloving skin injury +/- fascial dehiscence; solid organ, hollow viscus perforation or hematoma, mesenteric bleeding, bladder and/or great vessel injuries; dislocation, fractures, and/or subluxation of iliac wings and lumbar, sacral, and thoracic spine. [1]

Skeletal injuries

Musculoskeletal injuries are rarely life-threatening in pediatric patients – unless associated with ongoing severe hemorrhage – and rarely require concurrent surgical intervention with abdominal, head or thoracic injuries.[1] The ACS Committee on Trauma has, however, recommended definitive treatment of femoral fractures early in the trauma course as long as the patient is hemodynamically stable.[1] Urgent or emergent surgical interventions for skeletal injuries in children are usually associated with vascular damage, limb ischemia, neurologic dysfunction, open fractures, compartment syndrome, or nonreducible joint dislocations.[1]

Pain out of proportion to a limb injury should raise suspicion of compartment syndrome in pediatric patients.[1] Definitive therapy for compartment syndrome is surgical fasciotomy of all involved compartments in the affected limb/area.[1] Injuries most commonly associated with compartment syndrome include fractures of the tibia and forearm.[1]

Vascular injuries in conjunction with limb fractures are rare in children: most vascular injuries are associated with supracondylar fractures of the distal humerus, but may also occur in association with fractures of the pelvis, distal femur, and proximal tibia as well as dislocations of the knee.[1] Angiograms may be needed for evaluation of vascular injuries in children, just as in adults.[1]

References

1. Reynolds P, Scattoloni J, Ehrlich P, Cladis F, Davis P. Anesthesia for the pediatric trauma patient. In Davis P, Cladis F, Motoyama E, eds. *Smith's Anesthesia for Infants and Children.* 8th edn. Philadelphia, PA: Elsevier/Mosby; 2011. pp. 971–1002.
2. National Trauma Data Bank Subcommittee. National Trauma Data Bank 2010: Pediatric Report. 2010: 1–66.
3. McClain C, Soriano S. Neurosurgery and Neurotraumatology: Anesthetic considerations. In Bissonette B, ed. *Pediatric Anesthesia: Basic Prinicples, State of the Art, Future.* 1st edn. Shelton, CT: People's Medical Publishing House; 2011. pp. 1569–88.
4. Young D, Wesson D. Trauma. In Coté C, Lerman J, Anderson B, eds. *A Practice of Anesthesia for Infants and Children.* 5th ed. Philadelphia, PA: Saunders/ Elsevier; 2013. pp. 789–803.
5. Guffey P, Andropoulos D. Anesthesia for burns and trauma. In Gregory G, Andropoulos D, eds. Gregory's Pediatric Anesthesia. 5th edn. Blackwell; 2012. pp. 896–918.
6. Terry S, Kaplan L. Near-drowning. In Wilson L, Grande C, Hoyt D, eds. *Trauma, Volume 1: Emergency Resuscitation Perioperative Anesthesia Surgical Management.* 1st edn. New York, NY: Informa Healthcare; 2007. pp. 685–97.

Chapter 23

Burns

Terry G. Fletcher, James E. Hunt, and Joe R. Jansen

Burns

1. Types, mechanisms, locations, and implications of injuries
2. Inhalation injuries/airway management
3. Fluid resuscitation and calculating burn surface area
4. Anesthetic and pain management of the burn patient

Types, mechanisms, locations, and implications of injuries

The American Burn Association maintains a National Burn Repository for data collected on acute burn admissions within the USA. Overall, pediatric burn patients account for approximately one-third of total burn admission volume.[1] Scald burns account for most of the pediatric burns in children under 4 years of age.[1] Flame burns account for most of the pediatric burns in children 5 years of age and older. [1] Burn trauma is the second leading cause of death in children between 1 and 4 years of age, and the third leading cause of death in children younger than 18 years of age.[1] Intentional injury/abuse is causative for approximately 1 in 6 pediatric burn injuries.[1]

More burn patients survive their wounds, and enjoy improved quality of life,[1] because of several advances in modern medical and surgical care, including: improved access to emergency and initial care; better understanding of the pathophysiology of burn and inhalation injury; targeted resuscitation initially and perioperatively; advanced ventilation modalities and respiratory care protocols; improved infection control practices; advanced surgical and wound care technologies and techniques such as early burn wound excision and grafting; improved nutritional support and attenuation of the hypermetabolic response. [1]

Burn injuries must be described by the percent total body surface of injury incurred, as well as the depth of tissue involved (e.g., superficial or first-degree, partial-thickness or second degree, full-thickness or third degree, or fourth degree) (Table 23.1).[1]

First-degree burns are classified as superficial burns and have the following characteristics: only the epidermal layer is involved and barrier functions are preserved, associated with mild–moderate pain, no blistering, and no scarring. These types of burns are commonly seen in sunburns.[1]

Second-degree or partial-thickness burns involve the epidermal layer with varying degrees of dermal extension. These burns can have a wet or dry appearance and are usually classified as superficial/partial-thickness or deep/partial-thickness, respectively. Wet-appearing partial-thickness burns are common with scald injuries and are associated with: localized hyperemia, edema, blistering, and moderate to severe pain. These burns typically heal in 7–10 days with appropriate care, and scar formation is uncommon. Dry appearing partial-thickness burns are common with flame or chemical exposure. These wounds may appear red or pale, usually exhibit moderate to severe blistering and are less painful (secondary to more significant nerve injury) versus superficial partial thickness-injuries. Dry partial-thickness burns may advance to full thickness injury, and usually require 2 to 8 weeks to heal without intervention; scar formation is probable without surgical intervention.[1]

Third-degree burns are classified as full-thickness injuries. These burns are the result of prolonged chemical, friction, or thermal exposure causing complete damage to epidermal and dermal tissue layers. Third-degree burns are painless (secondary to

Essentials of Pediatric Anesthesiology, ed. Alan David Kaye, Charles James Fox and James H. Diaz. Published by Cambridge University Press. © Cambridge University Press 2015.

Table 23.1 Thermal injury characteristics

Designation	Involvement (example source of injury)	Examination signs
First degree	Superficial (e.g.,sunburn)	Epidermal layers only Barrier functions remain intact Mild to moderate pain No scarring
Partial-thickness (Second degree)	Superficial partial-thickness (e.g., scald burn)	Epidermal layers + extension into dermis Barrier functions impaired Wet appearance Hyperemic Edematous Mild to moderate blistering Moderate to severe pain Heals in 7–10 days Scar formation unlikely
	Deep partial-thickness (e.g., prolonged scald, flame or chemical injury)	Epidermal layers + significant extension into dermis Barrier functions impaired/lost Dry appearance Edematous Moderate to severe blistering Moderate pain Heals in 2–8 weeks; may progress to full-thickness injury Scar formation likely
Third degree	Full thickness (e.g., prolonged thermal/flame, or chemical contact)	Complete epidermal and dermal involvement Barrier functions lost Dry appearance Eschar with waxy or leathery appearance No edema in eschar +/– sloughing of skin or presence of charring on eschar Minimal pain Requires surgical excision + scarring
Fourth degree	Full-thickness (e.g., electrical injury)	Complete epidermal and dermal loss + involvement of fascia, muscle, tendon, bone Barrier functions lost Muscle/bone necrosis Extensive surgical intervention/reconstruction required

Source: Modified from *Smith's Anesthesia for Infants and Children*. 8th edn. Elsevier; 2011.

complete nerve destruction) and very often have a dry, waxy white or leathery appearance. Excision and grafting is required of these types of burns.[1]

Fourth-degree burns are full-thickness injuries that include not only complete epidermal and dermal tissue, but involve fascia, muscle, and bone as well. These types of burns can often be seen with prolonged flame exposure or electrical injury. Such injuries will require extensive surgical intervention.[1]

Burn injuries that meet American Burn Association (ameriburn.org) criteria should be transferred to an appropriate burn center for definitive care as soon as medically feasible. Those ten criteria include:[2]

1. Partial thickness burns greater than 10% total body surface area (TBSA).
2. Burns that involve the face, hands, feet, genitalia, perineum, or major joints.
3 Third-degree burns in any age group.

4. Electrical burns, including lightning injury.
5. Chemical burns.
6. Inhalation injury.
7. Burn injury in patients with pre-existing medical disorders that could complicate management, prolong recovery, or affect mortality.
8. Any patient with burns and concomitant trauma (such as fractures) in which the burn injury poses the greatest risk of morbidity or mortality. In such cases, if the trauma poses the greater immediate risk, the patient may be initially stabilized in a trauma center before being transferred to a burn unit. Physician judgment will be necessary in such situations and should be in concert with the regional medical control plan and triage protocols.
9. Burned children in hospitals without qualified personnel or equipment for the care of children.
10. Burn injury in patients who will require special social, emotional, or rehabilitative intervention.

Pathophysiological changes that occur with burn injuries are quite significant and include hypermetabolism, loss of thermal insulation, septicemia, and increased inflammatory responses. The increased inflammatory responses contribute directly to multi-organ system changes.[3]

Table 23.2 Systemic effects of major burn injury

System	Acute phase	Chronic phase
Neurologic	Encephalopathy Seizures ↑ ICP Post-traumatic stress Acute pain	Encephalopathy Seizures ICU Delirium Post-traumatic stress Acute + chronic pain
Cardiovascular	Myocardial depression ↓ Cardiac output	Hypertension Tachycardia ↑ Cardiac output
Pulmonary	↑ & ↓ airway obstruction ↓ FRC ↓ Pulmonary compliance ↓ Chest-wall compliance	Pneumonia Tracheal stenosis ↓ Chest-wall compliance
Hepatic	↓ Synthetic function	↑ Synthetic function Hepatitis Heaptic dysfunction
Renal	↓ GFR	↓ GFR Tubular dysfunction
Skin	↑ Temperature, fluid, and electrolyte loss ↑ Infection risk	Contractures Scarring
Hematopoietic	↓ Red cell mass Thrombocytopenia ↑ Fibrin split products/fibrinolysis Coagulopathies	Thrombocytosis Transfusion reactions Coagulopathies
Metabolic	↓ Ionized calcium	↓ Ionized calcium ↑ O_2 consumption ↑ CO_2 production
Pharmacokinetic	Altered Vd Altered protein binding Altered pharmacodynamics Altered pharmacokinetics	↑ Opioid/sedative tolerance Drug interactions Altered receptor function Enzyme induction

Source: Modified from *Smith's Anesthesia for Infants and Children*. 8th edn. Elsevier; 2011.

Acute phase pathophysiological changes can last from a few hours to several days. Characteristics of the acute phase of major burn injury include: hemoconcentration, decreased cardiac ouput and myocardial depression, decreased FRC, marked inflammatory response, and increased fluid and electrolyte loss.[1] Conversely, characteristic pathophysiologic changes that occur after resolution of the acute phase (i.e., chronic phase changes) of a major burn injury include: increased cardiac output, increased oxygen consumption, hypermetabolic state, and hypertension.[1] Acute and chronic phase changes are summarized in Table 23.2.[1]

Inhalation injuries/airway management

Burn injuries occurring in closed spaces significantly increase the risk of a patient obtaining inhalation injury from exposure to particulate matter and toxins in smoke or chemical vapors.[3] Evidence of a possible inhalational injury may include: burns noted on face, lips, nares, or intraoral cavities; carbonaceous debris in naso- or oropharynx or sputum; mucosal sloughing; voice changes or stridor; dyspnea or respiratory distress (if not intubated); hypoxia; confirmed carboxyhemoglobin toxicity; and presenting history.[1] Initially, a chest radiograph (CXR) may appear normal following an inhalational injury, but results may change over time as inflammatory and infectious complications arise. However, the CXR often underestimates the severity of an inhalational injury.[4] Treatment modalities for an inhalational injury may include aerosolized heparin, mucolytics, serial bronchoscopy, and pulmonary suctioning.[1]

Worsening airway compromise due to increased swelling and edema of the glottic opening is expected over the course of the acute phase fluid resuscitation; therefore early intubation may be needed.[3] Stridor can be an ominous sign of impending airway obstruction due to swelling and edema, and warrants immediate evaluation with preparation for definitive airway management.[3] Patients with circumferential burns of the torso are a concern during acute injury phase and initial fluid resuscitation as well. These patients may rapidly develop abdominal and thoracic compartment syndromes which restrict ventilation, and may thereby require abdominal and thoracic escharotomies to improve ventilation.[3]

Progressive edema can distort facial and tracheal anatomy.[1] Adhesive tape which may work well on most patients does not adhere well on patients with facial burns because of constant fluid weeping from tissue. Methods to prevent dislodgement may include suturing or wiring to teeth, securing with umbilical or trach tape and frequent reassessments and secondary confirmation by chest radiographs.[1]

Although fluid restriction may help minimize pulmonary edema in other patients, burn patients require large volumes of fluid in the initial resuscitation to maintain perfusion and minimize end-organ damage; fluid restriction in the setting of large surface area or major burns will contribute to worsening metabolic and hemodynamic function.[1] Physiological effects of inhalational injury are numerous but include ciliary dysfunction, leukocyte aggregation and increased endothelial permeability.[1] Bronchial sloughing and edema may contribute to increased airway pressures.[1]

Carbon monoxide has a binding affinity to hemoglobin 200 times greater than that of oxygen, and exposure will rapidly lead to carboxyhemoglobin toxicity.[1] As a result, there is a leftward shift of the oxygen–hemoglobin dissociation curve. Signs and symptoms of carbon monoxide poisoning include: agitation, dizziness, lethargy, seizures, chest pain, dyspnea, and noncardiogenic pulmonary edema.[1] Pulse oximetry readings often show 100% due to overlapping of carbon monoxide with oxygen in the absorption spectrum. Therefore, arterial blood gas analysis or co-oximetry should be utilized when CO poisoning is suspected. The half-life of carboxyhemoglobin on room air is approximately 4 hours. The half-life reduces to approximately 1 hour on 100% oxygen.[1]

Cyanide toxicity diminishes mitochondrial oxidative phosphorylation by inactivating cytochrome oxidases, effectively shutting down the electron transport system. When this occurs, oxygen is not utilized (PaO_2 increases) and lactic acidosis ensues from anaerobic metabolism.[4] Patients may exhibit signs and symptoms similar to carbon monoxide poisoning; supplemental oxygen will not improve the developing acidosis. Treatment for cyanide toxicity includes sodium thiosulfate, sodium nitrite, and hydroxocobalamin. Nitrites such as amyl nitrite or sodium nitrite induce methemoglobin, which then competes directly with cytochrome-binding sites for cyanide, resulting in formation of less toxic cyanomethemoglobin.[1] Use of nitrites in younger pediatric patients must take into consideration subsequent production of methemoglobin and potential for associated worsening of tissue oxygenation.[1]

Fluid resuscitation and calculating burn surface area

Patients with major burns require fluid resuscitation. Large volumes of fluids are needed following a major burn injury, due to increased microvascular permeability, increased tissue osmotic pressure, rapid reduction of plasma volume and interstitial fluid accumulation.[3] Even nonburned tissue is affected and becomes edematous for the same reasons. Plasma volume is lost most rapidly during the 4–6 hours immediately postinjury.[3]

Traditional formulas such as the Parkland and Modified Brooke formulas were developed for adults. These burn resuscitation formulas can be of great value in guiding fluid resuscitation in older children; however, serious underestimation of the necessary fluid volume may occur if applied to infants and toddlers weighing less than 10–20 kg.[3] Adding maintenance requirements to the Parkland formula of 4 ml/kg/% TBSA helps to minimize under-resuscitation during the first 24 hours.[5] The Modified Brooke formula is also used on pediatric patients, and gives an additional 2–3 ml/kg/% for patients weighing less than 20 kg.[3] The Galveston formula is the only formula developed specifically for children and takes into account body surface area for both burn and maintenance fluid requirements, as well as incorporating management of protein, dextrose, and electrolyte needs.[3]

Targeting appropriate clinical endpoints during volume resuscitation will include monitoring for: hemodynamic stability, absence of protein or glucose in urine, base deficit less than two, minimal systemic acidosis, intact sensorium, normothermia, and urine output 1–2 ml/kg dependent on child's age.[1]

Traditionally, the rule of nines has been used for estimating the body surface area involved with burns in adults. Charts derived from Lund and Browder are often utilized to estimate body surface area of burns in children at different ages of development. These charts take into account the relatively larger head and smaller lower extremities in estimating body surface area.[2] The palm and fingers of the patient's hand represent about 1% of the patient's total body surface area; this estimation can be used to calculate the surface area of small and scattered burns (Figure 23.1).[6]

Anesthetic and pain management of the burn patient

Standard monitor placement is often problematic in the burn patient. Strategies to combat these problems include: placement and monitoring of arterial lines in place of unreliable blood-pressure cuff; placement of pulse oximeter on tongue, ear, nose, scrotum, or vulva in the presence of poor signal transduction of an extremity; and placement of needle probes when ECG pads do not adhere to burned tissue.[1]

One of the most significant challenges during major excision and grafting procedures of burn patients is heat conservation.[3] Both total intravenous anesthesia and inhalational anesthesia techniques impair hypothalamic thermoregulation in a dose-dependent manner to cause vasodilation and redistribution of core body temperature.[3] Methods to prevent perioperative heat loss include: increased ambient temperature, forced air warming devices, conductive and radiant warmers, fluid warmers, humidity and moisture exchange devices, warm linens/blankets and moisture barriers. Effective communication between the surgeon and the anesthesiologist is imperative when it comes to hypothermia. Preoperatively, both should agree on a patient temperature threshold at which the case will be terminated. The anesthesiologist should remind the surgeon to cover as much of the patient as possible when they are not working on an area.[3]

Blood loss can be rapid and life-threatening during burn wound excision – especially during tangential excision: for every 1% of body surface excised, up to 3.5–5% of total blood volume can be lost.[3] Placement of large-bore intravenous catheters is advantageous for rapid administration of blood products in burn patients when significant blood loss is anticipated. Additional vascular access is also advantageous in the event the central line were to become nonfunctional.[4] Generally, the area of tissue excised should not exceed 10–15% of total body surface area during any one procedure. Blood transfusion should not be based on a set hemoglobin concentration trigger value but should instead be based on hemodynamic considerations, patient history, and the likelihood of ongoing bleeding.[3]

Burn patients tend to be chronically hypocalcemic, and administration of $CaCl_2$ may be needed to aid formation of the platelet plug as well as progression of the coagulation cascade in order that wound hemostasis is achieved.[3] Epinephrine soaked

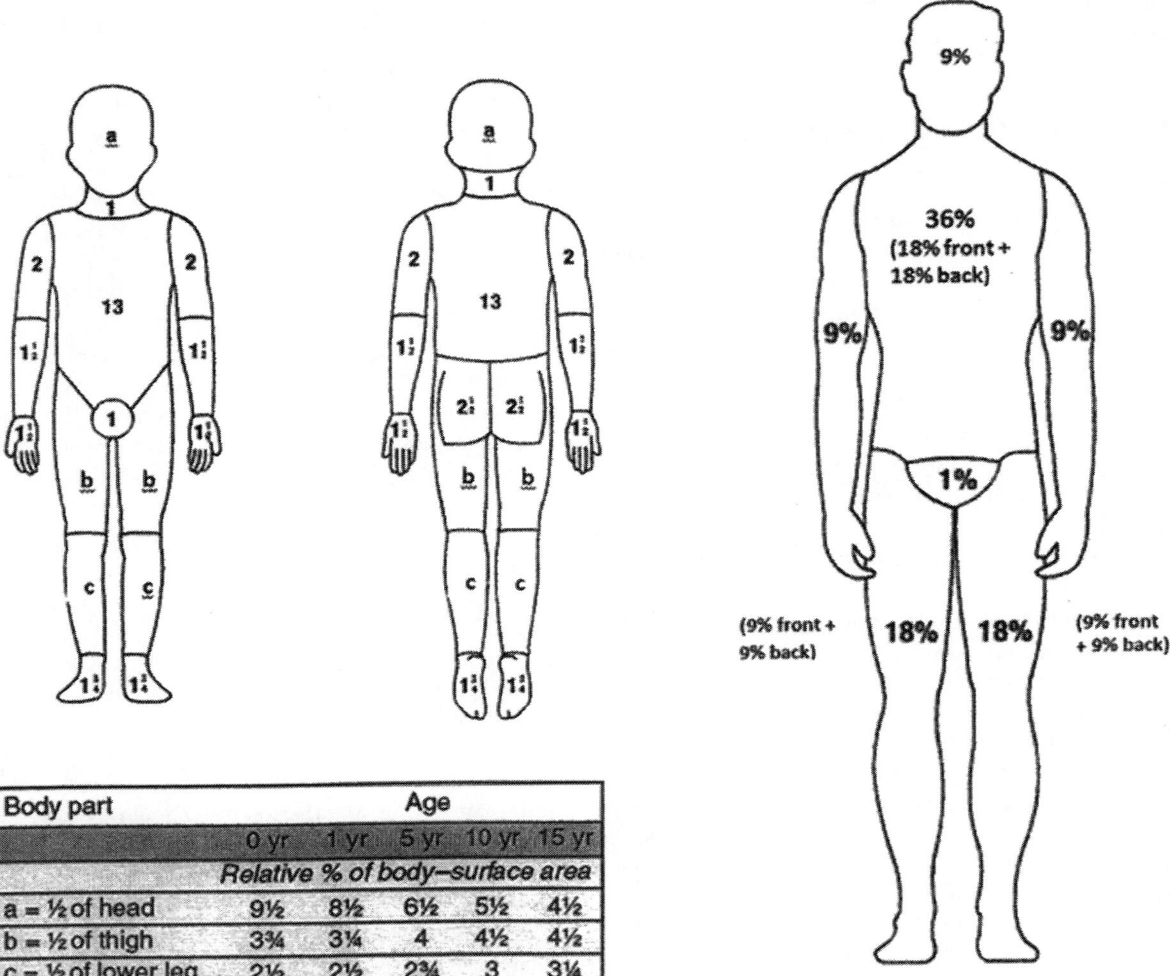

Body part	Age				
	0 yr	1 yr	5 yr	10 yr	15 yr
	Relative % of body–surface area				
a = ½ of head	9½	8½	6½	5½	4½
b = ½ of thigh	3¾	3¼	4	4½	4½
c = ½ of lower leg	2½	2½	2¾	3	3¼

Figure 23.1 *Source:* Modified from *Smith's Anesthesia for Infants and Children*. 8th edn. Elsevier; 2011.

sponges (1:10 000 dilution) are commonly used to produce small-vessel vasoconstriction and limit blood loss. Intravascular absorption of epinephrine is rarely a concern.[5] Extremity tourniquets are also useful in minimizing blood loss, as is spray-on thrombin and kaolin-impregnated gauze. Albumin may be beneficial in treating hypovolemia, although it has no effect on minimizing or reducing blood loss.

Cardiac output and tissue blood flow can be significantly decreased in the acute phase. Clearance and metabolism of many drugs are also diminished during this period.[3]

Succinylcholine causes an increased response in burn patients due to up-regulation of acetylcholine receptors. The increase is the result of an increase in acetylcholine receptor on the muscle membrane and not just the neural junction.[1] After approximately 24 hours, succinylcholine is contraindicated in burn patients due to potential massive release of potassium. Complications resulting from hyperkalemia may initially be seen as peaked T-waves on ECG, but can rapidly progress to dysrhythmias and hemodynamic instability. Treatment includes giving calcium to stabilize the myocardium, D50, and insulin to drive excess potassium intracellularly, bicarbonate to decrease acidosis, and hyperventilation to induce a respiratory alkalosis.[5]

Maintaining urine output greater than 1–1.5 ml/kg/h is desirable for pediatric burn patients and is usually a good sign of adequate volume resuscitation and hemodynamic function.[4] Patients with electrical burns may appear to have minor superficial skin damage, but can have significant internal injuries. Damage to muscle tissue – whether from electrical injury or deep thermal injury – can result in hemoglobinuria and myoglobinuria, which increase the risk of renal injury and failure. Treatment goals seek to minimize renal damage by maintaining renal tubule patency. Alkalization of urine with sodium bicarbonate prevents precipitation of proteins in renal tubules. Giving mannitol to promote an osmotic diuresis can also aid in flushing out tubule debris.[5]

Resistance to nondepolarizing muscle relaxants is thought to occur because of an increase in the number of extrajunctional receptors located on muscle membrane of burn patients. The degree of resistance is related to the size and severity of the burn wound and can begin to be evident within a week of the initial burn injury.[3]

Muscle relaxant antagonists are unaffected by these changes, therefore dosing remains unchanged.[3]

Sevoflurane, desflurane, and isoflurane are acceptable for maintenance of anesthesia. Sevoflurane is suitable for induction, while isoflurane has cost advantages.[4]

Ketamine is considered an anesthetic and analgesic of choice in treatment of burn patients. Ketamine is a noncompetitive antagonist of NMDA receptors.[1] It can be administered via the intramuscular, oral, or rectal routes in addition to the intravenous route. Advantages of ketamine include: anesthesia, analgesia, rapid onset, short duration, bronchial dilation, minimal respiratory depression, reduction of systemic inflammation, and direct central sympathetic stimulation.[4] However, ketamine can act as a direct myocardial depressant, especially in hypovolemic and catecholamine-depleted patients. Concurrent administration of benzodiazepines can significantly minimize risk of dysphoria associated with ketamine use.[1]

During the hypermetabolic phase of a burn injury, there is a reduced affinity for agonist to the myocardial β-adrenergic receptors, causing diminished receptor-mediated signal transduction, leading to a reduction in adenylate cyclase activity and production of cAMP. The net result is a diminished cardiovascular response to adrenergic agents such as epinephrine.[3]

Metabolic needs increase to 1.2–1.7 times the normal basal rate for burned children.[6] Because of the need for frequent surgeries and sedations associated with wound care and the increased nutritional and caloric intake required for healing in burn patients, some burn centers use modified NPO guidelines for burn patients. Enteral nutrition is continued during surgery or sedation for intubated patients. Enteral feeding is discontinued for nonintubated patients up to 4 hours prior to the procedure. In order to improve the nutritional status burn patients, preoperative fasting down to 1 hour has been advocated and considered safe.[4]

The severity of pain is dictated by the size of the injury.[5] Burn injuries induced experimentally cause local inflammatory changes that are discernible as allodynia, hyperemia, and hyperalgesia.[2] Scheduled and per need opioids are often used to treat pain in the pediatric burn patient. Other methods have also been successfully used to manage burn pain in children including: patient controlled analgesia (PCA), anxiolytics, acetaminophen, NSAIDs, NMDA antagonist (ketamine), alpha-2 agonists (clonidine and dexmedetomidine), and anticonvulsants (gabapentin). Nonpharmacologic approaches include immersive virtual reality and music therapy.[5] Dose requirements of opioids are higher in burn patients compared to nonburn patients due to rapidly developed tolerance.[2] In the past there was concern of opioid addiction in treating burn pain in children; however, addiction from therapeutic uses of opioids in pediatric burn patients has not been reported.[5] Problems associated with the use of PCA include risk of under treatment of pain in patients not able to use their hands or understand PCA usage principles, and risk of over-treatment from family members.[4] Wound closure is the most effective analgesic and opioid requirement decreases rapidly once this has taken place.[5]

Unfortunately, procedural associated pain is often poorly managed in children.[4] Approximately 30% of patients with major burns will experience post-traumatic stress disorder.[4] Facilities routinely treating burned children should develop pain and anxiety guidelines. These guidelines should focus on safety and efficacy reflective of the diversity of patient ages as well as range of patient acuities. Further, the guideline should advise specific pharmacotherapies – including dosing and acceleration of treatment. Finally the guide should include a narrow group of pharmacologic agents in effort to maintain staff familiarity and reduce the risk of untoward events related to subtherapeutic or unintentional overdosing.[5] Developing anxiety and pain management guidelines based on assessment scales improves outcomes while minimizing sleep disturbance and post-traumatic psychological disturbances.[4]

Pain from a freshly harvested donor site tends to be the most intense pain associated with burn injuries.[1] When preparing a donor site for harvest, surgeons often utilize tumescence (infiltrating subdermal saline) with bupivacaine or lidocaine. The infiltrated saline stretches the skin to facilitate skin harvest and the local anesthetic helps with pain. A lateral femoral cutaneous nerve block helps – particularly with anterolateral thigh pain.[1] Adjuvants such as gabapentin, NSAIDs, and ketamine are also helpful in combating donor site pain.

References

1. Romanelli T. Anesthesia for burn injuries. In Davis P, Cladis F, Motoyama E, editors. *Smith's Anesthesia for Infants and Children*. 8th edn. Philadelphia, PA: Mosby; 2011. pp. 1003–22.
2. Burn Center Referral Criteria as excerpted from *Guidelines for the Operation of Burn Centers (pp. 79 –86), Resources for Optimal Care of the Injured Patient, Committee on Trauma, 2006. American College of Surgeons.* Available from http://www.ameriburn.org/BurnCenterReferralCriteria.pdf (accessed September 14, 2013).
3. Guffey PJ, Andropoulos DB. Anesthesia for burns and trauma. In Gregory G, Andropoulos D, editors. *Gregory's Pediatric Anesthesia.* 5th edn. Wiley-Blackwell; 2012. pp. 896–918.
4. Bernath M, Stucki P, Berger MM. Burns and post-burn care: Anesthetic considerations. In Bissonnette B, editor. *Pediatric Anesthesia: Basic Principles – State of the Art – Future.* 1st edn. Shelton, CT: People's Medical Publishing House; 2011. pp. 2049–70.
5. Shank ES, Cote CJ, Martyn JAJ. Burn injuries. In Coté C, Lerman J, Anderson B, editors. *A Practice of Anesthesia For Infants And Children*. 5th edn. Saunders; 2013. pp. 712–31.
6. Clarke HM, de Chalain TMB. Burns and post-burn care: Surgical considerations. In Bissonnette B, editor. *Pediatric Anesthesia: Basic Principles – State of the Art – Future.* 1st edn. Shelton, CT: People's Medical Publishing House; 2011. pp. 2031–48.

Chapter 24

Evaluation and preoperative preparation of the pediatric patient

Rahul Dasgupta and Hani Hanna

Developmental milestones (age)	Motor skills	Social and cognitive
2 MONTHS	Regards objects Follows 180° Lifts head and shoulders off bed when prone	Smiles socially Coos Makes reciprocal vocalizations
4 MONTHS	Steady head control while sitting Holds head up Bears weight on forearms in the prone position Pushes with feet when in standing position Reaches for objects	Laughs out loud Squeals Initiates social interaction
6 MONTHS	Transfers object from one hand to the other Rolls over in both directions Sits with support	Turns directly to sound and voice Babbles consonant sounds Imitates speech sounds
9 MONTHS	Feeds self with fingers Plays gesture games (pat-a-cake) Bangs two objects together Holds two objects at one time Sits without support	Says "mama" and "dada" Understands his/her own name Recognizes common objects (e.g., bottle) Recognizes common people (e.g., daddy)
12 MONTHS	Pulls to a stand and cruises Takes a few independent steps Neat pincer grasp of raisin or pellet	Says "mama" and "dada" with specific meaning Says at least one specific word
15 MONTHS	Plays ball gives and takes a toy Drinks from a cup Makes a line with a crayon Makes two-cube tower Walks independently	Says three to six specific words; Follows simple commands Uses jargon
18 MONTHS	Feeds self with spoon Stacks tower of three cubes Runs Walks up steps with hand held	Imitates household tasks Says seven to ten words Identifies one or more body parts
24 MONTHS	Washes and dries hands, removes clothing Stacks tower of four to six cubes Feeds self with spoon and fork Runs well Kicks ball	Combines words into two- or three-word phrases Points to pictures named Uses vocabulary of 50+ words Uses "I," "me," and "mine" in speech

Essentials of Pediatric Anesthesiology, ed. Alan David Kaye, Charles James Fox and James H. Diaz. Published by Cambridge University Press. © Cambridge University Press 2015.

Evaluation of coexisting disease

a. Cerebral palsy

- Spastic, hypotonic, dystonic, athetotic or mixed monoplegia diplegia or quadriplegia.[1]
- Seizures and cognitive disorders are common.
- Phenytoin causes gum hyperplasia.
- Abrupt discontinuation of baclofen causes withdrawal seizures, hallucinations, and pruritis.
- Valproic acid: hepatotoxicity, bone marrow suppression, and platelet dysfunction.
- Anticonvulsants use causes resistance to NDMR due to hepatic-enzyme induction; even with absence of anticonvulsants, CP patients shows resistance to NDMR-like vecuronium (unknown mechanism).[2]
- High incidence of latex allergies.
- Scoliosis patients may have pulmonary impairment (restrictive) and are more liable to blood loss and platelet dysfunction.
- Most surgical cases require general anesthesia with tracheal intubation.
- Presence of GERD, poor function of laryngeal and pharyngeal reflexes.
- Inhalational agents are safe as there is no increased risk of MH.
- Proconvulsants methohexital, etomidate and meperidine are best avoided in the presence of seizures.
- Succinylcholine doesn't produce abnormal potassium release.[3]
- More liable to hypothermia.
- Delayed emergence from brain abnormalities or hypothermia.[4]
- Delay extubation until fully awake.
- Epidural and caudal are used for intra and postoperative pain.
- Postoperative muscles spasms may be treated by diazepam.
- More liable to postoperative pulmonary complications.[5]

b. Cystic fibrosis

- AR mutation single gene CFTR defect in chromosome 7.
- Abnormal chloride transport in exocrine glands, increase chloride in sweat(> 80 meq/l) leads to decrease sodium and water transport in various glands and mucous plugging.[6]
- Lungs, viscous mucous, impaired ciliary clearance leads to COPD obstructive pattern (high FRC low FEV1 low VC low PEFR) repeated lung exacerbation by infection and longstanding leads to corpulmonale.[7]
- Meconium ileus at birth, pansinusitis, DM, biliary obstruction, absent vas deferens obstructive azospermia.
- Pancreatic insufficiency ADEK — II, VII, IX and X.
- Management include vigorous CPT, humidification(7% Nacl), bronchodilators, antibiotics, Dornase alpha (pulmozyme) (recombinant DNAse cleaves dNA in sputum decreasing its viscosity).[8]
- Delay elective surgery to optimize chest conditions.
- Maintain humidified inspired air.
- Vitamin K supplementation.
- Inhalational induction may be prolonged.[9]
- Avoidance of anticholinergic agents.

c. Gastroesophageal reflux

- More common in cerebral palsy and after repair of TEF.
- Parents describe spitting up after meals, recurrent URI, wheezing, or esophagitis.
- Diagnosis is by upper GI series, nuclear scan, upper endoscopy, and esophageal pH probe.
- Patients with GERD are liable to aspiration on induction of anesthesia.[12]
- Medical treatment consists of thickened feeding, H2 blockers, and Cisapride (a dopamine antagonist) as motility agent.
- Surgery is by Nissen Fundoplication and Thal–Nissen Partial wrap.

d. Latex allergy

- Most common cause of intraoperative anaphylaxis reactions in children (muscle relaxants in adults).
- Lip swelling when a child put a toy balloon to the lips or tongue swelling when the dentist put a rubber dam in the mouth is suggestive of latex allergy.
- Patients with spina bifida meningeomyelocele, urinary tract anomalies with frequent bladder

- Avoidance of anticholinergic agents

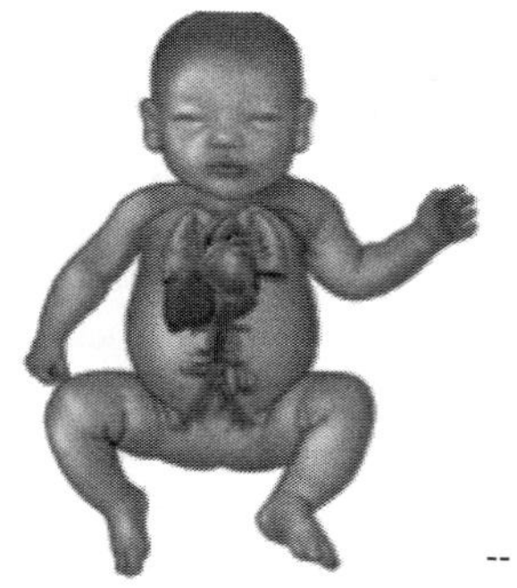

Figure 24.1 Down syndrome © *Nucleus*.

catheterizations, history of multiple surgeries (more than 6), atopic skin and those with allergy to tropical fruits (banana, chestnut, avocado, kiwi, pineapple) are at higher risk.[13]

- Latex free environment is the most important measure for prevention of latex anaphylaxis.

e. Down syndrome

f. Mediastinal masses

- The anterior mediastinum includes the thymus, lymph nodes, and occasionally the parathyroid/ thyroid glands.
- Note position of the mass (anterior/posterior/ middle mediastinum as airway obstruction is more common with anterior masses.[14]
- The most common anterior mediastinal masses include lymphomas (Hodgkin and non-Hodgkin), teratomas, angiomatous tumors, and thymic lesions.[15]
- Airway obstruction can occur emergently at any time during the anesthetic, as the mass can compress the heart and decrease ventricular filling and ejection.
- In the preoperative history and physical the following items should be noted: a history of a night cough, syncope, a "refusal to lie down," and examination findings as cyanosis, wheezing, jugular venous distention, head/neck swelling.[16]
- Reducing the mass with steroid and/or radiation therapy prior to the procedure being performed is a common occurrence.
- Notable findings on radiologic studies include: compressed/deviated trachea on chest X-ray and a compressed airway and cardiac/great vessels on CT scan.
- Common findings on echocardiogram include compression of heart chambers and pericardial involvement by the mass.

- Flow volume loops are useful and the exact reduction of expiratory flow rate should be noted. A reduction of 50% or more is significant as well as if the tumor is intra or extrathoracic.[14]
- Make sure blood is available for rapid transfusion as significant blood loss is possible.
- Premedication is not recommended if one is concerned about airway obstruction.
- Prior to induction of anesthesia a range of ETTs, stylets, laryngoscope blades should be ready, as well as a surgeon available for emergent rigid bronchoscopy.

g. Reactive airway disease

- Asthma affects 5–10% of children in USA and is a chronic inflammatory disease of the airways.[17]
- Symptoms are secondary to bronchoconstriction and edema/secretion in the large and small airways.[15]
- Asthma is thought to be caused by several factors which include environmental allergens, emotional stress, exercise.[15]
- Treatment for mild asthma consists of b-adrenergics such as albuterol. In more severe cases corticosteroids (inhaled and oral) along with leukotriene antagonists may be utilized.
- Routine medications should be given to the patient with asthma on the day of surgery. Consider an IV stress dose of hydrocortisone on induction of anesthesia for children who are on high dose inhaled or oral steroids.
- Prior to an elective surgery patients with asthma should not have had an acute attack within the past month.
- If a Viral URI is present surgery should be deferred for at least 4–6 weeks.[15]
- Note frequency and severity of attacks on the preoperative consult and a history of ICU admissions/intubations for management of asthma.[17]
- Type and frequency of use of medications should be recorded. If b-adrenergics are used frequently it is likely they may be necessary in the perioperative period.[17]
- Check for wheezing or shortness of breath on the physical exam. If necessary a bronchodilator may be needed. If the wheezing does not resolve s/p bronchodilator administration consider rescheduling elective surgeries.
- Midazolam is a good choice for premedication, and one may consider atropine as well for its properties as an antisialagogue and bronchodilator.

h. Upper respiratory tract infections

- Upper respiratory tract infections (URTIs) in children are fairly common and a risk factor for respiratory complications as laryngospasm, bronchospasm, and desaturation of oxygen saturation of hemoglobin.[18]
- Symptoms that may encourage an anesthesiologist to cancel include: fever > 38C, purulent nasal discharge/productive cough, lethargy, and wheezing.[18]
- URTIs are predominantly due to viral infections however one should be aware of the differential diagnosis which includes non-infectious rhinitis (as seasonal allergies), viral infections (as influenza) and bacterial infections (as pneumonia).
- Noted risk factors that contribute to morbidity in the setting of URTI include: age < 1 year old, history of prematurity (< 37 weeks old), asthma, history of parental smoking, and children with congenital heart disease.[18]
- If a surgery is deemed emergent or urgent surgery may progress regardless of the presence of URTI. However for elective surgery cancellation may be more prudent.[18]
- Ear, nose, and throat and airway procedures carry a higher risk of respiratory complications in children with and without a URTI.
- Facemask anesthesia has the lowest incidence of airway complication in patients with URTI, followed by usage of a laryngeal mask airway. Endotracheal intubation has been noted to increase the risk of respiratory complication up to 11 times.[19]
- Cancellation has a profound social impact on a child and his or her family and an informed discussion involving the anesthesiologist, parents, and surgeon is best and the final decision should be documented in the chart.[18]
- There is no consensus among experts regarding the optimal time to delay surgery after a simple

URTI but a period of 2–4 weeks following resolution of symptoms has been adopted by many centers.[19]

- According to some studies preoperative administration of bronchodilators can be of some benefit in reducing intraoperative bronchospasm.[20]
- Children with rhinorrhea may benefit from oxymetazoline or synephrine administration to clear up dry secretions during anesthesia.[17]

i. Congenital heart disease

- As preoperative considerations for specific cardiac lesions will be detailed in the chapter focused on congenital heart disease, this section will outline general considerations in this group of children.
- Review all pertinent studies/consultations for children with CHD prior to a procedure, including electrocardiograms, echocardiography, cardiology consultations, and cardiac catheterization reports.
- Make special note of the child's cardiac anatomy and physiology, repaired vs. palliated vs unrepaired cardiac lesions, functional status, need for anticoagulation, and risk of endocarditis.[18]
- As the presence of pacemakers and automatic implantable cardiac defibrillators is common in this group of children, checking for the indication for, mode, and date of last device check is warranted. Note the risk for electrocautery interference in the particular procedure to be performed.[18]
- Children with CHD can present early in life with respiratory distress, cyanosis, or failure to thrive.[21]
- Congestive heart failure is common as well in this group and can be precipitated by severe obstruction to blood flow (as found in stenotic lesions) and abnormally increased blood flow via intracardiac or extracardiac shunts.[21]
- It is common to find children with CHD having reduced exercise tolerance, increased incidences of respiratory infections, chest pain or syncope. Oftentimes they are below average on age-based weight and height percentiles.[21]
- Children with CHD that is associated with increased pulmonary blood flow may have reduced pulmonary function due to increased pulmonary vascular resistance, decreased compliance, and obstruction to small airways. Over time chronic increases in pulmonary blood flow can cause smooth muscle hypertrophy in the pulmonary arterioles leading to pulmonary hypertension.[21]
- On the other hand children with decreased pulmonary blood flow may encounter problems with dead space ventilation and have gradients in end-tidal and arteriolar carbon dioxide levels and an increase in the time necessary for an inhalational induction of general anesthesia.
- Obstructive lesions cause concentric hypertrophy of the affected ventricle and thus become it becomes subject to arrhythmias and myocardial ischemia. Large shunts or incompetent valves cause eccentric hypertrophy and result in dilated ventricles that are vulnerable to increases in preload and anesthetics that depress the myocardium.[21]
- Children who have cyanotic CHD undergo compensatory changes in their blood which include polycythemia and increased blood volume. Side effects of these changes include renal and cerebral thrombosis, and coagulopathy due to thrombocytopenia and decreased coagulation factors.[21]
- Renal and hepatic function in this subset of children is frequently impaired and can cause delayed clearance of medications.

j. Autism spectrum disorders

- Autism spectrum disorder (ASD) encompasses several neurodevelopmental disorders of empathy including autism, Asperger syndrome, pervasive developmental disorder.[22]
- ASD is characterized by impaired social communication and interaction as well as repetitive/restricted behaviors and decreased ability to form imaginative thoughts.[22]
- Males are affected four times as much as females.
- Contacting parents prior to an anesthetic to delineate the degree of ASD and particular behaviors and interactions to avoid can be useful.
- Outpatient surgery and ensuring an expedient return of the patient to his/her home environment and routines are important to the patient with ASD.
- Premedication with PO midazolam and/or ketamine have been found to be effective in this population.[22]

- Commonly performed procedures in the ASD population include various ENT procedures, dental restorations and brain MRI scans.[22]
- Scheduling these patients as the first case of the day, limiting the time between admission and induction of anesthesia, allowing parental presence during induction of anesthesia, recovering patients in a low-stimulation environment, removing intravenous catheters when possible, and discharging home as soon as possible have all been noted to reduce behavioral disturbances in the ASD population.[22]

Physical examination

- Performing a physical examination in a calm, non-threatening manner is best when dealing with children.
- General appearance: note presence of cyanosis, pallor, jaundice, dysmorphic features, and developmental delay. Assess overall nutritional state, level of consciousness, abnormal posture, or movement disorders. Vitals and SPO_2 should be recorded along with current bodyweight.
- A formal airway exam in children may be difficult or impossible to perform in younger children. Instead assessment should be focused on identifying certain predictors of difficult intubation: limited mouth opening, breathing through the mouth instead of the nares (possible indicator of adenoid hypertrophy), loose teeth, mandibular hypoplasia or retrognathia, large tongue, decreased cervical spine flexion or extension, and scars from prior neck or tracheal surgery.[18]
- The cardiac exam should include checking peripheral pulses (brachial/femoral), evaluating cardiac murmurs and looking for signs of heart failure as cyanosis, tachypnea, crackles on auscultation of the lungs, and hepatomegaly.[18]
- The respiratory exam should include an assessment of work of breathing, presence of a (productive) cough, tracheal position (midline or shifted to either side), chest wall deformities, and auscultation of the lungs to detect wheezes, rhonchi, or crackles.
- Noting peripheral veins sites for application of topical local anesthetic cream is prudent. Indwelling vascular access devices and arteriovenous fistulas should be localized and examined for patency and site infection and to ensure they are adequately padded to prevent compression perioperatively.[18]
- Identifying other implanted devices as feeding tubes and electronic devices such as pacemakers is important as electronic devices can malfunction in the setting of surgical electrocautery or the MRI suite.[18]
- Spinal anatomy should be examined prior to performing neuraxial anesthetics. Spinal malformations/deformities, prior surgery, or local skin infection may be a contraindication to the anesthetic. Pre-existing neurological deficits should be documented prior to neuraxial or regional techniques to provide a description of the patient's baseline neurologic status.[18]

Laboratory testing

- Routine testing is not indicated for most elective procedures in children.[23]
- Preoperative hemoglobin is ordered for those who will undergo procedures with the potential for blood loss, hemoglobinopathy, former preterm infant, and those younger than 6 months of age.
- Coagulation studies are indicated in major reconstructive surgery.
- A type and cross-match is indicated in preparation for potential blood transfusions in procedures with high expected blood loss.
- Pregnancy testing: the literature is insufficient to inform patients or physicians on whether anesthesia causes harmful effects on early pregnancy. Pregnancy testing may be offered to female patients of childbearing age and for whom the result would alter patient's management.[23]

Fasting requirements

- Preoperative fasting requirements are straightforward and similar to those found in adults.
- Clear fluids: 2 hrs.
- Breast milk: 4 hrs.
- Formula/cow's milk/ "Light Meal": 6 hrs
- Solids: 8 hrs.[24]
- Clear fluids include water, carbonated beverages and other fluids free of particles. Orange juice

with pulp has particles and thus should not be considered clear.

- A light meal is typically considered toast and clear fluids. A meal that includes fried/fatty foods and or meat should be considered as "solids."[24]

Age-related differences in anesthetic risk

- Age-related differences in anesthetic risk can be correlated with a general decrease in cardiac and pulmonary reserve and well as an increased likelihood of anesthetic complications (such as difficulty in intubation, medication errors, incidence of malignant hyperthermia) in children when compared to adults. This difference is most noted in neonates and infants. The remainder of this section will serve to elucidate some of the more pertinent differences between children (particularly neonates and infants) in comparison to older children and adults which can lead to higher anesthetic risk.
- Neonates and infants have weaker intercostal muscles and diaphragms and more compliant ribcages and larger abdomens which lead to less efficient ventilation in comparison to older children and adults.[25]
- Decreased type I muscle fibers in the diaphragm leads to quicker fatigue in this group. In addition since ventilatory drive is not developed in this age group hypoxia and hypercapnia may not increase respiratory rate and may in fact depress respiration.[25]
- Smaller and decreased airways (increasing airway resistance), decreased functional residual capacity (FRC), and increase, oxygen consumption limits oxygen reserve and predisposes this group to hypoxemia during periods of apnea or hypoventilation. This in turn significantly reduces the period of time one can safely intubate patients in these age.[25]
- Neonates and infants have many anatomical differences when compared to older children and adults. These include a relatively larger head/tongue and smaller nasal passages, a larynx that is more cephalad and anterior, a longer and more floppy epiglottis, and a trachea and narrower and neck that is shorter. Also of note neonates are obligate nasal breathers until around 5 months. The significance of these smaller and narrower airways is that mucosal edema will have proportionally larger effect on air flow obstruction in neonates and infants versus adults.[25]
- Neonates and infants have ventricles that are less compliant/more fibrous than adults. This leads to a fixed stroke volume and a cardiac output more dependent on heart rate. Neonates and infants are also more prone to bradycardia as their sympathetic nervous systems and baroreceptor reflexes are not fully developed, their myocardium is less sensitive to exogenously administered catecholamines (IV epinephrine) and is more sensitive to depression by volatile anesthetics. Finally of note since baroreceptor reflexes are underdeveloped hypovolemia may not be accompanied by tachycardia.[25]
- The ratio of surface area to weight is greater in this group, which potentiates heat loss in the operating room environment. It is important to realize mild hypothermia (34–35 degrees Celsius) can cause significant perioperative issues as delayed awakening cardiac and respiratory depression and a deranged response to anesthetic agents. While neonates have mechanisms to overcome their inability to shiver as the metabolism of brown fat stores, volatile anesthetics inhibit this mechanism.[25]
- Neonates and infants have immature kidneys (kidney function usually reaches adult levels by 6 months of age) and thus may exhibit decreased reatinine clearance, sodium retention, and bicarbonate reabsorption along with relative hyposthenuria. These differences are exaggerated in the premature infant and put these patients at risk for volume overloading and pulmonary edema with resulting heart failure.[25]
- In terms of the gastrointestinal system neonates have an increased incidence of gastroesophageal reflux, and their immature liver metabolizes drugs less readily leading to prolonged duration of certain anesthetic drugs. Also neonates have decreased glycogen stores and are at risk for perioperative hypoglycemia. The risk of hypoglycemia is higher in neonates who are premature, receiving total parenteral nutrition, or born to mothers with uncontrolled diabetes.[25]

Informed consent

- *Informed consent*:
  - Adequate provision of information including the nature of the ailment or condition, the nature of proposed diagnostic steps or treatment and the probability of their success; the existence and nature of the risks involved; and the existence, potential benefits, and risks of recommended alternative treatments (including the choice of no treatment).[26]
  - Assessment of patient understanding of the above information.
  - Assessment, if only tacit, of the capacity of the patient or surrogate to make the necessary decisions.
  - Assurance, insofar as it is possible, that the patient has the freedom to choose among the medical alternatives without coercion or manipulation.
- *Assent:*
  - Helping the patient achieve a developmentally appropriate awareness of the nature of his or her condition.
  - Telling the patient what he or she can expect with tests and treatment.
  - Making a clinical assessment of the patient's understanding of the situation and the factors influencing how he or she is responding (including whether there is appropriate pressure to accept testing or therapy).[26]
  - Soliciting an expression of the patient willingness to accept the proposed care.
- Children younger than 7 years have insufficient decision making capacities to effectively participate in the informed consent process. In this situation, the best interest standard guides decision making and the best interest lies with the parents who want the best for their children.[27]
- Anesthesiologists should seek to resolve disagreement without resorting to legal intervention. However the state has an interest in protecting those who cannot protect themselves. If other options have failed, anesthesiologists should report parents they believe to be choosing unacceptable treatments to child welfare authorities for possible legal action.
- **Informed assent:** Children ages of 7 to 13 years should participate in decision making to the extent their development permits.
- **Emancipated minors:** are minors who have a statutory right to legally consent for their own health decisions (military, married, have children, or economically independent).
- **Mature minor**: the patient must be determined by a judge to be legally and ethically capable of giving legal consent in a specific situation.
- **Disclosure** should be based on the reasonable person standard; information disclosed must satisfy the hypothetical reasonable person the amount disclosed should be based through patient-driven interaction.
- **Children of Jehovah's witnesses:** Inform patient and family that, as with all patients, attempts will be made to follow the family's wishes within the standard of care. Because refusal of transfusion therapy is deemed a "matter of conscience" the anesthesiologist should clarify acceptable interventions like deliberate hypotension, deliberate hypothermia, hemodilution, use of colloids, erythropoietin, iron. Some Jehovah's witnesses will accept blood via cell saver if it remains in a closed continuous loop.[27]
- The family should be informed that in critical situations, the anesthesiologist will transfuse while concomitantly seeking legal authorization with help of hospital. In instances where likelihood of requiring blood is high an anesthesiologist may choose to obtain the court order preoperatively.

References

1. Miller RD. Anesthesia for orthopedic surgery. In Miller RD, editor. *Miller's Anesthesia*. 7th edn. Elsevier Health Sciences Publishing; 2010. p. 2248.
2. Bissonnette B. Anesthesia for the Patient with Coexisting Diseases. In Bissonnette B, editor. *Pediatric Anesthesia*. People's Medical Publishing House; 2011. p. 950.
3. Dierdorf SF, McNiece WL, Rao CC. Effect of succinylcholine on plasma potassium in children with cerebral palsy. *Anesthesiology* 1985; **62**: 88–90.
4. Hines RL. Pediatric diseases. In Hines RL, Marschall KE, editors. *Stoelting's Anesthesia and Co-existing Diseases*. 5th edn. Elsevier Health Sciences Publishing; 2008. p. 603
5. Litman RS. Neurologic and neuromuscular diseases. In

Litman RS, editor. *Basics of Pediatric Anesthesia.* Tablet edition. Publisher; 2013. p. 56.

6. Andropoulos DB, Mann D, Garcia PJ. Anesthesia for transplantation. In Gregory GA, Andropoulos DB, editors. *Gregory's Pediatric Anesthesia.* West Sussex, UK: Blackwell Publishing; 2012. p. 706.

7. Konstan MW, Morgan WJ, Butler SM, *et al.* Risk factors for rate of decline in forced expiratory volume in one second in children and adolescents with cystic fibrosis. *J Pediatr* 2007; **151**: 134–9.

8. Davis PJ, Cladis FP, Motoyama EK. Anesthesia for genetic metabolic and dysmorphic. In Davis PJ, Cladis FP, Motoyama EK, editors. *Smith's Anesthesia for Infants and Children.* 8th edn. Elsevier Health Sciences Publishing; 2010. p. 1123.

9. Cote CJ, Lerman J, Steward DJ. Essentials of pulmonology: Expert consult. In Cote CJ, Lerman J, Anderson B, editors. *A Practice of Anesthesia for Infants and Children: Expert Consult.* 5th edn. Elsevier Health Sciences Publishing; 2013. pp. 233–4.

10. Shott SR. Down syndrome: common otolaryngologic manifestations. *Am J Med Genet Part C Semin Med Genet* 2006; **142C**: 131–40.

11. Kraemer FW, Stricker PA, Gurnaney HG *et al.* Bradycardia during induction of anesthesia with sevoflurane in children with Down syndrome. *Anesth Analg* 2010; **111**(5): 1259–63.

12. Davis PJ, Cladis FP, Motoyama EK. Respiratory physiology in infants and children. In Davis PJ, Cladis FP, Motoyama EK, editors. *Smith's Anesthesia for Infants and Children.* 8th edn. Elsevier Health Sciences Publishing; 2010. p. 284.

13. Bissonnette B. Anesthesia for the patient with coexisting diseases. In Bissonnette B, editor. *Pediatric Anesthesia.* China: People's Medical Publishing House; 2011. p. 919.

14. McFadyen G, Budac S, Richards M, Martin LD. Anesthesia for thoracic surgery. In Gregory GA, Andropoulos DB, editors. *Gregory's Pediatric Anesthesia.* 5th edn. West Sussex, UK: Blackwell Publishing; 2012. pp. 569–86.

15. Cote CJ, Todres D, Ryan JF. Preoperative evaluation of pediatric patients. In Cote CJ, editor. *A Practice of Anesthesia for Infants and Children.* 3rd edn. Philadelphia, PA: Saunders; 2001. pp. 49–50.

16. Cote CJ, Todres D, Ryan JF. General and thoracoabdominal surgery. In Cote CJ, Lerman J, Steward DJ, editors. *Manual of Pediatric Anesthesia.* 6th edn. Philadelphia, PA: Churchill Livingstone Elsevier; 2010. pp. 375–7.

17. Cote CJ, Lerman J, Steward DJ. Medical conditions influencing anesthetic management. In Cote CJ, Lerman J, Steward DJ, editors. *Manual of Pediatric Anesthesia.* 6th edn. Philadelphia, PA: Churchill Livingstone Elsevier; 2010. pp. 174–77.

18. Davidson A, Howard K, Browne W, Habre W, Lopez U. Preoperative evaluation and preparation, anxiety, awareness, and behavior change. In Gregory GA, Andropoulos DB, editors. *Gregory's Pediatric Anesthesia.* 5th edn. West Sussex, UK: Blackwell Publishing; 2012. pp. 282–3.

19. Von Ungern-Sternberg BS. Risk assessment for respiratory complications in pediatric anesthesia: a prospective cohort study. *Lancet* 2010; **376**(9743): 773–83.

20. Von Ungern-Sternberg BS, Boda K, Schwab C, *et al.* Larygeal mask airway is associated with an increased incidence of adverse respiratory events in children with recent upper respiratory tract infections. *Anesthesiology* 2007; **107**(5): 714–19.

21. Cote CJ, Lerman J, Steward DJ. Cardiovascular surgery and cardiologic procedures. In Cote CJ, Lerman J, Steward DJ, editors. *Manual of Pediatric Anesthesia.* 6th edn. Philadelphia, PA: Churchill Livingstone Elsevier; 2010. pp. 399–402.

22. Andropoulos DB, Mann D, Garcia PJ. Anesthesia for the patient with a genetic syndrome. In Gregory GA, Andropoulos DB, editors. *Gregory's Pediatric Anesthesia.* 5th edn. West Sussex, UK: Blackwell Publishing; 2012. pp. 1000–1.

23. Roy WL, Lerman J, McIntyre BG. Is preoperative haemoglobin testing justified in children undergoing minor elective surgery? *Can J Anaesth* 1991; **38**: 700–3.

24. American Society of Anesthesiologists. Practice guidelines for preoperative fasting: applications to healthy patients undergoing elective procedures. *Anesthesiology* 2011; **114**(3): 495–511.

25. Butterworth J, Mackey DC, Wasnick J. Pediatric anesthesia. In Butterworth J, Mackey DC, Wasnick J, editors. *Morgan and Mikhail's Clinical Anesthesiology.* 5th edn. London: McGraw-Hill Medical; 2013. pp. 877–906.

26. Committee on Bioethics, American Academy of Pediatrics. Informed consent, parental permission, and assent in pediatric practice. *Pediatrics* 1995; **95**: 314–17.

27. Andropoulos DB, Mann D, Garcia PJ. Ethical considerations. In Gregory GA, Andropoulos DB, editors. *Gregory's Pediatric Anesthesia.* West Sussex, UK: Blackwell Publishing; 2012. pp. 2–5.

Chapter 25

Pediatric fluid management

Kelly A. Machovec and B. Craig Weldon

In children greater than 6 months old, total body water (TBW) equals 60% of body weight (BW). For term infants up to 6 months, TBW equals 75% of BW, and for preterm and low birth weight infants, TBW is 80% of BW.[1,2] The TBW gradually decreases with age as a result of a decrease in extracellular fluid (ECF).

The TBW is divided into intracellular and extracellular spaces (see Figure 25.1). In infants over 6 months old, ICF is about 2/3 of TBW, and ECF is 1/3 of TBW. In infants younger than 6 months, ECF volume predominates, with the ECF space comprising up to 60% of total body water. Extracellular fluid volume, as a percentage of body weight, is 45% in the term neonate, 30% in a one year old, and 20% in an adult.[3] The intracellular fluid space contains high concentrations of potassium, phosphorus, and magnesium. The ECF is subdivided into plasma and interstitial fluid compartments. The predominant electrolytes in ECF are sodium and chloride. The plasma component of ECF contains blood cells, platelets, and proteins. The interstitial fluid compartment is similar in composition to the ICF compartment, and fluid movement between these compartments is determined by Starling forces according to the following relationship:

$$J_v = K_f([P_c - P_i] - \sigma[\prod_c - \prod_i]),$$

where J_v describes net movement of fluid between compartments, K_f is a constant, and $([P_c - P_i] - \sigma[\prod_c - \prod_i])$ describes the net driving force of fluid. In this equation, P_c and P_i describe capillary and interstitial hydrostatic pressures, respectively, σ is a coefficient, and $\prod_c$ and $\prod_I$ describe capillary and interstitial oncotic pressures, respectively.

Blood volume varies with age, decreasing from birth to adulthood on a milliliter/kilogram basis (see Table 25.1).

Renal physiology

Twenty-five percent of cardiac output supplies the kidneys, with 90% of renal blood flow going to the cortex and 10% to the medulla. Renal blood flow (RBF) is autoregulated, maintaining constant flow for systolic blood pressures of 80–180 mmHg. Glomerular filtration rate is also constant over this range due to changes in renal vascular resistance. Renal autoregulation occurs in denervated kidneys, suggesting that it is not dependent on external factors. Instead, autoregulation occurs according to the "myogenic hypothesis": increases in intraluminal pressure result in vascular smooth muscle contraction, reducing blood flow to basal levels. It is unclear whether the low blood pressures present in preterm infants and neonates exceed the limits of autoregulation.

The functional unit of the kidney is the glomerulus, responsible for plasma filtration. The glomerular filtration rate (GFR) is governed by hydrostatic pressure and renal blood flow. Glomerular–tubular balance describes the phenomenon by which changes in GFR affect tubular resorption rates, adjusting solute and water excretion to preserve ECF volume and solute composition. Volume expansion, diuretics, and conditions such as the syndrome of inappropriate antidiuretic hormone (SIADH) disrupt this glomerular–tubular balance and may lead to fluid and electrolyte derangements.

Clearance, defined as the volume of plasma cleared of a substance over a time interval, estimates glomerular filtration rate (GFR). Creatinine clearance (CrCl) can be calculated after 24-hour urine collection using the following formula:

$$\text{CrCl (ml/min / 1.73 m}^2) = U \times V \times SA\ m^2 / \min \times P_{cr} \times 1.73\ m^2,$$

Essentials of Pediatric Anesthesiology, ed. Alan David Kaye, Charles James Fox and James H. Diaz. Published by Cambridge University Press. © Cambridge University Press 2015.

where U is urine creatinine concentration, V is volume of urine, SA is surface area in meters squared, and P_{cr} is plasma creatinine. In children, in whom urine collection may not be possible, CrCl can be estimated using Schwartz's formula:

$$\text{CrCl (ml/min/1.73 m}^2) = (\text{Height cm}/P_{cr}) \times k,$$

where P_{cr} is plasma creatinine concentration, K is a constant related to muscle mass (0.33 in preterm infants, 0.45 in full-term infants through one year of age, 0.55 in 2 years and older and in adolescent girls, and 0.70 in adolescent boys).[4] The GFR estimates based on creatinine concentration may overestimate true GFR in children with impaired renal function, who experience increases in both tubular and gastrointestinal secretion of creatinine. Thus, their serum creatinine does not accurately reflect activity at the glomerulus.

Renal maturation and tubular function

The kidneys begin development at 5 weeks gestational age, with the first nephrons appearing at 8 weeks of gestation. One-third of nephrons are present by 20 weeks gestation, and by 36 weeks, all nephrons are formed. After 20 weeks gestation, kidney growth is proportional to gestational age. Premature infants will continue to develop new nephrons until about 35 weeks postconceptual age. Once the full number of nephrons is present, further growth is due to increases in glomerular and tubular size. Renal development in extrauterine life is characterized by hypertrophy of existing neurons.

Neonates exhibit both reduced RBF and GFR. The low RBF is due to increased renal vascular resistance in utero, which rapidly changes at birth.[5] The low GFR is due to low systemic blood pressure, high renal vascular resistance, and a smaller capillary surface area for filtration. The GFR is a function of both gestational age and postnatal age. Neonates double GFR by 2 weeks of age and triple it by 3 months in the absence of acquired renal insufficiency. The GFR reaches adult levels by 2 years of age. Premature infants have a low GFR at birth that increases more slowly than in their full-term counterparts but, renal maturation occurs rapidly out of necessity when the infant is separated from the placenta.

Full-term infants are able to conserve sodium despite a low GFR. As GFR and the filtered sodium load increase, the proximal tubule is able to increase sodium absorption.[6] However, preterm infants exhibit prolonged glomerular--tubular imbalance, with GFR exceeding the ability of the tubules to reabsorb sodium.[5] This is due to immaturity of the proximal convoluted tubules. In addition, the distal convoluted tubule does not respond to aldosterone.[6] The result is that preterm infants are at risk for excessive sodium excretion and hyponatremia. Sodium reabsorption increases with age:

Table 25.1 Blood volume

Age	Estimated blood volume (ml/kg)
Premature infants	90–100
Term infants	80–90
Infants < 1 year	75–80
Children	70–75
Adults	65–70

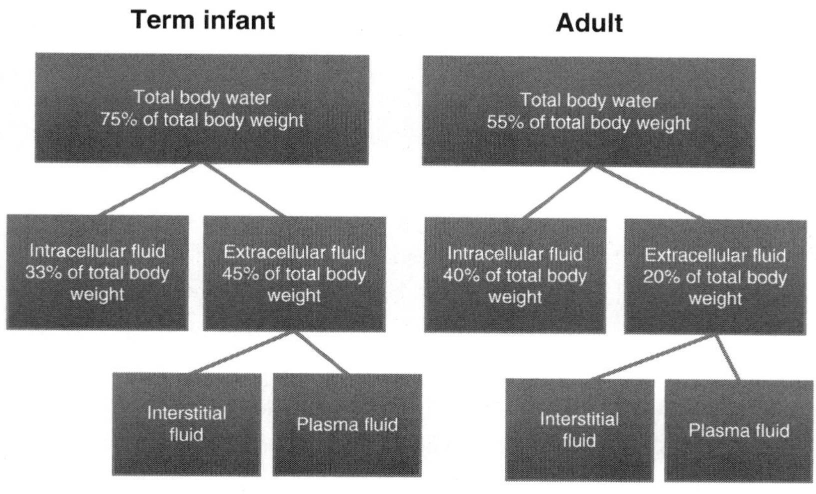

Figure 25.1 Infant (< 6 months of age) and adult body fluid compartments as a function of total body water. With age, total body water decreases to 60% of total body weight as a result of loss of extracellular fluid.

Table 25.2 The 4-2-1 rule for maintenance fluid requirements

Weight	Fluid requirement
Up to 10 kg	4 ml/kg
10–20 kg	40 ml + 2 ml/kg above 10 kg
>20 kg	60 ml + 1 ml/kg above 20 kg

a neonate at 30 weeks postconceptual age excretes 5% of a filtered sodium load, while a full-term neonate excretes only 0.2% of a filtered sodium load.[7]

Both full-term and preterm infants have reduced urinary concentrating ability.[5] The newborn renal medulla is relatively hypotonic due to poor urea accumulation in the medullary interstitium, leading to reduced function of the countercurrent concentrating mechanism. In addition the collecting duct is not as sensitive to ADH at this age. Infants reach adult levels of urine concentrating ability by 3–5 weeks. As a result, the maximal urine concentration of a preterm infant is 300 mOsm/l, compared to 700 mOsm/l in a ful-term infant and 1300 mOsm/l in an adult. Renal diluting capacity matures by 3–5 weeks of age.

Control of fluid volume

Antidiuretic hormone

Antidiuretic hormone (ADH), synthesized in the hypothalamus and transported to the posterior pituitary gland, is stored as arginine vasopressin. The most important stimulant for its release is plasma osmolality – a 1–2% increase in ECF osmolality causes release of ADH. ADH binds to V_2 receptors in the renal collecting ducts, resulting in increased cAMP levels and expression of aquaporin-2 channels, to increase water reabsorption. A secondary stimulant for ADH release is perceived decrease in intravascular volume, as sensed by arterial baroreceptors in the carotid sinus, and left atrial stretch receptors. This hypotension or hypovolemia stimulates nonosmolar release of ADH. The ADH serves to maintain plasma osmolality and sodium concentration within a very narrow range. Pathologic release of ADH (i.e., from tumors or surgical stress) results in decreased urine output and hypervolemia. Very high levels of ADH, as caused by trauma, stress, or critical illness, result in renal cortical vasoconstriction, redistributing blood flow to the medulla. Other stimulants for ADH release include low urine output, increased uric acid excretion, and urine sodium concentration >20 meq/l.

Table 25.3 NPO guidelines

Clear liquids	2 hours
Breast milk	4 hours
Infant formula	6 hours
Light meal	6 hours
Heavy or fatty meal	8 hours

Renin–angiotensin–aldosterone system

The renin–angiotensin–aldosterone (RAA) system is responsible for control of sodium and potassium hemostasis as well as vascular tone. Renin is released from the juxtaglomerular apparatus, located at the distal tubule and the afferent arteriole. Low chloride delivery to the distal tubule near the JGA causes renin release. Renin cleaves circulating angiotensinogen, forming angiotensin I, which is converted to angiotensin II by angiotensin converting enzyme (ACE). Angiotension II is the active molecule of the RAA system. Angiotensin II causes efferent arteriole vasoconstriction, increased ADH release, increased sodium absorption in the proximal tubule, and aldosterone release. Aldosterone increases active sodium and water reabsorption in the proximal tubule and promotes intravascular volume expansion. Aldosterone promotes hydrogen and potassium loss and high levels may lead to hypokalemia and metabolic alkalosis.

Perioperative fluid management

Fluid therapy in pediatric patients must consider maintenance requirements, insensible losses, and fluid deficits. The goal of perioperative fluid therapy is to maintain tissue perfusion. The classic calculation of maintenance fluid requirements using the "4–2–1" rule was adapted from Holliday and Segar[8] in 1957 (Table 25.2). Holliday and Segar's recommendations were based on the metabolic requirements for patients at rest, whereby 1 ml of water is required to metabolize 1 kcal.[8] However, subsequent studies have questioned the application of this rule to surgical patients, as children have reduced energy expenditure under general anesthesia.[3] Further, this rule does not address fluid deficit or abnormal (i.e., surgical) fluid losses. Furman and Berry proposed a method of fluid replacement assuming a prolonged, 6–8 hour NPO time, but this has come under scrutiny with the newer ASA NPO Guidelines (Table 25.3).[9] In addition, the idea of "third-space losses" – extracellular fluid that does not equilibrate with the intravascular space – has been questioned.[10] Energy expenditure and fluid requirements increase with stress. However, ADH levels also increase with stress, leading to reduced water excretion.

Infants have higher fluid needs than adults for three reasons: higher metabolic and growth rates, higher surface area to body weight ratio resulting in increased insensible losses, and higher urinary excretion of solutes with lower tubular concentrating ability, resulting in higher obligatory fluid losses. The immature, thin skin and large surface area of very low birth weight infants puts them at increased risk of evaporative heat loss. Neonates, both premature and full term, have a greater total body water to body weight ratio, allowing more fluid loss before showing symptoms of dehydration.

Intraoperative fluid management

Intraoperative fluid management must address fluid deficits and ongoing losses in addition to maintenance requirements. Furman *et al.* developed a strategy of fluid replacement whereby one half of the calculated deficit is replaced in the first hour of the procedure, and one half is replaced in the subsequent 2 hours.[11] The idea of "deficit" is being challenged, as many patients are now adequately hydrated preoperatively due to more liberal fasting guidelines.[9] Replacement of insensible losses is also an area of debate. Estimates of fluid loss vary with the type of surgical trauma, with minor procedures losing 6 ml/kg/h and severe trauma losing 10 ml/kg/h; one group estimates that neonates being treated for necrotizing enterocolitis have third-space losses up to 50 ml/kg/h.[3] A practical strategy when treating presumed hypovolemia is to administer 10–20 ml/kg of crystalloid (normal saline or Ringer's lactate) and assess hemodynamic parameters. This may be repeated if there is a laudable response to the initial bolus or when persistent hypovolemia is suspected. Numerous crystalloid boluses without improvement suggest the need for blood/colloid replacement or consideration of a pathophysiology other than hypovolemia causing the hemodynamic anomaly.

Choice of fluids

The crystalloid versus colloid debate remains active in pediatric anesthesiology. Crystalloid fluids are cheap, of a nonhuman source, and replace third-space and insensible losses. Colloid fluids have the advantage of superior volume expansion and improved plasma oncotic pressure, but have significant side effects depending on the colloid chosen, including coagulation abnormalities, anaphylaxis, renal impairment, and risk of disease transmission, including prion disease.

Human albumin (HA) is a plasma product, heat treated to 60 degrees Celsius and then sterilized to reduce the risk of disease transmission,[12] though it may carry a risk of prion disease. Human albumin is available in 5% and 25% solutions; albumin 5% is osmotically equivalent to plasma on a 1:1 ml basis. Studies in hypotensive neonates suggest that normal saline resuscitation is equivalent to HA in maintaining normotension and even preventing fluid retention.[13,14] Despite the lack of evidence to support the practice, administration of HA appears to be popular in the neonatal period for volume expansion.[15] Albumin's anticoagulant effects are limited until administration of > 25% blood volume,[16] but at this point it may inhibit platelet aggregation[17] and antithrombin III activity,[18] thus producing a hypocoagulable state. Anaphylaxis is rare with albumin administration but can be fatal. A review of crystalloid versus HA management in children with severe infection and septic shock suggests an advantage to colloid use in children with malaria, but overall evidence was weak.[19] The SAFE trial (Saline versus Albumin Fluid Evaluation Study), conducted in adults, found no difference between saline and albumin administration between groups in terms of mortality, length of stay, mechanical ventilation, or renal failure;[20] however, these authors subsequently found a disadvantage to using albumin in patients with traumatic brain injury.[21] More quality studies are needed to address the efficacy of albumin in pediatric populations.

Synthetic colloids include gelatins, dextran, and hydroxyethyl starches (HES). Gelatins are not available in the USA due to the risk of anaphylactic reactions[22] and will not be discussed further. Dextran is a glucose polymer synthesized by bacteria from sucrose. Dextran is available as 10% dextran 40 and 6% dextran 70. These products differ in molecular weight (40 000 Da versus 70 000 Da, respectively), which confers differences in renal excretion, with dextran 70 remaining in the intravascular space for a longer period due to reduced renal excretion.[23] Dextrans may increase bleeding by decreasing platelet adhesion and decreased levels of Factor VIII; dextrans also increase fibrinolysis[24] and interefere with red blood cell cross matching.[23] Anaphylaxis to dextran may be avoided by pretreatment with a hapten inhibitor. The dose of dextran should be limited to 20 ml/kg in pediatric patients.[10]

The HES are synthetic colloids classified by concentration, molecular weight, molar substitution (MS, ratio of hydroxyethyl groups to glucose units), and C2:C6 ratios (indicates hydroxyethylation pattern on the glucose molecule).[25] High molecular weight, high MS, and high C2:C6 ratios confer longer time in the intravascular space. However, high MW and MS also confer more side effects, including hypocoagulability (decreased function of vWF, platelets, and factor VIII), renal impairment, and pruritis.

Third-generation HES (HES 130/0.4) have become very popular in recent years due to excellent volume expansion, and lack of disease transmission. Two studies comparing HES to 5% albumin in pediatric patients show no difference in hemodynamic or coagulation abnormalities.[26,27] In addition, a small study examining use of HES versus 5% albumin versus isotonic saline in hypotensive neonates found that HES did not improve cardiac output better than albumin or saline.[28] Recent data from adult studies showed an increased risk of renal failure and mortality compared to crystalloid solutions in critically ill patients.[29–31] A meta-analysis of adult patients on cardiopulmonary bypass showed increased risk of bleeding in patients who received hydroxyethyl starch products.[32] In June 2013 the U.S. Food and Drug Administration issued a warning against use of this product in critically ill patients.[33]

Postoperative fluid management

Intraoperative hydration with crystalloid may reduce postoperative nausea and vomiting in patients undergoing minor surgical procedures. For patients undergoing major surgical procedures or those requiring postoperative NPO periods (i.e., abdominal surgery), intravenous hydration is recommended. Hyponatremia is a common electrolyte disorder in this population. Causes of hyponatremia include administration of hypotonic fluid, pituitary and adrenal insufficiency, central nervous system disorders associated with sodium wasting, and SIADH.[3] Postoperative levels of ADH are high due to hypovolemia, physiologic stress, and pain. When this situation is combined with hypotonic fluid administration, dilutional hyponatremia may develop. This can be circumvented by avoiding hypotonic fluids in the immediate postoperative period or maintenance fluids may be reduced through the first postoperative day.[34]

Role of glucose in parenteral fluids

Glucose metabolism is a function of glucose intake, glycogen conversion to glucose, and glycogenolysis. Term infants have liver glycogen stores to maintain a normal serum glucose (40–60 mg/dl) for a 10–12 hour fasting period. Glycogen storage and glycogenolysis ability develop in the third trimester, so preterm infants are more likely to be glycogen deficient. Gluconeogenesis does not take place in the fetal liver but the enzymes responsible for this process develop quickly after birth.[35,36] A dextrose infusion of 4–7 mg/kg/min is sufficient to maintain normoglycemia in this population. This is best achieved with 1% or 2.5% dextrose solutions, as higher concentrations of dextrose may result in hyperglycemia.

In addition to preterm infants, other children at risk for intraoperative hypoglycemia include newborns of diabetic mothers, infants with Beckwith–Weideman syndrome, patients undergoing resection of pheochromocytoma, certain patients with inborn errors of metabolism and patients with diabetes on insulin therapy. Symptoms of hypoglycemia include cyanosis, apnea, lethargy, seizures, and hypotonia; many of these symptoms are masked under general anesthesia. Causes of hypoglycemia include sepsis, hypoxia, and high insulin levels (e.g., from a mother with diabetes).[5] In otherwise healthy infants and children intraoperative dextrose infusion is not indicated.

References

1. Friis-Hansen B. Body composition during growth. In vivo measurements and biochemical data correlated to differential anatomical growth. *Pediatrics*. Jan 1971; **47**(1): Suppl 2: 264.
2. Kagan BM, Stanincova V, Felix NS, Hodgman J, Kalman D. Body composition of premature infants: relation to nutrition. *American Journal of Clinical Nutrition*. Nov 1972; **25**(11): 1153–64.
3. Murat I, Dubois MC. Perioperative fluid therapy in pediatrics. *Paediatric Anaesthesia*. May 2008; **18**(5): 363–70.
4. Schwartz GJ, Brion LP, Spitzer A. The use of plasma creatinine concentration for estimating glomerular filtration rate in infants, children, and adolescents. *Pediatric Clinics of North America*. Jun 1987; **34**(3): 571–90.
5. Murat I, Humblot A, Girault L, Piana F. Neonatal fluid

management. *Best Practice & Research. Clinical Anaesthesiology.* Sep 2010; **24**(3): 365–74.

6. Spitzer A. The role of the kidney in sodium homeostasis during maturation. *Kidney International.* Apr 1982; **21**(4): 539–45.
7. Vanpee M, Herin P, Zetterstrom R, Aperia A. Postnatal development of renal function in very low birthweight infants. *Acta Paediatrica Scandinavica.* Mar 1988; **77**(2): 191–7.
8. Holliday MA, Segar WE. The maintenance need for water in parenteral fluid therapy. *Pediatrics.* May 1957; **19**(5): 823–32.
9. Practice guidelines for preoperative fasting and the use of pharmacologic agents to reduce the risk of pulmonary aspiration: application to healthy patients undergoing elective procedures: an updated report by the American Society of Anesthesiologists Committee on Standards and Practice Parameters. *Anesthesiology.* Mar 2011; **114**(3): 495–511.
10. Bailey AG, McNaull PP, Jooste E, Tuchman JB. Perioperative crystalloid and colloid fluid management in children: where are we and how did we get here? *Anesthesia and Analgesia.* Feb 2010; **110**(2): 375–90.
11. Furman EB, Roman DG, Lemmer LA, *et al.* Specific therapy in water, electrolyte and blood-volume replacement during pediatric surgery. *Anesthesiology.* Feb 1975; **42**(2): 187–93.
12. McClelland DB. Safety of human albumin as a constituent of biologic therapeutic products. *Transfusion.* Jul 1998; **38**(7): 690–9.
13. So KW, Fok TF, Ng PC, Wong WW, Cheung KL. Randomised controlled trial of colloid or crystalloid in hypotensive preterm infants. *Archives of Disease in Childhood. Fetal and Neonatal edition.* Jan 1997; **76**(1): F43–46.
14. Oca MJ, Nelson M, Donn SM. Randomized trial of normal saline versus 5% albumin for the treatment of neonatal hypotension. *Journal of Perinatology: Official Journal of the California Perinatal Association.* Sep 2003; **23**(6): 473–6.
15. Greenough A. Use and misuse of albumin infusions in neonatal care. *European Journal of Pediatrics.* Sep 1998; **157**(9): 699–702.
16. Tobias MD, Wambold D, Pilla MA, Greer F. Differential effects of serial hemodilution with hydroxyethyl starch, albumin, and 0.9% saline on whole blood coagulation. *Journal of Clinical Anesthesia.* Aug 1998; **10**(5): 366–71.
17. Jorgensen KA, Stoffersen E. On the inhibitory effect of albumin on platelet aggregation. *Thrombosis Research.* Jan 1980; **17**(1–2): 13–18.
18. Joorgensen KA, Stoffersen E. Heparin-like activity of albumin. *Thrombosis Research.* 1979; **16** (3–4): 569–74.
19. Akech S, Ledermann H, Maitland K. Choice of fluids for resuscitation in children with severe infection and shock: systematic review. *BMJ.* 2010; **341**: c4416.
20. Finfer S, Bellomo R, Boyce N, *et al.* A comparison of albumin and saline for fluid resuscitation in the intensive care unit. *New England Journal of Medicine.* May 2004; **350**(22): 2247–56.
21. Myburgh J, Cooper DJ, Finfer S, *et al.* Saline or albumin for fluid resuscitation in patients with traumatic brain injury. *New England Journal of Medicine.* Aug 2007; **357**(9): 874–84.
22. Barron ME, Wilkes MM, Navickis RJ. A systematic review of the comparative safety of colloids. *Archives of Surgery.* May 2004; **139**(5): 552–63.
23. Mitra S, Khandelwal P. Are all colloids same? How to select the right colloid? *Indian Journal of Anaesthesia.* Oct 2009; **53**(5): 592–607.
24. de Jonge E, Levi M. Effects of different plasma substitutes on blood coagulation: a comparative review. *Critical Care Medicine.* Jun 2001; **29**(6): 1261–7.
25. Westphal M, James MF, Kozek-Langenecker S, *et al.* Hydroxyethyl starches: different products–different effects. *Anesthesiology.* Jul 2009; **111**(1): 187–202.
26. Standl T, Lochbuehler H, Galli C, *et al.* HES 130/0.4 (Voluven) or human albumin in children younger than 2 years undergoing non-cardiac surgery. A prospective, randomized, open label, multicentre trial. *European Journal of Anaesthesiology.* Jun 2008; **25**(6): 437–45.
27. Liet JM, Bellouin AS, Boscher C, Lejus C, Roze JC. Plasma volume expansion by medium molecular weight hydroxyethyl starch in neonates: a pilot study. *Pediatric Critical Care Medicine.* Jul 2003; **4** (3): 305–7.
28. Liet JM, Kuster A, Denizot S, *et al.* Effects of hydroxyethyl starch on cardiac output in hypotensive neonates: a comparison with isotonic saline and 5% albumin. *Acta Paediatrica.* May 2006; **95**(5): 555–60.
29. Guidet B, Martinet O, Boulain T, *et al.* Assessment of hemodynamic efficacy and safety of 6% hydroxyethylstarch 130/0.4 vs. 0.9% NaCl fluid replacement in patients with severe sepsis: The CRYSTMAS study. *Critical Care.* May 2012; **16**(3): R94.
30. Perner A, Haase N, Guttormsen AB, *et al.* Hydroxyethyl starch 130/0.42 versus Ringer's acetate in severe sepsis. *New England Journal of Medicine.* Jul 2012; **367** (2): 124–34.

31. Myburgh JA, Finfer S, Bellomo R, *et al.* Hydroxyethyl starch or saline for fluid resuscitation in intensive care. *New England Journal of Medicine.* Nov 2012; **367**(20): 1901–11.

32. Navickis RJ, Haynes GR, Wilkes MM. Effect of hydroxyethyl starch on bleeding after cardiopulmonary bypass: a meta-analysis of randomized trials. *Journal of Thoracic and Cardiovascular Surgery.* Jul 2012; **144**(1): 223–30.

33. Aubron C, Bellomo R. Infusion of hydroxyethyl starch-containing fluids. *Minerva Anestesiologica.* Sep 2013; **79**(9): 1088–92.

34. Holliday MA, Ray PE, Friedman AL. Fluid therapy for children: facts, fashions and questions. *Archives of Disease in Childhood.* Jun 2007; **92**(6): 546–50.

35. Kalhan SC, Parimi P, Van Beek R, *et al.* Estimation of gluconeogenesis in newborn infants. *American Journal of Physiology, Endocrinology, and Metabolism.* Nov 2001; **281**(5): E991–7.

36. Kalhan S, Parimi P. Gluconeogenesis in the fetus and neonate. *Seminars in Perinatology.* Apr 2000; **24**(2): 94–106.

Chapter 26

Pediatric transfusion therapy and blood conservation

Kelly A. Machovec and B. Craig Weldon

The perioperative period is associated with a high risk of blood product transfusion. Blood conservation and the avoidance of allogeneic transfusion are imperative given the major impacts of transfusion on mortality and morbidity.[1] Improvements in donor screening and blood collection and processing have drastically lowered the infectious risks of blood transfusion while there is growing concern over the noninfectious consequences of transfusion.

Risks of transfusion

Infectious complications

The risk of contracting HIV from a blood transfusion in the USA is approximately 1 in 1.5 million donations[2] due to donor screening and viral nucleic acid testing. Increasingly, infections such as the West Nile Virus and prion diseases continue to threaten our blood supply and challenge the screening process. Table 26.1 demonstrates a summary of viral transfusion complications.

Bacterial contamination of blood and platelet packs remains a common problem, accounting for 10% of U.S. and U.K. transfusion-related fatalities.[3] Bacterial contamination of packed red blood cells (PRBCs) occurs uncommonly (< 1:1000000 units) but is associated with nearly 100% mortality. The most common organism is *Yersinia enterolitica*. Platelets, which cannot be refrigerated, are more likely to suffer contamination, but the clinical course of the infected recipient is variable, with a mortalty of 25%.

Noninfectious complications

Known noninfectious risks of transfusion include acute hemolytic reactions, alloimmunization, anaphylaxis, febrile reactions, hyperkalemia, graft versus host disease, circulatory overload, transfusion-related lung injury (TRALI),[4] transfusion-related immunomodulation (TRIM),[5] and transfusion-related gut injury (TRAGI).[6] Noninfectious complications are responsible for 87–100% of fatal transfusion complications.[2] It should be noted that children have a higher incidence of transfusion reactions than adults. The majority of events include clerical errors, including blood bank procedures, and actual product administration.[7]

Hemolytic transfusion reactions are due to preexisting antibodies in the recipient that attack donor blood cells.[2] Symptoms include fever, chills, rigors, chest and abdominal pain, hypotension, hemoglobinuria and diffuse bleeding. Other causes of hemolysis, including bacterial contamination, a dysfunctional blood warmer, infusion through a small gauge catheter, and red blood cell hemolysis due to mixture with hypotonic fluid should be ruled out.

Febrile reactions are nonhemolytic and may be diagnosed when there is a one degree Celsius increase in temperature during or soon after a transfusion after excluding other possible etiologies of fever.[2] Leukoreduction has resulted in a decreased incidence of febrile reactions.

Table 26.1 Risk of viral disease transmission from blood product transfusion in the USA.

Virus	Incidence of transmission
Hepatitis B	1:137 000
Hepatitis C	< 1:1 000000
Human immunodeficiency virus (HIV)	< 1:900 000
Human T lymphotropic virus types I and II	1:250 000–1:2 000 000

Essentials of Pediatric Anesthesiology, ed. Alan David Kaye, Charles James Fox and James H. Diaz. Published by Cambridge University Press. © Cambridge University Press 2015.

Hyperkalemia leads to cardiac arrest in children more often than adults, due to a smaller blood volume and immature renal function. The potassium load in a given unit of packed red cells increases directly with the storage time of the unit. Therefore, the freshest blood should be given to patients with the smallest blood volumes (neonates and infants). Other strategies to avoid hyperkalemia include washing older red cell units and avoiding rapid infusion through very small-gauge intravenous catheters.

Transfusion-related lung injury (TRALI) is defined as a new lung injury within 6 hours of a transfusion.[8] Pathophysiologically, donor antibodies attack and activate recipient white blood cells in the lung microcirculation, which then damage the pulmonary capillary endothelium, leading to pulmonary edema. Mediators in transfused plasma also activate neutrophils that are readied by trauma or surgical stress. While reports of TRALI in pediatric patients[9] are rare, TRALI is responsible for a large number of overall transfusion related deaths in the USA and Great Britain.[3] Since the American Red Cross has limited plasma distribution from multiparous female donors (whose plasma contains large amounts of antibodies directed at white blood cells), the incidence of TRALI has decreased.[10]

Transfusion-related immunomodulation (TRIM) describes the process whereby allogeneic blood transfusion influences the recipient's immune function. There is an association between perioperative transfusion of aging, stored red blood cells (RBC) and the progression of cancer,[11] an increased incidence of postoperative infections, and increased mortality, but these associations do not explain the mechanism of immune modulation. Other factors resulting from red blood cell storage, including decreased RBC deformability,[12] changes in microvascular blood flow,[13,14] reduced oxygen delivery to tissues,[15] and organ dysfunction[16] could potentially contribute to poor outcomes. Avoiding transfusion of older red blood cells does not necessarily prevent TRIM. A recent analysis of over 400 000 transfusions found a very weak association between old red blood cell administration and mortality.[17] Leukoreduction may help to decrease TRIM by reducing the inflammatory response and, hence, the immune disturbance associated with RBC transfusion.

Transfusion-related gut injury (TRAGI) is a newly described entity in premature infants in which RBC transfusion has been associated with the development of necrotizing enterocolitis.[6] The mechanism for this is still under investigation but may be related to changes in intestinal blood flow induced by stored blood transfusion.

Indications for transfusion

Whole blood

To be considered fresh, whole blood must be stored for less than 48 hours but cold storage adversely affects platelet function, leading the military to advocate for warm, fresh whole blood in combat victims. Mandatory viral nucleic acid testing may delay the administration of this product beyond the optimal 48-hour period. Reconstituted whole blood is a mixture of stored red cells and fresh frozen plasma but provides no platelets, and results in more donor exposures. Reconstituted whole blood is only indicated in three scenarios: exchange transfusion to treat hemolytic disease of the newborn in order to avoid severe hyperbilirubinemia with kernicterus, after cardiopulmonary bypass, and during massive transfusion.

Red blood cells

The only indications for red blood cell (RBC) transfusion are to increase oxygen carrying capacity of the blood, or to dilute concentration of abnormal hemoglobin moieties in patients with sickle cell disease or thalassemia. Transfusion triggers for patients less than 4 months old are more liberal, due to this population's limited ability to produce erythropoietin, increase cardiac output, and release oxygen to tissues. For patients older than 4 months, the American Society of Anesthesiologists (ASA) Task Force on Blood Component Therapy provides recommendations for adult patients that can be applied to pediatric patients. These guidelines state that transfusion is rarely needed for hemoglobin greater than 10 g/dl, is often needed for hemoglobin less than 6 g/dl, and that no one transfusion trigger should be employed.[18] In fact, in critically ill but stable children, a transfusion threshold of 7 g/dl has been found to decrease transfusion requirements without increasing negative outcomes.[19] It is important to monitor for ongoing anemia as well as other markers of oxygen delivery such as lactate levels and mixed venous oxygen saturation. The transfusion of 5 to 10 ml/kg of packed RBCs is expected to raise the hemoglobin by 1–2 g/dl.[20]

Two populations deserve special consideration. First, children with cyanotic congential heart disease require higher hemoglobin concentrations to maintain adequate oxygen delivery in the presence of mixing lesions. In this population, a hemoglobin target of 13–18 g/dl is acceptable. Second, children with sickle cell disease occasionally require preoperative red blood cell transfusion both to correct anemia and to dilute the concentration of hemoglobin S to less than 30%.

Fresh frozen plasma

Indications for the transfusion of FFP are taken from the ASA Task Force on Blood Component Therapy and are identical to those of adult patients. The criteria for transfusion are limited to emergency warfarin reversal, correction of coagulopathy with INR > 1.5, or correction of coagulopathy after massive transfusion (defined as replacement of more than one blood volume).[18] Five to 10 ml/kg of FFP is an adequate starting dose for FFP administration.

Platelets

Indications for platelet transfusion are similar to those for adults. A platelet count of 50×10^9/l is adequate for most procedures.[18] Ideally, platelet count should be obtained prior to transfusion, but platelets may be given empirically during massive transfusion with evidence of microvascular bleeding if there is insufficient time to obtain laboratory values.

Surgical procedures and perioperative transfusion

Perioperative cardiac arrest in children is often due to inadequate fluid resuscitation as well as consequences of massive transfusion, including electrolyte disturbances.[21,22] Among pediatric populations, neonates are at highest risk for allogenic blood transfusion.[23,24] Reasons for this include an immature coagulation system that is disrupted by surgical trauma resulting in higher blood loss,[25] a relatively smaller blood volume leading to post transfusion dilutional coagulopathy that may exacerbate blood loss, and a poor tolerance for anemia due to an altered Frank–Starling relationship, decreased myocardial compliance, and reduced oxygen tissue delivery by fetal hemoglobin.

Perioperative blood conservation strategies

The American Society of Anesthesiologists,[26] the Society of Thoracic Surgeons, and the Society of Cardiovascular Anesthesiologists[27] do not include pediatric patients in developing guidelines for transfusion because of the paucity of evidence in this population. Therefore, we must apply evidence from adult populations in pediatric transfusion and blood conservation decisions. Lowering transfusion triggers, employing blood-sparing surgical techniques, use of antifibrinolytic agents, preoperative autologous donation, cell savage, deliberate hypotension, acute normovolemic hemodilution, hypervolemic hemodilution, and preoperative erythropoietin administration are options for blood conservation planning.

Lowering transfusion triggers

Reducing the lowest acceptable hemoglobin reduces blood product transfusion rates.[28,29] A randomized controlled trial (RCT) of critically ill adults demonstrated that these patients could tolerate lower hemoglobin levels without negatively influencing outcomes.[30] A trial of nonbleeding pediatric intensive care patients also found that no harm came from lowering the transfusion threshold.[19] The results in the pediatric study held true in children who had both cardiac[31] and general surgical[32] procedures. Studies in premature neonates examining lower transfusion threshold have produced conflicting results.[33,34]

Decreased transfusion thresholds can become part of institutional transfusion guidelines in an effort to lower transfusion rates.[35,36] There is evidence in scoliosis repair[37] and, possibly, craniofacial procedures [38] that program guidelines can reduce allogenic transfusion. Even in neonatal intensive care populations, monitored compliance with moderate transfusion guidelines reduced transfusion without affecting patient outcomes.[39]

Blood-sparing surgical innovations

Electrocautery and topical thrombin are two examples of surgical innovation resulting in reduced blood loss. In pediatric surgery, the advent of minimally invasive craniosynostosis repair has decreased the formerly nearly universal need for transfusion after cranial vault reconstruction[40–42] While several minimally invasive approaches to craniosynostosis repair in infants have appeared in the literature,[40] endoscopic strip craniectomy[43] and spring-mediated cranioplasty[44] are the techniques most focused on transfusion reduction. Both methods lower transfusion, lower intensive care admission rates, shorten length of stay, and reduce costs.[43,45,46]

Antifibrinolytic agents

The coagulation system is balanced between thrombosis and fibrinolysis. Tissue injury due to surgery or trauma activates both the coagulation system, resulting in thrombin generation and clot, as well as the fibrinolytic system, activating plasmin which cleaves fibrin and lyses clot. Excessive or inappropriate fibrinolysis may result in further bleeding and coagulopathy.[47] This system can be manipulated pharmacologically with three agents designed to inhibit thrombolysis, reduce blood loss, decrease transfusion: aprotinin, epsilon-aminocaproic acid (EACA) and tranexamic acid (TXA). Aprotinin will not be discussed further as it was removed from the U.S. market in 2008 due to increased mortality in adult cardiothoracic surgery patients.[48] Of note, studies in pediatric surgical patients found aprotinin to be as efficacious as EACA and TXA in reducing blood loss[49–51] and a qualitative review[51] of studies in pediatric surgical patients have found these drugs to be equally efficacious in reducing surgical blood loss. Both EACA and TXA are lysine analogs that inhibit the conversion of plasminogen to plasmin, thus preventing activation of plasmin and decreasing fibrinolysis.[2]

Epsilon aminocaproic acid

Clinical experience with EACA is mostly in cardiac and orthopedic procedures. A meta-analysis of EACA in scoliosis surgery showed no difference in blood transfusion compared to those who did not receive antifibrinolytic therapy, but those who received antifibrinolysis experienced less blood loss and lower volume of transfusion.[49] Several retrospective studies in infants and children undergoing cardiac surgery show no difference in transfusion avoidance between EACA and TXA.[52–55]

Tranexamic acid

A recent RCT of TXA given to adult trauma patients who were actively bleeding or at risk for hemorrhage showed reduced mortality and fatal hemorrhage in the group who received TXA.[56] In children, TXA is utilized in cardiac surgery, spinal surgery, and more recently, cranial vault reconstructions. Two RCTs demonstrated reduced blood transfusion in craniofacial surgery with use of TXA.[57,58]

While the overall safety profile of TXA in pediatric populations is encouraging,[49,50] there is concern of increased seizures with use of TXA. This concern is based on results of two retrospective studies in children comparing TXA to aprotinin[52] and EACA[53] that found a nonstatistically significant increase in seizures in the patients receiving TXA. Evidence in the adult cardiac surgery patients from large retrospective studies does show a significant increase in the postoperative incidence of seizures with TXA compared with EACA.[59,60] Given this association, high-dose TXA ($\geq$ 100 mg/kg) should be used cautiously until further data emerge.

Preoperative autologous donation

Preoperative autologous donation (PAD) avoids allogenic blood transfusion with the most obvious advantage being avoidance of alloimmunization.[61] However, no randomized, controlled trials in children compare PAD alone with other management techniques during high blood-loss procedures. The evidence that exists combines PAD with other blood conservation measures, confounding the effects of PAD itself. While PAD avoids alloimmunization, it does not avoid the risks of bacterial contamination or clerical error leading to incorrect transfusion.

Preoperative autologous donation is associated with special problems in children, including their smaller blood volume, which limits the amount able to be donated, and their inability to tolerate repeated vascular accesss and donation procedures.[62] Further, the compensation after donation must be considered: adults compensate for intravascular volume loss after donation by increasing stroke volume and heart rate to maintain cardiac output. School-aged children may be able to compensate in this way; but infants with immature myocardium have a limited ability to increase stroke volume, and may not compensate as easily.[63] Finally, use of this strategy must consider the cost of PAD and mandatory waste of unused PAD units (30–50% of donated units).[64] If PAD is utilized, a longer interval between donation and surgery maximizes compensatory erythropoiesis.[2]

Evidence suggests that, although PAD reduces ABT,[65–67] it increases the overall incidence of both autologous and allogeneic transfusion, thus predisposing patients to other transfusion risks.[61] The same guidelines for transfusing allogeneic blood should be applied for transfusing autologous blood.

Cell salvage techniques

Intraoperative cell salvage (ICS) involves collecting, purifying, and concentrating blood cells salvaged from the operative field.[68] Cell salvage is a proven effective method of blood conservation in adult populations, with a meta-analysis finding an absolute risk reduction of ABT of 21%.[69]

Randomized trials of ICS in pediatric populations are lacking. Technological advances using collecting bowls with volumes as low as 55 ml [2] allow this technique to be used in smaller patients, thus avoiding ABT.[70] Intraoperative cell salvage reduces ABT in infants and children having cranial vault econstruction,[71,72] cardiac procedures,[73] and orthopedic procedures[74] compared with controls. A disadvantage of ICS is that blood cells but not coagulation factors or platelets are replaced.[63]

Transfusing unwashed salvaged blood may reduce ABT in adults but safety concerns exist surrounding retransfusion of inflammatory mediators, fat particles, activated leukocytes, and contaminants.[75] Pediatric applications of this technique have been developed[76,77] but evidence is not strong enough to recommend this technique in children.

Deliberate hypotension

Deliberate hypotension (DH) is the use of pharmacologic agents to reduce blood pressure, which may potentially reduce blood loss. This method of blood conservation is effective in adults having orthopedic and orthognathic procedures in terms of reduced blood transfusion.[78] Deliberate hypotension in healthy patients has minimal impact on organ perfusion and is associated with rare serious complications.[79]

In pediatric populations, little evidence supports DH use as a sole intervention to reduce ABT. However, DH is routinely used in adolescent scoliosis and orthognathic surgery. One study reported less blood loss in the DH group compared to controls, but the overall blood loss was minimal and neither group required transfusion.[80] A study of DH in infants having craniofacial reconstruction found a significant reduction in blood loss in the study group.[81] Deliberate hypotension is often used in combination with other blood conservation techniques, including PAD, ICS, and acute normovolemic hemodilution (ANH). The combination of DH with normovolemic anemia has been reported in pediatric patients[82,83] but should be used cautiously due to the risk of organ hypoperfusion.[84]

Acute normovolemic and hypervolemic hemodilution

Acute normovolemic hemodilution (ANH) involves removing blood from the patient and replacing with crystalloid or colloid solution in the postinduction period of anesthesia; the goal being to lower the patient's hematocrit while maintaining normal intravascular volume.[85] Surgical bleeding then occurs at a lower hematocrit and blood loss is replaced with crystalloid. When blood loss has ceased or the transfusion threshold is reached the collected blood is returned to the patient. Advantages of this technique are that blood collected from the patient remains in the operating room, avoiding the risk of clerical transfusion error, and contains functional platelets and clotting factors.

Studies in healthy children and adolescents indicate that they tolerate ANH well. Nadir hematocrits of 9% in adolescents[86] and 17% in children[87] found no negative impact on oxygen delivery before retransfusion of collected blood; ANH has been successfully used as the sole blood sparing modality in children undergoing bone marrow harvest,[88] craniosynostosis,[87,89] and scoliosis surgery[90,91] but there have been no RCTs in pediatric patients.

Young infants may not tolerate acute normovolemic anemia due to their reduced ability to maintain oxygen delivery to tissues.[63] The normal physiologic response to ANH is an increase in cardiac output by increasing stroke volume and an increase in the oxygen extraction ratio.[92] Young infants (less than 4 to 6 months old) rely on increases in heart rate to increase cardiac output as they have a limited ability to increase stroke volume. These infants also have varying amounts of Hgb F, which does not release oxygen to peripheral tissues as well as Hgb A.[62] Thus, ANH should probably be avoided in this population.

Another group that does not tolerate normovolemic hemodilution is infants and children having cardiac surgery. Hemodilution to hematocrit of 16% significantly decreased regional cerebral oxygenation in one group of children having cardiac surgery.[93] A second RCT of infants undergoing cardiac surgery found that hemodilution to a hematocrit of 21.5% correlated with poor psychomotor testing at one year of age.[94]

Hypervolemic hemodilution

Hypervolemic hemodilution (HH) is an alternative to ANH that avoids blood collection. It involves infusing a colloid solution to reach a target hematocrit; it is particularly useful for anticipated blood losses of less than 40% of the patient's blood volume.[95] As with ANH, surgical blood loss occurs at a lower hematocrit. One RCT examining this technique in children having scoliosis surgery demonstrated a reduced volume of allogeneic transfusion in the HH group, although the overall blood loss was not different between groups.[96]

Preoperative erythropoietin administration

Erythropoietin, produced by the kidneys, controls the differentiation of progenitor cells into red blood cells.[63] Human recombinant erythropoietin (EPO) has been used for the past two decades to increase red blood cell mass perioperatively.[97] Early reports in pediatric patients demonstrated the blood-sparing potential of EPO in neurosurgical,[98] craniofacial,[99] and spinal surgery[100] cases. However, these studies demonstrated that EPO cannot be used a sole blood conservation technique.

Drawing on experiences in adult blood conservation, EPO was combined with PAD in pediatric cardiac,[101,102] scoliosis,[103] and craniofacial[101] surgeries. The use of EPO improved compliance rates for donation and resulted in a higher hematocrit on the day of surgery, thus reducing ABT.[102,103] Human recombinant erythropoietin has also been used in combination with ANH, as it raises the preoperative hematocrit.[104,105] Again, EPO is a useful adjunct to other blood conservation techniques. Of note, 2 weeks of EPO therapy are required for maximum efficacy, although the rate of hematocrit increase is not easily predictable for a given patient.[63]

References

1. Glance LG, Dick AW, Mukamel DB, *et al.* Association between intraoperative blood transfusion and mortality and morbidity in patients undergoing noncardiac surgery. *Anesthesiology.* Feb 2011; **114**(2): 283–92.
2. Lavoie J. Blood transfusion risks and alternative strategies in pediatric patients. *Paediatr Anaesth.* Jan 2011; **21**(1): 14–24.
3. Vamvakas EC, Blajchman MA. Transfusion-related mortality: the ongoing risks of allogeneic blood transfusion and the available strategies for their prevention. *Blood.* Apr 2009; **113**(15): 3406–17.
4. Silliman CC, McLaughlin NJ. Transfusion-related acute lung injury. *Blood Rev.* May 2006; **20**(3): 139–59.
5. Vamvakas EC, Blajchman MA. Transfusion-related immunomodulation (TRIM): an update. *Blood Rev.* Nov 2007; **21**(6): 327–48.
6. Christensen RD, Lambert DK, Henry E, *et al.* Is "transfusion-associated necrotizing enterocolitis" an authentic pathogenic entity? *Transfusion.* May 2010; **50**(5): 1106–12.
7. Stainsby D, Jones H, Wells AW, Gibson B, Cohen H. Adverse outcomes of blood transfusion in children: analysis of UK reports to the serious hazards of transfusion scheme 1996–2005. *Br J Haematol.* Apr 2008; **141**(1): 73–9.
8. Toy P, Popovsky MA, Abraham E, *et al.* Transfusion-related acute lung injury: definition and review. *Crit Care Med.* Apr 2005; **33**(4): 721–6.
9. Church GD, Price C, Sanchez R, Looney MR. Transfusion-related acute lung injury in the paediatric patient: Two case reports and a review of the literature. *Transfus Med.* Oct 2006; **16**(5): 343–8.
10. Eder AF, Herron RM, Jr., Strupp A, *et al.* Effective reduction of transfusion-related acute lung injury risk with male-predominant plasma strategy in the American Red Cross (2006–2008). *Transfusion.* Aug 2010; **50**(8): 1732–42.
11. Atzil S, Arad M, Glasner A, *et al.* Blood transfusion promotes cancer progression: a critical role for aged erythrocytes. *Anesthesiology.* Dec 2008; **109**(6): 989–97.
12. Barshtein G, Manny N, Yedgar S. Circulatory risk in the transfusion of red blood cells with impaired flow properties induced by storage. *Transfus Med Rev.* Jan 2011; **25**(1): 24–35.
13. Tsai AG, Cabrales P, Intaglietta M. Microvascular perfusion upon exchange transfusion with stored red blood cells in normovolemic anemic conditions. *Transfusion.* Nov 2004; **44**(11): 1626–34.
14. Reynolds JD, Ahearn GS, Angelo M, *et al.* S-nitrosohemoglobin deficiency: a mechanism for loss of physiological activity in banked blood. *Proc Natl Acad Sci U S A.* Oct 23 2007; **104**(43): 17058–62.
15. Kiraly LN, Underwood S, Differding JA, Schreiber MA. Transfusion of aged packed red blood cells results in decreased tissue oxygenation in critically injured trauma patients. *J Trauma.* Jul 2009; **67**(1): 29–32.
16. Gauvin F, Spinella PC, Lacroix J, *et al.* Association between length of storage of transfused red blood

cells and multiple organ dysfunction syndrome in pediatric intensive care patients. *Transfusion*. Sep 2010; **50**(9): 1902–13.

17. Edgren G, Kamper-Jorgensen M, Eloranta S, *et al*. Duration of red blood cell storage and survival of transfused patients (CME). *Transfusion*. Jun 2010; **50**(6): 1185–95.
18. Practice guidelines for blood component therapy. A report by the American Society of Anesthesiologists Task Force on Blood Component Therapy. *Anesthesiology*. Mar 1996; **84**(3): 732–47.
19. Lacroix J, Hebert PC, Hutchison JS, *et al*. Transfusion strategies for patients in pediatric intensive care units. *N Engl J Med*. Apr 19 2007; **356**(16): 1609–19.
20. Davies P, Robertson S, Hegde S, *et al*. Calculating the required transfusion volume in children. *Transfusion*. Feb 2007; **47**(2): 212–16.
21. Bhananker SM, Ramamoorthy C, Geiduschek JM, *et al*. Anesthesia-related cardiac arrest in children: update from the Pediatric Perioperative Cardiac Arrest Registry. *Anesth Analg*. Aug 2007; **105**(2): 344–50.
22. Flick RP, Sprung J, Harrison TE, *et al*. Perioperative cardiac arrests in children between 1988 and 2005 at a tertiary referral center: a study of 92,881 patients. *Anesthesiology*. Feb 2007; **106**(2): 226–37.
23. Strauss RG. Transfusion therapy in neonates. *Am J Dis Child*. Aug 1991; **145**(8): 904–11.
24. Keung CY, Smith KR, Savoia HF, Davidson AJ. An audit of transfusion of red blood cell units in pediatric anesthesia. *Paediatr Anaesth*. Apr 2009; **19**(4): 320–8.
25. Guzzetta NA, Miller BE. Principles of hemostasis in children: models and maturation. *Paediatr Anaesth*. Jan 2011; **21**(1): 3–9.
26. Practice guidelines for perioperative blood transfusion and adjuvant therapies: an updated report by the American Society of Anesthesiologists Task Force on Perioperative Blood Transfusion and Adjuvant Therapies. *Anesthesiology*. Jul 2006; **105**(1): 198–208.
27. Ferraris VA, Brown JR, Despotis GJ, *et al*. 2011 update to the Society of Thoracic Surgeons and the Society of Cardiovascular Anesthesiologists blood conservation clinical practice guidelines. *Ann Thorac Surg*. Mar 2011; **91**(3): 944–82.
28. Carson JL, Hill S, Carless P, Hebert P, Henry D. Transfusion triggers: a systematic review of the literature. *Transfus Med Rev*. Jul 2002; **16**(3): 187–99.
29. Hill SR, Carless PA, Henry DA, *et al*. Transfusion thresholds and other strategies for guiding allogeneic red blood cell transfusion. *Cochrane Database Syst Rev*. 2002(2): CD002042.
30. Hebert PC, Wells G, Blajchman MA, *et al*. A multicenter, randomized, controlled clinical trial of transfusion requirements in critical care. Transfusion Requirements in Critical Care Investigators, Canadian Critical Care Trials Group. *N Engl J Med*. Feb 1999; **340**(6): 409–17.
31. Willems A, Harrington K, Lacroix J, *et al*. Comparison of two red-cell transfusion strategies after pediatric cardiac surgery: a subgroup analysis. *Crit Care Med*. Feb 2010; **38**(2): 649–56.
32. Rouette J, Trottier H, Ducruet T, *et al*. Red blood cell transfusion threshold in postsurgical pediatric intensive care patients: a randomized clinical trial. *Ann Surg*. Mar 2010; **251**(3): 421–7.
33. Bell EF, Strauss RG, Widness JA, *et al*. Randomized trial of liberal versus restrictive guidelines for red blood cell transfusion in preterm infants. *Pediatrics*. Jun 2005; **115**(6): 1685–91.
34. Kirpalani H, Whyte RK, Andersen C, *et al*. The Premature Infants in Need of Transfusion (PINT) study: a randomized, controlled trial of a restrictive (low) versus liberal (high) transfusion threshold for extremely low birth weight infants. *J Pediatr*. Sep 2006; **149**(3): 301–7.
35. Mallett SV, Peachey TD, Sanehi O, Hazlehurst G, Mehta A. Reducing red blood cell transfusion in elective surgical patients: the role of audit and practice guidelines. *Anaesthesia*. Oct 2000; **55**(10): 1013–19.
36. Ansari S, Szallasi A. Blood management by transfusion triggers: when less is more. *Blood Transfus*. Jun 15 2011; **4**(1): 1–6.
37. Hassan N, Halanski M, Wincek J, *et al*. Blood management in pediatric spinal deformity surgery: review of a 2-year experience. *Transfusion*. Oct 2011; **51**(10): 2133–41.
38. Stricker PA, Cladis FP, Fiadjoe JE, McCloskey JJ, Maxwell LG. Perioperative management of children undergoing craniofacial reconstruction surgery: a practice survey. *Paediatr Anaesth*. May 20 2011.
39. Baer VL, Henry E, Lambert DK, *et al*. Implementing a program to improve compliance with neonatal intensive care unit transfusion guidelines was accompanied by a reduction in transfusion rate: a pre-post analysis within a multihospital health care system. *Transfusion*. Feb 2011; **51**(2): 264–9.
40. Di Rocco C, Tamburrini G, Pietrini D. Blood sparing in craniosynostosis surgery. *Semin Pediatr Neurol*. Dec 2004; **11**(4): 278–87.
41. Faberowski LW, Black S, Mickle JP. Blood loss and transfusion practice in the perioperative

management of craniosynostosis repair. *J Neurosurg Anesthesiol.* Jul 1999; **11**(3): 167–72.

42. Stricker PA, Shaw TL, Desouza DG, *et al.* Blood loss, replacement, and associated morbidity in infants and children undergoing craniofacial surgery. *Paediatr Anaesth.* Feb 2010; **20**(2): 150–9.

43. Barone CM, Jimenez DF. Endoscopic craniectomy for early correction of craniosynostosis. *Plast Reconstr Surg.* Dec 1999; **104**(7): 1965–73; discussion 1974–65.

44. Lauritzen C, Sugawara Y, Kocabalkan O, Olsson R. Spring mediated dynamic craniofacial reshaping. Case report. *Scand J Plast Reconstr Surg Hand Surg.* Sep 1998; **32**(3): 331–8.

45. Jimenez DF, Barone CM, Cartwright CC, Baker L. Early management of craniosynostosis using endoscopic-assisted strip craniectomies and cranial orthotic molding therapy. *Pediatrics.* Jul 2002; **110**(1 Pt 1): 97–104.

46. Shah MN, Kane AA, Petersen JD, *et al.* Endoscopically assisted versus open repair of sagittal craniosynostosis: the St. Louis Children's Hospital experience. *J Neurosurg Pediatr.* Aug 2011; **8**(2): 165–70.

47. Levy JH, Dutton RP, Hemphill JC, 3rd, *et al.* Multidisciplinary approach to the challenge of hemostasis. *Anesth Analg.* Feb 2010; **110**(2): 354–64.

48. Fergusson DA, Hebert PC, Mazer CD, *et al.* A comparison of aprotinin and lysine analogues in high-risk cardiac surgery. *N Engl J Med.* May 2008; **358**(22): 2319–31.

49. Tzortzopoulou A, Cepeda MS, Schumann R, Carr DB. Antifibrinolytic agents for reducing blood loss in scoliosis surgery in children. *Cochrane Database Syst Rev.* 2008(3): CD006883.

50. Schouten ES, van de Pol AC, Schouten AN, *et al.* The effect of aprotinin, tranexamic acid, and aminocaproic acid on blood loss and use of blood products in major pediatric surgery: a meta-analysis. *Pediatr Crit Care Med.* Mar 2009; **10**(2): 182–90.

51. Eaton MP. Antifibrinolytic therapy in surgery for congenital heart disease. *Anesth Analg.* Apr 2008; **106**(4): 1087–100.

52. Breuer T, Martin K, Wilhelm M, *et al.* The blood sparing effect and the safety of aprotinin compared to tranexamic acid in paediatric cardiac surgery. *Eur J Cardiothorac Surg.* Jan 2009; **35**(1): 167–71; author reply 171.

53. Martin K, Breuer T, Gertler R, *et al.* Tranexamic acid versus varepsilon-aminocaproic acid: efficacy and safety in paediatric cardiac surgery. *Eur J Cardiothorac Surg.* Jun 2011; **39**(6): 892–7.

54. Martin K, Gertler R, Sterner A, *et al.* Comparison of blood-sparing efficacy of epsilon-aminocaproic acid and tranexamic acid in newborns undergoing cardiac surgery. *Thorac Cardiovasc Surg.* Aug 2011; **59**(5): 276–80.

55. Martin K, Gertler R, Liermann H, Mayr NP, *et al.* Switch from aprotinin to varepsilon-aminocaproic acid: impact on blood loss, transfusion, and clinical outcome in neonates undergoing cardiac surgery. *Br J Anaesth.* Dec 2011; **107**(6): 934–9.

56. Shakur H, Roberts I, Bautista R, *et al.* Effects of tranexamic acid on death, vascular occlusive events, and blood transfusion in trauma patients with significant haemorrhage (CRASH-2): a randomised, placebo-controlled trial. *Lancet.* Jul 2010; **376**(9734): 23–32.

57. Dadure C, Sauter M, Bringuier S, *et al.* Intraoperative tranexamic acid reduces blood transfusion in children undergoing craniosynostosis surgery: a randomized double-blind study. *Anesthesiology.* Apr 2011; **114**(4): 856–61.

58. Goobie SM, Meier PM, Pereira LM, *et al.* Efficacy of tranexamic acid in pediatric craniosynostosis surgery: a double-blind, placebo-controlled trial. *Anesthesiology.* Apr 2011; **114**(4): 862–71.

59. Martin K, Knorr J, Breuer T, *et al.* Seizures after open heart surgery: comparison of epsilon-aminocaproic acid and tranexamic acid. *J Cardiothorac Vasc Anesth.* Feb 2011; **25**(1): 20–5.

60. Keyl C, Uhl R, Beyersdorf F, *et al.* High-dose tranexamic acid is related to increased risk of generalized seizures after aortic valve replacement. *Eur J Cardiothorac Surg.* May 2011; **39**(5): e114–121.

61. Lauder GR. Pre-operative predeposit autologous donation in children presenting for elective surgery: a review. *Transfus Med.* Apr 2007; **17**(2): 75–82.

62. Weldon BC. Blood conservation in pediatric anesthesia. *Anesthesiol Clin North America.* Jun 2005; **23**(2): 347–61, vii.

63. Verma S, Eisses M, Richards M. Blood conservation strategies in pediatric anesthesia. *Anesthesiology Clinics.* Jun 2009; **27**(2): 337–51.

64. Bess RS, Lenke LG, Bridwell KH, Steger-May K, Hensley M. Wasting of preoperatively donated autologous blood in the surgical treatment of adolescent idiopathic scoliosis. *Spine.* Sep 2006; **31**(20): 2375–80.

65. Forgie MA, Wells PS, Laupacis A, Fergusson D. Preoperative autologous donation decreases allogeneic transfusion but increases exposure to all red blood cell transfusion: results of a meta-analysis. International Study of Perioperative Transfusion

(ISPOT) Investigators. *Arch Intern Med.* Mar 1998; **158**(6): 610–16.

66. Henry DA, Carless PA, Moxey AJ, *et al.* Pre-operative autologous donation for minimising perioperative allogeneic blood transfusion. *Cochrane Database Syst Rev.* 2002(2):CD003602.

67. Carless P, Moxey A, O'Connell D, Henry D. Autologous transfusion techniques: a systematic review of their efficacy. *Transfus Med.* Apr 2004; **14**(2): 123–44.

68. Ashworth A, Klein AA. Cell salvage as part of a blood conservation strategy in anaesthesia. *Br J Anaesth.* Oct 2010; **105**(4): 401–16.

69. Carless PA, Henry DA, Moxey AJ, *et al.* Cell salvage for minimising perioperative allogeneic blood transfusion. *Cochrane Database Syst Rev.* 2010(4):CD001888.

70. Jimenez DF, Barone CM. Intraoperative autologous blood transfusion in the surgical correction of craniosynostosis. *Neurosurgery.* Dec 1995; **37**(6): 1075–9.

71. Dahmani S, Orliaguet GA, Meyer PG, *et al.* Perioperative blood salvage during surgical correction of craniosynostosis in infants. *Br J Anaesth.* Oct 2000; **85**(4): 550–5.

72. Fearon JA. Reducing allogenic blood transfusions during pediatric cranial vault surgical procedures: A prospective analysis of blood recycling. *Plast Reconstr Surg.* Apr 2004; **113**(4): 1126–30.

73. Golab HD, Scohy TV, de Jong PL, Takkenberg JJ, Bogers AJ. Intraoperative cell salvage in infants undergoing elective cardiac surgery: a prospective trial. *Eur J Cardiothorac Surg.* Aug 2008; **34**(2): 354–9.

74. Nicolai P, Leggetter PP, Glithero PR, Bhimarasetty CR. Autologous transfusion in acetabuloplasty in children. *J Bone Joint Surg Br.* Jan 2004; **86**(1): 110–12.

75. Munoz M, Garcia-Vallejo JJ, Ruiz MD, *et al.* Transfusion of post-operative shed blood: laboratory characteristics and clinical utility. *Eur Spine J.* Oct 2004; **13** Suppl 1: S107–113.

76. Blevins FT, Shaw B, Valeri CR, Kasser J, Hall J. Reinfusion of shed blood after orthopaedic procedures in children and adolescents. *J Bone Joint Surg Am.* Mar 1993; **75**(3): 363–71.

77. Orliaguet GA, Bruyere M, Meyer PG, *et al.* Comparison of perioperative blood salvage and postoperative reinfusion of drained blood during surgical correction of craniosynostosis in infants. *Paediatr Anaesth.* Nov 2003; **13**(9): 797–804.

78. Paul JE, Ling E, Lalonde C, Thabane L. Deliberate hypotension in orthopedic surgery reduces blood loss and transfusion requirements: a meta-analysis of randomized controlled trials. *Can J Anaesth.* Oct 2007; **54**(10): 799–810.

79. Choi WS, Samman N. Risks and benefits of deliberate hypotension in anaesthesia: a systematic review. *Int J Oral Maxillofac Surg.* Aug 2008; **37**(8): 687–703.

80. Precious DS, Splinter W, Bosco D. Induced hypotensive anesthesia for adolescent orthognathic surgery patients. *J Oral Maxillofac Surg.* Jun 1996; **54**(6): 680–3; discussion 683–4.

81. Diaz JH, Lockhart CH. Hypotensive anesthesia for craniectomy in infancy. *Brit J Anaesth.* 1979; **51**(3): 233–5.

82. Schaller RT, Jr., Schaller J, Furman EB. The advantages of hemodilution anesthesia for major liver resection in children. *J Pediatr Surg.* Dec 1984; **19**(6): 705–10.

83. Schaller RT, Jr., Schaller J, Morgan A, Furman EB. Hemodilution anesthesia: a valuable aid to major cancer surgery in children. *Am J Surg.* Jul 1983; **146**(1): 79–84.

84. Han SH, Bahk JH, Kim JH, *et al.* The effect of esmolol-induced controlled hypotension in combination with acute normovolemic hemodilution on cerebral oxygenation. *Acta Anaesthesiol Scand.* Aug 2006; **50**(7): 863–8.

85. Monk TG. Acute normovolemic hemodilution. *Anesthesiol Clin North America.* Jun 2005; **23**(2): 271–81, vi.

86. Fontana JL, Welborn L, Mongan PD, *et al.* Oxygen consumption and cardiovascular function in children during profound intraoperative normovolemic hemodilution. *Anesth Analg.* Feb 1995; **80**(2): 219–25.

87. Hassan AA, Lochbuehler H, Frey L, Messmer K. Global tissue oxygenation during normovolaemic haemodilution in young children. *Paediatr Anaesth.* 1997; **7**(3): 197–204.

88. Desa VP, Bekassy AN, Schou H, Werner MU, Werner O. Hemodilution during bone-marrow harvesting in children. *Anesth Analg.* May 1991; **72**(5): 645–50.

89. Hans P, Collin V, Bonhomme V, *et al.* Evaluation of acute normovolemic hemodilution for surgical repair of craniosynostosis. *J Neurosurg Anesthesiol.* Jan 2000; **12**(1): 33–6.

90. Du Toit G, Relton JE, Gillespie R. Acute haemodilutional autotransfusion in the surgical management of scoliosis. *J Bone Joint Surg Br.* May 1978; **60**-B(2): 178–80.

91. Olsfanger D, Jedeikin R, Metser U, Nusbacher J, Gepstein R. Acute normovolaemic haemodilution and idiopathic scoliosis surgery: effects on homologous blood requirements. *Anaesth Intensive Care.* Aug 1993; **21**(4): 429–31.

92. Vaniterson M, Vanderwaart FJM, Erdmann W, Trouwborst A. Systemic hemodynamics and oxygenation during hemodilution in children. *Lancet.* Oct 28 1995; **346**(8983): 1127–9.

93. Han SH, Kim CS, Kim SD, Bahk JH, Park YS. The effect of bloodless pump prime on cerebral oxygenation in paediatric patients. *Acta Anaesthesiol Scand.* May 2004; **48**(5): 648–52.

94. Jonas RA, Wypij D, Roth SJ, *et al.* The influence of hemodilution on outcome after hypothermic cardiopulmonary bypass: results of a randomized trial in infants. *J Thorac Cardiovasc Surg.* Dec 2003; **126**(6): 1765–74.

95. Singbartl K, Schleinzer W, Singbartl G. Hypervolemic hemodilution: an alternative to acute normovolemic hemodilution? A mathematical analysis. *J Surg Res.* Oct 1999; **86**(2): 206–12.

96. Chen YQ, Chen Y, Ji CS, Gu HB, Bai J. Clinical observation of acute hypervolemic hemodilution in scoliosis surgery on children. *Zhonghua Yi Xue Za Zhi.* Nov 2008; **88**(41): 2901–3.

97. Goodnough LT, Rudnick S, Price TH, *et al.* Increased preoperative collection of autologous blood with recombinant human erythropoietin therapy. *N Engl J Med.* Oct 1989; **321**(17): 1163–8.

98. Schiff SJ, Weinstein SL. Use of recombinant human erythropoietin to avoid blood transfusion in a Jehovah's Witness requiring hemispherectomy. Case report. *J Neurosurg.* Oct 1993; **79**(4): 600–2.

99. Helfaer MA, Carson BS, James CS, *et al.* Increased hematocrit and decreased transfusion requirements in children given erythropoietin before undergoing craniofacial surgery. *J Neurosurg.* Apr 1998; **88**(4): 704–8.

100. Vitale MG, Stazzone EJ, Gelijns AC, Moskowitz AJ, Roye DP, Jr. The effectiveness of preoperative erythropoietin in averting allogenic blood transfusion among children undergoing scoliosis surgery. *J Pediatr Orthop B.* Jul 1998; **7**(3): 203–9.

101. Sonzogni V, Crupi G, Poma R, *et al.* Erythropoietin therapy and preoperative autologous blood donation in children undergoing open heart surgery. *Br J Anaesth.* Sep 2001; **87**(3): 429–34.

102. Komai H, Naito Y, Okamura Y, *et al.* Preliminary study of autologous blood predonation in pediatric open-heart surgery impact of advance infusion of recombinant human erythropoietin. *Pediatr Cardiol.* Jan-Feb 2005; **26**(1): 50–5.

103. Franchini M, Gandini G, Regis D, *et al.* Recombinant human erythropoietin facilitates autologous blood collections in children undergoing corrective spinal surgery. *Transfusion.* Jul 2004; **44**(7): 1122–4.

104. Polley JW, Berkowitz RA, McDonald TB, *et al.* Craniomaxillofacial surgery in the Jehovah's Witness patient. *Plast Reconstr Surg.* May 1994; **93**(6): 1258–63.

105. Meneghini L, Zadra N, Aneloni V, *et al.* Erythropoietin therapy and acute preoperative normovolaemic haemodilution in infants undergoing craniosynostosis surgery. *Paediatr Anaesth.* Jun 2003; **13**(5): 392–6.

Chapter

27 Preoperative anxiolysis and sedation

Paul A. Tripi

Introduction

Preoperative anxiety is common in children. According to one study, as many as 60% of children undergoing surgery experience preoperative anxiety.[1] By extrapolation from U.S. National Health Statistics Report data, this places as many as 3 000 000 children at risk for preoperative anxiety every year.[2] The adverse consequences of such anxiety include emotional distress and dissatisfaction, lack of cooperation during induction of anesthesia, and negative postoperative behavioral changes. Approaches for mitigating distress are built on three major strategies: psychosocial preparation, avoidance of separation from parents or guardians, and premedication.

The problem of preoperative anxiety

No child wants to be "stuck with needles," have an operation, or visit a doctor's office rather than engage in play or a favorite activity. These attitudes develop early in life as children make frequent visits to medical facilities for well-care, which sometimes include intramuscular injections for immunization or needle insertions for phlebotomy. It is likely that an aversion to needles and health care providers develop during these unavoidable experiences early in a child's life. Most children develop separation anxiety from parents by 8 to 10 months of age, and as preschoolers (18 months to 6 years) have well-developed fears of the unknown, which certainly would include unfamiliar surgical facilities staffed with unfamiliar people. Young children also have imaginary fears, such as monsters, which can amplify the more reality-based fears they are experiencing. By the school-age years (6–12 years old), fears become more realistic, and can include pain and awareness under anesthesia. Adolescents (over 12 years) also may experience fears of death and loss of privacy. Anesthesiologists must consider the developmental level of children when addressing the fears and anxiety they may be experiencing in the preoperative period (see Table 27.1).[3]

Children may manifest their anxiety in a variety of ways. The most obvious manner is to behave poorly and to be uncooperative. It is not uncommon for children to cry, scream, kick or hit others, breath hold, resist placement of an anesthesia mask, or even attempt to flee during the transition from waiting in preoperative holding to the start of anesthesia care. Insertion of an intravenous line or placement of a mask over a child's face during inhalational induction of anesthesia can be met with a great deal of resistance and lack of cooperation. Children may scream and flail during such interventions, which lengthens the procedure time, increases the chance of injury to the child, and often produces anxiety in family members with the child. Children may also exhibit negative behaviors following surgery, which are thought to be related to anxiety. Such behaviors can include poor eating, sleep disturbance, withdrawal, enuresis, and separation anxiety, which may last for months following the surgery.[1,4–6]

Some children are more at risk than others for preoperative anxiety. Perhaps the most obvious risk factor is previous surgery, since negative experiences with prior surgery will sensitize a child to a repeat of the surgical experience, even if the planned surgery is minor with little or no associated pain. Although age as an independent risk factor is controversial, one study in young children found that repeat surgery, withdrawn or dependent behavior, and lack of preoperative preparation placed children at risk for perioperative anxiety.[7] Children with a history of temper tantrums or clingy, dependent behavior are more likely to manifest emergence distress behaviors.[8] Another large study that examined 1250 children

Essentials of Pediatric Anesthesiology, ed. Alan David Kaye, Charles James Fox and James H. Diaz. Published by Cambridge University Press. © Cambridge University Press 2015.

Table 27.1 Developmental considerations for the preparation of children for anesthesia and surgery

Young infants (0–9 months)	Older infants and toddlers (9–18 months)	Preschool and young children (18 months–6 years)	School age children (6–12 years)	Adolescents (over 12 years)
Considerations: Parent anxiety likely to be higher than infants' anxiety	*Considerations:* Stranger anxiety present	*Considerations:* Anxiety reactions prevalent	*Considerations:* Anxiety and fears better managed by child	*Considerations:* Better understanding of anesthesia and surgery experience
Rarely need premedication or parental presence during induction		Oral premedication and parental presence often necessary	Can be much variability among children's reactions	Fears may include that dignity, modesty, or sexuality will be violated, being injured or dying
Helpful strategies: Speak softly, wrap in blanket, avoid unnecessary delays	*Helpful strategies:* Playing simple games to gain trust, parental presence or premedication	Helpful strategies: Playing, providing simple explanations, distraction, give choices	*Helpful strategies:* Discuss fears honestly and give reassurances, increase role in decisions regarding anesthesia	*Helpful strategies:* Direct explanations to the adolescent, do not exclude from discussions of their care

from 3 to 12 years old found the following factors to be associated with high anxiety: younger age, previous behavioral problems in the health care setting, greater than five previous hospital admissions, longer duration of procedure, and anxious parents at induction.[9] Parental anxiety may adversely influence child anxiety, which is discussed in the section on parent presence during induction of anesthesia.

Identifying children who are at risk for preoperative anxiety and recognizing manifestations of such anxiety are the first steps to managing this problem effectively. Anesthesiologists must construct an effective strategy for addressing fears and reducing anxiety in every child they manage. Psychosocial preparation, avoidance of parental separation, and premedication are the three major interventions to combat preoperative anxiety in children.

Psychosocial preparation

Psychosocial preparation is the mainstay of managing preoperative anxiety in children, and it is utilized at least to some degree for every child facing surgery. The term refers to the need to address both the psychological development of the child and social interactions taking place between the patient and family members as well as caregivers. The anesthesiologist should present herself to the child in a way that is appropriate for the child's age and developmental level, with a special emphasis on assessing and addressing the child's fears. At the same time, it is important to be friendly and to gain the trust of the child, while observing closely the interaction of the child with his family members and/or guardians. Such observations are critical to understanding how the family can help to reduce the child's anxiety.

Psychosocial preparation begins prior to the day of surgery. Once surgery is scheduled, it is important that parents are truthful with children about the upcoming visit to the hospital or surgical center. The level of detail provided to the child and the timing of a discussion is often left to the parent, and will depend upon the child's developmental level and anticipated level of anxiety regarding the surgery. As a general guideline, younger children are informed with less detail and a shorter timeframe before surgery, while adolescents may be very involved with the planning of a surgery from the moment a surgeon schedules a procedure. There is no place for a "surprise" visit to the hospital rather than an anticipated visit to the zoo or favorite museum. Support should be provided by the surgical center staff, in the form of family-friendly brochures and/or videos to educate the child and family about the upcoming experience. Many pediatric surgical centers have a dedicated child-life staff that can provide tours of the facility, provide on-phone counseling, and answer questions from the child and family. With recent advances in computer technology, virtual tours and online information is often available to families.

Most anesthesiologists meet the patient and family on the day of surgery. The initial visit to the bedside is a critical period to assess a child's developmental level, identify and address fears, and observe interactions between the child and family members. The anesthesiologist should present herself in a child-friendly manner that gains trust and puts the patient and family at ease. Especially in young children, it is important that hospital attire is nonthreatening. To the extent allowed by the operating room dress code, anesthesiologists often wear brightly colored caps or jackets to camouflage their underlying scrubs. Medical equipment can include animal flashlights, clip-on figures for stethoscopes, and cartoon stickers for anesthesia masks. Distraction techniques are useful to make the hospital environment less threatening and to make a connection with the child. Good examples of such techniques include use of storytelling, magic tricks, juggling, and coloring books. Many institutions have programs in place to assist anesthesiologists with psychosocial preparation of patients for anesthesia and surgery. Interactive computer games, video games, clown doctors, low sensory stimulation, hypnosis, parental acupuncture, comprehensive behavioral programs, and cartoon/video clips have all been shown to benefit children.[10–19] Following careful psychosocial preparation, many patients will allow an IV insertion or mask induction of anesthesia without premedication or parent presence during induction of anesthesia.

Parent presence during induction of anesthesia (PPI)

Parent presence during induction of anesthesia (PPI) is another intervention for reducing child anxiety. One can think of PPI as an extension of psychosocial interventions into the operating room (OR) or induction room. A parent or guardian is placed in a clean hospital jumpsuit and cap, along with a mask when necessary, and then is allowed to stay with the child until inhalational induction of anesthesia is completed. The main goal of the intervention is to reduce separation anxiety in the child and improve cooperation during induction. Other advantages may include increased parent satisfaction and avoidance of premedication, while purported disadvantages include decreased O.R. efficiency, diminished sterility, distraction or disruption of the anesthesia team, adverse parent outcome, and medicolegal concerns. Before using PPI, anesthesiologists should be aware of parent/patient attitudes regarding PPI, be aware of any institutional policies regarding PPI, understand data concerning effectiveness of the intervention in reducing child anxiety and improving cooperation, and establish proper procedures for performing PPI.

Anesthesiologists' attitudes regarding the effectiveness of PPI vary, but parents and patients generally have positive attitudes regarding this intervention. In one study in children having a repeated surgery, more than 80% of parents chose PPI regardless of whether or not they experienced PPI during the prior surgery.[20] When given a choice, children are almost uniformly in favor of having a parent accompany them during induction (author's personal observation). There is great variation in the frequency with which anesthesiologists utilize PPI. In a 2004 survey of ASA anesthesiologists, approximately 50% of respondents never used PPI, while 10% allowed PPI in more than 75% of cases.[21] Among respondents, 26% reported a hospital policy that did not allow PPI and 23% reported that there was no policy in place. The variation in attitudes regarding PPI among parents and anesthesiologists can occasionally lead to dissatisfaction when a parent who desires PPI is matched with an anesthesiologist who does not utilize the intervention.

Since there are strong and variable opinions regarding PPI, it is important to have guidelines in place for a surgery center or hospital. The current guidelines at the author's institution include the following elements: 1. A parent, guardian, or family member may sometimes be allowed to accompany a child to the operating room for induction of anesthesia, 2. During the preoperative evaluation just prior to surgery, the anesthesiologist caring for the child will determine if this is appropriate, 3. If presence is permitted, only one individual may accompany the child to the operating room, and 4. Presence is not permitted, except under unusual circumstances, if the child is less than 1 year old, a rapid sequence induction is needed, or the child is medically unstable. Such guidelines clearly define the anesthesiologist as the final decision-maker regarding PPI, help to maintain patient safety, afford flexibility, and minimize the chance for miscommunication among care providers. Anesthesiologists should play a central role in establishing guidelines at their institutions.

Evidence for benefit of PPI on patient and parent outcomes is mixed. At least eight randomized, controlled trials have examined the effectiveness of PPI on outcomes such as child anxiety at induction, child cooperation at induction, parent anxiety, and parent satisfaction.[22–29] Such studies have generally not shown a benefit to PPI on these outcomes, except a study by Kain in 2000 showing reduced parent anxiety and increased satisfaction, but they all included randomization of patients to PPI or no PPI prior to an assessment of an anesthesiologist as to whether the child would benefit from PPI. Evidence and experience is convincing that an anxious parent is not beneficial to the child during induction, and may increase child anxiety.[16,30] Kain performed much of the aforementioned research on PPI, and he was able to re-examine his data on the basis of four possible pairings of patient and parent: calm parent and calm child, calm parent and anxious child, anxious parent and calm child, and anxious parent and anxious child.[30] He found that anxious children benefited from calm parents, but overly anxious parents increased children's anxiety during induction of anesthesia. The author's experience with thousands of patients suggests that the pairing of a calm parent or guardian with an anxious child often decreases anxiety and improves cooperation, while an anxious parent is less likely to benefit a child and may add to the child's anxiety. Calm children generally do well with an inhalational induction, with or without the presence of a parent.

If an anesthesiologist does choose PPI, she must perform the intervention appropriately, and avoid common pitfalls. Most important, a parent must be properly prepared for PPI. The parent should be forewarned that the child may object to placement of the anesthesia mask, make involuntary movements, and develop noisy breathing and jerky eye movements. The parent should be coached about providing supportive and positive comments during the induction, while avoiding scolding of the child at any point. Proper attire must be given to the parent, along with instructions about avoiding sterile trays and instruments. A nurse or assistant must be available to take the parent back to the waiting room once the induction is completed. Parents often find the experience quite emotional and they may develop increased heart rate during PPI,[27] so they may wish to speak with the escort for a few moments before being left in the waiting room. Because the experience can be very stressful for a parent, pregnant mothers and overly anxious parents should not be offered PPI. Anesthesiologists should be aware that families often compare experiences, so they must be prepared to explain why PPI was offered to one family and not another. Finally, it is of paramount importance that the anesthesiologist, and no other care provider, makes the final decision regarding the offering of PPI to a family. When done right, PPI can be a tremendously powerful and satisfying experience for child, parent, and the anesthesia providers.

Preoperative sedation

Despite the best efforts of the perioperative care team to reduce anxiety, it is sometimes necessary to administer preoperative sedation to achieve adequate anxiolysis. This should not be viewed as a failure, but rather a reflection of the reality that some children will be anxious no matter how much effort is provided by the anesthesiologist, other staff, and family to address fears and provide reassurance. Numerous studies have shown that premedication facilitates separation of children from parents and improves cooperation during induction of anesthesia.[31,32] Patients most often requiring sedation include children who are: preschoolers, school aged, having repeat surgery, chronically ill, developmentally delayed, behaviorally impaired, or unusually attached to the primary caregiver. Parents are often able to accurately predict a child's level of distress in response to medical interventions, so it is useful to ask them whether they feel their child would benefit from premedication. In some institutions sedation is routinely administered to a population of patients (e.g., all patients 1 to 10 years old); however, this is not cost effective and it may result in unnecessary pharmacologic adverse effects. In addition, at least one study found an increased incidence of adverse postoperative behavioral changes in children receiving preoperative oral midazolam versus placebo.[33] The decision to premedicate a child should be based upon the unique qualities and needs of that child.

With the increases in ambulatory and same-day admission cases, children often come to the preoperative holding area without prior consultation with an anesthesiologist and without intravenous (IV) access. This provides special challenges regarding the administration of preoperative sedation. Children should not receive sedation at home for many reasons,

Table 27.2 Advantages and disadvantages associated with different routes of premedicant delivery

	IV	Oral	IM	Rectal	Nasal
Advantages	Fast onset, reliable, allows for titration	Least painful and threatening, reliable sedation	Useful for uncooperative patients	Can be useful for children under 3 years	Reliable absorption, easy to administer
Disadvantages	Catheter insertion is painful, invasive, time-consuming, induces anxiety	Bitter tasting, child may refuse or spit out	Painful, induces anxiety	Erratic absorption, discomfort on administration	Bitter tasting, cooperation from child necessary

including the lack of appropriate monitoring, absence of skilled personnel to deal with an adverse response, and variability in the response of children to sedative agents. Insertion of an intravenous catheter in the preoperative holding area is painful, induces anxiety, and can be time consuming. Therefore, anesthesiologists will often be confronted with unpremedicated children during the immediate preoperative period, and must be familiar with administration of premedicants via nonintravenous routes.

There are multiple routes of nonintravenous delivery, each with advantages and disadvantages (see Table 27.2). Intramuscular (IM) injection was once a popular method for delivery of sedation; however, it is painful and induces anxiety. This route is still sometimes used for sedation of infants or combative older patients (e.g., a developmentally delayed teenager). Transmucosal routes of delivery include rectal, buccal, and nasal approaches. Rectal administration of medications is best tolerated by children less than 3 years old. It is not commonly used because of erratic absorption, discomfort on administration, and occasional parental anxiety. Buccal delivery requires cooperation from the patient, and the medication may be swallowed before transmucosal delivery has occurred. The nasal route provides reliable absorption and less discomfort than intramuscular injections, however many children feel threatened and will not cooperate during application of nose drops. Oral administration of premedicants is the least painful and threatening of all choices, and reliable sedation can be achieved by this route. One limitation of this approach is that commonly used oral premedicants (midazolam and ketamine) are bitter, which induces some children to either refuse to drink the premedicant or spit it out.

The ideal premedicant has the following properties: 1. minimal discomfort on administration, 2. rapid onset of action, 3. no prolongation of emergence and postoperative recovery, 4. reliable anxiolysis to achieve smooth induction, 5. no respiratory depression, cardiac depression, or other adverse effects, and 6. ease of administration. Midazolam, ketamine, opioids, and alpha-2-adrenoreceptor agonists can be administered by the nonintravenous routes and fulfill many of the above criteria. Anesthesiologists should also consider the costs associated with giving a premedicant. Costs of premedicants will vary between institutions, so it is important for anesthesiologists to become familiar with costs within their institutions.

Midazolam is the most commonly administered premedicant, and it is considered the gold standard in children. It is a short-acting, water soluble benzodiazepine with anxiolytic, anterograde amnestic, and hypnotic properties, with minimal or no pain on intravenous injection due to its water solubility and no prolongation of recovery times following use for premedication.[34,35] When intravenous access is unavailable, it is usually administered either orally or nasally. The oral dose is 0.5 mg/kg, with onset of action within 10 minutes, anxiolysis within 20 minutes, and peak serum levels at about 50 minutes.[36] A large dose is necessary because bioavailability following oral administration is about 36%, reflecting extensive first-pass hepatic and intestinal metabolism. In clinical practice, optimal levels of sedation are achieved between 20 and 30 minutes after administration. It is formulated as a cherry-flavored syrup in a concentration of 2 mg/ml, and is supplied as a multiuse bottle. In healthy children, significant cardiac and respiratory depression do not occur, but a parent or nurse must remain with the child since unsteadiness and head instability is common.[37]

If the child refuses to drink the oral preparation, then the nasal route of delivery is often selected, especially in young children. A dose of 0.2 to

0.3 mg/kg delivered via an atomizer provides effective anxiolysis within 10 minutes of administration, which coincides with the time at which peak plasma concentrations are achieved.[38] Bioavailability is about double that found for orally administered midazolam, which accounts for the smaller doses. Nasally administered midazolam is very bitter and irritating, which often produces a brief period of crying in the child. Theoretical concerns of neurotoxicity, due to direct tracking of the midazolam along olfactory nerves, have been expressed by some clinicians, however there have been no reports of such a complication. Midazolam used in this way has a safety profile that is similar to oral midazolam. Other routes of administration include intravenous, intramuscular, rectal, and jet injection. The latter three are rarely used since the oral and nasal routes are so effective. The intravenous route of administration is optimal if it is available to the anesthesiologist. Small doses (e.g., 0.05 mg/kg) are injected painlessly and titrated to the desired effect, while the patient is clinically monitored.

Ketamine is a phencyclidine derivative with amnestic, hypnotic, and analgesic properties. An oral dose of 6 mg/kg reliably produces sedation within 20 to 25 minutes and is not associated with significant cardiorespiratory depression or dysphoria.[39] It is especially useful in children who must undergo a painful procedure, such as insertion of an intravenous catheter, prior to induction of anesthesia. Disadvantages include a bitter taste and a high incidence of minor adverse effects including nystagmus, random limb movements, and tongue fasciculations.[39] Intramuscular ketamine is useful in combative patients who will not cooperate with administration of sedation by any other route. A dose of 2–4 mg/kg produces sedation within a few minutes, although it may prolong recovery from anesthesia in some children.[40] Patients should be closely monitored after administration of ketamine.

Compared to midazolam, opioids are much less commonly used to achieve preoperative sedation. Nasally administered sufentanil in a dose of 1.5 to 3.0 mcg/kg achieves sedation and smooth separation from parents within 10 minutes. However, adverse effects in some patients include oxygen desaturation, chest rigidity, and prolongation of emergence from anesthesia.[41] Oral transmucosal fentanyl citrate is delivered by allowing a child to lick a lozenge (oralet) attached to a plastic holder. Various dose lozenges are available to deliver a dose of 5–15 mcg/kg, which achieves sedation within 10 minutes and peak sedation within 30 minutes. Adverse effects include pruritus, nausea/vomiting, respiratory depression, and delayed emergence, which mandates that patients receive careful monitoring including pulse oximetry.[42] Although opioids may occasionally be indicated for sedation in patients, they are usually avoided because of these side effects. Many anesthesiologists limit use to careful titration of small doses via an intravenous line just prior to transport to the operating room.

Alpha-2-adrenergic agonists may also be used to provide preoperative sedation in children, while providing other benefits such as analgesia and reduced anesthesia requirements. Although oral clonidine 5 mcg/kg has been used successfully for premedication,[43,44] dexmedetomidine is gaining popularity for this purpose. Dexmedetomidine has approximately eight times the alpha-2 selectivity when compared to clonidine, and can be delivered for premedication by orogastric, nasal, buccal, and intramuscular routes. The bioavailability of dexmedetomidine by each of these routes is 16%, 65%, 82%, and 104%.[45] Dexmedetomidine premedication produces sedation, anxiolysis, analgesia, and decreases in heart rate and blood pressure, while maintaining ventilation and airway reflexes. It is odorless and tasteless, which confers an advantage over midazolam in children who are resistant to the latter's bitter taste. The most likely routes of administration are nasal and intramuscular, because the orogastric route is associated with low bioavailability and the buccal route requires cooperation of the child to avoid swallowing the medication. A nasal dose of 1 mcg/kg generally produces satisfactory sedation within 30 minutes and maximal sedation about 1 hour after administration, without significant respiratory or cardiac depression.[46,47] Intramuscular dexmedetomidine has been used to provide sedation in children having MRI or CT.[48] In a dosage range of 1–4 mcg/kg, time to adequate sedation was 13 minutes, no patients developed bradycardia or oxygen desaturation, and 14% of patients developed hypotension (defined as > 20% awake normal value) which did not require treatment. As clinical experience increases, anesthesiologists may increase their use of dexmedetomidine to provide preoperative sedation.

Conclusion

It is crucial that anesthesiologists appreciate that children and parents commonly experience anxiety during the preoperative period. The amount of anxiety experienced by children varies because of differences in age, developmental level, fears, prior experiences, and social situations. Negative consequences of anxiety and psychologic distress may include negative behaviors that can last well into the postoperative period, lack of cooperation during transport to the operating room and induction of anesthesia, and dissatisfaction. Interventions to decrease anxiety and improve cooperation include psychoprophylaxis, parent presence, and premedication. The end result of these efforts is a smooth, positive, and controlled preoperative experience that is rewarding for patients, families, and the care team.

References

1. ZN Kain, LC Mayes, TZ O'Connor, *et al.* Preoperative anxiety in children. Predictors and outcomes. *Arch Pediatr Adolesc Med* 1996; **150**(12): 1238–45.
2. KA Cullen, MJ Hall, A Golosinskiy. Ambulatory surgery in the USA, 2006. *Natl Health Stat Report* 2009; **28**(11): 1–25.
3. PA Tripi, TM Palermo. Psychosocial preparation of children for anesthesia and surgery. *Progr Anesthesiol* 1999; **12**: 195–204.
4. R Stargatt, AJ Davidson, GH Huang, *et al.* A cohort study of the incidence and risk factors for negative behavior changes in children after general anesthesia. *Paediatr Anaesth* 2006; **16**(8): 846–59.
5. LH Kotiniemi, PT Ryhanen, J Valanne, *et al.* Postoperative symptoms at home following day-case surgery in children: a multicentre survey of 551 children. *Anaesthesia* 1997; **52**(10): 970–6.
6. JE Eckenhoff. Relationship of anesthesia to postoperative personality changes in children. *Am J Dis Child* 1959; **86**: 587–91.
7. TR Vetter. The epidemiology and selective identification of children at risk for preoperative anxiety reactions. *Anesth Analg* 1993; **77**: 96–9.
8. PA Tripi, TM Palermo, S Thomas, *et al.* Assessment of risk factors for emergence distress and postoperative behavioural changes in children following general anaesthesia. *Paediatr Anaesth* 2004; **14**: 235–40.
9. AJ Davidson, PP Shrivastava, JK Huang, *et al.* Risk factors for anxiety at induction of anesthesia in children: a prospective cohort study. *Paediatr Anaesth* 2006; **16** (9): 919–27.
10. C Campbell, MT Hosey, S McHugh. Facilitating coping behavior in children prior to dental general anesthesia: a randomized controlled trial. *Paediatr Anaesth* 2005; **15**(10): 831–8.
11. A Patel, T Schieble, M Davidson, *et al.* Distraction with a hand-held video game reduces pediatric preoperative anxiety. *Paediatr Anaesth* 2006; **16**(10): 1019–27.
12. L Vagnoli, S Caprilli, A Robiglio, *et al.* Clown doctors as a treatment for preoperative anxiety in children: a randomized, prospective study. *Pediatrics* 2005; **116**(4): e563–7.
13. F Agostini, F Monti, E Neri, *et al.* Parental anxiety and stress before pediatric anesthesia: a pilot study on the effectiveness of preoperative clown intervention. *J Health Psychol* 2013 (epub ahead of print).
14. ZN Kain, SM Wang, LC Mayes, *et al.* Sensory stimuli and anxiety in children undergoing surgery: a randomized, controlled trial. *Anesth Analg* 2001; **92**(4): 897–903.
15. S Calipel, MM Lucas-Polomeni, E Wodey, *et al.* Premedication in children: hypnosis versus midazolam. *Paediatr Anaesth* 2005; **15**(4): 275–81.
16. S Wang, I Maranets, ME Weinberg, *et al.* Parental auricular acupuncture as an adjunct for parental presence during induction of anesthesia. *Anesthesiology* 2004; **100**: 1399–404.
17. ZN Kain, AA Caldwell-Andrews, LC Mayes, *et al.* Family-centered preparation for surgery improves perioperative outcomes in children: a randomized controlled trial. *Anesthesiology* 2007; **106**(1): 65–74.
18. J Lee, J Lee, H Lim, *et al.* Cartoon distraction alleviates anxiety in children during induction of anesthesia. *Anesthe Analg* 2012; **115**(5): 1168–73.
19. KA Mifflin, T Hackmann, JM Chorney. Streamed video clips to reduce anxiety in children during inhaled induction of anesthesia. *Anesth Analg* 2012; **115**(5): 1162–7.
20. ZN Kain, AA Caldwell-Andrews, LC Mayes, *et al.* Parental intervention choices for children undergoing repeated surgeries. *Anesth Analg* 2003; **96**: 970–5.
21. ZN Kain, AA Caldwell-Andrews, DM Krivutza, *et al.* Trends in the practice of parental presence during induction of anesthesia and the use of preoperative sedative premedication in the USA, 1995–2002: Results of a follow-up national survey. *Anesth Analg* 2004; **98**: 1252–9.
22. ZN Kain, LC Mayes, LA Caramico, *et al.* Parental presence during induction of anesthesia. A randomized controlled trial. *Anesthesiology* 1996; **84**: 1060–7.

23. ZN Kain, LC Mayes, S Wang, *et al.* Parental presence during induction of anesthesia vs. sedative premedication: Which intervention is more effective? *Anesthesiology* 1998; **89**: 1147–56.

24. JC Bevan, C Johnston, MJ Haig, *et al.* Preoperative parental anxiety predicts behavioral and emotional responses to induction of anesthesia in children. *Can J Anaesth* 1990; **37**: 177–82.

25. ZN Kain, LC Mayes, SM Wang, *et al.* Parental presence and a sedative premedicant for children undergoing surgery: A hierarchical study. *Anesthesiology* 2000; **92**: 939–46.

26. TM Palermo, PA Tripi, E Burgess. Parental presence during anesthesia induction for outpatient surgery of the infant. *Paediatr Anaesth* 2000; **10**: 487–91.

27. ZN Kain, AA Caldwell-Andrews, LC Mayes, *et al.* Parental presence during induction of anesthesia: physiological effects on parents. *Anesthesiology* 2003; **96**: 970–5.

28. ZN Kain, AA Caldwell-Andrews, LC Mayes, *et al.* Family-centered preparation for surgery improves perioperative outcomes in children: a randomized controlled trial. *Anesthesiology* 2007; **106**(1): 65–74.

29. YC Arai, N Kandatsu, S Kurokawa, *et al.* Parental presence during induction enhances the effect of oral midazolam on emergence behavior of children undergoing general anesthesia. *Acta Anaesthesiol Scand* 2007; **51**(7): 858–61.

30. ZN Kain, LC Mayes, AA Caldwell-Andrews, *et al.* Predicting which children benefit most from parental presence during induction of anesthesia. *Paediatr Anaesth* 2006; **16**: 627–34.

31. LH Feld, JB Negus, PF White. Oral midazolam preanesthetic medication in pediatric outpatients. *Anesthesiology* 1990; **73**: 831–4.

32. RM Brustowicz, DA Nelson, EK Betts, *et al.* Efficacy of oral premedication for pediatric outpatient surgery. *Anesthesiology* 1984; **60**: 475.

33. T McGraw, A Kendrick. Oral midazolam premedication and postoperative behaviour in children. *Paediatr Anaesth* 1998; **8**: 117–21.

34. PJ Davis, FX McGowan, IT Cohen, *et al.* Preanesthetic medication with intranasal midazolam for brief pediatric surgical procedures. Effect on recovery and hospital discharge times. *Anesthesiology* 1995; **82**: 2–5.

35. KK Brosius, CF Bannister. Oral midazolam premedication in preadolescents and adolescents. *Anesth Analg* 2002; **94**(1): 31–6.

36. K Payne, FJ Mattheyse, D Liebenberg, *et al.* The pharmacokinetics of midazolam in pediatric patients. *Eur J Clin Pharmacol* 1989; **37**: 267.

37. CO McMillan, IA Spahr-Schopfer, N Sikich, *et al.* Premedication of children with oral midazolam. *Can J Anaesth* 1992; **39**: 545–50.

38. EJ Walbergh, RJ Wills, J Eckhert. Plasma concentrations of midazolam in children following intransal administration. *Anesthesiology* 1991; **74**: 233–5.

39. H Gutstein, KL Johnson, MB Heard, *et al.* Oral ketamine preanesthetic medication in children. *Anesthesiology* 1992; **76**: 28–35.

40. R Hanallah, RI Patel. Low-dose intramuscslar ketamine for anesthesia pre-induction in young children undergoing brief outpatient procedures. *Anesthesiology* 1989; **70**(4): 598–600.

41. HW Karl, AT Keifer, JL Rosenberger, *et al.* Comparison of the safety and efficacy of intransal midazolam or sufentanil for preinduction of anesthesia in pediatric patients. *Anesthesiology* 1992; **76**: 209–15.

42. PS Nelson, JB Streisand, SM Mulder, *et al.* Comparison of oral transmucosal fentanyl citrate and an oral solution of meperidine, diazepam, and atropine for premedication in children. *Anesthesiology* 1989; **70**: 616–21.

43. S Inomata, S Kihara, M Miyabe, *et al.* The hypnotic and analgesic effects of oral clonidine during sevoflurane anesthesia in children: a dose–response study. *Anesth Analg* 2002; **94**(6): 1479–83.

44. HT Bergendahl, PA Lonnqvist, S Eksborg, *et al.* Clonidine vs. midazolam as premedication in children undergoing adeno-tonsillectomy: a prospective, randomized, controlled clinical trial. *Acta Anaesthesiol Scand* 2004; **48**(10): 1292–300.

45. KP Mason, J Lerman. Dexmedetomidine in children: Current knowledge and future applications. *Anesth Analg* 2011; **113**(5): 1129–42.

46. VM Yuen, TW Hui, MG Irwin, *et al.* A randomised comparison of two intranasal dexmedetomidine doses for premedication in children. *Anaesthesia* 2012; **67**: 1210–16.

47. ZS Cimen, A Hanci, GU Sivrikaya, *et al.* Comparison of buccal and nasal dexmedetomidine premedication for pediatric patients. *Pediatr Anesth* 2013; **23**: 134–8.

48. KP Mason, NB Lubisch, F Robinson, *et al.* Intramuscular dexmedetomidine sedation for pediatric MRI and CT. *AJR Am J Roentgenol* 2011; **197**: 720–5.

Chapter 28

Regional anesthesia and analgesia

Sean H. Flack, Lizabeth D. Martin, and J. Grant McFadyen

Mechanism of action

The conduction of nerve impulses requires a flow of sodium ions into the nerve, in response to depolarization of the nerve membrane. During the passage of a nerve impulse, or action potential, the permeability of the membrane to sodium ions increases transiently, and sodium flows into the nerve. A local anesthetic (LA) drug acts by binding to voltage-gated sodium channels and altering the relative stability of their resting, open, and inactivated conformations. Sodium channels and other ion channels are present early in the fetal development of peripheral nerves (1).

Types of local anesthetics

All LAs have a lipophilic (unsaturated aromatic ring) moiety and a hydrophilic (hydrocarbon chain) moiety, connected by an ester or amide linkage. Esters include procaine, chloroprocaine, cocaine, tetracaine and benzocaine. Amides include lidocaine, etidocaine, prilocaine, mepivacaine, bupivacaine, levobupivacaine, ropivacaine and dibucaine. Bupivacaine, levobupivacaine and ropivacaine are long-acting LAs.

Pharmacokinetics

Absorption

Regional blocks, either neuraxial or peripheral, require the injection of a large volume of a concentrated solution of LA into a confined anatomical space, which retains the solution for a prolonged period of time. Amide LAs are considered to have a bioavailabilty of 1 (2). Systemic uptake competes with entry into the effect site, and there is a parallel relationship between the central circulation and the effect site. When radiolabeled LA is injected outside nerves in animal models, less than 3% of the injected dose enters a nerve, and over 80% of an injected dose leaves the surrounding tissues within 30 minutes. This imposes structural requirements on drugs for local anesthesia: they must dissolve well and diffuse rapidly in both aqueous and lipid microenvironments. Factors that influence local blood flow and diffusion of drug into nerves can dramatically alter LA efficacy (3,4).

After injection into the epidural space, absorption of LA into the bloodstream follows a biphasic process. The buffering properties of the epidural space prevent a rapid rise in serum concentration. After epidural injection of bupivacaine, the time to reach maximum serum concentration (t_{max}) is similar in adults, children and infants, i.e., the bupivacaine concentration peaks about 30 minutes after injection. However, the ropivacaine t_{max} is much longer in infants and young children than in older children and adults (5). The t_{max} of ropivacaine varies from 115 minutes in children aged 1–2 years, to 62 minutes in 3–4-year-olds, to 30 minutes (the adult value) in children aged 5–8 years (6). Ropivacaine has intrinsic vasoconstrictive properties. This may contribute to this delayed t_{max}, in a manner similar to that caused by epinephrine added to bupivacaine (7).

Distribution

The volume of distribution of ropivacaine is smaller than that of bupivacaine in adults (8). A large volume of distribution is an important factor in lowering the peak concentration (C_{max}) of a drug. When the dose is similar, ropivacaine C_{max} is higher than bupivacaine C_{max} (9). The volume of distribution of ropivacaine is slightly smaller in younger children than in older children (6,10). Together with the lower clearance of LAs seen at a younger age, this may explain why higher ropivacaine C_{max} values are seen in younger children.

Essentials of Pediatric Anesthesiology, ed. Alan David Kaye, Charles James Fox and James H. Diaz. Published by Cambridge University Press. © Cambridge University Press 2015.

Table 28.1 Dosage guidelines for long-acting LAs

Local anesthetic	Single dose mg/kg	Continuous infusion rate mg/kg/h	Continuous infusion < 6 months mg/kg/h
Bupivacaine	2.5	0.4	0.2
Levobupivacaine	3	0.4	0.2
Ropivacaine	3	0.4	0.2

Metabolism

Esters are metabolized by plasma cholinesterases. Amides are metabolized in the liver by cytochrome P450 enzymes. These enzymes are not fully mature at birth (11), and mature during the first few years of life.

Elimination

Lidocaine has a relatively high hepatic extraction ratio (0.65–0.75), and is considered flow-limited for its elimination. Therefore, a drop in cardiac output may decrease hepatic clearance of lidocaine, resulting in toxicity (12). Monoethylglycinexylidide (MEGX), the major metabolite of lidocaine, impairs microsomal activity, leading to a decrease in intrinsic clearance. As a result, lidocaine infusion is not recommended in children.

Bupivacaine and ropivacaine have a relatively low hepatic extraction ratio (0.3–0.35) and are considered rate-limited for their elimination. Thus, protein binding is the major factor that may change total clearance. The main protein that binds LAs is α1-acid glycoprotein (AAG). This is an acute-phase protein, so its concentration rises rapidly during inflammatory processes, particularly during the postoperative period. Neonates and infants have a lower AAG concentration than adults, therefore their free fraction of LA is increased accordingly (13). Because the free fraction of LA is responsible for its toxicity, neonates and infants may be at greater risk of LA systemic toxicity (LAST).

For both bupivacaine and ropivacaine, clearance is low at birth and increases during the first year of life (10,14). Although ropivacaine clearance continues to increase from the age of 1 to 8 years (6), the difference is not clinically relevant because ropivacaine has a markedly lower toxic potential (15). Furthermore, while bupivacaine and levo-bupivacaine are equipotent (16), ropivacaine is only 60% as potent as bupivacaine (17). Thus, the use of ropivacaine is acceptable in neonates and young infants (5,18).

Toxicity of local anesthetics in children

Local anesthetic systemic toxicity (LAST)

The main mechanism of action of LAs is to block sodium channels, thereby interrupting the propagation of nerve impulses. However, this action is not limited to the sodium channels of nerves involved in pain transmission. The LAs will have an effect on any tissue containing sodium channels. If there is rapid absorption into the systemic circulation, or if LA is inadvertently injected into a blood vessel, significant blockade of sodium channels in other tissues may occur, and serious complications may ensue. The two most important organs associated with systemic toxicity of LA are the central nervous system and the heart. Toxicity may lead to seizures, tachyarrhythmias, and ultimately death from apnea and cardiovascular collapse (19).

It is an essential part of good practice of regional anesthesia to prevent LAST from occurring, especially if more than one block is being performed. Choice of LA and avoiding excessive doses of LA is very important, particularly in infants and neonates. Ropivacaine and levobupivacaine have been shown in animal studies to be less toxic than bupivacaine (20).

Dosage guidelines for long-acting local anesthetics (19,21):

Using LA with epinephrine delays systemic absorption of bupivacaine, and decreases peak plasma concentration (17).

Epinephrine can aid in detection of intravascular injection of LA. Signs include:

- 10 bpm increase in heart rate
- 25% change in T-wave amplitude
- > 15 mmHg increase in BP

Bear in mind that an epinephrine test dose is not 100% sensitive in detecting intravascular injection (22), and is less sensitive when total intravenous anesthesia (TIVA) rather than inhalational anesthesia is used to maintain anesthesia (23). Using real-time ultrasound to visualize spread of local anesthetic can aid in ruling out intravascular injection of LA. Whenever a large volume of LA is injected as a bolus, slow, incremental injection with frequent aspiration of the syringe, to check for blood return, should always be employed.

Babies and children who are given continuous infusions of LA via epidural or peripheral nerve catheters should be closely observed for symptoms and signs of LA toxicity such as:

- Ringing in ears
- Circumoral numbness
- Disorientation
- Double vision
- Seizures

A child who becomes restless, uncooperative, agitated or combative, or drowsy, obtunded or apneic may be exhibiting signs of LA toxicity!

If local anesthetic toxicity does occur, stop the infusion or injection of LA and start resuscitation:

- Airway
  - Endotracheal intubation
- Breathing
  - 100% oxygen
  - Maintain normocarbia
- Circulation
  - Establish good IV access
  - Strongly consider placement of an arterial line, for monitoring and drawing blood for arterial blood gasses (ABGs) and drug levels

Lipid emulsion (Itralipid®) has become a mainstay of treatment of severe LAST. There is ongoing debate concerning the optimal timing of administration. Evidence from animal research indicates that high-dose epinephrine may impair lipid resuscitation (24). Please refer to www.asra.com to obtain the most up-to-date practice advisory.

Local tissue toxicity

Use of LAs may cause muscle necrosis (25). It has been speculated that premature neonates may be a population at specific risk for this complication (19). Transient neurological symptoms have been reported after spinal lidocaine and bupivacaine, and after epidural administration in children (26). There are concerns that epinephrine added to epidural solutions could be responsible for permanent neurological injury due to decreased spinal cord blood supply (27). It has been suggested that epidural epinephrine be limited to the test dose, so as not to exceed 5 mcg/kg in 0.1 ml/kg (28).

Central neuraxial blockade: indications, contraindications, techniques, adjuvants and controversies

Introduction

Neuraxial blockade for anesthesia and analgesia in children has been described since the early 1900s, initially with the development of spinal anesthesia shortly after the discovery of local anesthetics. Caudal and epidural anesthesia in children came into use much later (29). Since that time, indications, techniques and medications for neuraxial blockade have evolved. Caudal anesthesia is now considered one of the most widespread techniques utilized in pediatric anesthesia (30).

Indications and benefits

All types of surgery on the lower part of the body can be covered by caudal block, which is most commonly employed for urologic, orthopedic and general pediatric surgical procedures. Caudals provide postoperative pain relief, and duration of the block depends on the local anesthetic type, volume and adjuvants that are utilized (31–33). Caudals are most often used in conjunction with general anesthesia, and typically decrease the concentration of inhaled anesthetic required to achieve surgical anesthesia. Some anesthesiologists use caudals as the primary anesthetic in a fully awake or lightly sedated patient. This technique may be particularly useful when avoiding exposure to general anesthesia or airway manipulation is desired. Examples may include neonates, patients with neuromuscular disease, or those with recent respiratory infections or pulmonary pathology. In addition to single injection caudal techniques, caudal epidural catheters may be placed for extended intraoperative and postoperative analgesia.

Continuous epidural analgesia is indicated for open thoracic surgery, major intra-abdominal or pelvic surgery, or bilateral lower extremity procedures. Beyond the humane provision of pain control and patient satisfaction, there may be additional reported benefits to epidural analgesia. Physiologic benefits, include decreased catecholamine release, improved ventilation and earlier return to gut function (34). Opioids are the most common alternative for managing perioperative pain, and avoiding well-known opioid related side effects including respiratory depression, sedation, hypotension, pruritus, nausea, vomiting and constipation is favorable. Epidural analgesia has been shown to decrease hospital and PICU length of stay (35). The benefit of reducing volatile anesthetic exposure with regional anesthesia is also an important consideration. The effect of volatile anesthetics on the developing brain remains controversial. Animal models suggest that dose-dependent toxicity may occur, particularly in the immature developing brain, although data in humans remain inconclusive (36).

Use of spinal block in pediatric patients remains limited, and is mainly utilized as an awake technique for ex-premature infants at risk for postoperative apnea (37). The duration of spinal anesthesia in children is < 60–75 minutes, which requires close coordination between anesthesia and surgery as well as short surgical times (38). That being said, spinal anesthesia provides a reliable, dense block and is useful for surgeries on the lower body in select patients.

Contraindications and risks

Contraindications to neuraxial blockade include patient refusal, infection at the insertion site, systemic infection, spina bifida, increased intracranial pressure, local anesthetic allergy and coagulopathy. In patients with degenerative neurologic conditions, spine abnormalities or spine hardware, and hypovolemia, the increased risk of complications should be carefully weighed against the benefits.

Neuraxial pediatric anesthesia is associated with risks, which have been described in several large multicenter trials. The UK pediatric epidural audit of 10 633 epidurals from multiple centers over 5 years, showed 1:2000 serious complication rate and 1:10 000 persistent complication rate. All five reported nerve injuries resolved (39). The French-Language Society of Pediatric Anesthesiologists described a seven times higher complication rate for neuraxial versus peripheral regional techniques in a 1-year prospective multicenter evaluation (40). There were no long-term sequelae.

More recently the multicenter Pediatric Regional Anesthesia Network (PRAN) reported on 14 917 regional blocks (41). No long-term sequelae were reported. There were no complications reported in 6210 single injection caudal blocks; 2,946 neuraxial catheters were placed, 3 (0.1%) reported paresthesias postoperatively, all of which resolved without sequelae. Dural puncture rate was 1% during epidural and caudal catheter placement. Despite the extremely low reported serious complication rates in all of these studies, case reports of permanent neurologic injury including paralysis exist in the literature (42). Careful risk/benefit analysis, meticulous technique and experience is recommended prior to placing high lumbar or thoracic epidurals, where damage to the spinal cord can lead to devastating complications.

The most common complications in children following spinal anesthesia include postdural puncture headache (4%), backache (5–10%), transient neurological symptoms (3–4%) (38). As in adults, risk of developing postdural puncture headache is decreased by using small-gauge, atraumatic spinal needles.

Anatomic considerations and techniques

There are several important anatomic considerations when performing neuraxial anesthesia in children. The spinal cord may end as low as L3 in infants, rather then L1 in adults. A conus medullaris (terminal end of the spinal cord) that extends below L3 may suggest a tethered spinal cord. The dural sac may extend as low as S4 in young infants, which should be carefully considered during needle placement for caudal blocks. The spinous processes in young children are more parallel and horizontal, thus facilitating a midline approach to the epidural space. The largest intervertebral space is usually at the level of T12–L1. The ossification of the sacrum in children is incomplete into the teenage years, making sacral intervertebral block possible. The CSF volume in infants is relatively high compared to adults and older children. Also CSF production is increased, which may explain why infants require more local anesthetic for a spinal block. The nerves in neonates and young infants are thinner and not fully myelinated until the second year of life, which allows a lower concentration of local anesthetic to be effective.

Most neuraxial techniques in children are performed under general anesthesia. In adults, concern has been raised about safety of performing regional procedures on unconscious patients who are incapable of reporting paresthesia (43). In children, however, most agree that risk of needle placement in uncooperative patients who may be cognitively incapable of reporting paresthesia outweighs the benefit.

Safety data from large multicenter studies are further supportive of this practice (39–41).

Caudal

After induction of general anesthesia, the patient is positioned in the left lateral decubitus position with the knees and hips flexed. If performing the technique in an awake neonate, the prone position is preferred. Landmarks are then identified. The sacral hiatus forms an equilateral triangle with the posterior superior iliac spines. The bony protuberance of the sacral cornu can often be identified on either side of the hiatus. Sterile technique should be employed. Sterile prep with chlorhexidine taking care to swab in a cranial to caudal direction is recommended. Needle insertion occurs at 60–70 degree angle at the proximal most cranial portion of the sacral hiatus until a characteristic "pop" or change in resistance is appreciated as the needle passes through the sacrococcygeal membrane. After puncture of the sacrococcygeal membrane, the needle should only be advanced several millimeters to avoid dural trespass. Commonly used needles include 25G butterfly, 22–25G caudal needle or 22–24G angiocatheter (44). For single-shot caudal blocks, 1 ml/kg of 0.2% ropivacaine or 0.25% bupivacaine is recommended dosing. The dose should be administered with intermittent aspiration and injection to monitor for possible intravascular, interosseous or intrathecal injection. Continuous ECG monitoring and blood pressure cycling should be employed during dosing. If epinephrine is added to the local anesthetic, this may provide an added safety benefit of test dosing for intravascular injection. Real-time ultrasound can be employed to confirm appropriate placement in the caudal space.

Epidural

Communication with the surgical team to identify the location of the surgical incision is essential for successful epidural placement. Appropriate dermatomal level selection allows for selective blockade of surgical area while avoiding undesired side effects such as motor blockade. We often use a 5 cm 20G Tuohy needle with a 24G epidural catheter in patients younger than 2 years. A 5 or 10 cm 18G Tuohy needle and a 20G epidural catheter are typically used in older children. Loss of resistance is the most common technique for identifying the epidural space. Techniques with air and saline have been described. If air is used, a small volume (< 1 ml total) is recommended to avoid introduction of venous air embolism. Typically, 1 mm of depth per kilogram of body weight is used to approximate the depth of the epidural space, although this can vary considerably from individual to individual. Ultrasonography can be used to identify the anatomy and measure approximate distance to the epidural space. Once the epidural space is located, 3–4 cm of catheter length is left in the space, predicting catheter tip placement within 2 segments higher or lower than the needle entry point. In small children, ultrasound can be used to visualize catheter position. Other methods including radiology and ECG guidance have been described to confirm catheter placement. For thoracic and high lumbar epidural placement, typically 0.6 ml/kg of 0.2% ropivacaine is used for initial bolus dosing. In teenagers, 0.5% ropivacaine may be used for low thoracic and lumbar epidurals to achieve surgical anesthesia. Hemodynamic change with epidural dosing in children is atypical, and should by promptly investigated. At our institution infusions are typically maintained with 0.2% ropivacaine; 0.1% ropivacaine is used in neonates and young infants. Clonidine is added in patients who weigh more than 10 kg. Maximum infusions rates are 0.4 mg/kg/h for patients over 6 months and 0.2 mg/kg/h for patients younger than 6 months (45). Additional training is recommended to safely perform pediatric epidural placement, particularly high lumbar or thoracic epidurals in infants and neonates.

Spinal

Spinal needles size 25–27 gauge are recommended. Spinal puncture is associated with minimal pain and can be performed in awake children; however, topical anesthetics are advised to minimize patient discomfort. Light sedation may also be utilized during the procedure. The patient is typically positioned sitting or lateral decubitus. The end of the spinal cord is more caudal in infant and young children, so a lower approach is preferred. Bupivacaine or ropivacaine 0.5 mg/kg are commonly used. Higher doses (up to 1 mg/kg) may be used in neonates or young infants < 5 kg (37,38).

Adjuvants

Adjuvants may be used to enhance the quality or duration of caudal or epidural block.

Epinephrine may be used as an additive to prolong the duration of a caudal block. It has additional benefit of serving as a test marker for intravascular or intraosseous injection, and is commonly used to test epidural catheters for intravascular placement.

Concern has been raised about neuraxial epinephrine and risk of spinal cord ischemia (18), and controversy exists about its role in neuraxial anesthesia. Epinephrine use should be reserved for test dosing with single-shot caudal or higher neuraxial catheters, and should be avoided as an additive in infusions.

Opioids prolong the duration and may improve the quality of the block (46); however, it has been demonstrated that epidural opioids are associated with significant side effects including respiratory depression, nausea, pruritus and urinary retention (47,48). It remains an area of debate as to whether or not benefits of caudal epidural opioids outweigh the risks (44,48). Some patients may not require opioid in addition to a good epidural block with local anesthetic. Minimizing opioid-related side effects postoperatively may be best achieved by starting with opioid-free epidural infusions and supplementing with intermittent intravenous or oral opioids if needed.

Clonidine has been shown to prolong the duration of epidural blocks with minimal side effects (49,50). The dose is typically 1–2 mcg/kg. Sedation, hypotension and bradycardia have been observed with higher doses. Young infants seem particularly sensitive and apnea may occur. Caution should be observed in the outpatient setting. Our current epidural practice is to dose with local anesthetic +/− clonidine in patients > 10 kg, and administer IV opioids as a rescue technique only as needed.

Safety data for neuraxial use of ketamine, midazolam and neostigmine remain insufficient to support their use as epidural adjuvants (44).

Controversies

Neuraxial anesthesia in children has come into widespread use in pediatric centers worldwide. Datasets from large multicenter studies have shown very low complication rates, and the safety profile of these techniques is favorable. There remain several important controversies, largely pertaining to rare but devastating complications.

Acute compartment syndrome occurs when there is increased pressure in a closed muscle compartment. Early recognition and treatment is essential to avoid ischemia, limb loss and even death. There is concern that use of regional anesthesia in children at risk for postoperative compartment syndrome may confuse the clinical presentation and delay diagnosis. If regional techniques are elected in high-risk patients, close monitoring and increased index of suspicion are key to a timely diagnosis. In this setting, pain must not be erroneously attributed to inadequate analgesia from failed block. Using less concentrated local anesthetics in high-risk patients (≤ 0.25%) and closely matching the block to cover the most appropriate surgical dermatomes are also recommended (43).

Paralysis after epidural placement is a rare but devastating complication. There is concern that use of epinephrine-containing local anesthetics, particularly near the lumbar and thoracic region could lead to vasospasm of the vasculature supplying the spinal cord and result in irreversible ischemia. It is difficult to draw conclusions from case reports of rare events; epinephrine has a long track record of being used for test dosing in epidural and caudal techniques, and may add safety benefit by alerting the proceduralist of intravascular placement if the test dose is positive. Recent recommendations suggest limiting epinephrine to test dosing, and avoiding its use as an additive in continuous infusions (46).

Peripheral nerve blockade: indications, contraindications and techniques

Indications

Peripheral nerve blocks are underutilized in children, perhaps related to longstanding safety concerns about performing nerve blocks in anesthetized patients. However, large multicenter databases have demonstrated that this is indeed safe and that both success and complication rates should not differ from published adult data (41). Keys to successful nerve blocks in children include intimate knowledge of relevant anatomy, use of appropriately sized equipment, ultrasound guidance whenever visualization of nerves and/or anatomic landmarks is possible and effective procedural sedation/anesthesia. Indications for peripheral nerve blocks include surgical and other painful procedures on the head and neck, trunk, and upper and lower extremities. Potential procedural settings include operating or procedural rooms, emergency departments, intensive care units and outpatient clinics (51).

Contraindications

Absolute contraindications to peripheral nerve blockade include parental or patient refusal, local infection and allergy to local anesthetics. Relative contraindications include pre-existing neurologic deficits and coagulation disorders.

Table 28.2 Supraorbital and supratrochlear nerve blocks

Indications	Frontal craniotomy VP shunt Ommaya shunt placement Dermoid cyst excision
Complications	Intravascular injection Hematoma Orbital injury
Equipment	1–2 ml 0.5% ropivacaine 27–30 gauge needle attached to syringe via T-piece connector
Patient position	Supine, head neutral
Technique	In midline, palpate supraorbital foramen in roof of orbital rim Advance needle to bone, then withdraw 1 mm and inject Apply pressure and massage site

Techniques

For successful block placement, attention to ergonomics is important, particularly when ultrasound guidance is used. If required, the ultrasound (US) machine should be positioned such that visualization of the screen, probe, needle and operator's hands are achieved without the operator needing to turn his/her head. A high-frequency linear probe is ideal for most nerve blocks in children. Sterility is ensured by application of a sterile transparent dressing or sleeve cover over the probe. Air trapping between probe and cover must be avoided to preserve image quality. For transparent dressings, this is achieved by stretching the dressing over the probe. Gel is placed inside sleeve covers to achieve the same result. Gel-free sleeve covers are also commercially available. Needle selection is determined by the observed depth of the nerve on US as well as the need for simultaneous stimulation. Alcohol-based chlorhexidine is the antiseptic of choice for skin preparation and individual sterile packs of gel should be preferred over multiuse bottles.

Head and neck blocks

These blocks are simple to perform and involve terminal sensory branches; consequently the risk for nerve injury is small. Small volume of local anesthetic and fine needles are used, usually without ultrasound guidance (52).

Table 28.3 Infraorbital nerve block

Indications	Cleft lip surgery Endoscopic sinus surgery Rhinoplasty
Complications	Intravascular injection Hematoma Orbital injury Damage to numb lip if child inadvertently bites lip
Equipment	1–2 ml 0.5% ropivacaine 27–30 gauge needle attached to syringe via T-piece connector
Patient position	Supine, head neutral
Technique	*Extraoral approach*: In midline, palpate supraorbital foramen in floor of orbital rim Advance needle to bone, then withdraw 1 mm and inject Apply pressure and massage site *Intraoral approach*: In midline, palpate supraorbital foramen in floor of orbital rim Place finger over foramen to prevent needle injury to globe Evert upper lip Insert needle at level of first premolar and advance toward foramen

Supraorbital and supratrochlear nerve blocks

These two nerves are terminal branches of the ophthalmic division of the trigeminal nerve and innervate the scalp, forehead and upper eyelid (Table 28.2).

Infraorbital nerve block

The maxillary branch of the trigeminal nerve becomes the infraorbital nerve once it exits the infraorbital fossa. It then divides into sensory branches to the lower eyelid and upper lip, teeth and gums, nasal mucosa as well as palate and roof of the mouth. Care must be taken to avoid injury to the globe by inadvertent puncture (Table 28.3).

Superficial cervical plexus block

Formed by the ventral rami of C1–C4, these nerves wrap around the posterior border of the sternocleidomastoid muscle to form four branches:

Table 28.4 Superficial cervical plexus block

Indications	Tympanomastoidectomy Otoplasty Cochlear implant Thyroid surgery (bilateral block)
Complications	Intravascular injection Hematoma Horner's syndrome (due inadvertent deep cervical plexus block) Phrenic nerve paralysis (due to excessive volume administration)
Equipment	0.1–0.2 ml/kg 0.5% ropivacaine 27 gauge needle attached to syringe via T-piece connector Linear high-frequency ultrasound probe
Patient position	Supine, head turned to contralateral side
Technique	At the level of cricoid cartilage, identify posterior border of sternocleidomastoid muscle (SCM) Insert needle along border of muscle and inject If US guided, transverse probe placement, then IP or OOP needle insertion to place needle tip alongside posterior border of SCM

lesser occipital, great auricular, transverse cervical and supraclavicular nerves (Table 28.4).

Greater occipital nerve block

Derived from the posterior ramus of C2, this nerve lies lateral to the occiput and medial to the occipital artery and its blockade is useful for posterior craniotomies and occipital neuralgia (Table 28.5).

Truncal blocks

These blocks are useful for abdominal or chest procedures that do not require neuraxial analgesia. Procedures in older children that would warrant caudal analgesia in infants are also suitable. Small 27 gauge hypodermic needles attached to a syringe

Table 28.5 Greater occipital nerve block

Indications	Posterior craniotomy VP shunt Occipital neuralgia
Complications	Intravascular injection Hematoma
Equipment	2–3 ml 0.5% ropivacaine 27 gauge needle attached to syringe via T-piece connector Linear high-frequency ultrasound probe
Patient position	Prone or supine with head turned to contralateral side
Technique	Palpate artery below and lateral to occipital protuberance, insert needle immediately medial to palpation and inject. If US guided, transverse probe placement. Identify pulsatile artery, then IP or OOP needle insertion to position needle tip alongside artery

Table 28.6 Pectoralis block

Indications	Gynecomastia procedures Breast lump excisions
Complications	Intravascular injection Hematoma
Equipment	0.2–0.4 ml/kg 0.5% ropivacaine 27 gauge needle attached to syringe via T-piece connector Linear high-frequency ultrasound probe
Patient position	Supine
Technique	Transverse probe placement parallel to clavicle Identify artery and adjacent nerve in fascial layer between pectoralis major and pectoralis minor at the level of the 3rd rib. Use Doppler if necessary Use an IP medial-to-lateral needle trajectory to place needle tip next to artery Aspirate to exclude intravascular placement Observe for fascial plane hydrodissection upon injection

Table 28.7 Rectus sheath block

Indications	Umbilical hernia repair Epigastric hernia repair Mini-laparotomy via midline, vertical incision Laparoscopic procedures
Complications	Bowel injury
Equipment	0.2 ml/kg 0.5% ropivacaine bilaterally (0.4 ml/kg total) 27 gauge needle attached to syringe via T-piece connector Linear high-frequency ultrasound probe
Patient position	Supine
Technique	Transverse probe placement immediately above umbilicus Identify hypoechoic muscle surrounded by hyperechoic fascia Identify hyperechoic peritoneum immediately deep to posterior fascia Standing on patient's right, needle is advanced IP and lateral-to-medial for the right side The probe is then moved to the left side and an IP medial-to lateral-approach utilized for blocking the left rectus sheath Needle tip should abut but not pierce the posterior sheath With correct needle placement, clear separation of muscle from posterior sheath will be seen

Table 28.8 Ilioinguinal block

Indications	Inguinal hernia repair Hydrocele repair Orchiopexy Orchiectomy
Complications	Bowel injury
Equipment	0.1–0.2 ml/kg 0.5% ropivacaine 27 gauge needle attached to syringe via T-piece connector Linear high-frequency ultrasound probe
Patient position	Supine
Technique	Stand on contralateral side to block Position US probe such that its lateral edge rests just above ASIS and the medial edge is directed toward the umbilicus The operator's hypothenar eminence rests on the patient's iliac crest while holding the US probe between thumb and index finger Hypoechoic nerves are visualized in fascial layer between internal oblique and transversus abdominis Small vessels are often present and may look like nerves. Use Doppler to differentiate nerves from vessels Insert the needle using an IP medial-to-lateral approach Observe for fascial plane hydrodissection upon injection If advanced too far, the needle will impact iliac crest rather than perforating peritoneum and risking bowel injury

via a T-piece connector are ideal for accurate needle tip placement within the narrow fascial planes containing the respective nerves.

Pectoralis block

This interfascial block is an alternative to a paravertebral block or thoracic epidural for analgesia following anterior chest wall procedures (53). The lateral pectoral nerve arises from the lateral cord of the brachial plexus and innervates the pectoralis major muscle and overlying skin. It is visualized within the layer between pectoralis major and minor muscles next to the pectoral branch of the thoracoacromial artery. An additional injection in the fascial layer between pectoralis minor and serratus anterior extends analgesia into the axilla.

Rectus sheath block

This block anesthetizes the ventral rami of the intercostal nerves as they traverse the potential space between rectus muscle and posterior rectus sheath to innervate the anterior abdominal wall.

Some innervation of the muscle may also be blocked resulting in relaxation of the rectus sheath (54). It is most popular for umbilical hernia repair but may also be useful for anesthetizing midline ports placed for laparoscopic surgery (Table 28.7).

Table 28.9 Transversus abdominis plane block

Indications	Open appendectomy Ostomy closure Pfannenstiel incision (bilateral block necessary) Lateral laparoscopic ports
Complications	Bowel injury Renal injury
Equipment	0.2 ml/kg 0.5% ropivacaine 27 gauge needle attached to syringe via T-piece connector In larger patients a longer needle may be needed such as a 10 cm short-bevel needle Linear high-frequency ultrasound probe
Patient position	Supine
Technique	Stand on contralateral side to block Place US probe transversely between the costal margin and iliac crest in the midaxillary line Identify abdominal muscle layers (external oblique, internal oblique, transversus abdominis) Internal oblique is usually the most prominent layer and the transversus abdominis is the thinnest and deepest muscle Needle is inserted IP using an anterior-to-posterior approach Place needle tip deep to the fascial layer separating internal oblique and transversus abdominis Observe for fascial plane hydrodissection upon injection

The rectus abdominis muscle is surrounded by a fibrous sheath formed from the aponeuroses of the external oblique, internal oblique and transversus abdominis muscles. A midline raphe, the linea alba divides the muscle in half necessitating bilateral injections for complete anesthesia. Three transverse fibrous bands are adherent anteriorly and divide the muscle into smaller compartments. As these bands only traverse the anterior half of the muscle, a potential space exists posteriorly within which local anesthetic may spread.

Table 28.10 Interscalene block

Indications	Shoulder surgery
Complications	Horner's syndrome Phrenic nerve palsy Nerve injury
Equipment	0.1–0.2 ml/kg 0.5% ropivacaine 22 gauge short-bevel needle Linear high-frequency ultrasound probe
Patient position	Supine, head turned to contralateral side Bolster between scapulae
Technique	Stand at patient's head Rest probe on upper border of clavicle; identify subclavian artery deep to lateral border of sternocleidomastoid muscle. Brachial plexus lies immediately superficial and lateral to artery Slide probe up neck until nerve roots are seen separately within interscalene groove (ISG), usually at the level of the cricoid cartilage Needle is inserted IP using a posterior-to-anterior approach until needle tip is positioned within ISG, then inject Continuous visualization of entire needle is essential to avoid inadvertent injury to plexus or surrounding structures

Ilioinguinal block

Ilioinguinal and iliohypogastric nerve blocks are useful for surgeries performed via an inguinal incision. These nerves are branches of the primary ventral ramus of L1 and also receive contributions from T12. Superomedial to the anterior superior iliac spine they lie between internal oblique and transversus abdominis muscles (Table 28.8).

Transversus abdominis plane block

This block is most suitable for abdominal surgery below the umbilicus. At the midaxillary line, the anterior rami of the T9–12 and first lumbar nerves are found in the intermuscular plane between internal oblique and transversus abdominis muscle, deep to the fascial layer separating the two muscles. Blockade of these nerves provides unilateral analgesia to the skin, muscle and parietal peritoneum of the anterior abdominal wall (Table 28.9).

Table 28.11 Supraclavicular block

Indications	Upper limb surgery below the shoulder
Complications	Intravascular injection Pneumothorax Nerve injury
Equipment	0.1–0.2 ml/kg 0.5% ropivacaine 22 gauge short-bevel needle Linear high-frequency ultrasound probe
Patient position	Supine, head turned to contralateral side Bolster between scapulae
Technique	Stand at patient's head Rest probe on upper border of clavicle in a midclavicular position Identify subclavian artery deep to lateral border of sternocleidomastoid muscle Brachial plexus lies immediately superficial and lateral to artery ("2 o'clock position") Needle is inserted IP using a posterior-to-anterior approach until the needle tip is positioned next to plexus

Table 28.13 Radial nerve block

Indications	Rescue block for incomplete brachial plexus block Trigger thumb release
Complications	Intravascular injection
Equipment	2–3 ml 0.5% ropivacaine 27 gauge needle attached to syringe via T-piece connector Linear high-frequency ultrasound probe
Patient position	Supine
Technique	Transverse probe placement in antecubital fossa Identify hypoechoic, oval nerve lateral to biceps tendon lying in the intermuscular groove between brachialis and brachioradialis muscles IP lateral-to-medial or OOP needle trajectory

Upper limb blocks

Arising in the neck from spinal nerve roots C5–T1, the brachial plexus may be blocked by a variety of approaches and the site of surgery dictates which is

Table 28.12 Axillary block

Indications	Elbow, forearm and hand surgeries
Complications	Intravascular injection Nerve injury
Equipment	0.1–0.2 ml/kg 0.5% ropivacaine 22 gauge short-bevel needle In neonates and infants, a short 27 gauge needle attached to syringe via T-piece connector is preferred Linear high-frequency ultrasound probe
Patient position	Supine 90 degree abduction and external rotation of the arm
Technique	Stand on lateral side of arm Transverse probe position Identify neurovascular structures Block individual nerves using an IP lateral-to-medial approach Start with deepest nerve first Redirection of needle will be necessary An OOP approach may be substituted, particularly in neonates and infants Circumferential spread of LA around the artery will ensure success The musculocutaneous nerve should be identified (and separately blocked) lateral to the axillary bundle either within coracobrachialis or in the hyperechoic plane between biceps and coracobrachialis muscles

most appropriate. As an alternative to brachial plexus blocks, individual forearm nerve blocks may be performed for distal procedures.

Interscalene block

This is not commonly used in children and its performance in sedated or anesthetized patients has been discouraged by some. Nevertheless, it may be appropriate in older teenagers or young adults having shoulder surgery. The anterior and middle scalene muscles form the interscalene groove within which the C5–C7 roots are usually visualized, though some anatomic variability exists between individuals including intramuscular positioning of nerve roots (Table 28.10).

Table 28.14 Ulnar nerve block

Indications	Rescue block for incomplete brachial plexus block
Complications	Intravascular injection
Equipment	2–3 ml/ 0.5% ropivacaine 27 gauge needle attached to syringe via T-piece connector Linear high-frequency ultrasound probe
Patient position	Supine
Technique	Transverse probe placement at wrist Identify ulnar artery with nerve lying immediately medial Trace nerve proximally until no longer adjacent to artery thereby minimizing risk for intra-arterial injection IP or OOP needle trajectory may be used

Table 28.15 Median nerve block

Indications	Rescue block for incomplete brachial plexus block Carpal tunnel release Trigger thumb release
Complications	Rare
Equipment	2–3 ml 0.5% ropivacaine 27 gauge needle attached to syringe via T-piece connector Linear high-frequency ultrasound probe
Patient position	Supine
Technique	Transverse probe placement in antecubital fossa Identify hyperechoic nerve immediately medial to anechoic brachial artery Trace nerve to midforearm IP or OOP needle trajectory may be used

Table 28.16 Lumbar plexus block

Indications	Pelvic osteotomy Femoral osteotomy ORIF femoral fracture SCFE repair
Complications	Local anesthetic toxicity Puncture of vital organs Retroperitoneal hematoma Total spinal Epidural spread
Equipment	0.4 ml/kg 0.5% ropivacaine 22 guage short-bevel, stimulating needle (5 or 10 cm length)
Patient position	Lateral decubitus with hips and knees flexed 90 degrees as for epidural placement Operative side up
Technique	The iliac crests are palpated and the intercristal line (ICL) delineated The posterior superior iliac spine (PSIS) is then palpated and a perpendicular line drawn to intersect the ICL (PSIS–ICL line) The length of this line is defined as PSIS–ICL distance The distance from midline, defined as the line drawn between the spinous processes of the L3–5 vertebrae to the PSIS–ICL line, is also noted The needle is inserted at the intersection of the ICL and PSIS line, perpendicular to the skin in all planes Quadriceps stimulation at ≤ 0.8 mA is sought at the depth of the PSIS–ICL distance If quadriceps stimulation is not achieved, the needle should be withdrawn and redirected medially Local anesthetic is injected after negative aspiration and test dose Immediate loss of twitch and lack of resistance confirm accurate placement For adolescents, if the distance from midline to the intersection is greater than 5 cm, the needle should be inserted at a more medial point, three quarters of the distance from midline to the PSIS line

Supraclavicular block

This is the most common US-guided approach to the brachial plexus due to its relative ease and ability to provide comprehensive analgesia for the entire arm. Consequently, this block has been called "the spinal of the arm." Within the supraclavicular fossa, the divisions of the brachial plexus lie close together and superolateral to the subclavian artery. Visualized with ultrasound, they are often described as resembling a bunch of grapes or a cut pomegranate (Table 28.11).

Table 28.17 Femoral nerve block

Indications	Femur fracture Knee arthroscopy Anterior cruciate ligament reconstruction Patellar ligament realignment Vastus lateralis muscle biopsy
Complications	Intravascular injection Nerve injury
Equipment	0.2 ml/kg 0.5% ropivacaine 22 gauge short-bevel needle Linear high-frequency ultrasound probe
Patient position	Supine
Technique	Stand on the side of the patient where the nerve is to be blocked Place US probe along femoral crease and identify pulsing femoral artery Insert block needle at a flat angle to the skin in an IP lateral-to-posteromedial direction Pierce fascia lata and fascia iliaca lateral to the nerve and advance needle until the tip is immediately lateral to the nerve Inject local anesthetic above and below the nerve, taking care to avoid intraneural injection

Table 28.18 Lateral femoral cutaneous nerve block

Indications	Skin grafting Vastus lateralis muscle biopsy Prevention of tourniquet pain Treatment of myalgia paresthetica Adjunct to femoral nerve block for knee surgery
Complications	Rare
Equipment	0.1–0.2 ml/kg 0.5% ropivacaine 22 gauge short-bevel needle Linear high-frequency ultrasound probe
Patient position	Supine
Technique	Stand on the side of the patient where the nerve is to be blocked Place US probe along femoral crease and identify pulsing femoral artery Trace hyperechoic fascia iliaca laterally toward the ipsilateral anterior superior iliac spine (ASIS) until the round hyperechoic nerve is identified IP lateral-to-medial or OOP approaches may be used If the nerve is not visualized, successful blockade may be achieved by local anesthetic deposition deep to fascia iliaca, immediately medial to ASIS

Axillary block

Within the axilla, the axillary artery is surrounded by a fascial sheath containing the median nerve anteriorly, the ulnar nerve anteromedially and the radial nerve posterolaterally. Anatomic variations are common, particularly multiple axillary veins. Generally, the best views are obtained in the apex of the axilla (55) (Table 28.12).

Radial nerve block

This nerve supplies sensation to the radial side of the dorsum of the hand and the proximal dorsum of the thumb and index finger (56). It also innervates the posterior compartments of the arm and forearm (Table 28.13).

Ulnar nerve block

This nerve supplies sensation to the little finger and ulnar side of the ring finger and innervates most intrinsic muscles of the hand (Table 28.14).

Median nerve block

This nerve is easily identified in the midforearm where it is located deep to flexor digitorum superficialis and on the surface of flexor digitorum profundus. It supplies sensation to the palm and palmar aspect of the medial three and a half digits as well as innervating the thenar muscles, lateral two lumbricals and most muscles in the anterior forearm compartment (Table 28.15).

Lower extremity blocks

Procedures amenable to lower extremity (LE) blocks are mostly orthopedic, but not exclusively so. Analgesia for LE procedures frequently requires blockade of at least two peripheral nerves. For example, foot surgeries of ten demand saphenous (or femoral) nerve blocks in addition to a sciatic block. A femoral nerve block may be sufficient for most knee procedures; however, obturator nerve block may be required for medial coverage of the knee, while lateral femoral cutaneous nerve blockade is advised when the lateral aspect of the knee is involved. Similarly, if surgery involves the posterior aspect of the knee, such as in the case of anterior cruciate ligament (ACL) repair with hamstring allograft, supplementary sciatic nerve block is advised.

Lumbar plexus block

Derived from the ventral rami of L1–4 (and sometimes including a branch from T12), the lumbar plexus travels within the dorsal 2/3 portion of the psoas muscle. Relevant nerves derived from this plexus include femoral, lateral femoral cutaneous and obturator nerves and its value lies in the ability to successfully block all these branches with a single injection. Although rewarding, this is a technically challenging block and its use should be preceded by thoughtful risk–benefit analysis. Complications are usually due to inserting the block needle too medial or too deep. Consequently, LPB is underutilized, particularly in growing children, in whom plexus depth varies with age and body habitus (57). Unlike in adult practice, the transverse process in children is not a reliable landmark to use when advancing one's needle as it does not fully develop until adolescence (58) (Table 28.16).

Femoral nerve block

The femoral nerve supplies sensation to the anterior and lower medial portion of the thigh, femur and knee. The saphenous nerve (terminal branch of the posterior division of the femoral nerve) supplies sensation to the medial aspect of the leg below the knee down to the foot. The position of the femoral nerve immediately lateral and slightly posterior (deep) to the artery is well known and easily remembered by use of the mnemonic NAVEL (from lateral to medial the structures are nerve, artery, vein, empty space and lymphatics) (59). At the level of the femoral crease, the nerve lies underneath two fascial layers – fascia lata and fascia iliaca – and above the hypoechoic psoas and iliacus muscles. The iliopectineal ligament separates nerve from femoral artery and vein.

Lateral femoral cutaneous nerve block

This purely sensory nerve innervates lateral buttocks below the greater trochanter and anterolateral aspect of the thigh. Beneath the inguinal ligament, it runs immediately medial to the anterior superior iliac spine, between fascia lata and fascia iliaca (60).

Saphenous nerve block

This sensory nerve innervates anteromedial and posteromedial aspects of the lower extremity from distal thigh to foot. It descends lateral to the femoral artery within the adductor canal. Distal to the canal, it separates from the artery to lie superficial at the medial aspect of the knee. A subsartorial ultrasound-guided approach in the distal thigh is preferred. In combination with a sciatic nerve block for foot and ankle surgeries, selective blockade of the saphenous nerve is preferable to femoral nerve block as quadriceps muscle weakness is avoided (61). If the nerve is not well seen, a femoral nerve block may be substituted (Table 28.19).

Sciatic nerve block

This mixed motor and sensory nerve is the largest and longest peripheral nerve in the body and innervates posterior thigh and most of the lower leg below the knee. It comprises two divisions, the tibial nerve and the common peroneal nerve, contained within a common perineural sheath. These divisions typically diverge at the apex of the popliteal fossa, though interindividual variability exists (62). The tibial nerve supplies innervation to the dorsal leg and plantar surface of the foot. The common peroneal nerve is responsible for motor and sensory innervation to the lateral leg and dorsum of the foot. This block is useful for surgery of the tibia, fibula, posterior knee, ankle and foot and is most easily performed via an ultrasound-guided lateral popliteal approach (63).

A subgluteal approach with the patient in Sim's position is a useful alternative if the patient is already positioned laterally for a lumbar plexus block or when analgesia of the posterior thigh is required (64). The nerve, typically hyperechoic and flattened in shape, lies midway between the greater trochanter and ischial tuberosity. Depending on the expected depth, a linear or curved probe may be used.

An anterior approach to the SN may be substituted when movement of the femur in an awake patient is problematic. Consequently, it utility in anesthetized children is limited. The SN is visualized medial and posterior to the femur. Initial scanning

Table 28.19 Saphenous nerve block

Indications	ORIF ankle Ankle osteotomy
Complications	Intravascular injection
Equipment	0.1–0.2 ml/kg 0.5% ropivacaine 22 gauge short-bevel needle Linear high-frequency ultrasound probe
Patient position	Supine Mild external rotation of leg and slight knee flexion
Technique	Transverse probe placement at midthigh level Identify the hypoechoic, pulsatile femoral artery beneath sartorius muscle A small indentation of the posterior aspect of the muscle is typically created by the nerve and artery Scanning toward the knee, separation of artery and nerve is observed Position the probe such that the needle may be advanced IP, in an anteroposterior direction between vastus medialis and sartorius muscles to reach the hyperechoic, round nerve

in the transverse plane followed by a longitudinal scan and IP technique is recommended (65). Concomitant nerve stimulation may be required due to the deep nature of the block, but the associated discomfort may negate the reason for selecting this approach (Table 28.20).

Table 28.20 Sciatic nerve block

Indications	Tib-fib osteotomy ORIF ankle Ankle/foot osteotomy Plantar release Achilles tendon lengthening
Complications	Intravascular injection Nerve injury
Equipment	0.2 ml/kg 0.5% ropivacaine 27 gauge needle attached to syringe via T-piece connector Linear high-frequency ultrasound probe
Patient position	Supine Leg elevated on a stand or bolster
Technique	Place the US probe transversely in the popliteal fossa Simultaneous flexion and extension of the foot while scanning causes the nerves to move in a characteristic "seesaw" manner that greatly facilitates identification If the foot is immobile, locate the tibial nerve superficial and close to the anechoic, pulsatile popliteal artery The common peroneal nerve is observed lateral to the tibial nerve The block may be performed above or below the bifurcation, depending upon where nerve visualization is best Insert the needle in the groove between vastus lateralis and biceps femoris muscles and advance parallel to the US probe until its tip is positioned alongside the nerve Needle tip repositioning may be required to ensure circumferential spread

References

1. Wada A. Roles of voltage-dependent sodium channels in neuronal development, pain, and neurodegeneration. *Journal of Pharmacological Sciences*. 2006; **102**(3): 253–68.
2. Burm AG, de Boer AG, van Kleef JW, *et al*. Pharmacokinetics of lidocaine and bupivacaine and stable isotope-labelled analogues: a study in healthy volunteers. *Biopharmaceutics & Drug Disposition*. 1988; **9**(1): 85–95.
3. Cairns BE, Gambarota G, Dunning PS, Mulkern RV, Berde CB. Activation of peripheral excitatory amino acid receptors decreases the duration of local anesthesia. *Anesthesiology*. 2003; **98**(2): 521–9.
4. Masuda T, Cairns BE, Sadhasivam S, Dunning PS, Berde CB. Epinephrine prevents muscle blood flow: increases after perineural injection of tetrodotoxin. *Anesthesiology*. 2004; **101**(6): 1428–34.
5. Mazoit JX, Dalens BJ. Pharmacokinetics of local anaesthetics in infants and children. *Clinical Pharmacokinetics*. 2004; **43**(1): 17–32.
6. Lonnqvist PA, Westrin P, Larsson BA, *et al*. Ropivacaine pharmacokinetics after caudal block in 1–8 year-old children. *British Journal of Anaesthesia*. 2000; **85**(4): 506–11.
7. Burm AG, Van Kleef JW, Vermeulen NP, *et al*. Pharmacokinetics of lidocaine

and bupivacaine following subarachnoid administration in surgical patients: simultaneous investigation of absorption and disposition kinetics using stable isotopes. *Anesthesiology*. 1988; **69**(4): 584–92.

8. Morrison LM, Emanuelsson BM, McClure JH, *et al.* Efficacy and kinetics of extradural ropivacaine: comparison with bupivacaine. *British Journal of Anaesthesia*. 1994; **72**(2): 164–9.

9. Luz G, Innerhofer P, Haussler B, *et al.* Comparison of ropivacaine 0.1% and 0.2% with bupivacaine 0.2% for single-shot caudal anaesthesia in children. *Paediatric Anaesthesia*. 2000; **10**(5): 499–504.

10. Hansen TG, Ilett KF, Reid C, *et al.* Caudal ropivacaine in infants: population pharmacokinetics and plasma concentrations. *Anesthesiology*. 2001; **94**(4): 579–84.

11. Larsson BA, Lonnqvist PA, Olsson GL. Plasma concentrations of bupivacaine in neonates after continuous epidural infusion. *Anesthesia and Analgesia*. 1997; **84**(3): 501–5.

12. Tucker GT. Pharmacokinetics of local anaesthetics. *British Journal of Anaesthesia*. 1986; **58**(7): 717–31.

13. Lerman J, Strong HA, LeDez KM, *et al.* Effects of age on the serum concentration of alpha 1-acid glycoprotein and the binding of lidocaine in pediatric patients. *Clinical Pharmacology and Therapeutics*. 1989; **46**(2): 219–25.

14. Meunier JF, Goujard E, Dubousset AM, Samii K, Mazoit JX. Pharmacokinetics of bupivacaine after continuous epidural infusion in infants with and without biliary atresia. *Anesthesiology*. 2001; **95**(1): 87–95.

15. Santos AC, DeArmas PI. Systemic toxicity of levobupivacaine, bupivacaine, and ropivacaine during continuous intravenous infusion to nonpregnant and pregnant ewes. *Anesthesiology*. 2001; **95**(5): 1256–64.

16. Lyons G, Columb M, Wilson RC, Johnson RV. Epidural pain relief in labour: potencies of levobupivacaine and racemic bupivacaine. *British Journal of Anaesthesia*. 1998; **81**(6): 899–901.

17. Polley LS, Columb MO, Naughton NN, Wagner DS, van de Ven CJ. Relative analgesic potencies of ropivacaine and bupivacaine for epidural analgesia in labor: implications for therapeutic indexes. *Anesthesiology*. 1999; **90**(4): 944–50.

18. Kohane DS, Sankar WN, Shubina M, *et al.* Sciatic nerve blockade in infant, adolescent, and adult rats: a comparison of ropivacaine with bupivacaine. *Anesthesiology*. 1998; **89**(5): 1199–208; discussion 10A.

19. Lonnqvist PA. Toxicity of local anesthetic drugs: a pediatric perspective. *Paediatric Anaesthesia*. 2012; **22**(1): 39–43.

20. Guinet P, Estebe JP, Ratajczak-Enselme M, *et al.* Electrocardiographic and hemodynamic effects of intravenous infusion of bupivacaine, ropivacaine, levobupivacaine, and lidocaine in anesthetized ewes. *Regional Anesthesia and Pain Medicine*. 2009; **34**(1): 17–23.

21. Berde CB. Toxicity of local anesthetics in infants and children. *The Journal of Pediatrics*. 1993; **122**(5 Pt 2): S14–20.

22. Tobias JD. Caudal epidural block: a review of test dosing and recognition of systemic injection in children. *Anesthesia and Analgesia*. 2001; **93**(5): 1156–61.

23. Polaner DM, Zuk J, Luong K, Pan Z. Positive intravascular test dose criteria in children during total intravenous anesthesia with propofol and remifentanil are different than during inhaled anesthesia. *Anesthesia and Analgesia*. 2010; **110**(1): 41–5.

24. Hiller DB, Gregorio GD, Ripper R, *et al.* Epinephrine impairs lipid resuscitation from bupivacaine overdose: a threshold effect. *Anesthesiology*. 2009; **111**(3): 498–505.

25. Zink W, Graf BM. Local anesthetic myotoxicity. *Regional Anesthesia and Pain Medicine*. 2004; **29**(4): 333–40.

26. Bourlon-Figuet S, Dubousset AM, Benhamou D, Mazoit JX. Transient neurologic symptoms after epidural analgesia in a five-year-old child. *Anesthesia and Analgesia*. 2000; **91**(4): 856–7, table of contents.

27. Meyer MJ, Krane EJ, Goldschneider KR, Klein NJ. Case report: neurological complications associated with epidural analgesia in children – a report of 4 cases of ambiguous etiologies. *Anesthesia and Analgesia*. 2012; **115**(6): 1365–70.

28. Berde C, Greco C. Pediatric regional anesthesia: drawing inferences on safety from prospective registries and case reports. *Anesthesia and Analgesia*. 2012; **115**(6): 1259–62.

29. Brown TC. History of pediatric regional anesthesia. *Paediatric Anaesthesia*. 2012; **22**: 3–9.

30. Marhofer P, Ivani G, Suresh S, *et al.* Everyday regional anesthesia in children. *Paediatric Anaesthesia*. 2012; **22**: 995–1001.

31. Gunter JB, Dunn CM, Bennie JB, *et al.* Optimum concentration of bupivacaine for combined caudal–general anesthesia in children. *Anesthesiology*. 1991; **75**: 57–61.

32. Ansermino M, Basu R, Vandebeek C, Montgomery C. Nonopioid additives to local anaesthetics for caudal blockade in children: a systematic review. *Paediatric Anaesthesia*. 2003; **13**: 561–73.

33. Hong JY, Han SW, Kim WO, Cho JS, Kil HK. A comparison of high volume/low concentration and low volume/high concentration ropivacaine in caudal analgesia for pediatric orchiopexy. *Anesthesia and Analgesia*. 2009; **109**: 1073–8.

34. Bosenberg AT, Johr M, Wolf AR. Pro con debate: the use of regional vs. systemic analgesia for neonatal surgery. *Paediatric Anaesthesia.* 2011; **21**: 1247–58.

35. Moriarty A. Pediatric epidural analgesia (PEA). *Paediatric Anaesthesia.* 2012; **22**: 51–5.

36. Sun L. Early childhood general anaesthesia exposure and neurocognitive development. *British Journal of Anaesthesia.* 2010; **105**(Suppl 1): i61–8.

37. Puncuh F, Lampugnani E, Kokki H. Spinal anaesthesia in paediatric patients. *Current Opinion in Anaesthesiology.* 2005; **18**: 299–305.

38. Kokki H. Spinal blocks. *Paediatric Anaesthesia.* 2012; **22**: 56–64.

39. Llewellyn N, Moriarty A. The national pediatric epidural audit. *Paediatric Anaesthesia* 2007; **17**: 520–33.

40. Ecoffey C, Lacroix F, Giaufre E, *et al.* Epidemiology and morbidity of regional anesthesia in children: a follow-up, one-year prospective survey of the French Language Society of Paediatric Anaesthesiologists (ADARPEF). *Paediatric Anaesthesia.* 2010; **20**: 1061–9.

41. Polaner DM, Taenzer AH, Walker BJ, *et al.* Pediatric Regional Anesthesia Network (PRAN): A multi-institutional study of the use and incidence of complications of pediatric regional anesthesia. *Anesthesia and Analgesia.* 2012; **115**: 1353–64.

42. Meyer MJ, Krane EJ, Goldschneider KR, Klein NJ. Case report: neurological complications associated with epidural analgesia in children: a report of 4 cases of ambiguous etiologies. *Anesthesia and Analgesia.* 2012; **115**: 1365–70.

43. Mossetti V, Ivani G. Controversial issues in pediatric regional anesthesia. *Paediatric Anaesthesia.* 2012; **22**: 109–14.

44. Johr M, Berger TM. Caudal blocks. *Paediatric Anaesthesia.* 2012; **22**: 44–50.

45. Bosenberg AT, Thomas J, Cronje L, Lopez T, *et al.* Pharmacokinetics and efficacy of ropivacaine for continuous epidural infusion in neonates and infants. *Paediatric Anaesthesia.* 2005; **15**: 739–49.

46. Krane EJ, Tyler DC, Jacobson LE. The dose response of caudal morphine in children. *Anesthesiology.* 1989; **71**: 48–52.

47. Krane EJ. Delayed respiratory depression in a child after caudal epidural morphine. *Anesthesia and Analgesia.* 1988; **67**: 79–82.

48. Lonnqvist PA, Ivani G, Moriarty T. Use of caudal–epidural opioids in children: still state of the art or the beginning of the end? *Paediatric Anaesthesia.* 2002; **12**: 747–9.

49. Vetter TR, Carvallo D, Johnson JL, Mazurek MS, Presson RG, Jr. A comparison of single-dose caudal clonidine, morphine, or hydromorphone combined with ropivacaine in pediatric patients undergoing ureteral reimplantation. *Anesthesia and Analgesia.* 2007; **104**: 1356–63.

50. Singh R, Kumar N, Singh P. Randomized controlled trial comparing morphine or clonidine with bupivacaine for caudal analgesia in children undergoing upper abdominal surgery. *British Journal of Anaesthesia.* 2011; **106**: 96–100.

51. Suresh S, Frederickson M. Peripheral nerve blocks in children. In Hadzic A, ed. *Textbook of Regional Anesthesia and Pain Management.* New York: McGraw Hill, 2007: pp. 753–78.

52. Suresh S, Voronov P. Head and neck blocks in infants, children and adolescents. *Paediatric Anaesthesia.* 2012; **22**: 81–7.

53. Blanco R. The 'pecs block': A novel technique for providing analgesia after breast surgery. *Anaesthesia.* 2011; **66**: 847–8.

54. Karmakar MK, Kwok WH. Ultrasound-guided regional anesthesia. In Cote CJ, Lerman J, Todres ID, eds. *A Practice of Anesthesia for Infants and Children.* Philadelphia: Saunders, 2009: p.933.

55. Tsui BCH. Axillary block. In Tsui BCH, ed. *Atlas of Ultrasound and Nerve-stimulation-guided Regional Anesthesia.* New York: Springer, 2007: pp.99–107.

56. Polaner DM, Suresh S, Cote CJ. Regional anesthesia. In Cote CJ, Lerman J, Todres ID, eds. *A Practice of Anesthesia for Infants and Children.* Philadelphia: Saunders, 2009: p.899.

57. Rapp HJ, Grau T. Ultrasound-guided regional anesthesia in pediatric patients. *Techniques in Regional Anesthesia and Pain Management.* 2004; **8**: 179–98.

58. Walker BJ, Flack SH, Bosenberg AT. Predicting lumbar plexus depth in children and adolescents. *Anesthesia and Analgesia.* 2011; **112**: 661–5.

59. Katz J. *Atlas of Regional Anesthesia.* Norwalk: Appleton-Century-Crofts. 1985.

60. Ng I, Vaghadia H, Choi PT, *et al.* Ultrasound imaging accurately identifies the lateral femoral cutaneous nerve. *Anesthesia and Analgesia.* 2008; **107**: 1070–4.

61. Manickam B, Perlas A, Duggan E, *et al.* Feasibility and efficacy of ultrasound-guided block of the saphenous nerve in the adductor canal. *Regional Anesthesia and Pain Medicine.* 2009; **34**: 578–80.

62. Prasad A, Perlas A, Ramlogan R, *et al.* Ultrasound-guided popliteal block distal to sciatic nerve

bifurcation shortens onset time. *Regional Anesthesia and Pain Medicine*. 2010; **35**: 267–71.

63. Flack S, Anderson C. Ultrasound-guided lower extremity blocks. *Paediatric Anaesthesia*. 2012; **22**: 72–80.

64. Van Geffen GJ, Gielen M. Ultrasound-guided subgluteal sciatic nerve blocks with stimulating catheters in children: a descriptive study. *Anesthesia and Analgesia*. 2006; **103**: 328–33.

65. Tsui B, Ozelsel TJ. Ultrasound-guided anterior sciatic nerve block using a longitudinal approach: "expanding the view". *Regional Anesthesia and Pain Medicine*. 2008; **33**: 275–6.

Chapter 29

General anesthesia

Staci Cameron and Maria Matuszczak

Stages and signs of anesthesia

The stages of anesthesia were first described in 1847 by John Snow and Francis Plomley; however, in 1937 Arthur Guedel introduced the classification system which is widely known today consisting of stage I, II, III, and IV.[1] These stages describe the physiologic response to anesthesia and the signs the anesthesiologist can expect to observe during each stage in order to determine the anesthetic depth. They can be used to guide inhalational anesthesia. Historically, these stages were based on ether anesthesia. They do not apply when using neuromuscular blockers and intravenous anesthetics.

Stage I includes induction of anesthesia and loss of consciousness. Joseph Artusio divided stage I into three planes:

- plane I: no analgesia/amnesia
- plane II: partial analgesia and complete amnesia
- plane III: analgesia and amnesia

Stage II is the excitatory stage and starts with loss of consciousness until loss of eyelid reflex.

During stage II the patient may move or become combative requiring restrainment. Respirations become irregular and breathholding or even laryngospasm may occur. Coughing and vomiting have also been described. The pupils are dilated. The blood pressure and heart rate will increase. The degree of excitement may be blunted with premedication.

Stage III is deep anesthesia and encompasses the time when the patient's muscles are relaxed and ready for surgery. Onset of stage III is heralded by automatic respiration and return of blood pressure and heart rate toward normal. As the tongue and pharyngeal muscles relax, airway obstruction can ensue. Stage III has further been divided into four planes.

- Plane I: includes automatic respiration, loss of swallowing, and vomiting reflexes. Eyes may oscillate and pupils will become smaller while tearing decreases. The peripheral veins will dilate as cutaneous blood flow increases. This is an optimal time for intravenous cannulation in pediatrics.
- Plane II: the patient does not move with low-intensity stimulus such as skin incision. The tidal volumes begin to decline as intercostal muscles relax and respiratory rate increases. With CO_2 increase the pupils will dilate. Laryngeal and corneal reflexes disappear and eyes no longer move.
- Plane III: the patient is ready for surgery and does not move during strong surgical stimulus. Tidal volumes are further decreased and ventilatory assistance is indicated. The diaphragm will continue contracting such that asynchronous chest movements occur. The pupils become dilated with absent light reflexes.
- Plane IV: deep anesthetic plane in which the patient no longer initiates respirations.

Stage IV is anesthetic overdose causing apnea and shock resulting in death. The patient progressively becomes hypotensive and tachycardic until hemodynamic collapse occurs.

The BIS (bispectral index) monitor (Aspect Medical Systems, Newton, MA, USA) can be used to monitor the depth of anesthesia in older children and adolescents. On a scale from 0 to 100, values below 60 seem to decrease the risk of awareness.[2] The BIS monitor is based on an adult EEG algorithm, and its use in small children and infants is not yet validated. An age-specific algorithm is not available due to the rapid changes in the developing brain of the growing child and to the various EEG effects that different anesthetics cause in children.

Essentials of Pediatric Anesthesiology, ed. Alan David Kaye, Charles James Fox and James H. Diaz. Published by Cambridge University Press. © Cambridge University Press 2015.

Induction techniques

Selecting a technique for induction should be based upon the history and physical exam. Induction can be by inhalation, intravenous, intramuscular, or less commonly rectal. Regardless of the technique chosen, it is important to have the operating room warm and quiet for a more tranquil experience.

Inhalational induction with sevoflurane is the most common form and can be done with the child sitting or lying. In small infants it helps to allow a pacifier during induction. Older infants and toddlers can play with or hold a mask with scented oil or play with a favorite toy or blanket. Also, playing a movie or music, or telling a story can all be used as distractors during inhalational induction. Older children may enjoy blowing up the anesthesia balloon or playing a game on their phone or other gaming device. Many centers offer child life specialists who talk to the patient before going to the operating room and prepare them for general anesthesia. If parents are present during induction it is important to warn them of the side effects of general anesthesia beforehand. If the child does not like the face mask, they can breathe through the elbow of the circuit. If the child is sleeping prior to induction, simply apply the face mask gently, so as not to disturb it.

Seventy percent nitrous oxide can be used 1–2 minutes prior to titrating in sevoflurane. Nitrous oxide is odorless and thought to stun the patient so that the sevoflurane is better tolerated. Sevoflurane is dialed up quickly to 8%. Another quicker approach is to start with 8% sevoflurane.[3] Caution must be used in patients with cardiomyopathy and in neonates. Bradycardia can be treated by turning the sevoflurane down or off and/or giving intramuscular atropine 0.02 mg/kg.

In older children single-breath induction may be the better option. Start by explaining that they will blow out all of their breath, take the face mask and inhale as much as possible and hold their breath. When they can no longer hold their breath, they will blow out again as much as possible and inhale deeply again. Practice this once and then apply with a sevoflurane-primed circuit. Usually by the second breath, the patient will be asleep, but may need assisted ventilation at this point. Signs of stage II anesthesia may occur shortly thereafter.

Isoflurane and desflurane are not commonly used for mask induction due to their high pungency. Halothane has widely been replaced by sevoflurane but is still used in developing countries. The incidence of cardiac arrest due to volatile agents has significantly decreased since the introduction of sevoflurane due to its safe cardiovascular profile.[4,5] Sevoflurane also allows for tracheal intubation without the use of muscle relaxants.[6]

In patients with intravenous (IV) access, IV induction is the preferred method. Older children may allow an IV to be placed preoperatively with the aid of a topical anesthetic. Depending on the underlying pathology (example: congenital heart disease, malignant hyperthermia, acute abdomen, sepsis) IV access should be established before induction of anesthesia, independent of the child's age.

Agents which can be used for IV induction include propofol, ketamine, thiopental, methohexital, and etomidate.[7]

Propofol is most commonly used due to its quick onset and short half-life, as well as its antiemetic properties.[8] Techniques to prevent propofol burn on injection include: pretreatment with an opioid or lidocaine 0.5 mg/kg prior to or during injection (1–2 ml of lidocaine in Bier block fashion), choosing the most proximal IV site and a larger vein, gently scratching the skin near the injection site during injection so as to cause local nerve confusion, and diluting the propofol with normal saline or lactated Ringers and injecting slowly.[9] Induction doses vary depending on the age of the child, smaller children requiring sometimes a relatively high dose.[10]

Ketamine is an induction agent which maintains blood pressure and is recommended during states of hypovolemia and in those with cardiac disease requiring a normotensive state. Caution must be used in patients who are maximally compensated because it is a cardiodepressant and may cause cardiovascular collapse. Ketamine also has analgesic properties and inhibits bronchoconstriction. An antisialogogue and a benzodiazepine can be given to offset the oral secretions and psychomimetic effects of ketamine, respectively. An induction dose of 1–2 mg/kg of ketamine produces a dissociative state for about 10 to 20 minutes and analgesia for 30 to 60 minutes.[11]

Thiopental is not commonly used today. It has a very long half-life and precipitates many drugs. Neonates and ill patients require reduced doses.[12] Methohexital is a shorter-acting barbiturate,[13] but like propofol causes pain on injection and is associated with myoclonic movements.

Etomidate is known for its cardiovascular stability but is rarely used in pediatrics as it causes adrenal suppression. It is associated with myoclonic movements, pain on injection, and vomiting.

Intramuscular (IM) induction can be used in special circumstances, such as an extremely uncooperative patient who refuses inhalational induction, has no IV access, and refuses oral or nasal sedation. The IM use of ketamine induces a dissociated state within several minutes of injection. It is important to make sure that the previously uncooperative patient can be placed on a stretcher with monitors as soon as he relaxes from the IM injection.

Rectal induction may be better tolerated than IM or inhalation induction in an extremely fearful or uncooperative child. A 10% solution of thiopental or methohexital can be used for rectal induction. This type of induction is better suited for small children (less than 20 kg), since the volume of injectate is based per kilogram. It can also be used for older children with cognitive impairment and diaper use. Unfortunately, the rectal absorption of drugs is unpredictable making induction and emergence timing difficult.[14]

Rapid-sequence induction is indicated for patients who are considered to have full stomachs (fasting less than 2 hours for clears, 4 hours for breast milk, 6 hours for formula, or 8 hours for a meal,[15] traumatic injuries, presence of nausea and vomiting, abdominal distension, and intestinal obstruction). If the patient does not have IV access, it is best to place one preoperatively if time allows. The patient should be preoxygenated with 100% oxygen to reach an expired oxygen concentration of 0.9. If the child does not tolerate the mask, holding the circuit near the patient will enrich their environment with oxygen. An assistant can apply cricoid pressure during induction. The benefit of applying cricoid pressure in small children and infants has been questioned due to the airway distortion making intubation more difficult.[16] Styletted ETTs should be readily available with two functioning laryngoscopes and suction. Given the risk for undiagnosed myopathies in children, succinylcholine should be avoided if possible. Rocuronium 1–1.2 mg/kg can be given IV following 3–4 mg/kg of propofol or 1–3 mg/kg of ketamine. If succinylcholine is given, 0.02 mg/kg of atropine may be needed to avoid bradyarrythmias. If the child desaturates before the ETT is placed, gently ventilate with pressures less than 15 cmH_2O to avoid insufflating the stomach.

Airway management

Mask ventilation

a. **Indications** – Mask ventilation is used for oxygenation and ventilation, with and without anesthetic gases for induction and maintenance of anesthesia. It is typically used for short surgical cases, such as ear tubes or drainage of an abscess, and in patients who are not at risk for aspiration.
b. **Techniques** – The head must be in a neutral or slightly extended position. In young children and infants, a small shoulder roll may achieve this position. The face mask should allow the soft inflatable cuff to create a seal, covering the mouth just above the tip of the chin and bridge of the nose avoiding pressure on the eyes. Place fingers on the bony mandible so as not to compress the submandibular soft tissues which could cause airway obstruction. Using minimal pressure against the face mask, the thumb and forefinger should create a "C" shape around the top of the mask. The mouth should be slightly open to increase airflow, and the tongue should not be sticking to the roof of the mouth. Furthermore, the little finger can sublux the temperomandibular joint forward to displace the posterior pharyngeal structures and open the airway even more. This maneuver is referred to as "chin-lift-jaw-thrust." The other free hand can then be used to bag ventilate and increase airway pressure as needed to create the desired tidal volume. Tidal volumes of 10 ml/kg and peak pressures of 30 cmH_2O should not be exceeded. Avoid peak pressures above 15 cmH_2O so as not to insufflate the stomach and risk aspiration. For patients who are difficult to ventilate, use both hands on the face mask, with index fingers on the coronoids and thumbs on the mask while an assistant or the anesthesia machine ventilates the patient. Occasionally, a third person may be needed to apply jaw thrust. Difficulty in ventilation may be caused by airway obstruction due to a large tongue or soft tissue collapse, especially in patients with obstructive sleep apnea or tonsillar hypertrophy. Consider using an oropharyngeal airway or nasal airway during mask ventilation. The oropharyngeal airway should be measured against the side of the cheek and should extend from the corner of the mouth to the distal angle of the jaw. If the airway is too

short it will obstruct the airway, and if it is too long it may cause laryngospasm. Correct size nasal airways rarely precipitate laryngospasm but have to be introduced with care to avoid nasal bleeding.

c. **Limitations** – After induction of anesthesia, airway tone will decrease and may cause obstruction during ventilation. Gastric insufflation may occur during mask ventilation, especially with peak pressures greater than 15 cmH_2O, and the distended stomach may impair excursion of the diaphragm. Consider placing an orogastric tube to ventilate the stomach should this occur. Positioning may be difficult in infants due to their relatively large heads, a soft foam or towel ring may be placed around the head for stabilization. Children may be fearful of the mask, several techniques have been described above to coax the child into taking the mask.
d. **Devices** – These include a bag-valve mask and a face mask attached to an anesthesia circuit, but an ambu-bag with a mask, or a Jackson Rees T-piece breathing system can also be used to mask ventilate a child.[17]

Laryngeal mask airway (LMA)

a. **Indications** – The LMA can be used during spontaneous, assisted, or controlled ventilation and for any surgery or position that does not increase risk for aspiration. It is mostly used during procedures of less than 2 hours duration. This device is less traumatic to the airway and better tolerated in patients with recent upper respiratory tract infections or airway disease[18,19] and in those requiring frequent anesthesia. It can also be used as a conduit for fiber optic intubations and bronchoscopies.[20] In the anesthesia of difficult airway algorithm, placement of an LMA is indicated when unable to ventilate by face mask. Recently the LMA has been increasingly used for T&As.[21–23]
b. **Techniques** – Patient's head should be midline, in a neutral but slightly extended position. Choose an appropriate-sized LMA. The posterior surface of the LMA should be lubricated. Classically, it was taught to deflate the LMA prior to insertion; however, many find that a small amount of cuff inflation allows for easier insertion.[24] The LMA is inserted with the posterior surface in contact with the roof of the mouth. If room allows, the index finger can be positioned between the cuff and barrel to aid in gently pushing the LMA into place, always with pressure directed cephalad and toward the posterior pharynx. A common mistake is to apply pressure along the tongue, which makes the placement difficult. The orifice of the LMA should align with the vocal cords while the cuff is in contact with the surrounding tissues. The cuff pressure should not exceed 40 to 50 cmH_2O.[25,26] If unable to generate good tidal volumes with peak pressures of 20 cmH_2O or less, then the LMA may need to be repositioned or replaced with another size. Occasionally, placing the head back into a neutral position can create a good seal. Sometimes the tip or side of the cuff becomes folded on insertion and simply needs to be unfolded. In larger kids this can be done by placing a finger along the rim of the cuff. The LMA may not easily pass the posterior pharynx, may need to be placed upside down, and then rotated into position from the pharynx to the larynx. Another method is to have an assistant apply jaw thrust to open the posterior pharynx space and allow easier insertion.[27] The LMA is never to be forced into place. Commonly, the LMA size is too large and a smaller size will work better. Otherwise, if the problem is a large leak, consider using a larger-sized LMA.
c. **Limitations** – These include difficulty with troubleshooting LMA placement; although, it is considered much easier than intubation. The LMA does not isolate the airway and gastric distension can occur when peak inspiratory pressures exceed 17 cmH_2O in children. Intubation remains the safest method to protect against aspiration. Until further studies are done, the LMA should not be used in the prone position, but has been used in the lateral position.
d. **Devices** – The classic LMA (LMA North America, San Diego, CA) simply contains an inflatable cuff. The LMA supreme is a preformed LMA with a port allowing passage of an orogastric tube to suction gastric contents. Note, this LMA has not been proven to protect against aspiration. The fast-track LMA can be easily used for intubation. A wire-reinforced LMA can be used when the barrel must be repositioned to either side of the mouth. There are many other types of supraglottic devices[28,29] available with differences in texture, ease of placement, curvature, and ones that

Table 29.1 Pediatric ETT size and depth

Age	Preterm < 1000 g	Term 1000–2500 g	Term 0–1 month	Infant 1–6 months	Infant 6–12 months	Toddler 1–2 years	Children 2+
Uncuffed ETT	2.5	3	3	3.5	4	4.5	Age/4 + 4
Cuffed ETT			3	3	3.5	4	Age/4 + 3.5
Depth of insertion at alveolar ridge	6	6 + wt in kg	9	10	11	12	3 × size of uncuffed ETT age appropriate

contain a port which allows suctioning of secretions that fall next to the device.

Endotracheal Intubation

a. **Indications** – Endotracheal intubation is used to protect and secure the airway in patients with a full stomach or at risk for aspiration, emergencies, surgeries involving an intra-abdominal approach (including laparoscopies), surgeries of the thoracic cavity and all cases in which ventilation is difficult, surgery of the head or neck in which manipulation of the airway may be possible, and in surgeries involving prone positioning or when access to the airway is difficult.

b. **Techniques** – Select the correct-sized endotracheal tube (ETT) and laryngoscope blade. A formula to follow in children 2 years and older is age/4 then add 3.5 for cuffed tubes or add 4 for uncuffed tubes (Table 29.1). A half size smaller ETT should be readily available for smaller than anticipated airways. Cuffed ETTs are now regularly used in children of all ages.[30] The ETT cuff should be checked and deflated prior to insertion. The patient should be placed in a sniffing position. In neonates with relatively large heads, a small rolled towel can be placed beneath the shoulders. In older children a small folded blanket can be placed under the head for 5–10 cm elevation. The tragus should be slightly anterior to the sternum, while the head is slightly extended. This is referred to as a three-axis alignment (mouth, oropharynx, and trachea), or sniffing position, and allows visualization of laryngeal structures. In patients with extremely large heads, such as in hydrocephalus, the entire body may need to be elevated with folded towels or blankets to achieve this alignment. Alternatively, an assistant can manually elevate the shoulders using their hands. In infants and young children a Miller blade is favored by many. The Miller blade is positioned midline of the tongue and advanced into the vallecula. With the tip of the blade in the vallecula, pivot the blade such that the tongue is swept from right to left. Lifting the tip of the epiglottis with the blade may induce bradycardia. Also, never blindly advance a Miller blade past the epiglottis (with plans to withdraw the blade until the cords come into view) because this can and has caused severe airway trauma in pediatrics. Another approach is to turn the head slightly left; displacing the tongue left, and placing the blade into the far right of the mouth over the lateral bicuspids, aiming the tip of the blade to the midline while sweeping the tongue to the left. A Mac blade is also inserted to the far right of the tongue, sweeping the tongue to the left as the tip of the blade is inserted into the vallecula. The blade is then lifted slightly up and anterior to bring the cords into view. In either approach an assistant can be used to apply gentle anterior neck pressure or optimal external laryngeal manipulation (OELM), such that the cords are brought into view. With experience the laryngoscope handle can be held with the first three fingers (like a pencil would be held) so that the fourth and fifth fingers are free to wrap around the chin and anterior neck and apply pressure bringing the cords into view. Another approach is to use the right hand for OELM, and then holding this position, an assistant can place the ETT. The ETT should be placed just past the vocal cords so that the black indicator marker is aligned with the vocal cords. Before securing the ETT its position should always be confirmed by auscultation and the presence of $ETCO_2$. For very small neonates, a simple formula for depth of insertion is 6 + patient weight in kilograms. Secure the ETT at this depth. Breath sounds should be present during flexion of the head. If breath sounds disappear during flexion, withdraw the ETT by half a centimeter or until breath sounds reappear. This is especially important during cases in which the head may be repositioned. An air leak should be present at 20–25 cm H_2O to avoid ischemic damage to the tracheal mucosa and to decrease the risk of postintubation croup, if a cuffed ETT is used the cuff pressure should be checked with a manometer. One formula to calculate correct depth of insertion is three times the size of the age-appropriate calculated uncuffed ETT.

c. **Limitations** – Infants have relatively large tongues obstructing the view of the vocal cords. The larynx is more cephalad, making cord visualization challenging. The epiglottis is difficult to lift because it is narrower and angled away from the tracheal axis. Infant vocal cords are attached lower (caudad) and anteriorly making intubation difficult with hang-up at the anterior commissure of the vocal folds. The subglottic diameter becomes narrow, so that the ETT may pass the cords but not be advanced further. At 10–12 years of age the cricoid and thyroid cartilages reach adult size and complications with subglottic narrowing and cord angulation are less likely. There is little reserve and time for intubation in infants due to their higher metabolic rate and oxygen consumption.

d. **Devices** – The most commonly used tools for intubation are the Mac and Miller blades, which have already been discussed. Many other devices exist and have specific indications for their use. Most of them are used for the management of the difficult airway and will be discussed below. The video laryngoscopes are more commonly used for the normal airway, especially in the teaching environment where the instructor is able to share the direct view of the glottis.

   Video laryngoscopes

   1. C-Mac (Karl Stortz Endoscopy, Tuttlingen, Germany): consists of a Miller or Mac Blade connected to a camera that projects onto a video monitor and is used for direct videolaryngoscopy. After the blade is inserted in the mouth, look at the screen while slowly advancing the blade into the vallecula. Anterior neck manipulation by the assistant can bring the cords into view. A styletted ETT placed along the blade will be advanced into the trachea under video visualization. The available pediatric blades are Miller 0 and 1 and Mac 1.[31]
   2. Truview EVO2 (Truphatek International, Netanya, Israel): This is a blade with a prism at the tip that allows for a 46-degree view of the vocal cords. The blade is placed on a normal handle and can be used with its eye piece or with a connected video camera. The intubation can be performed without manipulation of the head or neck.[32] The Truview EVO2 has an oxygen insufflation port that can be used to give supplemental oxygen or blow away secretions during intubation. Place the blade midline along the curvature of the tongue and advance the blade while observing the video screen. Commonly, this blade is inserted too far, so advance the blade slowly over the tongue into the vallecula while looking on the video screen. The Truview comes with preformed stylets in different sizes. While looking into the mouth the styletted ETT should be placed parallel to the blade. Next, while looking at the video monitor, the tip of the ETT is advanced through the cords, the stylet is gently removed, and the ETT is advanced into position. The Truview comes with pediatric blades in four different sizes.
   3. Glidescope (Verathon Medical, Bothell, WA, USA): This is a video fiber optic baton that is placed into a sharply angled disposable plastic blade and allows intubation with minimal head or neck manipulation.[33] The blade comes in five different sizes: three pediatric and two adult. The blade is placed midline on the tongue and slowly advanced while watching the video monitor. The tip of the blade is placed in or near the vallecula, raising the epiglottis for vocal cord visualization. A styletted ETT is placed parallel to the blade and advanced under video monitor visualization. Once the ETT passes through the vocal cords, an assistant should slowly remove the stylet while gently advancing the ETT.

4. Airtraq indirect laryngoscope (Prodol Meditec, S.A., Vizcaya, Spain): disposable sharply angled blade with an eye piece that can be removed to connect a camera to share the view of the glottis. The device has a channel to guide the ETT into the trachea under video visualization.[34] The Airtraq comes in 4 different sizes; two are pediatric, size 0 for ETT 2.5 to 3.5, size 1 for ETT 3.5 to 5.5.

Management of the difficult airway

a. **Management plan** – The first step in management of a difficult airway is to perform a careful history and physical exam. Many congenital syndromes are associated with difficult airways, as well as patients with bilateral microtia, those with c-spine limitation due to trauma, and children with a small mouth opening, facial trauma, or facial and neck tumors. Second, formulate a plan that includes management of the airway should loss of the airway occur. The plan will include having airway equipment checked and ready for use, skilled help for positioning and monitoring, and a surgeon available to perform a surgical airway. In case of an unexpected difficult airway call for help immediately. If a difficult airway is anticipated, a safe approach is to have a cooperative, sedated, spontaneously breathing patient; however, in young children and infants, due to the lack of cooperation, general anesthesia is often used with assisted spontaneous ventilation. It is important to avoid neuromuscular blockade due to the possibility of airway obstruction upon pharyngeal and laryngeal muscle relaxation. Also, spontaneous breathing allows a visual guide for location of the vocal cords. Several combinations of drugs can be used: sevoflurane, fentanyl and versed, versed and ketamine, precedex, and topical or nebulized lidocaine, spray or jelly. Care must be taken to titrate the drugs slowly to effect and calculate the maximum dose of local that can be given. In small children sevoflurane has been successfully used for the management of the difficult airway under spontaneous ventilation. Sevoflurane can be administered through nasal cannula, a modified nasal trumpet with an ETT adapter, or a nasal ETT placed into the supraglottic space. At all times supplemental oxygen should be administered to the child during the instrumentation of a difficult airway.

In addition to the above described different video laryngoscopes, the following devices are used for the management of the difficult airway: fiberoptic scope, lighted stylet, Bullard blade, and Shikani and Bonfils stylet.[35] Note, experience must first be gained with normal airways prior to using any of these devices in a pediatric difficult airway. The fiberoptic scope is the gold standard and comes in sizes as small as 2.2 mm in diameter, which can pass through a 2.5 mm internal diameter (ID) ETT. These scopes use light and project images through an eyepiece or on a video screen for others to view. Smaller scopes do not have a supplemental oxygen port or a suction channel. Adapters exist that allow continuing mask ventilation while the scope passes through the adapter.

b. **Technique for fiberoptic** – The patient can be supine or sitting (if only sedated) with the head in a neutral position. For oral intubations, have an assistant hold the tongue with gauze or minimal suctioning from the end of suction tubing (no yankauer attached) and introduce the scope midline. For nasal intubations a small amount of vasoconstrictor spray helps to minimize bleeding prior to inducing the scope. Jaw thrust can be done by an assistant to help open the posterior pharynx for better visualization. As the scope is advanced, it is important to keep the fiber optic straight so as to allow precise manipulation of the tip. The scope should pass well into the trachea, close to the carina before advancing the ETT, so as to avoid retracting the scope out of the cords during ETT placement. When the scope is too large for the ETT, a cardiac guide wire can be passed through the working channel of the scope and into the trachea. The ETT can be passed over the guide wire or over a cardiac catheter or Cook exchange catheter that has been passed over the guide wire. If there is no working channel, load a larger ETT onto the fiberoptic scope and position the ETT in front of the vocal cords such that a wire can be passed through the ETT and into the trachea. A Cook exchange catheter can be placed over the wire to allow easier placement of the ETT. If an LMA is placed (with teeth of the LMA removed), advance the scope loaded with the ETT through the LMA into the trachea. The pilot cuff and the end adapter of the ETT may be removed to fit through the LMA. If the ETT is not long enough to remove the LMA safely, a second ETT can be used to hold the ETT in place while the LMA is removed. Use of lubrication will aid in passage of both the fiber optic and the ETT.

c. **Lighted stylet** – This is also called a light wand and is a malleable stylet with a light at the end. The ETT is positioned on the preformed stylet with the bevel at 12 o'clock and the stylet tip nonexposed. The device is then placed in the mouth and advanced along the curvature of the tongue. With the room lights dim, a ring of light will appear below the skin at the cricoid level when the stylet is through the cords. The ETT is then advanced over the stylet. This is a blind technique that does not require manipulation of the head and neck and is useful in C-spine immobility. Limitations include the need for larger ETT and several attempts. Hang up on the epiglottis may be overcome by moving the stylet to a more posterior position and creating more distance between the stylet and epiglottis or to rotate the ETT so that the bevel is up and is not caught on the arytenoids.
d. **Bullard** (ACMI Cooperation, Southborough MA) – This device has a 90-degree bend at the tip and uses fiberoptic and mirrors. It is used and positioned similar to a standard laryngoscope. It is helpful in difficult airways; minimal movement of the neck is needed, and requires only a very small mouth opening. Once the cords are visualized, the styletted ETT is placed along the scope and advanced through the cords. Limitations are hang-up at the right aryepiglottic fold and anterior vocal cord, as well as obstruction of the view by the ETT. The Bullard blade is available in three sizes: 'adult' for children over 10 years old, 'pediatric long' for children 3 to 10 years old and 'pediatric' for infants and small children.
e. **Shikani** (Clarus Medical, Minneapolis, MN, USA) and *Bonfils* (Karl Stortz Endoscopy, Tuttlingen, Germany) – While the Shikani is a malleable optical stylet with a light source fitting size 3.0 ETT, the Bonfils is not malleable but can be used with size 2.5 ETT.[36] These devices also use video fiber optics and can be used with or without direct laryngoscopy. They come with an ETT holder and can deliver oxygen during intubation. These optical stylets are helpful in the presence of a limited mouth opening by using a retromolar approach. This approach requires some training on a mannikin before use in a difficult airway.
f. **The difficult airway algorithm**[37] should be used in any patient who is difficult to ventilate, intubate, or both. Note that in any patient who is both difficult to intubate and ventilate, an LMA is the first next step. Percutaneous cricothyrotomy should only be used in emergency situations and be done by an experienced individual (one with training on simulators and animal models). Percutaneous cricothyrotomy has a high complication rate in children less than 5 years of age. It only allows oxygen insufflation and does not allow adequate ventilation. It is therefore a temporizing measure until a definitive airway is established. Many makes and models are available, and it is important to be familiar with one's own institutional device.
g. **Cricothyrotomy** – Position the patient such that the head is extended for good neck access. While stabilizing the trachea, locate and mark the cricoid membrane with fingernail (an experienced ultrasonographer can identify the cricoid membrane). A 12–14 gauge IV catheter with a 3 ml syringe attached is slowly inserted through the cricoid membrane until air is aspirated. Next insert the catheter and reconfirm placement by aspirating air again. Then remove the plunger from the 3 ml syringe, insert the adaptor from an 8 mm ETT, and connect to the breathing circuit.[38]

Methods for single-lung ventilation and lung separation

a. A simple approach to single-lung ventilation is by mainstemming a single lumen ETT. Left mainstem can be done by turning the patient's head to the right and advancing the ETT while turning 180 degrees and listening for loss of breath sounds on the right. Alternatively, a fiberoptic scope can confirm or guide placement of the ETT. An uncuffed tube may not protect the good lung from blood and pus, and may not allow the opposite lung to fully collapse. A cuffed ETT may obstruct the upper lobe orifice when placed into the right main bronchus.[39]

b. Bronchial blockers consist of a balloon-tipped catheter that can be placed in the bronchial lumen of the lung which needs to be collapsed. Several methods allow for placing a bronchial blocker:

   - perform an endobronchial intubation, placing a guide wire into the bronchus and remove the ETT. The blocker is then placed over the guide wire, the guide wire is removed, and the ETT replaced. A fiberoptic scope can be used for balloon positioning. When the balloon is inflated the lung will collapse over time. Some bronchial blocker catheters are hollow and allow suction to be used to deflate the lung, or allow CPAP with oxygen. If ventilation becomes difficult, the balloon may have been displaced into the trachea and needs to be repositioned.
   - a multiport adapter can also be used. These adapters allow placement of both a bronchial blocker and a fiberoptic scope through an ETT during continuous ventilation. The smallest ETT that can be used is a 5.0 mm ID tube. The bronchial blocker has a monofilament loop around which the fiberoptic is attached so that they move together into the bronchial lumen. Then, the bronchial blocker slides off the end of the fiber optic and the fiber optic can be removed.

c. The Univent ETT (Fuji Systems Corporation, Tokyo, Japan) has a bronchial blocker channel inside the ETT which makes balloon migration less likely during single-lung ventilation. Fiberoptic bronchoscopy is used for blocker placement. The smallest ID is 3.5 with outer diameter of 7.5 mm and cannot be used in children less than 6 years old. As with other bronchial blockers, the balloon is a low-volume, high-pressure balloon in which over inflation can cause mucosal injury. This blocker also has a hollow lumen for lung deflation or oxygen and CPAP.

d. Double-lumen tubes (DLT) are two tubes molded together such that the longer tube is for bronchial placement and the shorter tube is positioned in the trachea. This type of ventilation isolates the lungs from each other so that blood or pus does not contaminate the good lung. The DLTs come as small as 26 French or 8.7 mm OD and therefore these tubes can only be used in older children (age greater than 8–10 years). Double lumen tubes are placed under direct laryngoscopy. The tip of the tube is placed through the cords, and the stylet is removed. The tube is then rotated 90 degrees to the left or right and the tube is advanced gently (never forcefully). The depth of tube placement will vary and placement should always be guided by FOB and auscultation. The tracheal cuff pressure should not exceed 25 cm H_2O. Auscultate for breath sounds bilaterally then pass a fiberoptic scope through the tracheal lumen to check for tube placement. Note, a 3.6 mm OD FOB will pass a 35 F DLT, otherwise a smaller FOB will be needed for a smaller DLT. Inflate the bronchial cuff and observe that the bronchial cuff does not herniate into the tracheal lumen. If using a right-sided DLT listen to the right upper lobe to confirm no upper lobe occlusion occurred by the bronchial cuff. Once the patient is positioned for surgery, check tube placement again with FOB and auscultation. Continue ventilating both lungs for as long as possible. Note the tidal volumes during 20 cm peak pressure ventilation, and do not exceed this tidal volume on one-lung ventilation (generally 8–10 ml/kg). Also, do not exceed peak inspiratory pressures (PIP) of 40 cm H_2O. The respiratory rate can be increased and tidal volumes decreased to keep the PIP low. The CO_2 may increase to 45–60. Many recommend using FiO_2 of 1. Serial arterial blood gas analyses will monitor the PaO_2 and CO2 during single-lung ventilation. To deflate one lung, both cuffs need to be inflated. Clamp the ETT supplying the collapsed lung or disconnect this side of the ETT from the ventilator to allow lung deflation and then auscultate to confirm single-lung ventilation. If there is difficulty ventilating or increased peak pressures, check for tube migration, as the bronchial cuff may eventually migrate to occlude the tracheal lumen. Alternatively, pass a FOB to observe the patency of the upper lobe orifice. If needed, continuous positive airway pressure (CPAP) can be applied to the collapsed lung. Avoid overinflating the dependent lung, as high alveolar pressures can increase intrapulmonary shunt to the nondependent lung and worsen hypoxemia. If these methods are unsuccessful return to bilateral lung ventilation. If at the end of the case the DLT must be converted to an SLT, an exchange catheter with direct laryngoscopy should be used.

References

1. C. Langton Hewer. The stages and signs of anesthesia. *Br Med J* 1937; **2**(3996): 274–6.
2. I. Murat, I. Constant. Bispectral index in pediatrics: fashion or a new tool? *Paediatr Anaesth* 2005; **15**: 177–80.
3. M.-C. Dubois, V. Piat, I. Constant, O. Lamblin, I. Murat. Comparison of three techniques for induction of anesthesia with sevoflurane in children. *Paediatr Anaesth* 1999; **9**: 19–23.
4. R. Friesen, J. Wurl, G. Charton. Hemodynamic depression by halothane is age-related in pediatric patients. *Paediatr Anaesth* 2000; **10**: 267–72.
5. R.S. Holzman, M.E. van-der Velde, S.J. Kaus, *et al.* Sevoflurane depresses myocardial contractility less than halothane during induction of anesthesia in children. *Anesthesiology* 1996; **85**: 1260–7.
6. G.D. Politis, M.L. Frankland, R.L. James, *et al.* Factors associated with successful tracheal intubation of children with sevoflurane and no muscle relaxant. *Anesth Analg* 2002; **95**: 615–20.
7. R.D. Jones, A.R. Visram, M.M. Chan, *et al.* A comparison of three induction agents in pediatric anesthesia – cardiovascular effects and recovery. *Anesth Intensive Care* 1994; **22**: 545–55.
8. R.S. Hannallah, S.B. Baker, W. Casey, *et al.* Propofol: effective dose and induction characteristics in unpremedicated children. *Anesthesiology* 1991; **74**: 217–19.
9. L. Jalota, V. Kalira, E. George, *et al.* Prevention of pain on injection of propofol: systematic review and meta-analysis. *BMJ* 2011; **342**: d1110. doi: 10.1136/bmj.d1110.
10. E. Allsop, P. Innes, M. Jackson, M. Cunliffe. Dose of propofol required to insert the laryngeal mask airway in children. *Paediatr Anaesth* 1995; **5**: 47–51.
11. C. Lin, M.E. Durieux. Ketamine and kids: an update. *Paediatr Anaesth* 2005; **15**: 91–7.
12. K. O'Brian, D.N. Robinson, N.S. Morton. Induction and emergence in infants less than 60 weeks post-conceptual age: comparison of thiopental, halothane and desflurane. *Br J Anaesth* 1998; **80**: 456–9.
13. A. Beskow, O. Werner, P. Westrin. Faster recovery after anesthesia in infants after intravenous induction with methohexital instead of thiopental. *Anesthesiology* 1995; **83**: 976–9.
14. H. Alp, Z. Orbak, I. Gueler, S. Altinkaynak. Efficacy and safety of rectal thiopental, intramuscular cocktail and rectal midazolam for sedation in children undergoing neuroimaging. *Pediatr Int* 2002; **44**: 628–34.
15. The American Society of Anesthesiologists Committee on Standards and Practice Parameters. Practice guidelines for preoperative fasting and the use of pharmacologic agents to reduce the risk of pulmonary aspiration: application to healthy patients undergoing elective procedures. *Anesthesiology* 2011; **114**: 495–511.
16. D. Neuhaus, A. Schmitz, A. Gerber, M. Weiss. Controlled rapid sequence induction and intubation – an analysis of 1001 children. *Paediatr Anaesth* 2013; **23**: 734–40.
17. B.S. Von Ungern-Sternberg, S. Saudan, A. Regli *et al.* Should the use of the modified Jackson Rees T-piece breathing system be abandoned in preschool children? *Paediatr Anaesth* 2007; **17**: 645–60.
18. A.R. Tait, U.A. Pandit, T. Voepel-Lewis, *et al.* Use of laryngeal mask airway in children with upper respiratory tract infection: a comparison with endotracheal intubation. *Anesth Analg* 1998; **86**: 706–11.
19. B. Gharaei, H. Aghamohammadi, A. Jafari, *et al.* Use of laryngeal mask airway in children with upper respiratory tract infection, compared with face mask: randomized, single blind, clinical trial. *Acta Anaesthesiol Taiwan* 2011; **49**: 136–40.
20. M. Somri, C. Barna Teszler, R. Tome, *et al.* Flexible fiberoptic bronchoscopy through the laryngeal mask airway in a small premature neonate. *Am J Otolaryngol* 2005; **26**: 268–71.
21. D. Jr. Ranieri, A.G. Neugebauer, D.M. Ranieri, *et al.* The use of disposable laryngeal mask airway for adenotonsillectomies. *Rev Bras Anesthesiol* 2012; **62**: 788–97.
22. D.I. Sierpina, H. Chaudhary, D.L. Walner, *et al.* Laryngeal mask airway versus endotracheal tube in pediatric adenotonsillectomy. *Laryngoscope* 2012; **122**: 429–35.
23. K. Lalwani, S. Richins, L. Aliason, *et al.* The laryngeal mask airway for pediatric adenotonsillectomy: predictors of failure and complications. *J Pediatr Otorhinolaryngol* 2013; **77**: 25–8.
24. M.S. Kim, S.J. Bai, J.T. Oh, *et al.* Comparison of 2 cuff inflation methods before insertion of laryngeal mask airway for safe use without manometer in children. *Am J Emerg Med* 2013; **31**: 346–52.
25. A. Licina, N.A. Chambers, B. Hullett, *et al.* Lower cuff pressures improve the seal of pediatric laryngeal mask airways. *Paediatr Anesth* 2008; **18**: 952–6.
26. B. Schloss, J. Rice, J.D. Tobias. The laryngeal mask in infants and children: what is the cuff pressure? *Int J Pediatr Otorhinolaryngol* 2012; **76**: 284–6.
27. B. Ghai, J.K. Makkar, N. Bhardwai, J. Wig. Laryngeal mask airway insertion in children: comparison between rotational, lateral and standard technique. *Paediatr Anaesth* 2008; **18**: 308–12.

28. P. Szmuk, O. Gehlber, M. Matuszczak, *et al.* A prospective randomized comparison of cobra perilaryngeal airway and laryngeal mask airway unique in pediatric patients. *Anesth Analg* 2008; **107**: 1523–30.
29. S.D. Whyte, E. Cook, S. Malherbe. Usability and performance characteristics of the pediatric air-Q intubating laryngeal airway. *Can J Anaesth* 2013; **60**: 557–63.
30. R.S. Litman, L.G. Maxwell. Cuffed versus uncuffed endotracheal tubes in pediatric anesthesia: the debate should finally end. *Anesthesiology* 2013; **118**: 500–1.
31. A.L Vanderhal, G. Berci, C.F. Simmons, *et al.* A videolaryngoscopy technique for the intubation of the newborn: preliminary report. *Pediatrics* 2009; **124**: e339–46.
32. M.A Gomez, L.N. Serradilla, A.E. Alvarez. Use of the TruView EVO2 laryngoscope in Treacher Collins syndrome after unplanned extubation. *J Clin Anesth* 2012; **24**: 257–8.
33. J.H. Lee, Y.H. Park, H.J. Byon, *et al.* A comparative trial of the GlideScope(R) video laryngoscope to direct laryngoscope in children with difficult direct laryngoscopy and an evaluation of the effect of blade size. *Anesth Analg* 2013; **117**: 176–81.
34. F.S. Xue, H.P. Liu, X. Liao, *et al.* Endotracheal intubation with Airtraq® optical laryngoscope in the pediatric patients. *Paediatr Anaesth* 2011; **21**: 703–4.
35. J. Fiadjoe, P. Stricker. Pediatric difficult airway management: current devices and techniques. *Anesthesiol Clin* 2009; **27**: 185–95.
36. P.L. Krishnan, B.H. Thiessen. Use of the Bonfils intubating fibrescope in a baby with a severely compromised airway. *Paediatr Anaesth* 2013; **23**: 670–2.
37. The American Society of Anesthesiologists Task Force on Management of the Difficult Airway. Practice guidelines for management of the difficult airway: an updated report. *Anesthesiology* 2013; **118**: 251–70.
38. C.J. Coté, C.J. Hartnick. Pediatric transtracheal and cricothyrotomy airway devices for emergency use: which are appropriate for infants and children? *Paediatr Anaesth* 2009; **19** (Suppl 1): 66–76.
39. G.B. Hammer, B.G. Fitzmaurice, J.B. Brodsky. Methods for single-lung ventilation in pediatric patients. *Anesth Analg* 1999; **89**: 1426–9.

Chapter

30 Complications of anesthesia

Ranu Jain and Maria Matuszczak

Airway obstruction

Failure to manage the airway is a leading cause of death in pediatrics. In children airway obstruction occurs frequently during induction and emergence of anesthesia.[1]

Causes of airway obstruction

- *Anatomy*
- *Traumatic, burn*
- *Foreign body,*
- *Laryngospasm, bronchospasm*
- *Obstructive sleep apnea (OSA)*
- *Mechanical*

Anatomy

a. Large tongue: associated with several congenital syndromes, trisomy 21 being one of them, but can also be due to a hemangioma or neoplasm, or induced by burn or other trauma. Mask ventilation, intubation, and extubation can be a challenge and need to be planned carefully depending on the size of the tongue.
b. Micrognathia, retrognathia: associated with several syndromes, Pierre Robin sequence, Treacher Collins, and many more; mask ventilation, intubation, and extubation can be extremely difficult but are generally anticipated and the necessary preparation for the pediatric difficult airway must be taken (see Chapter 28).
c. Abscess: mask ventilation is generally not impaired but depending on the location of the abscess intubation can be difficult, trismus is often present. If located in the sublingual area the abscess can rupture during intubation and pus can obstruct the view of the glottis and the airway.
d. Laryngomalacia: can cause airway collapse during mask ventilation.
e. Tracheomalacia: depending on the location can cause obstruction even when patient is intubated.
f. Tracheal stenosis: due to scar tissue may be so severe that intubation is not possible and scar tissue will need to be removed under suspension laryngoscopy and spontaneous ventilation; team work with the ENT surgeon is very important. Most acquired subglottic stenoses are due to tracheal intubation, the culprit being: traumatic intubation, wrong size ETT, overinflated cuff, prolonged intubation, repeated intubation, sepsis, inflammation, gastric reflux, and other traumas.
g. Tumors:
    - Laryngotracheal papillomas (the most commonly found airway tumor in children) is caused by human papilloma virus (1:400 births), due to the availability of a HPV vaccine the incidence should decline. Papillomas are found on margins of vocal cords, epiglottis, pharynx or trachea, they are recurrent and need repeated treatments. Symptoms include stridor, airway obstruction, and hoarseness. The degree of obstruction can vary. The ENT surgeon should be present during induction. Surgical removal requires cryosurgery, CO_2 laser, and micro debridement. Anesthesiologist and ENT surgeon work as a team and decide together on the airway management. Spontaneous ventilation is generally maintained. Shielded laser tube or copper wrapped red rubber tube are used, the outer diameter of these tubes is larger than regular ETTs. Due to the risk of airway fire, FiO_2 should be minimal.[2]

Essentials of Pediatric Anesthesiology, ed. Alan David Kaye, Charles James Fox and James H. Diaz. Published by Cambridge University Press. © Cambridge University Press 2015.

- Mediastinal tumors (neurofibroma, lymphoma) can compress the trachea. Depending on the extent of the mediastinal tumor the availability of ECMO should be considered.
- Tumors of the mandible can significantly impair mouth opening and contribute to airway obstruction during induction.

Traumatic:

Facial trauma, fractures, lacerations, inhalational trauma, and burns depending on extent and location can cause airway obstruction. Lacerations on the face and blood in the airway may make mask ventilation impossible and also impairs visibility when needing video and fiberoptic devices. Airway management needs to be carefully planned.

Foreign body (FB) aspiration

Common in children, 1–3 years of age, tracheal obstruction and asphyxiation is the most severe complication causing the death of > 300 children/year in the USA. Most foreign bodies lodge in the right main bronchus, the left main bronchus being smaller and slightly angled. Chest X-rays with inspiratory, expiratory, and decubitus views may reveal the position of the foreign body. The FB may or may not cause any obstruction and chest X-ray may be normal, or may show hyperinflation of the ipsilateral side, or mediastinal shift. The treatment will be retrieval of the FB. Depending on the respiratory stress the case may be emergent and the child with full stomach. Call for help if child is in respiratory distress. Communication between the entire team is of utmost importance; the surgeon should be in the OR ready to place the rigid bronchoscope. All equipment needs to be ready and functional. Sevoflurane induction or gentle IV induction with maintained spontaneous ventilation, use of antisialogogue to decrease secretions and topical anesthetic to prevent coughing. The anesthesia circuit is connected to the rigid bronchoscope and $ETCO_2$ is often not measurable. Complete obstruction during retrieval of the trachea can make ventilation impossible and the FB may need to be pushed back into the main bronchus to allow for oxygenation. Hypercarbia, hypoxia, bradycardia, and hypotension are frequent adverse events and need symptomatic treatment. In the majority of cases the FB can be removed successfully. The decision to extubate will depend on the extent of airway manipulation, swelling and critical events during the procedure. In any case the child should be fully awake to be able to protect the irritated airway. Dexamethasone and racemic epinephrine should be administered.[3]

Laryngospasm, bronchospasm

a. Laryngospasm is due to reflex constriction of the laryngeal muscles, closing the glottis to air passage. Laryngospasm occurs at any time during anesthesia (unless intubated) but most frequently during induction and emergence. The younger the patient the higher is the risk. Laryngospasm is more frequent in children with recent or present URI, with manipulation of the airway during light anesthesia, and with an inexperienced anesthesiologist. The treatment consists of: deepen anesthesia, call for help (children have higher oxygen consumption and desaturate fast), apply jaw thrust and CPAP via mask, then give atropine and succinylcholine if bradycardia presents with increasing hypoxia.[4,5] Laryngospasm was the most common preceding event identified in the POCA (Pediatric Perioperative Cardiac Arrest) registry data; this may be due to failure to recognize laryngospasm before the onset of bradycardia and cardiac arrest.[6]
b. Sudden bronchospasm can be triggered by airway manipulation, and surgical manipulation under light anesthesia in children with a hyper-reactive airway. These children often suffer from asthma and treatment consists of inhaled albuterol and IV hydrocortisone. Volatile anesthetics and ketamine may help to reduce bronchospasm as well. Preoperatively children with asthma should continue their normal treatment including on the morning of surgery. In children with no history of reactive airway disease bronchospasm can be triggered by aspiration of gastric content or by anaphylaxis (see Section 8). In case of gastric aspiration bronchoscopic suctioning should be performed. Inhaled albuterol can be used. If the child breathes spontaneously and maintains normal SaO_2 on room air, extubation can be planned at the end of the procedure with a chest X-ray for documentation.

Obstructive sleep apnea (OSA)

Upper airway obstruction is the hallmark for children with obstructive sleep apnea undergoing anesthesia. Child obesity is a risk factor and exacerbates the disease. Mask ventilation can be difficult especially during induction of anesthesia, but postoperative upper airway obstruction is also increased. Opioids should be avoided or minimized as these children develop an increased sensitivity to opioids. Postoperatively children with moderate to severe OSA should be monitored overnight.[(7)]

Mechanical

Sudden airway obstruction during anesthesia can be due to mechanical problems. Kinked ETT, secretion or blood clot in ETT, anesthesia circuit trapped between OR table and other devices (e.g., surgical microscope). Check patency of the circuit and ETT, and suction ETT. If suction catheter can't be advanced the ETT is most likely totally occluded and needs to be exchanged. Auscultation is a valuable diagnostic tool if access to the chest is possible.

Signs and symptoms of airway obstruction

Awake or extubated child

a. Increased work of breathing, use of accessory muscles
b. Nasal flaring
c. Drooling
d. Grunting
e. Wheezing
f. Tachycardia if not treated eventually will lead to bradycardia
g. Tachypnea RR > 60 in infants; RR > 40 in child
h. Stridor: *Inspiratory* – Due to narrowing of airway above thoracic outlet. Supraglottic obstruction – macroglossia, laryngeal web, laryngomalacia,foreign body, vocal cord paralysis. *Expiratory* – Due to narrowing below the thoracic outlet, subglottic stenosis, vascular rings, hemangioma, foreign body, cysts. *Biphasic* – Due to midtracheal abnormalities, tracheomalacia, tracheal stenosis

Intubated child

a. Increased work of breathing, use of accessory muscles
b. Nasal flaring
c. Wheezing
d. Increased PIP pressures, decreased tidal volumes
e. Change, decrease or loss of $ETCO_2$ wave
f. Decrease or loss of chest excursion
g. Tachycardia if not treated eventually will lead to bradycardia
h. Tachypnea RR > 40 in infants; RR > 30 in children

Inadequate vascular access

Obtaining optimal intravenous access in children presents unique challenges that do not exist in the adult population. With the exception of minor procedures two IV catheters should be obtained before the child is prepped and draped. Inadequate vascular access contributes to morbidity by under-resuscitation. The Pediatric Perioperative Cardiac Arrest (POCA) registry emphasized the importance of adequate intravenous access. "Lack of good vascular access may contribute to the underestimation of fluid/blood loss and inadequate replacement of fluid/blood in anesthetized children."

These days PICC lines are commonly used especially in very small children, but they are not suitable for administration of viscous fluids (albumin, blood, FFP, platelets) due to their small diameter and their length. A second peripheral IV is needed for most procedures even if a PICC line is in place.

In a child with a history of difficult IV access several techniques improving visualization of the veins can facilitate IV placement including local warming, transillumination (different devices exist), and ultrasound. These techniques limit unnecessary punctures, hematomas, and bruises.

In an emergency or in a critically ill child, with dehydration and hypothermia causing peripheral vasoconstriction, the challenge becomes even more difficult. Pediatric Advanced Life Support (PALS) and Advanced Trauma Life Support (ATLS) now recommend placement of an intraosseous (IO) line if adequate IV access cannot be established within three attempts. Styletted intraosseous needles exist in sizes 14, 16, and 18 gauge. Access is typically obtained on the flat surface of the proximal tibia 1 to 2 cm below and 1 cm medial to the tibial tuberosity, avoiding the growth plate. The needle is inserted at a 90-degree angle to the skin surface using a twisting motion. A battery-operated drill for the IO placement is now available and less traumatic; needles are all 15 gauge but different lengths (15, 25, 45 mm). Once the needle is inserted the stylet is removed and aspiration of the bone marrow indicates proper placement. Fluids and medications for resuscitation can be given through the intraosseous needle. The IO needle can be difficult to secure; if displaced can cause infiltration leading to compartment syndrome. Other potential complications are damage to growth plate, infection, fracture, and fat, and bone marrow emboli.[8]

If the external jugular vein is visible IV access can be obtained by placing the child in the Trendelenburg position and by compressing the EJV with a tongue depressor at the level of the clavicle.

Femoral line placement, if no contraindication (e.g., abdominal trauma), can be done by landmarks or use of ultrasound.

Subclavian or internal jugular vein access can be obtained in patients with difficult IV access. Complications associated with these accesses, pneumothorax, infection, and perforation of the heart are highest with the subclavian approach.[9]

Iatrogenic trauma/positioning injury

The most common types of iatrogenic injury in pediatric anesthesia are:

- *Dental damage*
- *Airway injuries, vocal cords, trachea, mouth, nose*
- *Perforation, pneumothorax*
- *Positioning injuries, nerve injuries*
- *Postoperative visual loss*
- *Tourniquet damage*
- *Psychological trauma*

Dental damage

Knowledge about perioperative dental injuries is based on retrospective data and occurs between 0.02% and 0.05% of all general anesthetics.

Excoriation or laceration of the gum pads from direct laryngoscopy has been described in neonates.

Potential to injure the nondeciduous teeth is minimal, but a loose tooth risks being aspirated during anesthesia: it needs to be removed before intubation with written consent from the parents.

Damage can occur from laryngoscopy, suction catheters, and biting on oral airways; 50–70% of the injuries occur during intubation, 9–20% during extubation. Emergency procedures are associated with a higher incidence of dental injury. Pediatric patients are at lower risk for dental injuries than adults. The teeth most likely injured are the upper incisors. Only 2% of these injuries require intervention. If a tooth is avulsed, it should be reimplanted in its socket and a dentist should be consulted immediately, and the family informed.[10,11]

Airway injuries, vocal cords, trachea, mouth, nose

Most iatrogenic injuries to the pediatric airway are due to inadequate intubation technique, forceful intubation with a styletted ETT, oversized tube selection, overinflating the cuff. Many minor airway injuries heal without sequelae because the larynx and trachea of children tolerate considerable trauma. Sign of a tracheal injury is the development of a postoperative croup, most commonly due to a too large ETT, or an overinflated cuff. Tears in the mucosa can lead to scar formation, which in turn can cause obstruction of the airway requiring tracheostomy and airway reconstructive surgery. Early detection of the injury is sometimes difficult because stridor develops late when scar formation has occluded almost 50% of the airway.[12]

Perforation, pneumothorax

a. Perforation most likely occurs during central line placement. It can lead to significant morbidity and mortality. The highest incidence of perforation occurs with a subclavian approach. Perforation can cause a pneumothorax, laceration of the subclavian artery or the aorta with subsequent hematothorax. Perforation to the heart has also been described with lethal outcome. Central venous catheter-related complications in the POCA database are similar in profile to those reported from the Closed Claims Database. The conclusion of the Closed Claims study was that use of ultrasound guidance or pressure waveform analysis would prevent about 50 percent of complications related to CV catheter placement.
b. Perforation or laceration of the trachea occurs due to improper use of a styletted ETT, an oversized ETT or an overinflated cuff.[13]
c. Intrathecal perforation of an epidural catheter is rare but can occur even several days after its placement.

Positioning injuries, nerve injuries

The incidence of reported peripheral nerve injuries in children is 1% as compared to adults where it is 16%. This may be due to the fact that children are unable to describe sensory deficits as well as adults, and because they have less comorbidity (hypertension, diabetes, and tobacco smoking).

Table 30.1. Definition of hypotension by age group

Age	Systolic blood pressure
Term neonates (0 to 28 days)	< 60 mmHg
Infants (1 to 12 months)	< 70 mmHg
Children 1 to 10 years (5th BP percentile)	< 70 mmHg + (age in years x 2) mmHg
Children > 10 years	< 90 mmHg

Available recommendations are from adult data. Certain surgical specialties are more frequently associated with nerve injuries: neurosurgery, cardiac surgery, general surgery and orthopedic surgery. Upper extremity nerve injuries are more frequent than lower extremity, with ulnar nerve injury being the most common, and sensory deficits being slightly more common than motor deficits.

Other nerve injuries can be caused by overstretching extremities for long hours (especially in endoscopic or robotic surgery, sternotomy, thoracotomy, and the lithotomy position).[14,15]

Prolonged prone position can lead to pressure ulcers on the face, shoulders, and knees. Dependent edema can develop over time; significant swelling of the tongue has been described, needing prolonged intubation postoperatively.

Nerve injury can be induced by a compartment syndrome due to undiagnosed IV infiltration during surgery when extremities are not directly visible to the anesthesiologist. Urgent fasciotomy may be needed to prevent long-term nerve deficit

Nerve injuries can occur from direct needle trauma to the nerve while performing regional anesthesia; a perineural or intraneural hematoma can develop; case reports have been published but large data collection of regional anesthesia in children have not confirmed an increased risk.[16,17] While performing neuraxial blocks a devastating injury can be caused by accidental injection of neurotoxic drugs or by cord compression from hematoma. Cord ischemia has also been described from local or systemic hypotension. These are all extremely rare events.

Postoperative visual loss (POVL)

Multifactorial causes seem to be involved in POVL but are still poorly understood; POVL is a serious complication and is divided into:

a. ischemic optic neuropathy: both eyes are affected, the patient may have a normal postoperative course but then be readmitted for bilateral blindness, 40% may recover vision
b. central retinal occlusion (CRAO): mostly unilateral but recovery of vision is 0%
c. cortical blindness

Causes implicated in the development of POVL are: prolonged prone position, deep Trendelenburg position, hypotension, fluid balance, large blood loss with anemia, increased intraocular pressure with impaired perfusion of the eye, and direct pressure on the globe.[18]

Tourniquet damage

Potential problems associated with tourniquets include:

a. local skin damage under a poorly applied cuff
b. local tissue and nerve damage from overinflation
c. compromised circulation caused by extended use

The pneumatic tourniquet can cause muscle ischemia, edema, and congestion, leading to temporary or permanent damage. The most commonly reported complication is nerve paralysis followed by deep vein thrombosis.[19]

Hypotension

- *Definition*
- *Causes of intraoperative hypotension*
- *Shock*
- *Treatment*

Definition

Hypotension under anesthesia is defined as a > 30% drop in blood pressure.

Children maintain their blood pressures until 25–35% blood is lost; they compensate for inadequate circulation by catecholamine release and increased peripheral autonomic tone.

Preterm infants depend on heart rate for the cardiac output; the response to peripheral catecholamine is not yet fully developed and when anesthetized with inhalational agents these children are more prone to hypotension than older children[1,20] (see Table 30.1).

Tachycardia, narrow pulse pressure, low urine output, and slow capillary refill are precursors of hypotension.

Causes of intraoperative hypotension

- Equipment: size of blood pressure cuff, setting of monitor and transducer, arterial line tubing
- Decreased SVR: due to inhalational agents, IV anesthetics, vasodilators, sepsis, anaphylaxis, allergic reactions
- *Decreased preload*: Hypovolemia, acute blood loss, preoperative deficits, prolonged fasting times polyuria, burns
- *Increased intrathoracic pressures*: pneumothorax, hematothorax, excessive PEEP, tamponade, pulmonary embolism
- *Increased intra-abdominal pressure*: pneumoperitoneum, abdominal compartment syndrome
- *Increased venous capacitance*: high epidural, high spinal
- *Decreased contractility*: inhalational agents, myocardial depressants, hypocalcemia, metabolic acidosis, hypothermia
- *Dysrhythmias* (see below)

Shock

Shock is a late sign and defined as a condition in which perfusion of blood to vital organs, with oxygen and substrates, is inadequate to meet the body's metabolic demand.

Types: Hypovolemic, cardiogenic, septic, anaphylactic shock

Hypovolemia is the most common cause of shock in children; it can be due to acute blood and plasma loss (surgery, trauma), and water loss (burns, peritonitis).

Sepsis is a high cardiac output shock with V/Q mismatch; as a result there is compromised oxygen delivery to the tissues; the myocardial contractility is depressed, with later decline in cardiac output.

Cardiogenic shock is rare in children; severe hypoxemia, pulmonary venous embolism, and dysrhythmia in the perioperative setting can be the cause.

Anaphylactic shock see below in this chapter.

Treatment of hypotension

Check if:

- Blood pressure cuff size is appropriate for the child
- Arterial line is zeroed correctly
- No surgical instrument or heavy blanket is on child's extremity with BP cuff
- Decrease anesthetic depth
- Increase fluids, consider bolus of 10–20 ml/kg
- Direct treatment of hypotension at the underlying cause
- Communicate with surgeon
- Consider additional IV access
- Consider placement of invasive monitors: central venous pressure, arterial line placement
- Vasopressor support, inotropic support, and use antidysrhythmic drugs as needed

Hypertension

- *Definition*
- *Etiology*
- *Treatment*

Definition

Hypertension is defined as a blood pressure persistently greater than the 95th percentile for age, height, and gender in children.

Etiology

Essential hypertension is the most common cause of hypertension in children. Obesity is the primary cause of essential hypertension in the US. Hypertension is less frequent in children but nevertheless present in several disease processes and significantly contributes to perioperative morbidity:

- Cardiac: Coarctation of the aorta, aortoenteritis
- Renal: Chronic renal failure, Wilms tumor, renal artery stenosis, reflux nephropathy, glomerulonephritis
- Endocrine: Congenital adrenal hyperplasia, Conn's syndrome, Cushing's disease
- Hypo- or hyperthyroidism
- Oncologic: Neuroblastoma, pheochromocytoma,
- Genetic: Acute intermittent porphyria, Bardet – Biedl, von Hippel–Landau, Williams, Turner, neurofibromatosis, Guillain–Barré syndrome

Contributors to perioperative hypertension[(1)] are:

- Wrong size blood pressure cuff
- Wrong medication or overdose (including lidocaine with epinephrine infiltration by surgeon)

- Anticholinergic drugs
- Light anesthesia during elevated levels of stimulation
- Intravascular volume overload
- Increased intracranial pressure
- Catecholamine excess due to tumor manipulation
- Pain
- Anxiety

Treatment

- Ensure correct size blood pressure cuff
- Check for medication error or side effects
- Increase depth of anesthesia
- Treat of underlying disease processes
- Communicate with surgeon
- Consider beta blockade, alpha-2 agonist, or calcium channel blockade
- Consider invasive monitoring
- Treat pain, treat anxiety

Dysrhythmias

- *Definition*
- *Perioperative dysrhythmias*

Definition

Dysrhythmia means abnormal rhythm. Infrequent in children with anatomically normal hearts, the mechanisms of onset of the dysrhythmias is similar in adults and children.[(21)]

- *Sinus arrhythmia*: benign, normal variant, most common arrhythmia in children, the heart rate varies with breathing.
- ***Sinus tachycardia*:** HR > 100/min in older child or a teenager,
    - HR > 160–170/min in younger children.
- ***Sinus bradycardia*:** HR < 60/min for older children
    - HR < 80/min for infants
    - HR < 100/min for newborns.
- *Isolated premature atrial contractions*: benign in absence of heart disease, common in newborn. Early P wave, different morphology than the sinus P wave. Either conducted or not conducted to the ventricle.
- *Isolated premature ventricular contraction*: benign in absence of heart disease, wide QRS complex, T waves in opposite direction of QRS, incidence 0.3–2.2%.
- *First-degree AV block*: seen in 6% normal neonates, PR interval longer than normal. Seen in patients with rheumatic fever, rubella, mumps, cardiomyopathy, electrolyte disturbances, and cardiomyopathy
- *Second-degree AV block, also called Mobitz Wenckebach block*: presents with increasing P–QRS interval until one QRS is dropped. Rarely seen in children.
- *Third-degree AV block, also called complete heart block*: common cause of bradycardia in children with palliated or corrected CHD, there is complete dissociation between P waves and QRS. Pacemaker is needed and needs to be interrogated for correct functioning before anesthesia is induced.
- *Supraventricular tachycardia*: rapid regular narrow QRS rhythm originating above the ventricles, no P waves or P waves not associated with QRS, most common abnormal tachycardia in children.
- Paroxysmal sudden onset: in infants and toddlers heart rate may be > 240, while in older children HR may be between 180–250. Older children complain of palpitation, dizziness, shortness of breath, and chest tightness whereas newborns show hemodynamic instability.
- *Sick sinus syndrome*: electrical signals are either too slow or too fast or a combination of slow and fast. Rare in children, incidence increases with age.
- *Atrial flutter, atrial fibrillation, ectopic atrial tachycardia, junctional tachycardia*: not common in pediatric population with normal heart.
- *Ventricular tachycardia (VT)*: rare in childhood, benign form may resolve with exercise, but may also be induced by stress. Children with hypertrophic cardiomyopathy and long QT syndrome are more susceptible. Palpitations, shortness of breath, dizziness, and syncopies are common symptoms. If hemodynamically unstable cardioversion with 0.5–1 J/kg is the treatment of choice.
- *Ventricular fibrillation (VF)*: fast and erratic rate, ventricles unable to fill with blood and pump, life threatening, no pulse, loss of consciousness; CPR needs to be initiated immediately.

Perioperative dysrhythmias

The following causes (other than pre-existing dysrhythmias) contribute to dysrhythmia in the perioperative period:

- Surgical stress and light anesthesia
- Various medications, administered inadvertently or purposefully
- Hypoxia
- Hypercarbia
- Hypovolemia
- Anemia
- Acidosis
- Electrolyte abnormalities
- Hypo- and hyperthermia
- Head trauma with increased intracranial pressure

Dysrhythmias and arrhythmias are more likely to occur in children with CHD, myocarditis, and cardiomyopathy. Certain surgical manipulations can induce arrhythmias like strabismus surgery, laparoscopic insufflation, surgery close to the brain stem, endoscopic sinus surgery, and laryngoscopy. Bradycardia is the most frequent intraoperative arrhythmia in children and if persistent is treated with an anticholinergic agent. Removal of the cause is the first treatment. Severe persistent bradycardia may need administration of epinephrine and some chest compression to increase circulation of the drug. Sinus tachycardia is generally a normal physiological response to pain, stress, and fever; it is transient, and usually does not require treatment other than deepening the anesthesia and administering analgesic.

Cardiac arrest

- *Epidemiology*
- *Etiology*
- *Diagnosis*
- *Stages of CA*
- *Cardiopulmonary resuscitation guidelines, revised 2010*
- *Post cardiac arrest syndrome (POCS)*
- *Strategies for prevention of arrest*

Epidemiology

Pediatric cardiac arrest (PCA) is estimated to occur in 8–20/100 000 American children/year.

Of these, 50% occur in the hospital; 27% of children survive to hospital discharge as compared to 17% in adults.

Most data concerning the PCA in the perioperative period come from the Pediatric Perioperative Cardiac Arrest (POCA) Registry.

The POCA registry was created in 1994; reports were published in 2000 and 2007.[22,23] In the perioperative period PCA occurs at a rate of 2.8 per 10 000; 21% of PCAs occurred during induction; 67% during maintenance.

Death occurred in 43% within 24 hours and an additional 4% within 3 weeks; 55% of PCAs under anesthesia happened in children < 1 year of age, while 25% were < 1 month old.[15]

Etiology

Remember the 5 Hs: hypovolemia, hypoxia, hypothermia, hydrogen ion imbalance, hyper-/hypokalemia.

And remember the 5 Ts: supraventricular tachycardia, pulseless electrical activity, tension pneumothorax, tamponade, thromboembolism, and toxins.

The following etiologies have a higher risk of PCA under anesthesia:

a. Neonates
b. Hyperkalemia
c. Higher ASA
d. Emergency surgeries
e. Acidosis
f. Patients with congenital heart disease
g. Anaphylaxis; most common cause is latex, followed by antibiotics and neuromuscular blocking agents

Diagnosis

In the OR, standard ASA monitoring alerts the anesthesia provider to impending or actual PCA. The ECG may show dysrhythmias, or asystole; the $ETCO_2$ may show a rapid change and decrease in waveform secondary to decreased or no cardiac output; the pulse oximeter waveform will also change.

Anaphylaxis is identified by skin changes, bronchospasm, and cardiovascular collapse.

The ultimate clinical diagnosis of PCA depends on the palpation of a carotid, brachial or femoral pulse. Successful resuscitation usually depends on identifying the cause and correction of the underlying problem.

Stages of cardiac arrest

(a) No flow phase is the state of untreated CA. The key to improved outcome is to shorten this phase by early recognition and rapid initiation of life-support measures.

(b) Low-flow phase occurs during active cardiopulmonary resuscitation (CPR). According to the 2010 AHA guidelines, effective CPR is: push hard, and push fast, allow full chest recoil between compressions, avoid excessive ventilation, and minimize interruptions of chest compressions. Equally important is early detection and prompt defibrillation for ventricular fibrillation and pulseless ventricular tachycardia. The goal is to maximize myocardial perfusion.

Cardiopulmonary resuscitation guidelines, revised 2010

Initiate CPR for infants and children with chest compressions rather than rescue breaths.[24,25]

Change in CPR sequence (C-A-B rather than A-B-C)

The CPR should begin with 30 compressions (any lone rescuer; ratio 30/2) or 15 compressions (two healthcare providers; ratio 15/2) rather than with two ventilations.

(a) Chest compression 100/min. To achieve effective chest compressions the depth should be at least one-third of the AP diameter of the chest (about 4 cm in infants, 5 cm in children). In infants a circumferential compression is preferred to the focal sternal compression in older children.

If the infant or child is unresponsive take up to 10 seconds to feel for a pulse (brachial in an infant and carotid or femoral in a child) and begin chest compressions.

(b) Secure airway if needed, exhaled CO_2 detection is recommended in addition to clinical assessment to confirm tracheal tube position for neonates, infants, and children with a perfusing cardiac rhythm.

(c) Medications: Epinephrine; has alpha- and beta-adrenergic stimulating properties. Alpha increases the systemic and pulmonary vascular resistance, increasing the systolic and diastolic pressures, which increase the coronary blood flow.

(d) Defibrillation and use of the AED in infants. For infants, a manual defibrillator is preferred. If a manual defibrillator is not available, an AED equipped with a pediatric dose attenuator is preferred.

If neither is available, an AED without a pediatric dose attenuator may be used. Infant paddles should be used under 10 kg, and adult paddles for all children over 10 kg. Initial dose is 2 J/kg. The CPR should resume immediately for 2 minutes before the second shock at 4 J/kg should be delivered. The maximum dose is 10 J/kg or 200 J.

(e) Specific resuscitation guidance has been added for management of cardiac arrest in infants and children with single-ventricle anatomy, Fontan or hemi-Fontan/bidirectional Glenn physiology, and pulmonary hypertension. Single ventricle and obstructive lesions (particularly aortic stenosis) were the most common type of heart disease in the POCA registry.[26]

Post cardiac arrest syndrome (POCS)

Significant morbidity and mortality is largely due to the cerebral and cardiac dysfunction that results from prolonged whole-body ischemia. Anoxic brain injury, myocardial dysfunction, systemic ischemia, and reperfusion response can all manifest in the POCS.

Strategies for prevention of arrest

The cause-of-arrest profile from 1998–2003 suggests clinical strategies for the reduction of risk for anesthetized children.[27]

(a) The change from halothane to sevoflurane reduced incidence of PCA due to inhalational agents. Blood pressure and heart rate is maintained under sevoflurane anesthesia, sevoflurane being less cardio depressant than halothane.

(b) Local anesthetics with less potential for toxicity (including ropivacaine and the L isomer of bupivacaine) used for the regional anesthesia.

(c) Awareness of cardiac arrests from hypovolemia followed by massive blood transfusion and subsequent hyperkalemia.[28]

- Use the freshest packed red blood cells; avoid using whole blood.
- Do not irradiate the blood except when absolutely necessary (premature baby or

immunocompromised child). When irradiation is required, the time between irradiation and blood administration should be minimized.

- In high-risk situations (newborn, infant requiring > 1blood volume, or irradiated blood), measure the potassium in the blood to be transfused.

Anaphylactic and anaphylactoid reactions

- *Anaphylactic reaction*
- *Anaphylactoid reactions*
- *Symptoms*
- *Treatment*

Anaphylactic reaction

Anaphylactic reaction is IgE-mediated reaction in which the allergen binds to an IgE antibody on the surface of a mast cell and basophil. This interaction leads to the release of histamine into the systemic circulation.

Re-exposure of the allergen results in activation of IgE-bound mast cells and basophils with the resultant release of preformed mediators that are stored in cellular granules (histamine, tryptase, heparin, chymase, cytokines). In addition, arachidonic acid is metabolized to prostaglandins and leukotrienes are also released.[15]

Anaphylactoid reactions

Anaphylactoid reactions are nonIgE mediated reactions. Clinically, these reactions cannot be distinguished from anaphylactic reactions.

Allergic reactions can potentially occur at any time in the perioperative period.

Anaphylaxis often produces signs and symptoms within minutes of exposure but there are also biphasic reactions that can occur 1–72 hours after the initial exposure.

Children and adolescents with atopy, including asthma, eczema, and allergic rhinitis, are at higher risk of anaphylaxis. The severity of previous reactions does not necessarily predict the severity of a subsequent reaction. Individuals with a previous anaphylactic reaction are at a higher risk for recurrence.

In the perioperative scenario the most common culprit is latex followed by antibiotics and neuromuscular blocking agent.[29]

Symptoms

Allergic reactions can have either minimal symptoms such as a rash, or a life-threatening reaction involving multiple organ systems known as anaphylaxis. The symptoms can include the cardiovascular, respiratory, cutaneous, and gastrointestinal systems.

(a) Cardiovascular: may manifest as hypotension, bradycardia or tachycardia, cardiac arrhythmias.

Cardiovascular collapse may be the first sign of anaphylaxis; there is increased vascular permeability, which results in large amounts of intravascular fluid shift into the extravascular space causing severe hypotension.

(b) Respiratory: wheezing, bronchospasm; there is abrupt loss or decrease in the $ETC0_2$ waveform.

(c) Gastrointestinal: nausea, vomiting, and diarrhea (not appreciable during anesthesia).

Treatment

Treatment of anaphylactic reactions consists of removal of the causative agent; maintaining oxygenation (100% FiO_2), and ventilation; cardiovascular support by early administration of epinephrine and fluids. Bronchospasm can be treated with beta-2 agonists. Epinephrine administration will treat both hypotension (via alpha stimulation) and bronchospasm (via beta stimulation) and is therefore the drug of choice for severe anaphylactic reactions. Corticosteroids are given, H1 antagonists are also recommended, but have a longer onset time.

Histamine and tryptase levels are elevated during anaphylaxis. It is recommended to obtain levels of both chemical mediators during anaphylaxis due to their correlation with severity of disease. Skin testing remains a gold standard of diagnosis and is more sensitive than testing IgE-specific antibodies.

After experiencing an anaphylactic reaction the patient and their family need to be educated; this includes prescription of an epinephrine auto injector.

Awareness and recall under anesthesia

- *Definition*
- *Incidence*
- *Assessing awareness*
- *Preventive measures*
- *BIS monitor*

Definition

- Awareness is the explicit recall of sensory perceptions during general anesthesia.
- Explicit memory allows for conscious recall of stored information.
- Implicit memory is unconscious and unintentional.
- In terms of anesthesia, being awake means being conscious.

Incidence

The incidence of awareness under anesthesia in pediatric patients is 0.6–2.7%, whereas in adults it is 0.05%. Risk factors in adults are related to obstetric procedures, anesthesia in the very sick, trauma, cardiac surgery, bronchoscopy, and paralysis. Awareness can lead to anxiety and post-traumatic stress disorder.

The Joint Commission on Accreditation of Health-care Organizations (JCAHO) has recommended that stringent efforts be made to prevent awareness.

Although the incidence of awareness appears to be higher in children, the characteristics appear to be milder and the long-term effects less. Psychosocial complications seem to be rare.[30]

Assessing awareness

The ability of the pediatric population to communicate and the development of the process of memory in these patients, poses problems in defining and evaluating awareness under anesthesia. Due to the difficulty in assessing young children, most awareness studies have been done in children 5 years and older.

Under general anesthesia rate and volume of ventilation in spontaneously breathing children, as well as heart rate and blood pressure, when increased, may indicate a physiologic response to awareness.[31–33]

Preventive measures

The first step in reducing awareness in children is to acknowledge that it occurs.

Perioperative measures include patient and equipment assessment, adequate intraoperative use of medications and monitors, supplemental induction doses if difficult intubation. Repeated airway manipulation has been shown to be a risk factor. Monitor the end-tidal concentrations of volatile agents, maintained at 1 MAC, and minimize muscle relaxant. Nitrous oxide and opioid anesthesia may be combined with a volatile agent to decrease the incidence of awareness. Benzodiazepam or dexmedetomidine can be administered if the volatile agent can't be increased.

BIS monitor

The FDA states that the use of BIS (bispectral index) monitoring to guide anesthetic administration may be associated with a reduction in the incidence of awareness with recall in adults. However, studies have shown that awareness can occur at a BIS value < 65. Bispectral index monitoring has been used in adults and has shown reduced incidence of awareness, but no such studies have been performed in pediatric patients. The BIS monitor is based on an adult EEG algorithm, and its use in small children and infants is not yet validated. An age-specific algorithm is not available due to the rapid changes in the developing brain of the growing child.[34]

Until we can more fully understand the causes of awareness and recall under anesthesia preventing this adverse event remains a challenge. Meanwhile operating room behavior should be modulated since patients tend to remember auditory perceptions.

Psychosocial complications

- *Stress*
- *Fear and anxiety*
- *Preparation*
- *Emergence delirium*
- *Recovery*

Stress

The perioperative period can be terrifying for pediatric patients and their parents. The anxiety occurring during this period is manifested by increased stress, nervousness, and fear of the unknown. Minimizing this stress should be a priority of the perioperative staff.[35]

When possible, both parents and children should be encouraged to participate in making decisions regarding care.

Factors such as age, temperament, and anxiety of the child and parents in the perioperative period are predictors for behavioral changes. Extreme anxiety during induction of anesthesia is also associated with an increase of postoperative behavioral changes. Certain procedures (tonsillectomy, urological procedures) have been shown to have a higher incidence of behavioral changes.

Maladaptive behaviors in the postoperative period are agitation, increased muscle tone, deep breaths, frightened face expression, shivers, silence, cessation of playing, feeding difficulty, sleep disturbances, new onset enuresis, and unexplained crying. Depending on the study, between 15% and 60% of children undergoing surgery have been shown to present negative behavioral changes at 2 weeks postoperatively; these changes generally fade over time.

The stress response leads to increase in serum cortisol, catecholamine, cytokines, and natural killer cell activity, which in turn provoke catabolism, delayed wound healing and postoperative immunosuppression.

Children are particularly vulnerable to the global surgical stress response because of limited energy reserves, larger brain masses, and obligatory glucose requirements.

Fear and anxiety

Significant preoperative fear affects 40–60% of young children.

Younger children are afraid of separation from their parents. The separation anxiety can be present at 7–8 months of age and peaks at 1 year of age. Younger children have difficulty in verbalizing their fear. Older children are more anxious about the pain they will experience, the anesthetic, and the surgery.

Different factors affecting preoperative anxiety:

- younger age (1–5 years)
- shy, withdrawn, with difficulties in adaptation
- social issues at home
- high cognitive awareness
- divorced parents
- anxious parents
- previous negative experience with hospital environment

Children undergoing one-day surgical procedures have demonstrated markedly lower levels of anxiety compared to those staying in the hospital setting overnight.

The pharmacological premedication substantially reduces anxiety and fears in children.

Preoperative anxiety is likely to:

- prolong the induction of anesthesia
- increase the incidence of emergence delirium,
- increase postoperative pain

Preparation

- Various methods reduce preoperative anxiety in children when in the holding area but have not been shown to decrease the incidence of stress during induction. Nevertheless parents should be provided with information and instructions regarding the procedure. Different information material (booklet, videos, orientation tours) for parents and older children are found to be helpful to facilitate trust between the child, the parent, and the providers.
- If IV access is needed preoperatively, local anesthetic creams should be used to prepare the skin. In some cases intravenous access-related stress is unavoidable when inhalation induction of anesthesia is contraindicated.
- Various medications are used for the treatment of preoperative anxiety. The most commonly used drug is midazolam, memory is impaired in about 10 min, and anxiolytic effect is apparent in 15 min of administration.
- The benefit of the presence of parents during intravenous placement and induction of anesthesia is disputable. Children brought to the operating room with their parents show lower levels of anxiety and results in better patient and parent satisfaction. Parents should be prepared and asked whether they are able to manage emotional stress when seeing their child going to sleep. Voiced concerns are disruption of induction, crowding of the OR, and additional stress on the anesthesiologist.[36,37]

Emergence delirium

Emergence delirium (ED) is defined as nonpurposeful restlessness and inconsolability.[38]

Emergence delirium can be very stressful for parent and caregiver to witness; thrashing, screaming, and disorientation are the hall marks. It is often of short duration and self-limiting. Pharmacological control may be needed to decrease the risk of harm. Opioids, midazolam, propofol, and dexmedetomidine have all been used. The etiology is not well understood.

Recognized risk factors are:

- age 2–5
- preoperative anxiety
- inhalational agents

Recovery

Parents should be allowed early in the PACU when the child is recovering from anesthesia.

Proper management of the postoperative pain in children is still a serious problem and is undertreated. Some physicians wrongly believe that neonates and small children do not feel pain, as their nervous systems are immature due to incomplete myelinization of nerve fibers.

The adequate treatment of pain accelerates the healing process and reduces stress, which results in shorter recovery period and better patient satisfaction.

Prevention and treatment of postoperative nausea and vomiting should be initiated. The PONV causes discomfort, delays hospital discharge, and reduces the patient and parent satisfaction.

References

1. M. Salvadore, T. Engelhardt, J. Tobias. Acute complications during anesthesia. In: B. Bissonnette, ed. *Pediatric Anesthesia. Basic Principals – State of the Art – Future*. Shelton, People's Medical Publishing House, USA 2011; 910–12.
2. C.E. Collins. Anesthesia for pediatric airway surgery: recommendations and review from a pediatric referral center. *Anesthesiol Clin* 2010; **28**(3): 505–17.
3. O.A. Olutoye, M. F. Watcha. Eyes, ears, nose, and throat surgery. In: G.E. Gregory and D.B. Andropoulos, eds. *Gregory's Pediatric Anesthesia*. 5th Edition, Oxford, Wiley Blackwell, UK 2012; 792–5.
4. C. McDonnell. Interventions guided by analysis of quality indicators decrease the frequency of laryngospasm during pediatric anesthesia. *Paediatr Anaesth* 2013; **23**(7): 579–87.
5. A.A. Al-alami, M.M. Zestos, A.S. Baraka. Pediatric laryngospasm: prevention and treatment. *Curr Opin Anaesthesiol* 2009 Jun; **22**(3): 388–95.
6. S.M. Bhananker, *et al*. Anesthesia-related cardiac arrest in children: update from the Pediatric Perioperative Cardiac Arrest Registry. *Anesth Analg* 2007 Aug; **105**(2): 344–50.
7. I. Landsman, J.A. Werkhaven, E.K. Motoyama. Anesthesia for pediatric otorhinolaryngologic surgery. In: P.J. Davis, F.P. Cladis, E.K. Motoyama, eds. *Smith's anesthesia for Infants and Children*. 8th ed, Philadelphia, PA. Elsevier Mosby USA 2011; 792–6.
8. J. Voigt, M. Waltzman, L. Lottenberg. Intraosseous vascular access for in-hospital emergency use: a systematic clinical review of the literature and analysis. *Pediatr Emerg Care* 2012; **28**(2): 185–99.
9. S.M. Rupp, J.L. Apfelbaum, C. Blitt, *et al*. Practice guidelines for central venous access: a report by the American Society of Anesthesiologists Task Force on Central Venous Access. *Anesthesiology* 2012 Mar; **116**(3): 539–73.
10. H. Owen, I. Waddell-Smith, Dental trauma associated with anesthesia. *Anaesth Intensive Care* 2000; **28**(2): 133–45.
11. M.C. Vallejo, *et al*. Perioperative dental injury at a tertiary care health system: An eight-year audit of 816,690 anesthetics. *J Healthc Risk Manag* 2012; **31**(3): 25–32.
12. J. Holzki, M. Laschat, C. Puder. Iatrogenic damage to the pediatric airway. Mechanisms and scar development. *Paediatr Anaesth*. 2009; **19** Suppl 1: 131–46.
13. S.J. Stratton. Prehospital Pediatric Endotracheal Intubation *Prehosp Dis Med*. 2012; **27**(1): 1–2.
14. M.B. Welch, C.M. Brummett, T.D. Welch *et al*. Perioperative peripheral nerve injuries: a retrospective study of 380,680 cases during a 10-year period at a single institution. *Anesthesiology* 2009; **111**: 490–7.
15. R. Flick. Clinical complications in pediatric anesthesia. In: G.A. Gregory, D.B. Andropoulos eds. *Gregory's Pediatric Anesthesia*, Fifth Edition. Blackwell Publishing Ltd 2012: 11252–82.
16. C. Ecoffey, F. Lacroix, E. Giaufré *et al*. Epidemiology and morbidity of regional anesthesia in children: a follow-up one-year prospective survey of the French-Language Society of Pediatric Anesthesiologists (ADARPEF). *Paediatr Anaesth* 2010; **20**: 1061–9.
17. D.M. Polaner, A.H. Taenzer, B.J. Walker, *et al*. LD. Pediatric Regional Anesthesia Network (PRAN): a multi-institutional study of the use and incidence of complications of pediatric regional anesthesia. *Anesth Analg* 2012; **115**: 1353–64.
18. P. Szmuk, J.W. Steiner, R.B, *et al*. Pop Intraocular pressure in pediatric patients during prone surgery. *Anesth Analg* 2013; **116**(6): 1309–13.
19. S.J. Tredwell, M. Wilmink, K. Inkpen, J.A. McEwen. Pediatric tourniquets: Analysis of cuff and limb interface, current practice,

and guidelines for use. *J Pediatr Orthop* 2001; **21**: 671–6.

20. O.O. Nafiu, T. Voepel-Lewis, M. Morris, *et al.* How do pediatric anesthesiologists define intraoperative hypotension? *Paediatr Anaesth* 2009; **19**: 1048–53.
21. M.R. Jongbloed, S.R. Vicente, N.D. Hahurij, *et al.* Normal and abnormal development of the cardiac conduction system; implications for conduction and rhythm disorders in the child and adult. *Differentiation* 2012; **84**(1): 131–48.
22. J.P. Morray, J.M. Geiduschek, C. Ramamoorthy, *et al.* Anesthesia-related cardiac arrest in children: initial findings of the Pediatric Perioperative Cardiac Arrest (POCA) Registry. *Anesthesiology* 2000 Jul; **93**(1): 6–14.
23. S.M. Bhananker, C. Ramamoorthy, J.M. Geiduschek, *et al.* Anesthesia-related cardiac arrest in children: update from the Pediatric Perioperative Cardiac Arrest Registry. *Anesth Analg* 2007 Aug; **105**(2): 344–50.
24. M.D. Berg, S.M. Schexnayder, L. Chameides, *et al.* Pediatric basic life support: 2010 American Heart Association Guidelines for Cardiopulmonary Resuscitation and Emergency Cardiovascular Care. American Heart Association. *Pediatrics* 2010; **126**(5): e1345–60.
25. A. de Caen, F. Bhanji, What's new in pediatric resuscitation? A practical update for the anesthesiologist. *Can J Anaesth* 2012; **59**(4): 341–7.
26. C. Ramamoorthy, C.M. Haberkern, S.M. Bhananker, *et al.* Anesthesia-related cardiac arrest in children with heart disease: data from the Pediatric Perioperative Cardiac Arrest (POCA) registry. *Anesth Analg* 2010; **110**(5): 1376–82.
27. J.P. Morray. Cardiac arrest in anesthetized children: recent advances and challenges for the future. *Paediatr Anaesth* 2011 Jul; **21**(7): 722–9.
28. A.C. Lee, L.L. Reduque, N.L. Luban, *et al.* Transfusion-associated hyperkalemic cardiac arrest in pediatric patients receiving massive transfusion. *Transfusion* 2013 Apr 15. doi: 10.1111/trf.12192. [Epub ahead of print]
29. L. G. Maxwell, S.R. Goodwin, T. J. Mancuso, *et al.* In: P.J. David, F.P. Cladis, E.K. Motoyama eds. Associated Problems in Pediatric Anesthesia, *Miscellaneous Problems Smith's, Anesthesia for Infants and Children.* 8th ed, Elsevier Mosby USA 2011; 1165–72.
30. A. Davidson, K. Howard, W. Brown, *et al.*Preoperative Evaluation and Preparation, Anxiety, Awareness, and Behavior Change. In: G. Gregory, D.B. Andropoulos eds. *Gregory's Pediatric Anesthesia.* 5th ed, Blackwell Publishing Ltd 2012; 273–99.
31. A.J. Davidson, G. Huang, C. Czarnecki, *et al.* Awareness during anesthesia in children: a prospective cohort study. *Anesth Analg* 2005; **100**: 653–61.
32. U. Lopez, W. Habre, M. Laurencon, *et al.* Intra-operative awareness in children: the value of an interview adapted to their cognitive abilities. *Anaesthesia* 2007; **62**: 778–89.
33. S. Malviya, J. Galinkin, C. Bannister, *et al.* The incidence of intraoperative awareness in children: childhood awareness and recall evaluation. *Anesth Analg* 2009; **109**: 1421–7.
34. I. Murat, I. Constant. Bispectral index in pediatrics: fashion or a new tool? *Paediatr Anaesth* 2005; **15**: 177–80.
35. M.E. McCann, Z.N. Kain. The management of preoperative anxiety in children: an update. *Anesth Analg* 2001 Jul; **93**(1): 98–105.
36. J. Litke, A. Pikulska, T. Wegner. Management of perioperative stress in children and parents. Part I–the preoperative period. *Anaesthesiol Intensive Ther* 2012 Jul-Sep; **44**(3): 165–9.
37. J. Litke, A. Pikulska, T. Wegner. Management of perioperative stress in children and parents. Part II–anaesthesia and postoperative period. *Anaesthesiol Intensive Ther* 2012 Jul-Sep; **44**(3): 170–4.
38. I.T. Cohen, N. Deutsch, E.K. Motoyama. Induction, maintenance, and recovery, common problems in the postanesthetic care unit. In P.J. David, F.P. Cladis, E.K. Motoyama eds. *Smith's, Anesthesia for Infants and Children.* 8th ed, Elsevier Mosby USA 2011; 388–93.

Chapter

31 Special techniques and situations

Rahul Dasgupta and Hani Hanna

Controlled hypotension

- Controlled hypotension is generally used to reduce surgical blood loss or provide a "bloodless" operating field.[(1)]
- Typically it is accomplished with vasodilators, beta-blockers, deep inhalational anesthesia, or calcium channel blockers.
- Longer-acting medications (beta blockade, inhalation agent) may be suitable in procedures in which there is little risk for rapid blood loss; however, rapidly reversible medications (nitroglycerin/sodium nitroprusside) are more prudent to use in procedures that have a high risk for blood loss.[(1)]
- Controlled hypotension has disparate effects on each of the major organ systems.
- Neurologic:
  - Studies of adults have shown a MAP of 55 mmHg or higher with normocarbia ($PaCO_2$ 35–45 mmHg) results in mild or no decreases in cerebral metabolism. Some authors recommend the above as a standard; however, it appears children can tolerate lower pressures on an age-related basis. Normocarbia is extremely important to maintain as CBF is directly correlated with it (in adults it is noted that a 1 mmHg increase in $PaCO_2$ will increase CBF 2 ml/100 g/min).[(1)]
  - All volatile anesthetic agents decrease the cerebral metabolic rate and increase cerebral blood flow with isoflurane causing the largest decrease in cerebral metabolic rate.[(1)]
  - Calcium channel blockers and vasodilators (nitroglycerin/sodium nitroprusside) tend to cause regional increases in cerebral blood flow despite systemic hypotension and thus are not a good choice in children with ICP.[(1)]
  - Controlled hypotension had been shown to be safe in reduction of blood loss for posterior spinal fusion. If there is a risk of aortic dissection and commensurate decrease in spinal cord blood flow, hypotensive anesthesia may be contraindicated.[(1)]
- Cardiovascular:
  - All vasodilators will improve cardiac function as they reduce afterload. It also important to realize coronary blood flow autoregulates to some degree based on metabolic demand but is largely dependent on diastolic blood pressure.
  - Many authors feel vasodilating (sodium nitroprusside/nitroglycerin) drugs offer more control of blood pressure without negative inotropy as opposed to volatile agents or beta-blockers. Also the rapid reversibility of the these drugs is useful in procedures where large and rapid blood loss is common.[(1)]
- Renal:
  - Blood flow to the kidneys autoregulates between a MAP of 80–180 mmHg; however, general anesthesia may ablate this response to some degree.
  - Sodium nitroprusside, nitroglycerin, calcium channel blockers appear to maintain renal blood flow while causing systemic hypotension.[(1)]
  - Pulmonary: Pulmonary blood flow is usually decreased by all vasodilators secondary to increased pooling of blood in the peripheral circulation.[(1)]

Essentials of Pediatric Anesthesiology, ed. Alan David Kaye, Charles James Fox and James H. Diaz. Published by Cambridge University Press. © Cambridge University Press 2015.

- Hepatic:
  - The liver receives most of its oxygen from the hepatic artery but most of the blood flow to the liver comes from the portal vein; any changes in portal vein flow can have dramatic effects on hepatic function.
  - Studies have shown hepatic blood flow and oxygenation is maintained during controlled hypotension if the $PaCO_2$ is within normal physiologic range and a adequate blood volume is maintained.[2]
- Monitoring may change depending on the goals of the procedure in which controlled hypotension is used. If main objective is to lower perfusion pressure to improve operating conditions an arterial line may suffice but if the goal is to reduce surgical blood loss then CVP monitoring and an arterial line may be warranted.[1]
- The addition of a drug with vasodilating properties (e.g., morphine) may be useful in the premedication of a patient undergoing hypotensive anesthesia.
- A balanced mix of volatile agents and a vasodilating agent (nitroglycerin/sodium nitroprusside/short acting beta blocker or calcium channel blocker) is best as an anesthetic technique based purely on volatile agents may cause profound cardiac depression.[3]
- Short-acting beta blockers are not recommended in patients 2 years of age or younger, as cardiac output is heart rate dependent in this age group. Also beta blockers may cause hypoglycemia and thus glucose levels must be evaluated periodically.[1]
- Monitoring should include pulse oximetry, $etCO_2$, ECG, temperature, CVP, MAP, and ABGs at specific intervals to evaluate hematocrit, blood glucose, and acid–base status.
- Arterial line pressures are typically taken from the radial artery although femoral arterial lines are adequate as well. Dorsalis pedis arterial lines have been noted to be inaccurate in the literature and thus should be used with caution.[4]
- Once the desired MAP has been achieved, CVP should be recorded and maintained throughout the procedures to ensure the patient is normovolemic.
- Urine output should be monitored and be at least 0.5 to 1 ml/kg/h. Urine output is a simple way to determine if renal perfusion is adequate.[1]
- Once the patient's blood pressure is lowered and the surgical field is deemed bloodless by the surgeon the MAP should be raised slightly until bleeding develops. The MAP may then be reduced slightly until bleeding stops again. This method allows the anesthesia provider to maintain a MAP that is many times only 10–20% lower from the patient's baseline MAP.[1]
- It is important to position the patient so that the surgical field is the highest point so that one can take advantage of gravity to decrease blood entering the field. Also one must check to see that venous compression is minimal from positioning (i.e., abdominal pressure from padding) as this can raise venous pressure and contribute to increased bleeding.
- Hemoglobin levels must be maintained to ensure the patient's oxygen carrying capacity is not compromised. Although no conclusive studies have been done on children regarding optimal hemoglobin values, many authors recommend a level of no lower than 10 g/dl during controlled hypotension.[1]
- Relative contraindications to hypotensive anesthesia are presence of systemic disease-compromising organ function (atherosclerosis, autoimmune diseases, unrepaired cyanotic heart disease, etc.) and provider inexperience.

Controlled hypothermia

- Hypothermia (defined as a core body temperature less than 36 °C) has been shown to be beneficial in certain areas such as hypoxic ischemic brain injury, head trauma, CPB, deep hypothermic circulatory arrest, and neurosurgery.[5]
- Mild induced hypothermia (32–34 °C) has been associated with improved outcomes in adults suffering cardiac arrest and may improve patient outcomes in neonates afflicted with hypoxic–ischemic encephalopathy.[5]
- For every one degree Celsius decrease in body temperature the cerebral metabolic rate decreases about 7 percent, by nonspecifically slowing biochemical reactions as release of excitatory amino acids. This becomes useful in cardiac or intercranial vascular surgery where cerebral blood may be interrupted or deranged. In cardiac surgery moderate hypothermia is most often utilized (26–32 °C); however, patients are cooled to as low as 18–20 °C if total circulatory arrest is employed.[6]

- Of note while both hypothermia and hypocarbia may decrease cerebral blood flow, only hypothermia maintains the coupling of metabolism and cerebral blood flow. With hypocarbia cerebral blood flow is reduced below metabolic demand, which can lead to cerebral ischemia.[6]
- It is important to keep the negative effects of hypothermia in the perioperative period in mind as well. Intraoperative hypothermia has been associated with many adverse consequences, including cardiac complications (i.e., myocardial ischemia, arrhythmias), increased infection risk, impaired coagulation, and increased need for blood transfusions, electrolyte abnormalities, delayed drug clearance (particularly muscle relaxants), and high incidences of apnea and bradycardia in the neonatal population. Finally, it is well documented that children tend to lose heat more rapidly than adults.[6]

Management of laparoscopic surgery

- Advantages of the laparoscopic approach include minimizing the size of the incision, better visualization of the surgical area, more rapid recovery, early discharge from the hospital, better pain control and fewer postoperative pulmonary complications. Laparoscopic procedures are done in children of all ages and neonates. These include many procedures such as exploration for undescended testicles, hernias, pyloromyotomy, appendectomy, cholecystectomy, Nissen fundoplication, colectomy, pyeloplasty, bowel pull-through, nephrectomy, splenectomy, and staging cancer.[7]
- Carbon dioxide is the preferred gas because it does not support combustion, is rapidly cleared from the peritoneal cavity at the end of surgery, and does not expand bubbles or spaces. However it is rapidly absorbed from the peritoneum (infants > adults), and hypercapnea can occur, necessitating an increase in minute ventilation.
- Excess carbon dioxide may initiate a sympathetic response with increase in heart rate and blood pressure, causing an increase in cerebral blood flow, and may precipitate ventricular arrhythmias.
- Use of N_2O may not be ideal as it expands gas-filled cavities like bowel lumen and obscures the view of the surgical site.
- Intra-abdominal pressure created by the pneumoperitoneum ranges from 6 to 20 mmHg.
- The stomach must be decompressed with an orogastric or nasogastric tube after tracheal intubation to enhance the view of the upper abdominal contents.[7]
- **Pulmonary effects**
  - Increase in intra-abdominal pressure from insufflation coupled with head down-position causes cephalad displacement of the diaphragm, decreasing the FRC, compressing the lungs and causing collapse of the small alveoli, creating V/Q mismatch and hypoxemia. Keeping FIO_2 in excess of 30% together with a small amount of PEEP is desirable. The peak inspiratory pressure rises and lung compliance decreases following pneumoperitoneum.[8]
  - Gas tracking across the diaphragm may cause pneumomediastinum (subcutaneous emphysema) or pneumothorax.
- **Airway**
  - Requires tracheal intubation with cuffed ETT and controlled ventilation adjusted to the end-tidal carbon dioxide concentration.
  - Tip of the tube can migrate toward the carina leading to endobronchial intubation.
- **Cardiovascular effects**
  - Hemodynamic changes in response to pneumoperitoneum differ, depending on patient's volume status, cardiac status, and positioning
  - Pneumoperitoneum causes decrease in cardiac output, increase in afterload, systemic, and pulmonary vascular resistance especially with high intra-abdominal pressure (IAP) > 15, however with an IAP < 10 the impact on hemodynamics should be clinically insignificant.
  - Head up position (25–30 °) as in Nissen fundoplication reduces venous return, and cardiac output may lead to hypotension and hypoxemia.
  - High IAP decreases renal blood flow and diminishes urine output.
  - Intravenous access may be obtained above the diaphragm because a pneumoperitoneum can decrease the blood flow through the IVC and delay drug and fluid administration.[7]

- **Neurologic effects**
  - The intracranial pressure is increased following insufflation due to a combination of factors: increased IAP, high SVR, hypercapnea, and Trendelenberg position.
  - Patency of VP shunt should be assessed prior to surgery.[8]

Perioperative management of the intensive care unit patient

- The overarching aim of the PICU is to stabilize and treat critically ill patients. Frequently these patients may need surgical procedures and thus require anesthesia. While the breadth of pathology one encounters in the PICU patient population is vast there are frequently encountered disease states. Knowledge of appropriate management of these disease states can speed patient recovery whereas inappropriate management may negate or cause treatment efforts to stagnate.
- A thorough sign-out at the beginning of transport from and at the delivery back to the PICU is useful to the anesthesiologist and PICU team alike. Typically, important items as allergies, cardiorespiratory status, venous and arterial access, IV induction agents, intubation/mask ventilation information, fluid totals (blood products/urine output/estimated blood loss/crystalloids/colloids) medications administered/continued (antibiotics, inotropes), and intraoperative complications should be discussed.[9]
- Many critically ill patients are on inotropes and vasoconstrictors. Familiarity with correct dosing and mechanism of action and side effects of each drug is crucial.
- Understanding PALS and ACLS (should the child be a young adult) is important as perioperative malignant arrhythmias are not infrequent in PICU patients.
- Shock:
  - Shock can be defined as a mismatch between the oxygen demand by tissues and oxygen supply via tissue blood perfusion; it occurs when perfusion of blood to tissues is inadequate.
  - One common classification scheme for shock (with examples of each subtype in parentheses) is the following:
    - Hypovolemic (traumatic blood loss, severe GI losses as in intractable diarrhea)
    - Cardiogenic (myocardial infarction, stunning after CPB)
    - Extracardiac (pericardial effusion, mediastinal masses)
    - Distributive shock (sepsis, anaphylaxis, adrenal insufficiency)
  - Therapy goals for shock include quick recognition and rapid initial crystalloid replacement (20 cc/kg boluses up to 60 cc/kg). If it is refractory to fluid, central venous access should be established and dopamine infusion started up to 10 μg/kg/min.
  - If refractory to dopamine then epinephrine (cold shock) or norepinephrine (warm shock) is recommended, and hydrocortisone should be considered if adrenal insufficiency is a concern.
- Asthma:
  - Asthma is an inflammatory condition in which the airway submucosa is infiltrated with mast cells, eosinophils, and lymphocytes causing edema, mucus production, and plugging and leukocyte chemotaxis.
  - Asthma attacks have many triggers including viral and bacterial infections, allergens, and changes in weather conditions.
  - Treatment for asthma is multifactorial and can include many different drugs:
    - Supplemental oxygen (nasal cannula, facemask or BiPAP in selected patients), increasing FiO_2 in ventilated patients
    - Beta-receptor agonists: Inhaled (albuterol/xopenex) or IV (terbutaline)
    - Corticosteroids: Methylprednisolone preferred due to limited mineralocorticoid effects, but dexamethasone or hydrocortisone can be used
    - Methylxanthines: aminophylline
    - Magnesium (bronchial smooth muscle relaxant)
    - Helium (improves laminar flow around bronchial obstruction but since 70%

  helium/30% oxygen mixture required is limited by hypoxemia)
  - Ketamine (dissociative anesthetic that causes bronchodilation but increases secretions and may cause dysphoria)
  - Intubation and mechanical ventilation (patients needing intubation may have low pulmonary reserve and need to decompensate quickly, ketamine/ benzodiazepine and fluid boluses may be useful on induction, shorter-acting muscle relaxants preferred to allow patients to be reversible and return to spontaneous ventilation quickly)
  - Inhalational anesthetics: isoflurane is a potent bronchodilator, but technical aspects as ready access to vaporizers in the ICU may limit use
  - Extracorporeal life support: used in near fatal cases of asthma as a last resort

- Acute lung injury (ALI) and acute respiratory distress syndrome (ARDS):
  - ALI and ARDS are defined as the the acute occurrence of bilateral infiltrates on chest X-ray without evidence of left ventricle dysfunction/left atrial hypertension and a decreased PaO_2/FIO_2 (PF) ratio.
  - PF ratio of ≤ 300 is considered ALI.
  - PF ratio of ≤ 200 is considered ARDS.
  - Associated with significant mortality (> 22%).
  - Treatment guidelines include:
    - identifying underlying trigger (infection, pancreatitis) and requisite antibiotic therapy
    - tolerating hypercarbia/respiratory acidosis in ventilator management (pH 7.35–7.45 acceptable)
    - using tidal volumes less than 10 cc/kg and plateau pressures less than 30 cmH_2O in ventilator management
    - and incorporating fluid restriction after the patient is restored to euvolemia

- Intracranial pressure (ICP):
  - In the presence of closed cranial suture lines, ICP normally is determined by the total volume brain tissue, cerebral spinal fluid (CSF), and blood. Pathologic conditions such as tumors and foreign body also can contribute to ICP.
  - If there is obstruction to CSF or blood drainage ICP can rise. Compensatory mechanisms against the initial increase in ICP include redistribution of CSF to the spinal cord and increased absorption via the arachnoid villi.
  - ICP increase when the compensatory mechanisms are exhausted.
  - Symptoms of ICP may include nausea, vomiting, headache, and findings such as hypertension with reflex bradycardia.
  - Basic management of increased ICP involves:
    - Head elevation to 30 degress (improves venous drainage)
    - Adequate sedation, with the addition of muscle relaxants to avoid coughing (increases ICP)
    - If intubated, setting minute ventilation to ensure a $PaCO_2$ of 34–36 mmg and avoiding hypoxemia ($PaO_2 > 60$)
    - Cerebral perfusion pressure (CPP) is equal to mean arterial pressure (MAP) minus the ICP or the central venous pressure (CVP), whichever is higher. MAP may need to be increased through inotropes or intravascular volume replacement if either the ICP is increased.
  - As a 1 degree Celsius increase in temperature will cause the cerebral metabolism to increase 7%, temperature should be monitored and fever treated aggressively.
  - To limit large increases in CVP, IV fluids are decreased to 2/3 maintenance, and are isotonic. Hyperglycemia should be avoided and diuretics may be used to decrease intercranial volume.
- Status epilepticus:
  - Defined as a seizure > 30 min in duration or recurring seizures with such frequency that there is no noted return of consciousness between each seizure.
  - Initial care is supportive (monitoring vitals, maintaining the airway, intubation if necessary).

- Treatment with a benzodiazepine, such as lorazepam, is typically first-line therapy.
- Electrolyte levels including glucose, calcium, and magnesium should be measured and, if abnormal, treated.
- If seizures persist treatment with an additional dose of a benzodiazepine in combination with barbiturate and/or phenytoin may work. If seizures still continue to persist consultation with a pediatric neurologist is recommended.

- Sickle cell disease:
  - The most common hemoglobinopathy is hemoglobin S/sickle cell trait.
  - Hemoglobin S is caused by a mutation in the beta-chain which causes glutamine to be replaced by valine at a particular point in the chain. Abnormal beta-chains combine with alpha chains to form hemoglobin S.
  - If a patient is homozygous for the sickle cell disease it can cause loss of deformability or "sickling" in red blood cells in a deoxygenated state. These sickled cells can block blood vessels and infarct organ systems throughout the body. Most commonly the CNS, kidney, spleen, lungs, and bones are affected.
  - Sickle cell crises can be caused by infection, dehydration, acidosis, or hypoxia. Certain infections such as parvovirus b19 can also predispose one to crisis.
  - Acute chest syndrome is a particularly serious sickle cell crisis in which the pulmonary vasculature is affected by sickled RBCs.
  - Treatment of sickle crises focuses on supportive therapy with oxygen, IV hydration, and antibiotic treatment for infectious causes. If anemia is present a PRBC transfusion may help but exchange transfusions may be needed. Typically a hemoglobin of at least 10 g/dl is desirable.
- Stress hyperglycemia:
  - Hyperglycemia is quite common in critical illness and may result from illness-induced insulin resistance, increased production of glucose or undue administration of dextrose containing intravenous fluids.
  - As intensive insulin protocols appear to cause higher rates of hypoglycemia many PICUs have relaxed serum glucose targets of 80–180 mg/dL.
- Intrahospital transport of the PICU patient:
  - Intrahospital transport is defined as transport of patients within the hospital, as opposed to interhospital transport which refers to transport between different hospitals.
  - Risk/benefit ratio should be noted first; is transport of a critically ill patient worth the risk of the imaging or procedure to be done?
  - Generally the higher-risk patients include those who are intubated and have central/ arterial lines in situ.
  - Many times the transport team includes nurses, respiratory therapists, and patient care technologists in addition to the physician.
  - Transport monitors with the ability to monitor blood pressure, heart rate and rhythm, and SpO_2 are suggested for use while the patient is moved All medicine and equipment necessary to resuscitate the patient should be taken with the transport team.
  - If a patient is intubated the anesthesiologist should provide adequate sedation and avoid overaggressive hand ventilation during transport.[9]

References

1. Cote CJ, Dsida RM. Strategies for blood product management and transfusion reaction. In Cote CJ, editor. *A Practice of Anesthesia for Infants and Children*. 3rd edn. Philadelphia: Saunders; 2001. pp. 249–55.
2. Chauvin M, Bonnet F, Motembault C. Hepatic plasma flow during nitroprusside-induced hypotension in humans. *Anesthesiology*. 1985 Sep; **63**(3): 287–93.
3. Hersey SL, O'Dell NE, Lowe S. Nicardipine versus nitroprusside for controlled hypotension during spinal surgery in adolescents. *Anesthesia and Analgesia*. 1997 Jun; **84**(6): 1239–44.
4. Abou-Madi M, Lenis S, Archer D. Comparison of direct blood pressure measurements at the radial and dorsalis pedis arteries during sodium nitroprusside and isoflurane induced hypotension. *Anesthesiology*. 1986 Dec; **65**(6): 692–5.
5. Kilbaugh TJ, Topjian AA, Sutton RM, Nadkarni VM, Berg RA. Cardiopulmonary resuscitation.

In Gregory GA, Andropoulos DB, editors. *Gregory's Pediatric Anesthesia*. 5th edn. West Sussex, UK: Blackwell Publishing; 2012. pp. 262–4.

6. Brady KM, Easley B, Bissonnette B. Developmental physiology of the central nervous system. In Gregory GA, Andropoulos DB, editors. *Gregory's Pediatric Anesthesia*. 5th edn. West Sussex, UK: Blackwell Publishing; 2012. pp. 135–6.

7. Andropoulos DB, Mann D, Garcia PJ. Anesthesia for abdominal surgery. In Gregory GA, Andropoulos DB, editors. *Gregory's Pediatric Anesthesia*. 5th edn. West Sussex, UK: Blackwell Publishing; 2012. Pp. 736–8.

8. Davis PJ, Cladis FP, Motoyama EK. Respiratory physiology in infants and children. Davis PJ, Cladis FP, Motoyama EK, editors. *Smith's Anesthesia for General Abdominal, Thoracic, Urologic, and Bariatric Surgery*. 8th edn. Philadelphia. Elsevier Health Sciences Publishing; 2010. pp. 562–3.

9. Ross P, Bart R, Wetzel R. Pediatric intensive care. In Gregory GA, Andropoulos DB, editors. *Gregory's Pediatric Anesthesia*. 5th edn. West Sussex, UK: Blackwell Publishing; 2012. pp. 946–92.

Chapter 32

Anesthesia for remote locations

Joel A. Saltzman

The role of anesthesia outside the operating room has continued to grow exponentially, especially in the pediatric population.[1] While practitioners make the transportation of their expertise appear smooth and seamless, it can be fraught with danger, morbidity, and mortality unless due diligence is taken to assure safety in an uncommon location.[2–4] The usual control and comfort of the operating room setting must not be taken for granted when attempting to provide safe sedation or anesthesia in an off-site location. With appropriate preparation and education of the team, the practitioner can avoid the feeling of being alone on an island.

The nursing and specialty technicians in each location need to be familiar with the procedural plan, backup plan, and assumption of risks and benefits. Mock run-throughs with input from all team members will result in smoother procedures once the patient is on the table. Procedures outside the operating room require collaboration among the ordering physician, the physician, or technician providing the test, the team, and the anesthesia provider.[5] After a complete preanesthesia history and physical examination are performed, a gradation of sedation can be offered to optimize safe completion of the procedure. Based on the patient's medical condition and comorbidities, an anesthesia plan should be discussed with the provider and the family. Careful consideration must be taken to know when the risk-to-benefit ratio does not favor proceeding or requires rescheduling of the procedure. Similar consideration should be given to the efficacy of performing the procedure as an outpatient or inpatient procedure. While the procedure itself may not require overnight observation, the addition of anesthesia to the patient's medical condition might warrant it. The family, the ordering physician, and the anesthesia provider need to consider the effect of anesthesia on the patient's underlying medical conditions.

Educating the family and the patient (when age-appropriate) is essential to a successful outcome. Utilization of child life specialists to educate and calm the fears of the patient and family is an outstanding resource. Their training allows them to facilitate the placement of intravenous (IV) lines, assess levels of anxiety, and identify patients who may not require anesthesia for certain procedures. Families may not understand that their children are about to undergo anesthesia to allow for optimizing the test or procedure. They often believe or were told that their children would be in "twilight sleep," and they need to be educated for appropriate understanding. Each patient's plan should be individualized, and hence not perceived by the family as a protocol approach that may or may not apply to their child.

Extreme care must be taken to assure that providers do not find themselves in a "this is how they usually do it" situation. Adherence to hospital policy, society guidelines, and best practice guidelines are paramount. A range of sedation, from minimal medication and reassurance to full general anesthesia, should be an option. Regardless of the starting point, there needs to be the ability to advance to a higher level of care without risk to the patient, allowing for completion of the procedure or test.

The same diligence and concern provided for every anesthetic in the operating room must also be provided in an off-site location. Parents and ordering services need to understand the importance of the preanesthesia process, which includes adequate time for the preanesthesia history and maintenance of *nil per os* (NPO) standards. Immediate preprocedure assessment, consent, appropriate time out[6] (confirmation of correct patient, physician, procedure,

Essentials of Pediatric Anesthesiology, ed. Alan David Kaye, Charles James Fox and James H. Diaz. Published by Cambridge University Press. © Cambridge University Press 2015.

location), and adherence to monitoring standards are all equally important in the off-site setting. Prior to beginning any anesthetic or procedure, identification of the patient's recovery location is important. Some institutions require all patients undergoing sedation or anesthesia to recover in the postanesthesia care unit (PACU). This may require additional planning for patient transportation post-procedure, including identifying members of the transport team. Patients should be transported with appropriate monitors, oxygen, Ambu Bag or Jackson–Rees (bag/mask ventilation), and rescue medications. A transport box and a checklist should be included. An alternative is to create a recovery location in proximity to the procedure area. The post-procedure recovery area should maintain the same standards and quality as the PACU. This will require that nurses have the appropriate skills and training to function competently as PACU nurses in the immediate post-procedure period. All patients prior to discharge need to meet PACU standards based on Aldrete scores.[7,8] A postanesthesia evaluation is required, including but not limited to: cardiopulmonary status, mental status, temperature, pain, nausea and vomiting, and hydration.

A significant number of the procedures and studies will involve outpatients. A process to contact the families via telephone or email will provide an opportunity to resolve issues and provide reassurance.

Equipment and safety

Off-site locations introduce a cadre of challenges, especially regarding equipment and safety. Comprehensive planning and run-through before the patient arrives will promote increased safety and comfort for the patient and the team. With proper planning and anticipation of worst-case scenarios, one can avoid the "island effect" and the need to utter the words, "Quick, get me..." Each location will have special needs and restrictions that will be discussed in specific sections to follow.

A generalized approach to safety is universal with regard to monitors, equipment, and medication, whether in the operating room, MRI (magnetic resonance imaging) or CT (computed tomography) scanner laboratories, GI (gastrointestinal) laboratory, or other locations. In anticipation of the need to go to a higher level of care, all locations should have a full anesthesia set-up available.[9–11] Not every institution has an anesthesia machine at each location; this may limit the ability to provide the level of care needed to complete the procedure and result in cancellations. In order to increase comfort and familiarity, the anesthesia provider should have an anesthesia cart as similar as possible to the one routinely used in the operating room at each location. This does not eliminate the need for a crash cart, which also needs to be in each location. The provider and the team should identify the location of the emergency equipment prior to beginning any procedure.

The anesthesia cart should provide standard medications, airway equipment, fluids, syringes, needles, and the ability to advance to a higher level of care. Additional equipment may need to be added to allow for special needs. While a nasal cannula with end-tidal CO_2 measurement may not routinely be used in the operating room, it is standard airway equipment in an off-site location. Regardless of the level of sedation or anesthesia required, at the minimum monitors should include: pulse oximetry, end-tidal CO_2, temperature, pulse, and blood pressure.

Understanding the duration of the procedure and the anticipated position of the patient will allow for a better understanding of additional equipment needed. Thermoregulation in off-site locations can be difficult; however, it is very important, especially in the pediatric population. Each off-site location often presents interesting challenges to maintaining temperature, but general principles to avoid hypothermia by understanding and controlling heat loss remain constant. While the primary concern is hypothermia, some procedures and locations can lend themselves to hyperthermia. Prolonged MRIs can result in patients' temperatures increasing during the procedure. Well-insulated patients with minimal areas exposed during procedures can experience increases as well.

Positioning, duration, and exposure are additional safety factors to consider during off-site procedures. While the operating room staff may be accustomed to a patient in a prone or a lateral position, it is not standard in a CT scan, the catheterization laboratory, or the gastrointestinal procedure laboratory. A head-to-toe examination after patient positioning, prior to draping, must be completed and proper positioning confirmed to avoid injury. Many off-site procedures involve the use of X-rays, and care must be taken to provide safe conditions for the patient and the staff. Lead aprons can be placed over the patient as the procedure allows. All team members should be protected with lead aprons and thyroid shields and should wear badges to monitor exposure.

Practitioners with recurrent exposure should consider the addition of lead glasses. Location-specific safety issues will be discussed in each respective section.

The goal of obtaining a safe and successful study often hinges on management of the airway with minimal instrumentation. Unless indicated by the patient's medical condition or the requirements of the study, intubation and controlled ventilation is not routinely required. Delivery of supplemental oxygen and measurement of end-tidal CO_2 can be obtained by a nasal cannula designed to perform both tasks. Availability of nasal and oral airway adjuncts can assist with pharyngeal hypotonia causing airway obstruction. Simple airway repositioning and the addition of a jaw strap or tape may alleviate the obstruction. The ability to advance to a higher level of care, including but not limited to intubation and controlled ventilation, must always be considered and explained to the family prior to the start of the procedure. Preparing the family for the realistic probability of these events will allow for greater acceptance and understanding. Airway emergencies need equal consideration in the off-site location as in the operating room. The anesthesia provider may have a level of comfort in the operating room dealing with airway obstruction or laryngospasm that is more difficult to achieve in the off-site location. Early recognition of trouble and availability of equipment and medication will prevent patient harm. The possibility of laryngospasm at the beginning or end of the procedure should always be considered; however, it is equally possible they may occur during the procedure secondary to secretions. Standard techniques need to be rapidly available to override the spasm. The ability to deliver positive-pressure ventilation, medications for deepening the anesthetic and/or providing muscle relaxation, and suction should be included in standard preparations at any off-site location.

Personnel in all locations need the ability to handle unforeseen emergencies, including airway difficulties, allergic reactions, and malignant hyperthermia. Standardized laminated protocols and a malignant hyperthermia kit or cart will prevent unnecessary delays and increased complications. The ability to perform CPR or to follow pediatric advanced life support (PALS)[12] protocols takes on an entirely different dimension in an off-site location. Crash cart proximity and mock run-throughs will help prepare teams for emergencies and individuals to understand their roles, increasing teamwork, and optimal safety for the patient.

Medications

Medications should be chosen to safely optimize studies with minimal patient movement and anxiety. Numerous medication protocols in the literature involve administration of agents alone or in combination, and include protocols for chloral hydrate, propofol, pentobarbital, midazolam, ketamine, dexmedetomidine, and narcotics.[13–21] These protocols may be used as long as one individualizes the process to account for each patient's needs and keeps in mind that not moving is good, and not breathing is bad. Combination or "cocktail" anesthesia requires increased vigilance for unexpected reactions or changes in levels of anesthesia. Patients with developmental delays and other comorbidities may require decreased sedation dosages. Combinations of medications may allow for ideal conditions, decreases in total medication given, and rapid return to baseline when given carefully and judiciously. Significant literature compares and contrasts various cocktails of medications having the common goal of increasing effect and decreasing side effects.[22] As with any guidelines, individualizing for the patient's medical condition and titration to effect are key to safe administration. The following dosages are guidelines for medications delivered individually.

Chloral hydrate has a long history of use in the pediatric population. Although some respiratory depression has been reported at higher doses, it is considered a safe oral or rectal medication in young children. Unfortunately, recent shortages have made alternatives necessary. Dosage: 25–75 mg/kg orally or rectally; reports of up to 100 mg/kg with a maximum dosage of 2 grams have been reported.[16]

Midazolam, while an excellent anxiolytic, may not provide an adequate level of anesthesia to prevent movement during a procedure if given alone. Those patients requiring minimal medication and appropriate reassurance from their parents or child life specialist may do very well. Midazolam has been reported to decrease or eliminate the nightmares reported with ketamine and may be an appropriate premedication.[14] Dosage: 0.04–0.1 mg/kg IV; 0.5–1 mg/kg PO (bitter taste, flavored options available); 0.2–0.4 mg/kg nasal spray (burning sensation and bitter taste).

Ketamine is frequently used in patients with cardiovascular or respiratory concerns. Providing minimal respiratory depression and no drop in systemic vascular resistance, it is a common medication choice in patients with complex cardiopulmonary histories.

The trade-offs are increased salivation, post-procedure hypertension, tachycardia, emergence delirium, and nightmares. Most studies utilize midazolam and either glycopyrrolate or atropine when ketamine is used.[23] Dosage: 1–2 mg/kg IV; 5–10 mg/kg IM; 4–10 mg/kg oral; 3–8 mg/kg intranasal dosages.

Propofol appears to have become the most commonly used medication for nonpainful procedural or study anesthesia. The ability to titrate to effect and its rapid recovery profile make it ideal for a number of off-site locations. Numerous articles and studies use propofol as a comparison medication to the newest medication or combination of medications.[22,24,25] As with all medications, the addition of additional agents may have a synergistic effect, requiring a decrease in dosage to avoid respiratory depression. Some patients may become mildly hypotensive because of NPO guidelines and volume status, and IV fluids and appropriate decreases in dosage may be required. Dosage: 1–2 mg/kg to obtain optimum conditions, followed by an infusion of 5–10 mg/kg/h. Infusion rate may need to be increased or decreased in patients on other medications. Small doses of narcotic have been reportedly added in order to allow the infusion rate to be decreased; increased potential for respiratory depression may occur.

Pentobarbital sodium has been actively studied for use in infants and children. With the decrease in the availability of chloral hydrate, renewed interest in comparison efficacy has emerged. Studies suggest that, regardless of route of administration, pentobarbital may be equally efficacious as, or even, in some studies, preferred over chloral hydrate.[16,17] The ability to administer it orally and its suggested increased palatable acceptance offer families the option of not requiring intravenous access prior to administering the medication. Some articles suggest that oral administration has a lower rate of adverse respiratory events and therefore should be considered regardless of intravenous access.[17] Dosage: 1–6 mg/kg IV; 4–8 mg/kg PO. Consider starting at the lower end of dosage and repeating q 20 min for optimal effect and minimal events. The peak effect of an oral dose is at 20 minutes. Average time to discharge for patients treated with either the oral or intravenous form is similar.

Dexmedetomidine use in the pediatric population, both in the operating room and for non-pain procedures, has continued to grow. Initial studies appeared to have unpredictable results, but with continued study and modification of dosage a number of studies have shown predictable successful results.[15] As with the medications previously discussed, there is a volume of literature addressing combining dexmedetomidine with a number of other medications.[13,15,18,20,21,26,27] The route of administration, while initially intravenous, has also been studied and includes intranasal and intramuscular routes as well. Most studies, however, use the intravenous high-dose protocols to examine results compared with alternative medications or combinations of medications. Side effects associated with the higher-dose, initial intravenous bolus – hypotension and bradycardia – resolved spontaneously without adverse incident. Dosage for high-dose protocols: 2 mcg/kg intravenous followed by 1 mcg/kg/h.

Antisialagogue administration, used to prevent potential oral secretions, may commonly result in coughing and spasm. Atropine and glycopyrrolate have both been extensively studied and compared. Recent literature has shown less vomiting and agitation with atropine;[28] however, continued prospective examination of larger populations needs to be considered. Because of the benzyl alcohol, glycopyrrolate is not recommended for patients one month of age or younger. Potential concerns regarding administration of any antisialagogue in cystic fibrosis patients need to be considered. Dosage: atropine and glycopyrrolate 0.01 mg/kg.

Narcotics such as fentanyl have been added to many protocols, resulting in a decrease in overall dosage of medication and rapid return to baseline. Dosage: fentanyl 1–2 mcg/kg.

It is important to have a complete understanding of all medications that the patient has received prior to the administration of any anesthesia. There is a tremendous variation in the ways patients present for their studies. Patients may be receiving pain medications or other medications that will have a compounding effect on anesthesia. Confirming all medications and the last times of administration will allow for individualization of the patient's plan. Allowing the patient to continue to receive their pain medications and then titrating to effect the medications needed to complete the study results in a comfortable patient, the administration of less additional medication, and a smooth transition.

Magnetic resonance imaging (MRI)

Preparing to provide monitored anesthesia care or general anesthesia to a patient undergoing an MRI requires increased attention to environmental safety as well as to anesthesia concerns. Prior consideration of all equipment and personnel must involve a safety officer's evaluation and clearance. The smallest object remaining on the patient or team members can result in morbidity or mortality. There are a number of references that the MRI personnel and the anesthesia team can access to learn the MRI safety of devices and implants.[29] The Joint Commission Sentinel Event Alert describes a number of potential types of injury:[6] (1) Missile effect – objects rapidly pulled into the magnet; (2) dislodging of ferromagnetic objects, such as clips, pins, infusion devices; (3) burns – objects heating as a result of the MRI process, including tracheal tubes and reinforced endotracheal tubes; (4) device malfunctions – pumps, monitors, etc.; (5) support systems – equipment or supply shortage, replacement not available; (6) acoustic damage to the ears; (7) MRI contrast agent reactions; (8) MRI equipment – cryogen handling, storage.

With strict adherence to screening processes and the American College of Radiology (ACR) and Joint Commission on Accreditation of Hospital Organizations (JCAHO) zone recommendations, MRI safety can be assured.[29,30] Both organizations and many others have helped define areas of safe work by dividing the proximity to the MRI into four zones: *Zone I* – Free public access: no restrictions are placed on equipment and no screening is required. *Zone II* – Transition zone: this is reserved for patient histories, physicals, screening of the patient, and any family member planning to enter Zones III or IV; appropriate clothing is removed and provided. All members of the care team planning to enter Zones III and IV should be screened. *Zone III* – This zone is limited to the screened patient and accompanying personnel. Access is controlled by MRI personnel, because movement of unrecognized ferromagnetic objects can result in injury or death. *Zone IV* – The magnet. This zone is under constant direct supervision of trained MRI personnel; all nonMRI personnel need to be escorted while in Zones III or IV. Unexpected movement of ferromagnetic objects, as in Zone III, can result in injury or death.

While the patient and family are in Zone II, a complete anesthesia preoperative history and physical examination need to be completed. Two screenings need to be done in order to ensure MRI safety. An initial screening by the admitting nurse can alert the MRI personnel and anesthesia provider to special needs and concerns. The final screening must be performed by and ultimate permission to enter Zones III or IV granted by trained MRI personnel. A plan can then be discussed with the family, including the explanation that their child will be under anesthesia during the scan and the potential for the need to advance to a higher-care level. Questions and concerns regarding the patient's underlying condition and concerns regarding emergencies in the scanner should be addressed at this time. Families, the MRI staff, and the anesthesia team need to consider all of these factors prior to beginning the scan.

Creating a safe, monitored environment in the MRI laboratory requires preparation and planning by the entire team. The same anesthesia standards that apply in the operating room apply in this unique location. These standards include monitoring, the elimination of metallic objects, and careful examination of the patients and equipment. MRI-compatible monitors for electrocardiograms (ECGs), blood pressure, pulse oximetry, end-tidal CO_2, and temperature assure the same high standards and levels of monitoring. The majority of the patients will not be intubated; however, the use of a nasal cannula with end-tidal CO_2 measuring capabilities allows for consistent monitoring. An MRI-compatible anesthesia machine facilitates smooth transition to a higher level of care and is invaluable in an emergency situation. MRI-compatible pumps allow for continued infusion of medications, either for anesthesia or for other medications that the patient may require. The availability and location of an anesthesia cart will depend upon whether the cart is MRI compatible. An MRI-compatible equipment kit provides prompt access to emergency equipment and a level of comfort for the anesthesia provider.

Items often overlooked are potential missiles in the MRI laboratory, and include laryngoscopes, stethoscopes, pens, clipboards, paper clips, IV poles, medication pumps, pagers, badges, and many other items. Prior to entering Zone IV, an additional manual scan with a hand-held metal detector can detect a forgotten object on a patient, in a family member's pocket, or on a team member. Once the patient is under anesthesia, positioning and other patient safety concerns need to be addressed before they are moved into the scanner. A head-to-toe examination is done to ensure the integrity of the patient's airway, position in relation to the coil, ear protection, temperature regulation, padding, and intravenous access. In order to avoid injury from the MRI, associated equipment precautions include earplugs and/or head phones, padding between the patient and monitors, and padding between the scanner table or coil and the patient. Special attention to all emergency equipment is critical for MRI safety. In the urgency of resuscitating a patient, one does not want to endanger the patient or team with unsafe equipment.

Following the scan, the patient should be transported to a designated recovery area. The nursing team should be properly trained, and the equipment should meet all the standards of any postanesthesia recovery area. Once the patient meets the appropriate discharge criteria, Aldrete score, and a postanesthesia examination has been completed, the patient can be discharged. Discharge instructions and a resource phone number will help the family to participate in the process with decreased anxiety. A post-procedure phone call, either later that day or the following day, will help facilitate a positive experience for outpatients. Inpatients will also require a recovery period prior to returning to the floor or unit. A subgroup of patients will require coordination between services to allow them to move from the scanner to a second location for another procedure or for further care. The family needs to understand the plan to move their child while under anesthesia and where the secondary procedure will be performed. Prior to beginning the scan for these patients, all procedures should be discussed with the family and signed consent obtained for each procedure. Monitored transport and continued communication with the family will allow for a smooth transition.

Computed tomography

As with the majority of off-site locations, common anesthesia concerns during CT scans are compounded by the inherent procedural risks. The patient requiring a preoperative or decision-making scan can remain under anesthesia and be transported to the appropriate treatment area. By involving the ordering physician, nurses, and the radiology team in the planning of diagnostic studies and procedures in the CT laboratory, unexpected emergencies can be avoided. Mock run-throughs allow for a degree of comfort and assurance when a patient presents.

A complete anesthesia history and physical examination identifies potential risks and comorbidities. To facilitate better care, both the team and the patient's family should have a clear understanding of the scan's purpose, and there should be a plan for the postscan period. Not all institutions provide an anesthesia machine in the CT suite, but it may not be necessary because of the relatively short duration of most scans. As with all monitored anesthesia care or general anesthesia cases, American Society of Anesthesiologists (ASA)-recommended monitors should include: ECG, blood pressure, end-tidal CO_2, pulse oximetry, and temperature. Supplemental oxygen can be administered via specialized nasal cannula when intubation is not required. This does not eliminate the need for readily available anesthesia equipment if advancement to a higher level of care is necessary. Prior to the test, a team discussion that includes the radiologist, technician, and nurses will allow for the minimum individualized requirements to provide a safe and successful study. Some studies or patients' comorbid conditions may require intubation to provide necessary airway management and control chest wall movement. Regardless of intubation status, clear plans that include the location of the poststudy or procedure care should be in place.

Providing anesthesia during the CT scan can present logistical challenges. Appropriate protection of the patient and team from radiation should be implemented. Lead aprons, thyroid shields, and lead glasses are routine for the team and should be applied to accessible areas of the patient, study permitting. Equally important is temperature control. Contrary to conditions in the MRI scanner, the patients in the CT scanner may become cold through heat loss. Keeping the patient covered with warm blankets, procedural access permitting, will prevent rapid heat loss. Many CT scanners are located in proximity to the MRI scanner and will allow for a shared crash cart and a shared malignant hyperthermia cart. If the CT and MRI scanners are not located near each other, emergency equipment needs to be available for each location. Most CT scans are diagnostic and do not represent any direct stimulation to the patient. While some patients may be uncomfortable because of their injuries, lesions, or disease processes, these discomforts will be relieved by the anesthetic provided to perform the study. In the case of CT-guided needle biopsies or abscess drainage, additional medication will be required during the procedure. Care must be taken, while providing adequate pain control during the stimulation, that the patient continues to maintain an open airway when the procedure is complete and that a rescan is undertaken to assure proper placement of the biopsy needle or drain.

While some institutions will require post-procedure patients to return to the emergency room or to proceed to the operating room recovery area, many will have a postanesthesia recovery unit in the radiology department. Regardless of the location, the nursing staff need appropriate training to care for the patient and ensure that the patient meets Aldrete criteria. Transport from the CT scanner requires the patient to be monitored appropriately. At the minimum, a mask, oxygen, Jackson–Reese or Ambu bag, medications, and airway equipment should be included. Postoperative instructions for the family are important whether the patient is an inpatient or an outpatient. A poststudy or post-procedure phone call, especially for outpatients, will go a long way toward answering questions and eliminating residual concerns.

Gastrointestinal (GI) laboratory

Procedural sedation in the GI laboratory presents an increased layer of complexity because of the multiple diagnoses that present, the sharing of the airway, the range of potential procedures, and intermittent stimulation during the procedures. In addition to the routine preanesthesia history and physical examination, understanding of the patient's diagnosis and potential additional risks need to be addressed. Gastrointestinal patients can present with the concomitant physiologic concerns of electrolyte abnormalities, hypovolemia, anemia, pulmonary disease, and other comorbidities. Understanding the potential diagnostic and therapeutic indications for upper endoscopy and lower colonoscopy procedures will allow the anesthesia provider to provide a safe environment for the patient. All patients require full anesthesia monitoring and the same adherence to standards whether the procedure is performed in the operating room or the GI laboratory. Equally important are the availability of emergency equipment, crash carts, and trained personnel.

Upper endoscopy presents numerous anesthesia challenges. Sharing the airway with the gastroenterologist requires teamwork and communication to avoid airway compromise, aspiration, or laryngospasm. A majority of the endoscopic therapeutic procedures will present a significant increase in the risk of aspiration and/or laryngospasm, thereby requiring intubation and airway protection. A foreign body or an esophageal stricture can create a functional upper esophageal pouch filled with food and or secretions. Upper GI bleeding or esophageal varices are also associated with aspiration and spasm. Initiation of anesthesia, with the loss of gag reflex, will create a perfect setting for aspiration or spasm as well. Most endoscopic diagnostic procedures can be completed with careful control and monitoring of the shared airway. Delivery of supplemental oxygen via a nasal cannula with an end-tidal CO_2 port will provide increased safety. Significant stimulation can occur during initial passing of the scope through the oral pharynx into the esophagus. Careful timing of the initial bolus with placement of the scope will allow for a smooth beginning while sharing the airway. The entire team will benefit if scope monitors are arranged to allow the gastroenterologist and the team to observe each stage of the process. Most upper endoscopic procedures not requiring intubation can be completed with a preoperative dose of glycopyrrolate or atropine, followed by a bolus and infusion of propofol. An initial dose of 1–2 mg/kg of propofol will allow for a quiet field and ease of scope passing in most patients. Small incremental doses and/or infusion will allow for completion of the diagnostic study. In smaller children, infants, and those with airway concerns, ketamine has been effective in providing sedation. Following the study, the patient's stomach is suctioned to remove air and secretions. (Patients have complained of significant post-procedure abdominal pain, necessitating further X-rays and tests, when air was allowed to remain.) The patient is then transported to the recovery room and discharged once the Aldrete criteria have been met.

While colonoscopy does not require sharing the airway, diligence to deliver a safe anesthetic is equally important. Many of these patients may be significantly hypovolemic and have associated electrolyte abnormalities because of their disease processes, the bowel preparation procedure, or both. Patients with lower gastrointestinal bleeding may also present with significant anemia, which should be corrected prior to induction. Patients are usually positioned in the lateral decubitus position, and appropriate precautions need to be taken. Positioning a patient under anesthesia requires extreme care and the appreciation of potential risks. The entire team should be involved in the positioning, allowing the anesthesia provider to maintain the airway while directing the moving process. A head-to-toe inspection prior to beginning the procedure will prevent potential harm to the patient.

After positioning the patient with appropriate monitors in place, re-examination is needed to ensure that patients are not lying on any wires or monitor cables; the face, eyes, and ears are not under any pressure; extremities are padded; genitals are not under pressure; and there are no bone-on-bone pressure points. The initial medication dose is 1–2 mg/kg of propofol followed by an infusion. There are many cocktails that will allow for longer procedures, decreased total medication, and rapid recovery; the addition of 1–2 mcg/kg of fentanyl is not uncommon.

Some patients will require an upper endoscopy and colonoscopy while under anesthesia. This will require careful repositioning of the patient. Once the team is ready to proceed, a small bolus dose of propofol may be required to allow for introduction of the scope. Following the study or procedure the patient is transported to the recovery area until the Aldrete score is met for discharge. A postanesthesia assessment and documentation are required. As with other outpatient procedures, a follow-up phone call to the patient's family addressing questions and concerns will facilitate the family's confidence.

Starlight room

The anesthesia team can be proactive in individualizing patient care by providing a place to offer a gradation of sedation and anesthesia to patients requiring procedures outside the operating room. By allowing the patients to have a place where they can receive multiple layers of care, the negative psychological and physical effects of trying to perform some procedures at the bedside can be overcome. The patient and family need to know that their room is considered a safe area. A location in proximity to the operating room allows for shared resources, and allows the team to involve the parents in their child's care, as deemed appropriate. A number of potential procedures, ranging from burn debridement to dressing changes, abscess drainage, bone marrow biopsies, kidney biopsies, and others, can be considered and evaluated by the team in this specialized area, known as the starlight room (Figure 32.1a).

As with any off-site location, ASA guidelines for a complete preoperative assessment and NPO status need to be maintained. Families need to be informed that their children will be under anesthesia and full monitoring, and that the ability to go to a higher level of care is prepared for. Most procedures can be accomplished with nasal cannula delivery of supplemental oxygen and end-tidal CO_2 monitoring, pulse oximeter, blood pressure, ECG, and temperature monitoring. Some cases may require a mask, a laryngeal mask airway or an endotracheal tube, and all options need to be readily available. It may be necessary to alter the plan once the procedure has started and the dressings are removed. Having an anesthesia machine, crash cart, and a full operating room anesthesia set-up will alleviate the disruption of procedures and the unexpected need for emergency resources.

Contrary to procedures in many off-site locations, such as the MRI (Figure 32.1b) or CT scanner rooms, where the primary goal is to control movement, procedures in the starlight room location can and do result in significant stimulation. Care must be taken to utilize techniques that address stimulation as well as postoperative pain needs. It is equally important during the preoperative assessment to ascertain what medications the patient has received prior to arrival; this will allow the appropriate titration of medications without loss of spontaneous ventilation. Preprocedure midazolam can help alleviate the anxiety of the patient and, subsequently, that of the family. Patients without intravenous access can be assessed for a potential mask induction, and then for determining whether an IV should be established prior to or during the procedure. In patients with IV access, propofol or ketamine offer excellent induction and maintenance options. If propofol is used, it is important to appreciate the minimal analgesic effects and adding a narcotic should be considered. If ketamine is used, antisialagogue considerations can be addressed with glycopyrrolate and post-procedure delirium concerns can be reduced with midazolam. Other medications and techniques should be considered based on the procedure and the patient's co morbidities.

It is important to create a culture where the off-site location is considered an operating room. All procedures and policies should mirror operating room standards and practices, including but not limited to sterile technique, informed consent, and a time out. Following the procedure the patient needs to recover until Aldrete criteria are met. Proximity to the operating room allows the patient to recover in the PACU associated with the operating room. A postanesthesia assessment and note needs to be completed.

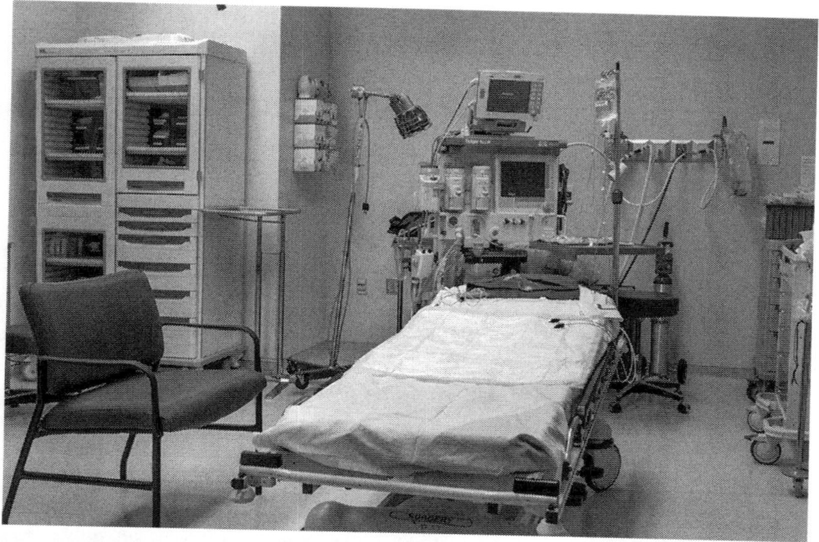

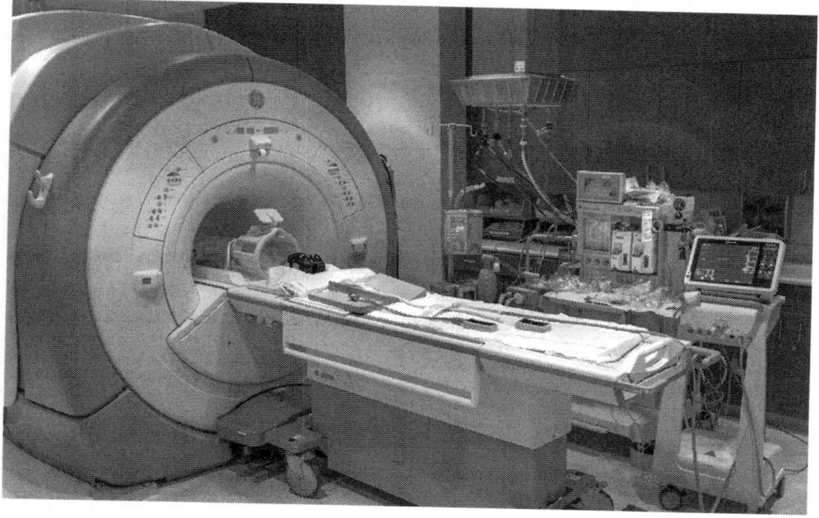

Figure 32.1 **(a)** The "starlight" room is a specialized area where a number of potential procedures, ranging from burn debridement to dressing changes, abscess drainage, bone marrow biopsies, kidney biopsies and others, can be considered and evaluated by the team. **(b)** The MRI (magnetic resonance imaging) scanner is used by radiologists to examine the soft tissues of the body. Sedation or general anesthesia may be necessary to keep the patient still during the procedure.

Vignettes

All vignettes involve hypothetical patients representing potential case scenarios. Each is designed to present one management approach; other options are acceptable and may be more appropriate. The patient's individual preoperative anesthesia assessment and requirements of the procedure or study must dictate the plan. The vignettes should also allow for a starting point for all members of the team to have a better understanding of the process and to allow for input and discussion.

GI vignette

A 6-year-old child with a history of weight loss and abdominal pain presents for an outpatient esophagogastroduodenoscopy with biopsies. After completion of the anesthesia assessment, baseline vital signs and NPO status, the plan is discussed with the family.

A peripheral IV line is established and the patient, with a parent, is escorted to the GI suite. Monitors, including pulse oximetry, ECG, and blood pressure, are attached; the patient has refused to allow the nasal cannula to be placed. Glycopyrrolate followed by propofol is given. The parent is escorted from the room as the nasal cannula is applied for oxygen delivery and end-tidal CO_2 measurement. Following a time out, the gastroenterologist and anesthesiologist agree to proceed with the introduction of the scope. Occasionally a small additional dose of propofol or lidocaine may be required. Once the scope passes, incremental doses of propofol are required to maintain an adequate level of anesthesia. Viewing monitors placed so the gastroenterologist and the anesthesiologist can observe the procedure allow for smoother understanding of the process. As the procedure is coming to an end, usually signaled by the removal of gas from the stomach or final esophageal biopsies, the propofol is discontinued. Careful and continuous airway monitoring during removal is critical, as secretions or the scope may trigger spasm. The patient is then transported to the recovery area. One should note that if the recovery area is not in direct proximity to the lab, the patient should be transported on monitors with emergency equipment and medications available. Report is then given to the recovery room nurse, and post-procedure vital signs are documented. The family returns to the recovery area, and the patient is discharged when they meet recovery room criteria and the postanesthesia assessment is completed. Although the family is given a number to call with any questions, a post-procedure phone call the next day assures the family and the team of a successful process.

A 4-year-old boy has swallowed a coin, is drooling, and will not eat. After its identification on X-ray, he presents for removal of the coin from the esophagus. An IV was placed while the patient was in the emergency room. Having been told that the procedure would be quick and that their son might need "twilight anesthesia," the family wants to know if "you can give a little something while they take it out." After the completion of the anesthesia assessment, baseline vital signs and NPO status, the family is informed of the risks of aspiration and agrees to a general endotracheal anesthetic. The monitors are then applied, a rapid-sequence induction is performed, and the airway is secured. A time out is completed, the scope is passed, and the process to remove the coin or coins begins. Following removal of the coin, the esophagus and stomach are inspected and suctioned and the scope is removed. Although the endotracheal tube has been secured at the lip, each removal or repositioning of the scope necessitates care directed at maintaining the tube placement to avoid unrecognized dislodgement. Following extubation, the patient is taken to the recovery room. A report is given to the recovery room nurse, and post-procedure vital signs are documented. The family returns to the recovery area, and the patient will be admitted or discharged when he meets the criteria and a postanesthesia assessment has been completed.

MRI vignette

An 11-month-old boy with a history of new-onset seizures requires an MRI with and without contrast. The patient was a full-term infant and was discharged home with mother. There have been no recent or current fevers or signs of illness, and no nausea or vomiting. The rest of the preanesthesia assessment is negative; NPO guidelines have been met. The plan is discussed with the parents and informed consent is obtained for an MRI scan with anesthesia. After the application of MRI-compatible standard ASA monitors, the patient is given glycopyrrolate and propofol. Supplemental oxygen is delivered via nasal cannula, also allowing for end-tidal CO_2 measurement. A propofol infusion is begun and the patient is positioned for the scan by the anesthesia, nursing, and MRI technician team. Acoustic protection along with proper padding must be applied before the scan begins. In addition to addressing standard anesthesia positioning concerns, care must be taken to ensure that monitors are padded, that there is no skin-to-skin contact, and that all digits and extremities are clear when moving into the MRI. Additional vigilance regarding the oxygen line and medication infusion lines is needed when moving the patient into the scanner. Most patients' temperatures will increase during prolonged MRI scans; however, small children and those with little muscle or body mass may require blankets or other warming measures. During the scan, the propofol infusion is titrated to prevent patient movement during the study but allow for normal vital signs. Patients may present with prolonged NPO times or other hypovolemic states requiring supplemental intravenous fluids. Occasionally patients will require additional airway support, including a shoulder roll, nasal or oral airway, laryngeal mask airway or intubation; the patient in this scenario requires only a shoulder roll. After completion of the noncontrast portion of the study, the patient remains on the bed, which is removed from the scanner in order to administer contrast. The contrast agent should be administered through the access port closest to the patient to avoid giving a bolus of propofol and to avoid the mixing of medications. While an allergic reaction to contrast is rare, close observation of the patient's response is necessary prior to continuing the scan. Reassessment of the airway and of the patient prior to moving back into the scanner, and equal vigilance regarding the oxygen tubing, medication lines, and extremities, are important. With constant vigilance, monitoring, and willingness to stop the procedure if the patient requires, a safe study is completed. Following the studies, the patient is taken to the recovery area, monitors are applied, and a report is given to the recovery nurse. The family is informed of the patient's status and reunited in the recovery area. An anesthesia postoperative assessment is completed and documented prior to discharge.

Starlight vignette

A 3-year-old girl with burns to the face and chest arrives for debridement and dressing change. The child had been seen in the emergency room the night before after having spilled a cup of soup on herself while removing it from the microwave. During completion of the anesthesia assessment, care must be taken in ascertaining the mechanism of the burn. While all burns have some common requirements for fluid resuscitation, pain management and temperature regulation, patients suffering burns from fire need further evaluation of potential airway involvement. Regardless of the process used to calculate fluid needs (by Parkland formula or other process), it is paramount to assure hemodynamic stability prior to the induction of anesthesia by assessing urine output, blood pressure, and heart rate. Understanding what medication the patient is currently receiving will be important in planning anesthesia for the procedure. Confirmation of the patient's current pain management and last dose will help prevent duplication or unexpected cardiopulmonary compromise. Families need to be aware that, though the plan is to begin the procedure with nasal cannula oxygen, it is not unexpected that the patient may require a higher level of care or airway management, and that these changes are considered an anticipatory part of the plan. Once the team agrees on the patient's status and the family understands the plan, the patient can be taken to the procedure room. Many of these patients are emotionally as well as physically traumatized, and a dose of midazolam will allow for smooth transport to the treatment room and will offer some coverage of the post-procedure delirium associated with ketamine. The treatment room should be warmed prior to the patient's arrival to prevent temperature loss from exposure. Care is taken in finding appropriate uninvolved areas to apply monitors, such as the pulse oximeter, blood pressure cuff, ECG leads, and nasal cannula oxygen with CO_2 monitoring. Glycopyrrolate followed by ketamine is often used; however, the family needs to be made aware of the post-procedure nystagmus and delirium they will observe. Families may ask that ketamine not be used during daily returns to dress the burns because of the frequently immediate post-procedure behavior seen in their children. Propofol can be used effectively, especially if combined with a narcotic, to allow for analgesia and an overall lower dose of medication. Following a time out, exposure and treatment of the burns can be undertaken. The entire team needs to participate in moving the patient in order to allow for a full exam and ease of access both during the procedure and while applying the dressings. Once the burns have been treated and dressed, the patient is transported to the recovery area, and a report is given to the nurse as a post-procedure set of vital signs is taken. Post-procedure pain medications need to be written by one service, either surgery or anesthesia, to avoid duplication and overdose. Following a postanesthesia assessment, the patient and family can be discharged from the recovery area to the appropriate unit.

CT vignette

A 4-month-old presents with stridor and trouble swallowing for a CT angiogram for work-up of a vascular ring. During completion of the preoperative anesthesia assessment, specific care to address airway and gastrointestinal symptoms must be taken. This study also requires teamwork between the radiologist, technician, and anesthesiologist to provide an optimal study. Controlled ventilation, either by mask or endotracheal tube, should be discussed to facilitate maximal results with maximal safety. A history of vomiting, gastroesophageal reflux disease, or significant stridor will require consideration of endotracheal tube control of the airway. Most patients, however, can have an excellent and safe study with mask ventilation or with a laryngeal mask airway if the respiratory rate is carefully controlled. Because of the vascular component of the study, discussion of size and location of the IV catheter should take place prior to placement. Once the radiologist, the family, and the anesthesia team are in agreement, the patient is placed on standard monitors, and a dose of glycopyrrolate followed by propofol is given. If there is an anesthesia machine in the CT scanner, the entire case can be completed with a mask or endotracheal tube anesthetic agent. Care to provide X-ray protection for the anesthesia team and the patient is also important. Lead aprons for the anesthesia team and to cover the patient allow for decreased exposure; lead glasses or other eye protection should be available. Following the study, the patient is transported to a recovery area until the Aldrete criteria are met. Alerting the recovery team to the possibility of postintubation croup and having the ability to treat it rapidly are important.

Off-site checklist

- Patient assessment
- Study assessment
- Team aware and agree
- Family aware and consents
- Monitors
  - pulse oximetry
  - end-tidal CO_2 ($ETCO_2$)
  - ECG
  - BP
  - temperature
- Anesthesia cart or equivalent
- Airway plan
  - nasal cannula with $ETCO_2$ port
  - other
- Medications
- Suction
- Higher level of care
  - oral/nasal airways
  - intubation equipment
  - positive-pressure ventilation
  - anesthesia machine
- Emergency medications

References

1. R. F. Kaplan, C. I. Yang. Sedation and analgesia in pediatric patients for procedures outside the operating room. *Anesthesiol Clin North America* 2002; **20**: 181–94, vii.
2. J. P. Cravero, G. T. Blike, M. Beach, *et al.* Incidence and nature of adverse events during pediatric sedation/anesthesia for procedures outside the operating room: report from the Pediatric Sedation Research Consortium. *Pediatrics* 2006; **118**: 1087–96.
3. J. Metzner, K. B. Domino. Risks of anesthesia or sedation outside the operating room: the role of the anesthesia care provider. *Curr Opin Anaesthesiol* 2010; **23**: 523–31.
4. R. Ramaiah, S. Bhananker. Pediatric procedural sedation and analgesia outside the operating room: anticipating, avoiding and managing complications. *Expert Rev Neurother* 2011; **11**: 755–63.
5. M. Mahmoud, B. Jones, D. J. Podberesky. Teamwork among pediatric anesthesia and radiology providers at a large tertiary-care children's hospital: past, present and future. *Pediatr Radiol* 2012; **43**: 460–3.
6. The Joint Commission. *Sentinel Event Alert*, Issue 38: Preventing accidents and injuries in the MRI suite. Feb 14, 2008.
7. J. A. Aldrete, D. Kroulik. A postanesthetic recovery score. *Anesth Analg* 1970; **49**: 924–34.
8. P. F. White, D. Song. New criteria for fast-tracking after outpatient anesthesia: a comparison with the modified Aldrete's scoring system. *Anesth Analg* 1999; **88**: 1069–72.
9. The American Society of Anesthesiologists. Standards for basic anesthetic monitoring. October 20, 2010.
10. C. J. Cote, S. Wilson. Guidelines for monitoring and management of pediatric patients during and after sedation for diagnostic and therapeutic procedures: an update. *Pediatrics* 2006; **118**: 2587–602.
11. J. Weaver. The latest ASA mandate: CO(2) monitoring for moderate and deep sedation. *Anesth Prog* 2011; **58**: 111–12.
12. M. E. Kleinman, L. Chameides, S. M. Schexnayder, *et al.* Part 14: Pediatric advanced life support: 2010 American Heart Association Guidelines for

Cardiopulmonary Resuscitation and Emergency Cardiovascular Care. *Circulation* 2010; **122**: S876–908.

13. B. S. J. S. A. Kulshrestha A, Kapoor V. Dexmedetomidine and fentanyl combination for procedural sedation in a case of Duchenne muscular dystrophy. *Anesth Essays Res* 2011; **5**: 224–6.

14. K. Lohit, V. Srinivas, S. Chanda Kulkarni. A clinical evaluation of the effects of administration of midazolam on ketamine-induced emergence phenomenon. *J Clin Diag Res* 2011; **5**: 320–3.

15. K. P. Mason, F. Robinson, P. Fontaine, R. Prescilla. Dexmedetomidine offers an option for safe and effective sedation for nuclear medicine imaging in children. *Radiology* 2013; **267**: 911–17.

16. K. P. Mason, P. Sanborn, D. Zurakowski, *et al.* Superiority of pentobarbital versus chloral hydrate for sedation in infants during imaging. *Radiology* 2004; **230**: 537–42.

17. V. J. Rooks, T. Chung, L. Connor, *et al.* Comparison of oral pentobarbital sodium (nembutal) and oral chloral hydrate for sedation of infants during radiologic imaging: preliminary results. *AJR Am J Roentgenol* 2003; **180**: 1125–8.

18. R. Siddappa, J. Riggins, S. Kariyanna, P. Calkins, A. T. Rotta. High-dose dexmedetomidine sedation for pediatric MRI. *Paediatr Anaesth* 2011; **21**: 153–8.

19. V. C. Slavik, P. J. Zed. Combination ketamine and propofol for procedural sedation and analgesia. *Pharmacotherapy* 2007; **27**: 1588–98.

20. J. D. Tobias. Dexmedetomidine and ketamine: an effective alternative for procedural sedation? *Pediatr Crit Care Med* 2012; **13**: 423–7.

21. Z. Tosun, A. Akin, G. Guler, A. Esmaoglu, A. Boyaci. Dexmedetomidine–ketamine and propofol–ketamine combinations for anesthesia in spontaneously breathing pediatric patients undergoing cardiac catheterization. *J Cardiothorac Vasc Anesth* 2006; **20**: 515–19.

22. S. Koruk, A. Mizrak, B. Kaya Ugur, *et al.* Propofol/dexmedetomidine and propofol/ketamine combinations for anesthesia in pediatric patients undergoing transcatheter atrial septal defect closure: a prospective randomized study. *Clin Ther* 2010; **32**: 701–9.

23. S. M. Green, M. G. Roback, B. Krauss. Anticholinergics and ketamine sedation in children: a secondary analysis of atropine versus glycopyrrolate. *Acad Emerg Med* 2010; **17**: 157–62.

24. W. M. A. Al Taher, E. E. Mansour, M. N. El Shafei. Comparative study between novel sedation drug (dexmedetomidine) versus midazolam-propofol for conscious sedation in pediatric patients undergoing oro-dental procedures. *Egypt J Anesth* 2010; **26**: 299–304.

25. S. Gottschling, S. Meyer, T. Krenn, *et al.* Propofol versus midazolam/ketamine for procedural sedation in pediatric oncology. *J Pediatr Hematol Oncol* 2005; **27**: 471–6.

26. C. M. Heard, P. Joshi, K. Johnson. Dexmedetomidine for pediatric MRI sedation: a review of a series of cases. *Paediatr Anaesth* 2007; **17**: 888–92.

27. V. Raman, D. Yacob, J. D. Tobias. Dexmedetomidine-ketamine sedation during upper gastrointestinal endoscopy and biopsy in a patient with Duchenne muscular dystrophy and egg allergy. *Int J Crit Illn Inj Sci* 2012; **2**: 40–3.

28. R. K. Mirakhur, J. W. Dundee. Comparison of the effects of atropine and glycopyrrolate on various end-organs. *J R Soc Med* 1980; **73**: 727–30.

29. F. G. Shellock. *Reference Manual for Magnetic Resonance Safety, Implants and Devices*. 2013 Edition. Los Angeles, CA: Biomedical Research Publishing; 2013.

30. E. Kanal, A. J. Barkovich, C. Bell, *et al.* ACR guidance document on MR safe practices: 2013. *J Magn Reson Imaging* 2013; **37**: 501–30.

Chapter

33 Anesthesia for pediatric organ transplantation

Naila A. Ahmad and Brenda C. McClain

Introduction

Approximately 123730 patients are waiting to receive organ transplants in the USA, according to the Scientific Registry of Transplant Recipients (SRTR); 2008 are children ranging in age from less than 1 year to 17 years. It is crucial for the pediatric anesthesiologist to understand the pathophysiological impact of end-stage organ disease since these children are often critically unstable at the time of presentation for transplantation. Communication between the surgeon and anesthesiologist is key to the success of these intricate procedures.

Liver transplantation milestones

History

The first human transplant was performed on a 3-year-old boy with biliary atresia in 1963 but the child did not survive due to fatal intraoperative hemorrhage from venous collateral vessels (1,2). Subsequently, six more attempts also failed. Dr. Thomas Starlz performed the first successful liver transplant in 1967 on a 1-year-old patient with hepatoblastoma who survived for 400 days (3). Thereafter, Dr. Starlz and colleagues transplanted 12 more patients and seven of those survived for more than 12 years (4). The survival rates remained low however, with subsequent improvement in surgical and anesthesia techniques and advancement in immunosuppression has led to better 1-year survival. Rates rose to greater than 90% and the 5-year survival rate rose to over 80% in many centers (3,4). The barriers to success had been failure to control intraoperative hemorrhage, poor organ preservation solutions and inadequate immunosuppression. The role of the immune system in organ rejection was discovered by Medawar in 1944 but it was not until 1967 that thymoglobulin, an antilymphocytic agent, was added to supplement the azathioprine and prednisone immunosuppression regimen. Cyclosporine was incorporated into the regimen in 1979 and was subsequently replaced with FK-506 (i.e., fujimycin or tacrolimus) in 1989 (5). The ideal preservation solution minimizes graft damage by inhibiting cellular changes during storage and at reperfusion upon re-establishment of blood supply (6). Initially, the preservative was a mixture of chilled Ringer's lactate and normal saline which preserved the organ approximately 4 to 6 hours. In 1987 the University of Wisconsin solution was developed which decreased cell swelling during hypothermic storage and increased preservation time toward 24 hours. In Europe, histidine–tryptophane–ketoglutarate (HTK) solution was developed for cardiac preservation and was subsequently used as a donor liver preservative and was found to have better penetration of the microcirculation; HTK was introduced in the USA in 2002 (2).

Epidemiology

According to the August 2013 report of the Scientific Registry of Transplant Recipients (SRTR), there are approximately 496 pediatric patients with chronic or ESLD waiting for liver transplantation. In 2012, 758 pediatric liver transplants were performed in the USA and this number has increased gradually from 509 pediatric donor recipients in 1990 (7).

Organ allocation

In the past, liver allocation for pediatric patients was done on the basis of geographic location and medical conditions as described by the Child Turcotte–Pugh (CTP) score, which ranked the child's status as 1, 2a, 2b, and 3 (8). Status 1 patients were of highest priority for transplant. These children presented in acute liver

Essentials of Pediatric Anesthesiology, ed. Alan David Kaye, Charles James Fox and James H. Diaz. Published by Cambridge University Press. © Cambridge University Press 2015.

failure of less than 6 weeks duration or had failed liver transplantation within 1 week of surgery and urgently required repeat transplantation. Status 2a, 2b, and 3 were defined by their CTP score plus their length of time on the waiting list. With the increasing success of liver transplants the number of children placed on the waiting list has increased and allocation is now done solely according to the severity of disease (8). In 2002 implementation of MELD (model for end-stage liver disease) scores for adults and PELD (pediatric end-stage liver disease) scores for children designated priority for organ allocation to the sickest patients rather than to those with the longest wait (4). The PELD score accurately estimates the 90-day waitlist mortality of children who are liver transplant candidates (9). The PELD score is based on age less than 1 year, height less than 2 standard deviations from the mean for age (in other words failure to thrive) and gender, total albumin, total billirubin and the international normalized ratio (INR). A retrospective review on pediatric post-transplant outcomes reveals that candidates with a pretransplant PELD score of < 3.6 or a score > 32.7 had 100% 1-year survival (10). The MELD score is used for adults and adolescents of 12–17 years of age and consists of INR, serum bilirubin, and serum creatinine. Renal failure is a predictor of increased mortality in adults with liver disease.

Indications for liver transplantation

Extrahepatic biliary atresia is the most common indication for liver transplantation in children (11). Biliary atresia accounts for over 60% of all indications for childhood liver transplantation. Alpha 1-antitrypsin deficiency is the diagnosis in 8% of pediatric transplant patients and is the next most frequently seen indication for pediatric liver transplantation (12); alpha 1-antitrypsin is a protease inhibitor that is made in the liver and acts to protect the lungs from inflammatory enzymes such as neutrophil elastase (13). Pulmonary symptoms in children include asthma-like symptoms that are nonresponsive to typical asthma treatment. Liver biopsy will show abundant PAS-positive globules within periportal hepatocytes with an eventual clinical picture of hepatic cirrhosis. The disease is variable in expression and, as a result, many people are misdiagnosed or receive late diagnosis.

Other indications for transplantation include biliary atresia as a coexisting disease as in Alagille syndrome. Alagille syndrome is characterized by cholestasis, cardiac disease, vertebral anomalies, ocular abnormalities and typical facial features. The cholestasis is the result of a paucity of interlobular bile ducts. Peripheral pulmonic stenosis is the most common cardiac problem seen in children with Alagille syndrome; however, complex intracardiac lesions such as tetralogy of Fallot, pulmonary atresia or ventricular septal defects significantly contribute to morbidity and mortality (14).

Wilson's disease is an autosomal recessive genetic disorder in which copper accumulates in tissues due to low ceruloplasmin; this manifests as neurological or psychiatric symptoms, Kayser–Fleischer rings of the iris and liver disease due to hepatolenticular degeneration (15). The disease can usually be controlled with medicines. Acute hepatic presentation is characterized by Coomb's negative hemolytic anemia and low alkaline phosphatase. Occasionally liver transplantation is required in childhood and most children who become transplant candidates present after 6 years of age. If the child presents with encephalopathy, prognosis is extremely poor.

Less frequently occurring causes of end-stage liver disease are numerous but rare. The remainder of pediatric cases is due to tumors, toxins, cirrhosis and other hepatic diseases. Regardless of the etiology, the common endpoint is liver failure leading to ESLD and the need for transplantation. Absolute contraindications to liver transplantation in children are few, except for the presence of severe pulmonary hypertension (PAP > 50 mmHg) or HIV/AIDS.

The manifestations of end-stage liver disease extend to nearly every organ system; ESLD causes loss of hepatocyte numbers and function leading to decreased synthetic function resulting in hypoalbuminemia, and the development of secondary hyperaldosteronism. Portal hypertension leads to the development of venous collaterals and esophageal varices; hemorrhage, ascites, spontaneous bacterial peritonitis, splenomegaly and thrombocytopenia ensue. Encephalopathy may represent azotemia and accumulation of ammonia. Electrolyte disturbances and cerebral edema with elevated intracranial pressure can cause mental status changes and coma. Deranged glucose metabolism may cause glucose intolerance or hypoglycemia since glycogen formation and gluconeogenesis are impaired (16).

Types of grafts

Pediatric liver transplants are mainly performed with cadaveric donor livers because of the scarcity of size-matched donors; however, reduced or split-liver grafts are becoming popular. One cadaveric donor liver is split into two and the right lobe is transplanted in an adult and the left is given to a pediatric recipient. The graft can also be obtained from a living related donor and the left lobe is transplanted into the child. Pediatric liver transplantation is likely the most successful of all solid organ transplant procedures (4).

Perioperative concerns

The clinical implications depend on how advanced the liver disease is and the presence of extrahepatic manifestations at the time of transplantation. It is very important for the anesthesiologist to understand the pathophysiology of ESLD for the management of anesthesia for transplantation. End-stage liver disease may have different etiologies but share the same final pathophysiology. Because of the complexity of the liver disease and other associated medical conditions, the patients require a multidisciplinary approach and communication among all involved specialists.

Preoperative assessment

Because ESLD affects nearly every organ system, it is imperative that a complete review of systems is performed. The assessment includes reported symptoms, review of pertinent labs and radiographs as well as a thorough history and physical examination. Attention to the pathophysiology of the following systems is mandatory. The impact of liver disease and multiorgan sequelae on anesthetic management are reviewed below.

Pathophysiology

Gastrointestinal

Raised intra-abdominal pressure from ascites places the patient at increased risk for aspiration from delayed gastric emptying. Respiratory compromise can arise from restrictive compression of the lungs by abdominal organomegaly (liver and spleen enlargement). Gastric and esophageal varices may bleed causing an increased bilirubin load and worsening azotemia. Portal hypertension and ascites is initially treated with sodium and water restriction (16).

Pulmonary function

Impaired respiratory function and hypoxemia are common in children with advanced liver disease. This is due to ascites, hepatosplenomegaly and pleural effusions causing reduced FRC, restricted alveolar exchange and ventilation/perfusion (V/Q) mismatch. This constellation of findings is known as hepatopulmonary syndrome, and is a common occurrence in children with biliary atresia or polysplenia syndrome. There is a fall in arterial oxygen levels upon sitting, which improves with lying supine. Patients display dyspnea and clubbing from chronic hypoxia. The syndrome is diagnosed by a technitium radiolabelled albumin scan or contrast echocardiography. Respiratory infections are common perioperatively, especially in patients with encephalopathy, poor gastric emptying or in patients requiring mechanical ventilation. Portopulmonary hypertension is the occurrence of pulmonary hypertension with a normal capillary wedge pressure yet elevated pulmonary vascular resistance (17). Portopulmonary hypertension can be seen in patients with Alagille syndrome and is associated with increased mortality; however, this comorbidity is otherwise a rare finding in children (12).

Cardiovascular function

A preoperative, hyperdynamic state results from an increase in cardiac output due to circulating angiotensin and catecholamines and from low systemic vascular resistance due to arteriovenous shunting. There is a resultant increase in mixed venous oxygen saturation. Because the systemic vascular resistance is low, children will be prone to hypotension after exposure to intravenous or volatile anesthetics and thus require dose reduction. The presence of intracardiac anomalies increases morbidity, in part due to enhanced vulnerability to the myocardial depressive effects of thromboxanes and prostaglandins that enter the circulation from the ischemic liver at the time of reperfusion (18).

Renal function

Renal function is well preserved in children with ESLD except in those presenting for retransplantation. Renal dysfunction may occur with sepsis, hypovolemia and drug toxicity. They may have prerenal azotemia from diuretic therapy for treatment of ascites. Hepatorenal syndrome is also less common in children but, when present, consists of impaired renal blood flow, low GFR, elevated serum creatinine, oliguria, low urinary sodium and a high urine to serum creatinine ratio (16).

Neurological function

Hepatic encephalopathy develops due to accumulation of ammonia, neuroactive peptides acting as false neurotransmitters, hyponatremia, hypoglycemia and alterations in cardiac output and cerebral metabolism (12). There can be cerebral edema and increased intracranial pressure.

Hematologic function

Concentrations of clotting factors II, VII, IX, and X may be low due to impaired synthesis or impaired absorption of vitamin K from the gut because of decreased bile acid secretion. There are decreased levels of antithrombin III, protein C and protein S, which predisposes to thrombosis (4). These patients are also anemic and thrombocytopenic because of sequestration of erythrocytes and platelets as a result of splenomegaly caused by portal hypertension. Anemia is exacerbated by poor nutritional status, repeated gastrointestinal blood loss and thrombocytopenia, which is often exacerbated by sepsis.

Anesthesia for liver transplant

Preoperative evaluation involves thorough history and physical examination to evaluate all organ systems. Familiarity with congenital syndromes associated with liver disease is mandatory. While all critical liver diseases share a common end, it is important to understand the primary cause of hepatic failure as well as other coexisting nonhepatic comorbidities (19). Adherence to infection control practices is important for the safety of the anesthesia provider as well, since these patients are often infected, and especially if the child presents with acute liver failure. NonA-E hepatitis is the most common cause of pediatric acute liver failure in the USA while hepatitis A predominates in South America. Hepatitis B is uncommon in children. The herpesvirus family can cause severe hepatic failure in neonates. Other hepatropic viruses in children include parvovirus, echovirus, Coxsackievirus and adenovirus (19).

A 12-lead ECG and echocardiogram should be performed to look for the presence of congenital heart disease, possible cardiomyopathy or rhythm disturbances. Cardiac catheterization may be indicated in patients with pulmonary hypertension as seen in Alagille syndrome and other complex congenital heart disease to evaluate the severity of cardiac pathology and its impact on the anesthetic plan. Liver transplantation is contraindicated if PAP > 50 mmHg is present. Patients must show response to medical treatment by reduction of the PAP to < 35 mmHg to be eligible for liver transplantation (20).

Preoperative arterial blood gas results help to evaluate the degree of hypoxia and acidosis. A chest radiograph is reviewed not only for the cardiac silhouette but for evidence of pleural effusions, pneumonia or pulmonary edema (19). Laboratory results should include a complete blood count, platelet count, PT, PTT, electrolyte panel and additional values for calcium, magnesium, glucose, albumin and ammonia.

Induction

Rapid-sequence induction is preferred because patients are considered as having a full stomach due to multiple factors including increased intra-abdominal pressure from ascites and organomegaly, delayed emptying from GI bleeding and hepatic encephalopathy and because of the urgent nature of the surgery. A rapid-sequence induction with propofol, etomidate or ketamine is the preferred technique. Muscle relaxation for intubation can be achieved with succinylcholine or rocuronium. Metabolism of succinylcholine may be delayed due to a reduced pseudocholinesterase concentration. The trachea should be intubated preferably with a cuffed endotracheal tube to ensure ventilation and to limit risks of aspiration. Attention to the cuff pressure is needed throughout the case to avoid excessive inflation and risk of tracheal ischemia, especially in small children. Some children who are properly NPO and without abdominal distension can even undergo an inhalational induction if no prior IV access has been established (21).

Maintenance of anesthesia is obtained by inhalation with sevoflurane, isoflurane or desflurane. Nitrous oxide should be avoided to prevent intestinal distension and the expansion of possible gas emboli. Analgesia is obtained with intermittent intravenous morphine administration or a fentanyl infusion and the latter can be continued postoperatively. Of note, fentanyl binds to alpha-1-acid glycoprotein, which is elevated during infections, making fentanyl less available to opioid receptors. Neuromuscular blockade can be achieved with any of the muscle relaxants but in cases where both hepatic and renal insufficiency exist, then cis-atracurium is the preferred agent since it does not depend on hepatic or renal elimination.

Because transplantation procedures are lengthy, eye lubrication is suggested as well as assurance that the eyes are closed and taped. All the pressure points should be padded (21,22).

Monitors should include a 3- or 5-lead ECG, noninvasive blood pressure and an arterial catheter, temperature monitor, nerve stimulator, pulse oximeter, CVP catheter, and urinary catheter. Transesophageal echocardiography (TEE) is used to assess filling of the heart and to estimate cardiac output (22). Pulmonary artery catheters are rarely used in children because of the size and risks of pulmonary complications.

At least two large-bore peripheral intravenous lines should be placed in the upper extremities for fluid resuscitation because of manipulation of the inferior vena cava during surgery. Teenage patients may accommodate a 6 FR catheter sheath placed centrally so that a rapid infusion device can be utilized. Ultrasound guidance is preferred for obtaining central vascular access because of coagulopathy and the risk of hematoma. Appropriately sized double-lumen central venous catheters should be placed in the upper half of the body. Central vascular access is needed for the infusion of ionotropes and other agents that may be harmful if extravasation were to occur during peripheral administration (e.g., $CaCl_2$, dopamine). The arterial pressure catheter should be placed in the upper extremity as well. Femoral artery catheters may not be reliable if aortic cross-clamp is used.

Children are prone to hypothermia because of their surface area to body mass ratio. This is compounded by heat loss from intra-abdominal exposure during liver transplantation. The operating room should be warmed before the patient enters. Every attempt should be made to keep the child warm during the preliminary steps of induction and while obtaining vascular access. Use warm blankets and forced hot air systems as well as radiant lamps. Intraoperatively, saline irrigation should be kept warm. Patients are also at risk of hypothermia when the cold liver graft is placed into the abdomen. All the intravenous fluids and blood products should be infused through fluid warmers and the patient should be draped in such a way as to avoid pooling of body fluids. Hypothermia can cause coagulation abnormalities, dysrhythmias, difficulty in cardiac resuscitation, impairment of renal function and delayed wound healing (23).

Hemodynamic stability is the focus throughout the procedure. The intravenous fluid of choice depends on the patient's renal status and the presence or absence of a metabolic imbalance. Normal saline and plasmalyte can be used while lactated Ringer's is usually avoided especially during the anhepatic phase when lactate cannot be metabolized; this causes further metabolic acidosis; 5% albumin needs to be given since these patients have hypoalbuminemia. Dextrose-containing solutions should be available in case hypoglycemia occurs. Fluid status is monitored by CVP and urine output. The CVP may not be a very reliable indicator of volume status because it is affected by changes in intra-abdominal pressure and transmitted pressure from surgical retractors. It is better to follow the CVP trend rather than the actual CVP value. The transesophageal echocardiogram (TEE) is a better guide of intravascular volume than is CVP because the former also gives information about cardiac function. Communication between the anesthesiologist and the surgeon is important at all times because of the dynamic nature of transplantation.

Maintenance

The impact of transplantation on anesthetic management

The liver transplantation procedure is divided into three stages: preanhepatic or dissection, anhepatic and postanhepatic or reperfusion. There are special requirements of anesthesia for these stages.

Dissection or preanhepatic stage

This phase lasts from skin incision to occlusion of the hepatic artery and portal vein. This phase is associated with significant blood loss due to coagulopathy and surgical bleeding especially in patients who have previously undergone the Kasai procedure (portoenterostomy) or prior liver transplantation. Maintaining hemodynamic stability can be challenging. Crystalloid administration may exceed totals of 100 ml/kg for the case. Adequate volume resuscitation fluids including colloids and blood products, and the correction of coagulopathy must be repeatedly assessed. Transfusion protocols vary as to the PRBC:FFP ratio administered. The ideal hematocrit is in the range of 26–30% and INR 1.5. Unless it is contraindicated, cell salvage techniques can be used to decrease the transfusion requirements (21). Cell savers are not used in patients with known malignancy. Serum glucose and electrolytes should be frequently checked and managed accordingly. Patients may develop citrate-induced hypocalcemia with rapid infusion of fresh frozen plasma.

Anhepatic stage

This stage begins with the clamping of the IVC and removal of the native liver up to the reanastomosis of the donor graft and its reperfusion. In the classic approach, the end-stage liver is removed en block after

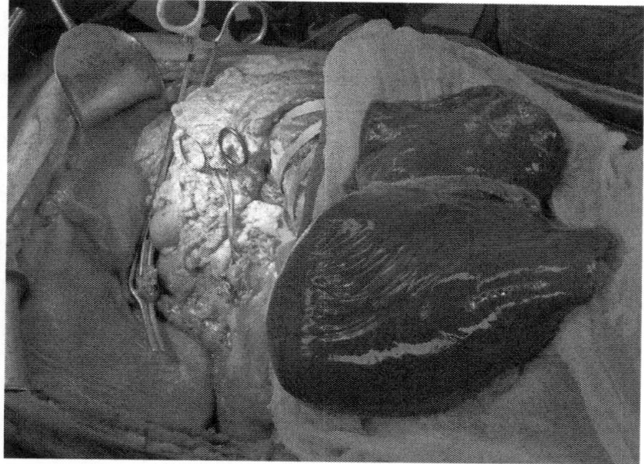

Figure 33.1 A new liver to go in, clamp on hepatic veins on cava (caval preservation). Anhepatic stage with partial clamping of the IVC. The potential for pre-load compromise is a major focus. Photograph courtesy of Dr. Janet Tuttle-Newhall, Director of Transplant Surgery, Saint Louis University School of Medicine.

dissecting it from its vascular supply and clamping the suprahepatic and infrahepatic vena cava, portal vein and hepatic artery (Figure 33.1). A reduction in preload occurs because the vena cava is cross-clamped. In pediatric liver transplantation a "piggy back" technique is preferred, which requires only partial clamping of the vena cava. The liver is separated away from the inferior vena cava, short hepatic veins, portal vein and the hepatic veins. The suprahepatic vena cava of the donor is anastomosed to the native hepatic veins and the infrahepatic vena cava is over sewn (Fig. 33.2). Some children may require a portocaval shunt if they are unable to tolerate clamping of the portal vein.

Since venous return is decreased with the clamping of the IVC, the goals during this stage are maintaining adequate preload and correction of metabolic abnormalities. Volume resuscitation is guided by CVP, blood pressure and urine output to maintain hemodynamic stability. Children with biliary atresia tolerate IVC clamping better than those with glycogen storage disease, presumably due to the presence of more collaterals. Thus, a lower systolic blood pressure and faster heart rate can be seen in children with glycogen storage disease during this stage of transplantation (24). Overhydration should be avoided because this can lead to congestion of the newly transplanted liver and excessive bleeding after reperfusion. Correction of hypoglycemia, acidosis, hypocalcemia, hyperkalemia and low hematocrit are required. During reperfusion, the inferior vena cava and portal vein are unclamped

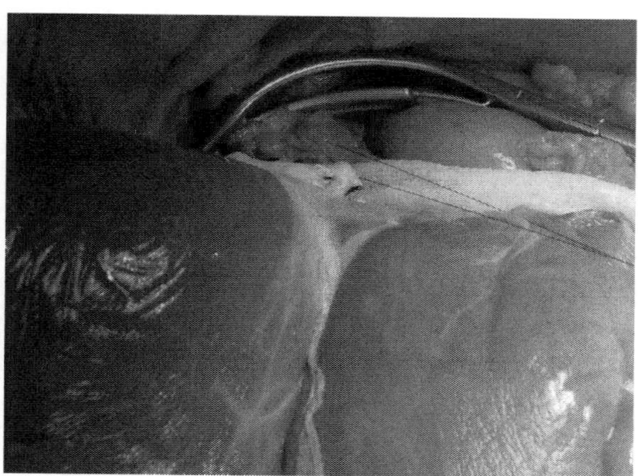

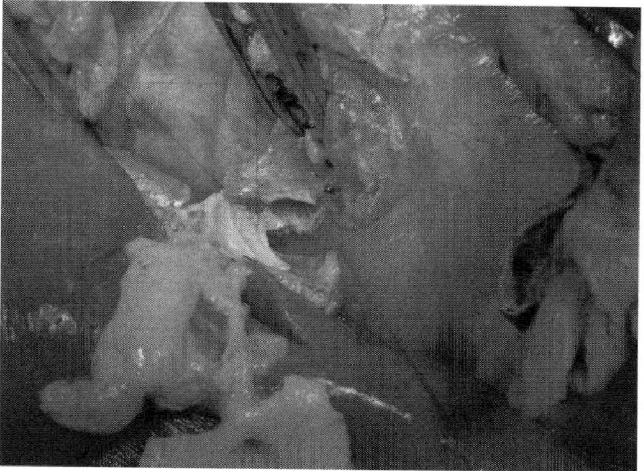

Figure 33.2 (a) Upper caval anastomosis. Suprahepatic vena cava of the donor graft anastomosis to the native hepatic vein. Photograph courtesy of Dr. Janet Tuttle-Newhall, Director of Transplant Surgery, Saint Louis University School of Medicine. **(b)** Portal vein anastomosis. To avoid future stricture, portal vein length is critical and should not be redundant. An everting suture technique is used to promote endothelium to endothelium growth between donor and recipient vessels. Photograph courtesy of Dr. Janet Tuttle-Newhall, Director of Transplant Surgery, Saint Louis University School of Medicine.

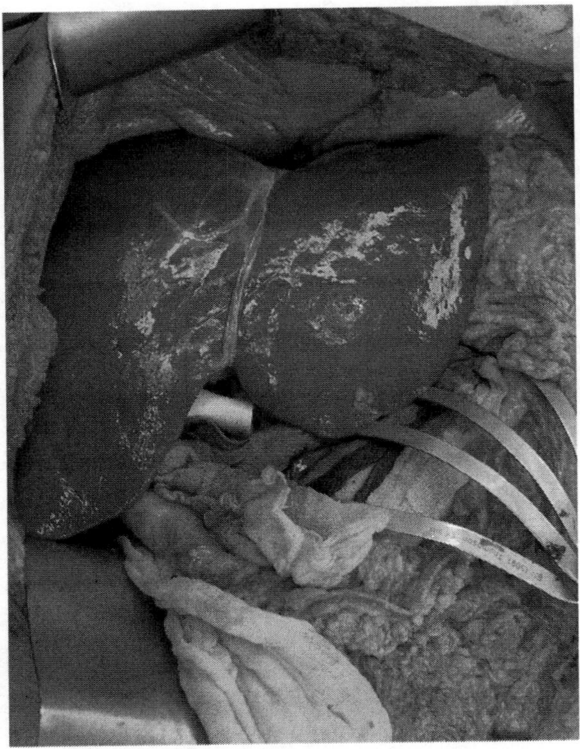

Figure 33.3 Reperfusion. Suprahepatic and infrahepatic clamps are removed and the donor liver is revascularized. Photograph courtesy of Dr. Janet Tuttle-Newhall, Director of Transplant Surgery, Saint Louis University School of Medicine.

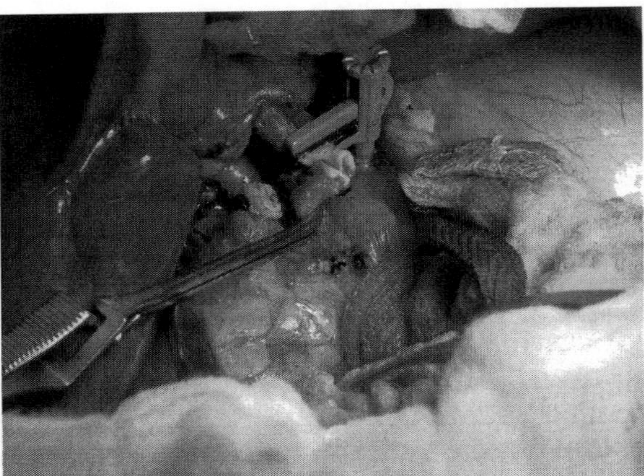

Figure 33.4 Hepatic artery anastomosis.Anastomosis is end to end. Length should provide just enough for a "lazy loop" to protect against kinking, which leads to thrombosis. Photograph courtesy of Dr. Janet Tuttle-Newhall, Director of Transplant Surgery, Saint Louis University School of Medicine.

and the donor graft is reperfused (Figure 33.3). Lastly, the hepatic artery is reanastomosed (Figure 33.4) All metabolic and electrolyte abnormalities should be corrected and intravascular volume should be restored prior to reperfusion to prevent hemodynamic instability. The surgical team should flush the liver with crystalloid or even the patient's blood to prevent a rise in potassium or lactate and to wash out debris and air emboli. The use of Wisconsin solution to flush the donor graft has shown some promise in limiting complications (25).

Despite all efforts for homeostasis, transient bradycardia, hypotension and dysrhythmias can occur in association with the unclamping of the IVC. Continued management of fluid and electrolyte disturbances and the use of inotropes will be essential.

Postanhepatic stage

Completion of the hepatic artery anastomosis and creation of biliary drainage define the postanhepatic stage. Many of the metabolic abnormalities start to autocorrect as the donor graft starts to function. There may be significant blood loss ongoing at this stage, especially with split-liver grafts, therefore fluid resuscitation and blood transfusion are continued but hematocrit is kept below 30% to decrease blood viscosity and to avoid hepatic artery thrombosis, which is the most common complication in pediatric hepatic transplantation (21).

Postoperative anesthetic concerns

Many patients remain intubated at the conclusion of surgery due to the required massive fluid resuscitation, changes in oncotic pressure and subsequent third spacing that occur. Airway edema may be present and a negative cuff leak test on deflation suggests significant laryngeal edema. Patients may be sedate from opioid administration, continued metabolic derangement or cerebral edema. Preventing blood loss and preserving renal function are important to postoperative stability (26).

Encephalopathy may be diminished or resolved as the donor graft function improves. Demonstration of a strong cough and gag reflexes and good cognition must be present if extubation is entertained. Pain control is generally managed with systemic opioids (Table 33.1).

Heart transplant

The first pediatric heart transplant was performed in 1967 by Kantrowitz on an 18-day-old neonate with

Table 33.1 Systems approach to anesthetic management for liver transplantation

Pathophysiologic changes	***Anesthetic implications***
Cardiac	*Cardiac*
Increased cardiac output	Hypotension with administration of anesthetics
Low systemic vascular resistance	Decreased sensitivity to catecholamines and vasopressors
Increased mixed venous oxygen saturation	
Decreased arteriovenous oxygen difference	
Pulmonary	*Pulmonary*
Hypoxemia	Adequate preoxygenation preinduction
Impaired hypoxic pulmonary vasoconstriction	Increased peak inspiratory pressure
Alveolar hypoventilation	PEEP
Decreased FRC	Consider cuffed ETT
Central nervous system	*Central nervous system*
Encephalopathy	Avoid sedatives
Cerebral edema	Fluid management may be complicated
Increased ICP	
Gastrointestinal	*Gastrointestinal*
Delayed gastric emptying	Rapid-sequence induction
Increased intra-abdominal pressure	
Liver	*Liver*
Portal hypertension	Impaired clearance of anesthetic drugs
Impaired synthetic and metabolic functions	Hypotension
Decreased intravascular volume	Glucose supplementation
Decreased glycogen stores	Large blood loss
Decreased clotting factors	Large-bore intravenous access
	Use ultrasound for central line placement
Renal	*Renal*
Prerenal azotemia	Monitor urine output
Hepatorenal syndrome	Monitor CVP

Adapted from Yudkowitz FS, Chietero M. Anesthetic issues in pediatric liver transplantation. *Pediatr Transplant* 2005; **9**: 666–72.

tricuspid atresia who survived for 6 hours (27). The 5-year survival rates have since improved to 70–80% for heart transplants due to advances in surgical technique, immunosuppression therapy and organ preservation. Early death occurs in less than 10% of recipients (28).

Demographics

In 2012, the number of pediatric transplants performed totaled 370 and included children from the neonatal period to 17 years of age. Over the past decade the annual number of procedures has remained constant. The number of infants less than 1 year of age receiving heart transplants also has remained relatively stable over the last decade at approximately 100 procedures per year. The 1-year infant survival rate is similar to that of older children (29).

Indications

The major indications for pediatric heart transplant are complex congenital heart disease, especially in children less than 1 year of age, cardiomyopathy in older children and retransplantation. Rare indications include unresectable cardiac tumors and sequelae of Kawasaki disease (30). Assessment for pre-existing comorbidities is required before a child is entered onto the transplant list. The United Network for Organ Sharing (UNOS) categorizes patients as 1A, 1B and 2 with 1A being the most critical. Children comprise less than 10% of the UNOS list for cardiac transplantation (31).

Complex congenital heart disease is the main indication for cardiac transplantation in infants and includes irreparable complex congenital cardiac conditions or lesions with end-stage heart failure after surgical repair. Hypoplastic left heart syndrome was once a major indication for transplantation but is no longer the case now with improvement in surgical technique. However, a failed Fontan is still an indication for heart transplant (32,33).

Dilated cardiomyopathy is the most common type of cardiomyopathy in children and is a reason for transplant in older children. Causes include viral myocarditis, neuromuscular disorders, chemotherapy, metabolic diseases, and genetic disorders. The primary abnormality is impairment of systolic function leading to congestive cardiac failure and the need for cardiac transplantation when medical therapy fails (34).

Hypertrophic cardiomyopathy is heterogeneous in its etiology and may be due to neuromuscular disease, inborn errors of metabolism and genetic disorders. There is a risk of sudden cardiac death. The left ventricular outflow tract obstruction can occur at rest and dynamically. The interventricular septum is often involved and there may be an abnormal mitral valve attachment. Concentric left ventricular hypertrophy in the absence of hypertension is seen.

Restrictive cardiomyopathy is rare in children. The disease is caused by infiltration of the myocardium as seen in mucopolysaccharoidosis, glycogen storage disease, amyloidosis, sarcoidosis and hemochromatosis. There is restrictive filling with diastolic dysfunction and pulmonary hypertension. It does not respond to medical or surgical treatment and cardiac transplant is necessary (34).

Retransplantation is performed in the management of post-transplant coronary vasculopathy and graft failure. Infants who had a transplant for congenital heart disease may need retransplantation in 10 years (31).

Contraindications

Relative contraindications include psychosocial issues, multiorgan failure, active malignancies, uncontrolled infection and severe organ dysfunction. Absolute contraindications include severe prematurity, low birth weight, hypoplasia of the pulmonary veins and arteries and irreversible pulmonary hypertension of greater than 6 Wood units (30).

Assessment of the donor

Availability of donors for children is limited but larger sized hearts can be transplanted with donor to recipient weight ratio of up to 3.0 without problems of chest closure, prolonged postoperative ventilation or increased duration of inotrope support (35). Larger-sized hearts are beneficial to the recipients who have pulmonary hypertension because a large right ventricle can better handle increased afterload (36).

Donors should be ABO blood group compatible but many centers are transplanting ABO-incompatible hearts into infants with success because of their poorly established immune system. To decrease the risk of graft rejection, plasma exchange should be done during cardiopulmonary bypass to reduce iso-hemaglutinin levels. ABO-compatible packed red blood cells matched to the recipient should be used for priming the CPB pump. There should be no anti-A or anti-B antibodies to the donor or recipient in all plasma components and platelets (37); HLA matching is time consuming and is not routinely done. Panel reactive antibodies (PRA) are circulating HLA alloantibodies which can cause graft rejection and so are assayed. Overall mortality is increased if PRA values are more than 10%. This is also important in further management for immunosuppression management (38).

Anesthesia for pediatric cardiac transplant

Preoperative assessment

It is very important to understand the basic pathophysiology as well as coexisting comorbidities in patients presenting for heart transplantation. These patients may have mild to moderate pulmonary hypertension, severely decreased cardiac function or renal insufficiency. A review of medications should be performed. The child may require preoperative inotropic support, which needs to be continued until cardiopulmonary bypass has been initiated.

Review of electrocardiogram, cardiac catheterization, echocardiogram and chest radiograph should be done. Laboratory investigations including complete blood count with differential, coagulation profile, serum electrolytes and metabolic panel should be done. The patient's NPO status and any recent change from the previous medical history and physical exam should be assessed in deciding the anesthetic plan.

Anesthetic management

Anesthetic management depends on the clinical status of the patient and indication(s) for the transplant. Some patients may be already intubated and receiving inotropes, pulmonary vasodilators or supported by a ventricular assist device (39). Other patients coming from home may not be properly NPO because of the unpredictable nature of donor availability which does not permit early notification. These patients may be very anxious and oral or intravenous midazolam may be required but should be carefully administered and monitored for any exaggerated response. Oxygen and airway equipment should be available at the time of premedication. Induction of anesthesia should be done only after noninvasive monitoring is established. Intravenous induction should be performed. If intravenous access is not already present then a catheter should be inserted. Inhalational inductions are to be avoided (12). Induction can be accomplished with ketamine, etomidate, midazolam and fentanyl or propofol and the latter should be given in small doses to avoid myocardial depression and hypotension. Ketamine is the agent of choice for many centers. If rapid-sequence induction is planned, then preoxygenation, succinylcholine or high-dose rocuronium should be given after administering the induction agent of choice. Maintenance of anesthesia may be accomplished with opioids, benzodiazepines and low-dose inhalational agent plus a nondepolarizing muscle relaxant.

After induction and intubation, more intravenous access should be obtained. Sites for arterial and central venous access should be discussed with the surgeon prior to bringing the patient to the operating room because of difficulties due to multiple cut downs and cardiac catheterizations from prior procedures. Ideally a large-bore double-lumen catheter is inserted into the left internal jugular vein and the right side is spared for obtaining future cardiac biopsies for assessment of rejection. The right groin is also spared in the event that the patient requires mini CPB emergently during the surgery. All catheters should be inserted with strict aseptic technique in anticipation of the effects of immunosuppressive therapy. A transesophageal echocardiography (TEE) probe is placed prior to transplantation. Inotrope infusions are continued until the initiation of bypass, if utilized. The potential for high-volume blood loss exists, especially if there is a coagulopathy or if the child has undergone multiple surgeries. Therefore, antifibrinolytic agents are indicated for control of any ongoing bleeding problem. There should be close collaboration with the donor organ retrieval team to avoid prolonged ischemia time.

Management of cardiopulmonary bypass is the same as for any open heart surgery. Dopamine and milrinone infusions are started before separating from CPB. Milrinone is used to decrease the pulmonary vascular resistance. Transesophageal echocardiography is done to evaluate the heart function. If the right heart appears distended then nitric oxide and hyperventilation are instituted to decrease pulmonary hypertension. The transplanted heart is denervated and therefore does not respond to atropine but will respond to epinephrine because of alpha and beta receptors within the donor heart (40). Temporary pacing may be needed if bradycardia does not respond to inotropes. If cardiac function is still poor then the patient may need extracorporeal membrane oxygenation (ECMO) or temporary support via a ventricular assist device (41).

Before termination from CPB, acid–base status, serum potassium and ionized calcium levels are corrected. After termination of CPB, protamine is given to reverse the anticoagulant effects of heparin. Platelets and fresh frozen plasma and cryoprecipitate are given as needed. Arterial blood gas, activated clotting time and complete coagulation profile should be checked. Immunosuppressive agents are started intravenously per protocol. The patient is transported to the intensive care unit for further management of ventilation, inotrope support, invasive monitoring and immunosuppressive therapy.

Renal transplantation

Renal transplantation in children has been so successful that it has been suggested as the treatment of choice for end-stage renal disease. Dialysis in children is associated with a greater than fourfold increase in mortality as compared to renal transplantation (42). In a Middle Eastern study, the overall 1- and 10-year actuarial survival rates were 99% and 98%, respectively for the recipients, and 88% and 84%, respectively, for the grafts (43). In the USA, 1-year survival of the grafts from living related donors is 89% and the 3-year survival is 80%. Survival data for cadaveric grafts are 74% and 62% for 1- and 3-year survival, respectively. Age at the time of transplantation is important as well as size and age match of donors. Those patients transplanted under 2 years of age have decreased survival. Children less than 10 kg are faced with a higher complication rate.

Indications and contraindications for renal transplantation

The causes of end-stage renal disease (ERSD) in children differ from adult ESRD; 40% of children present with congenital disease such as renal dysplasia or aplasia, obstructive uropathy, reflux nephropathy, congenital nephrotic syndrome or polycystic disease. Glomerulosclerosis accounts for about 25% of the cases presenting for transplantation. Hemolytic

Table 33.2 Diseases leading to renal transplantation in children

Alport syndrome
Prune belly syndrome
Nephrotic syndrome
Bladder extrophy
Renal aplasia/dysplasia
Glomerulosclerosis
Focal sclerosing glomerulonephritis
Hemolytic uremic syndrome (HUS)
Obstructive uropathy
Posterior urethral valves
Reflux nephropathy
Polycystic kidney disease
Systemic disease
Diabetes mellitus Lupus

Adapted from Uejima T. Anesthetic management of the pediatric patient undergoing solid organ transplantation. *Anesthesiol Clin N Am* 2004; **22**: 809–826.

uremic syndrome (HUS) is the cause of ESRD in less than 10% of pediatric patients (44,45).

Active malignancy is a contraindication for transplantation. Patient with Wilm's tumor must be disease free for 2 years before renal transplantation can be considered. HIV is controversial but in general is considered a contraindication (Table 33.2).

Preoperative assessment

Patients with ESRD should be carefully evaluated for concomitant disease. Postdialysis hypovolemia can contribute to hemodynamic instability at the time of induction. Hyperkalemia may contribute to rhythm disturbances at induction and throughout the case. Elevated serum calcium and phosphate may occur secondary to hyperparathyroidism. Assessment for glucose intolerance or frank diabetes mellitus should be evaluated and treated. Hypertension, congestive heart failure, pericardial effusions or cardiomyopathies may also compromise hemodynamic stability. Hematological concerns include anemia, thrombocytopenia and abnormal platelet function even if the count is normal. Neurologic symptoms may include somnolence, memory loss, seizures and even coma (12).

Anesthetic management

Induction

The use of sevoflurane in renal transplantation has been questioned because of the theoretical nephrotoxic effects of compound A that results from the agent's interaction with carbon dioxide absorbant used in the anesthesia circuit system. Human studies of sevoflurane show no untoward renal effects. Isoflurane, desflurane and sevoflurane have been shown to be safe anesthetics for patients with ESRD (46). Intravenous induction with propofol, barbiturates and ketamine are safe; however, etomidate is typically avoided because of its potential to induce adrenal insufficiency.

Neuromuscular blocking agents

Succinylcholine can be used for intubation; however, a predictable increase in serum potassium of 0.5 meq/L occurs in healthy patients and this response may not be tolerated in patients with renal failure. The patient should have a serum potassium less than 5.5 mEq/L if succinylcholine is felt to be required (47).

Long-acting nondepolarizing paralytics will have a prolonged effect thus, pancuronium should likely be avoided. Intermediate-acting agents such as vecuronium and rocuronium are eliminated independently of renal function but can be prolonged, in part due to active metabolites. Mivacurium is eliminated via hydrolysis by plasma cholinesterases; however, esterase levels may be lower than normal in this patient population. Atracurium and cis-atracurium are inactivated by Hoffman elimination and ester hydrolysis. Laudanosine is a potentially neurotoxic metabolite of the atracuriums and is excreted by the kidney. Since cis-atracurium is the more potent of the two, it produces a lower concentration of laudanosine. Both atracurium and cis-atracurium can be used for relaxation during renal transplantation (47).

Analgesics

Morphine has over six metabolites but there are two metabolites of note: morphine-3-glucuronide (M3G), which is neuroexcitatory, and morphine-6-glucuronide (M6G), an analgesic that has a longer half-life than the parent compound. Unpredictable accumulation and binding to opioid receptors places the renal patient at risk for oversedation, respiratory depression and untoward gastrointestinal effects from morphine. Therefore, morphine should be avoided. Hydromorphone has no active analgesic metabolites; however, the primary metabolite of hydromorphone, hydromorphone-3-glucuronide, has neuroexcitatory potential similar to or greater than the M3G metabolite of morphine (48). Short-term therapy with hydromorphone is acceptable for the perioperative period, provided that close observation for the respiratory and sedative effects are monitored.

Fentanil, alfentanil, and sufentanil have inactive metabolites and can be safely used for intraoperative or postoperative pain control. Remifentanil has a mildly active metabolite, GR90291, that is of no consequence to renal transplant patients. Remifentanil is metabolized by tissue esterases and elimination is via renal excretion; however, use of any of the fentanyl derivatives is acceptable since their pharmacokinetics are not altered by ESRD (47).

Epidural analgesia has been used successfully in children without major morbidity. Intraoperative hemodynamic instability has not been reported. Postoperatively, supplemental analgesics may be needed for renal transplant patients. Concern for risk of epidural hematoma and infection in the presence of coagulopathy and immunosuppression are reasonable; however, an adverse outcome is extremely rare. Preoperative coagulation profiles should be obtained. With daily epidural care, catheters placed by percutaneous insertion can safely remain for 4 days (45).

Intraoperative maintenance

Assurance of perfusion pressure is paramount to the success of the transplant. A central venous catheter is used for monitoring fluid balance not only during surgery but can be valuable in the postoperative period, yet every center does not employ this practice. Absolute CVP values may be less important than the trend of values; CVP–guided fluid therapy may help optimize hydration. Two large-bore peripheral intravenous catheters are essential since fluid administration totals may exceed 80 ml/kg. Albumin and hydroxyethyl starch can be used for severe volume deficits. Normal saline is the routine fluid of choice; however, metabolic acidosis can result from administration of large volumes of saline due to its chloride content and subsequent potassium shifts that result in worsened hyperkalemia. Dopamine, mannitol and furosemide may be used to increase diuresis. An arterial catheter provides hemodynamic monitoring and is a sampling source for close monitoring of electrolytes and the occurrence of anemia (45–47).

Postoperative management

Volume therapy to maintain urine output is essential. Pain control should be a balanced regimen with avoidance of nephrotoxic drugs. The NSAIDs are typically withheld; however, COX-2 inhibitors such as ketorolac have been administered for pediatric transplantation without adverse outcome (49). Continuance of immunosuppressive therapy and monitoring for early graft rejection are key. Perioperative demise is usually related to cardiovascular events or infection.

Summary

Organ transplantation in children has made significant advances due to improved surgical techniques, organ preservation and better immunosuppression regimens. Families and patients undergo significant duress from the pervasive effects of having a life-threatening illness control their lives. Social stigma may be experienced by adolescents. The wait list process is anxiety-provoking and is emotional by nature as the child and family go through the steps of waiting, preparing and then receiving a transplant. Support is invaluable to the families and anxieties must be allayed when possible. Assurances are best accomplished when families work with a unified transplant team whose common goal is the improvement of the child's chances for a full life.

References

1. Starzl TE, Marciaro TL, Vonkaula KN, *et al.* Homotransplantation of the liver in humans. *Surg Gynecol Obstet* 1963; **117**: 659–64.
2. Starzl TE. History of liver and other splanchnic organ transplantation. In Busutill RW, Klintmalm GB, eds. *Transplantation of the Liver.* Philadelphia, PA: W.B. Saunders; 1996, pp. 3–22.
3. Kamath BM, Olthoff KM. Liver transplantation in children: Update 2010. *Pediatr Clin N Am* 2010; **57**: 401–14.
4. Bennett J, Bromley P. Perioperative issues in pediatric liver transplantation. *Int. Anesthesiol Clin* 2006; **44**(3): 125–47.
5. Starzl TE, Todo S, Fung J, *et al.* FK506 for liver, kidney, and pancreas transplantation. *Lancet* 1989; **2**: 1000–4.

6. Eghtesad B, Aucejo F, Fung JJ. Preservation solutions in liver transplantation: what are the options? *Liver Transpl* 2005; **12**: 196–8.

7. Organ Procurement and Transplant Network. Based on OPTN data, Aug 23, 2013.

8. Freeman RB, Weisner RH, Harper A, *et al*: The new allocation system : moving toward evidence-based transplantation policy. *Liver Transpl* 2002; **8**: 851–8.

9. Barshes NR, Lee TC, Udell IW, Mahoney A, *et al.* The pediatric end-stage liver disease (PELD) model as a predictor of survival benefit and posttransplant survival in pediatric liver transplant recipients. *Liver Transpl* 2006; **12**: 475–80.

10. Bourdeaaux C, Tri TT, Gras J, Sokal E, *et al.* PELD score and posttransplant outcome in pediatric liver transplantation: a retrospective study of 100 recipients. *Transplantation* 2005; **79**: 1273–6.

11. Yudkowitz FS, Chietero M. Anesthetic issues in pediatric liver transplantation. *Pediatr Transpl* 2005; **9**: 666–72.

12. Uejima T. Anesthetic management of the pediatric patient undergoing solid organ transplantation. *Anesth Clin N Am* 2004; **22**: 809–26.

13. Gettins PG. Serpin structure, mechanism and function. *Chem Rev* 2002; **102**(12): 4751–804.

14. Emrick KM, Rand EB, Goldmunitz E, Krantz ID, *et al.* Features of Alagille syndrome in 92 patients: frequency and relation to prognosis. *Hepatology* 1999; **29**: 822–9.

15. Ala A, Walker AP, Ashkan K, Dooley JS, Schilsky ML Wilson's disease. *Lancet* 2007; **369** (9559): 397–408.

16. Vaja R, McNicol L, Sisley I. Anaesthesia for patients with liver disease. *Contin Educ Anaesth Crit Care Pain* 2010; **10**(1): 15–19.

17. Budhiraja R, Hassoun P. Portopulmonary hypertension: a tale of two circulations. *Chest* 2003; **123**: 562–76.

18. Hochhauser E, Alterman I, Weinbroum A, *et al.* Effects of vasoactive substances released from ischemic reperfused liver on the isolated rat heart. *Exp Clin Cardiol* 2001; **6**(1): 29–34.

19. Dhawan A. Etiology and prognosis of acute liver failure in children. *Liver Transpl* 2008; **12**: S80–4.

20. Saleemi S. Portopulmonary hypertension. *Ann Thorac Med* 2010; **5**(1): 5–9.

21. Yudkowitz FS, Chietro M. Anesthetic issues in pediatric liver transplantation. *Pediatr Transpl* 2005; **9**: 666–72.

22. Feierman DE, Yudkowitz FS, Hojsak J, Emre S. Management of a cadaveric orthotopic liver transplantation in a pediatric patient with complex congenital heart disease. *Pediatr Anesth* 2006; **16**: 669–75.

23. Kurz A, Sessler DJ, Lenhardt R. The study of wound infection, Temperature Group. Perioperative normothermia to reduce the incidence of surgical-wound infection and shorten hospitalization. *N Engl J Med* 1996; **334**: 1209–16.

24. Huang HW, Lu HF, Chiang MH, *et al.* Hemodynamic changes during the anhepatic phase in pediatric patients with biliary atresia versus glycogen storage disease undergoing living donor liver transplantation. *Transplant Proc* 2012; **44**(2): 473–5.

25. Mirza DF, Gunson BK, Khalaf H, *et al.* Effect of pre-reperfusion portal venous blood flush on early liver transplant function. *Transpl Int* 1996; **9**(Suppl 1): S188–90.

26. Feltracco P, Ori C. Anesthetic management of living transplantation. *Minerva Anestesiol* 2010; **76**(7): 525–33.

27. Kantrowitz A, Halter JD, Joos H, *et al.* Transplantation of the heart in an infant and an adult. *Am J Cardiol* 1968; **22**: 782–90.

28. Azeka E, Barbero-Marcial M, Jatene M, *et al.* Heart transplantation in neonates and children: intermediate-term results. *Aeq Bras Cardiol* 2000; **74**: 197–208.

29. Chinnock RE Bailey LL. Heart transplantation for congenital heart disease in the first year of life. *Curr Cardiol Rev* 2011; **7**(2): 72–84.

30. Huddleston CB. Indications for heart transplantation in children. *Prog Pediatr Cardiol* 2009; **26**: 3–9.

31. Williams GD, Ramamoorthy C. Anesthesia considerations for pediatric thoracic solid organ transplant. *Anesthesiol Clin North Am* 2005; **23**: 709–31.

32. Chen JM, Davies RR, Mital SR, *et al.* Trends and outcomes in transplantation for complex congenital heart disease: 1984 to 2004. *Ann Thorac Surg* 2004; **78**: 1352–61.

33. Bernstein D, Naftel D, Chin C, *et al.* Outcome of listing for cardiac transplantation for failed Fontan: a multi-institutional study. *Circulation* 2006; **114**: 273–80.

34. Lee KJ, McCrindle BW, Bohn DJ. Clinical outcomes of acute myocarditis in childhood. *Heart* 1999; **82**: 226–33.

35. Bailey LL. Heart transplantation techniques in complex congenital heart disease. *J Heart Lung Transplant* 1993; **12**: 168–75.

36. Doroshow RW, Ashwal S, Saukel JW. Availability and selection of donors for pediatric heart transplantation. *J Heart Lung Transplant* 1995; **14**: 52–8.

37. Foreman C, Gruenwald C, West L. ABO-incompatible heart

transplantation: a perfusion strategy. *Perfusion* 2004; **19**: 69–72.

38. Jacobs JP, Quintessenza JA, *et al.* Pediatric cardiac transplantation in children with high reactive antibody. *Ann Thorac Surg* 2004; **78**: 1703–9.

39. Schure AY, Kussman BD. Pediatric heart transplantation: demographics, outcomes, and anesthetic implications. *Pediatr Anesth* 2011; **21**: 594–603.

40. Murphy DA, Thompson GW, Ardell JL, *et al.* The heart reinnervates after retransplantation. *Ann Thorac Surg* 2000; **69**: 1769–81.

41. Mitchell MB, Campbell DN, Bielefeld MR, *et al.* Utility of extracorporeal oxygenation for early graft failure following heart transplantation in infancy. *J Heart Lung Transplant* 2000; **19**: 834–9.

42. McDonald SP, Craig JC. Australian and New Zealand Paediatric Nephrology Association. Long-term survival of children with end-stage renal disease. *N Engl J Med* 2004; **350**(26): 2654–62.

43. Otukesh H, Hoseini R, Rahimzadeh N, *et al.* Outcome of renal transplantation in children: a multi-center national report from Iran. *Pediatr Transpl* 2011; **15**(5): 533–8.

44. Giessing M, Muller D, Winkelmann B, Roigas J, Loening SA. Kidney transplantation in children and adolescents. *Transplant Proc* 2007; **39**: 2197–201.

45. Coupe N, O'Brien M, Gibson P, De Lima J. Anesthesia for pediatric renal transplantation with and without epidural analgesia – a review of 7 years experience. *Pediatr Anesth* 2005; **15**: 220–8.

46. Schmid S, Jungwirth B. Anaesthesia for renal transplant surgery: an update. *Eur J Anaesthesiol* 2012; **29**: 552–8.

47. SarnKapoor H, Kaur R, Kaur H. Anaesthesia for renal transplant surgery. *Acta Anaesthesiol Scand* 2007; **51**: 1354–67.

48. Smith HS. Opioid metabolism. *Mayo Clin Proc* 2009; **84**(7): 613–24.

49. Rocca GD, Costa MG, Bruno K, *et al.* Pediatric renal transplantation: anesthesia and perioperative complications. *Pediatr Surg Int* 2001; **17**: 175–9.

Chapter 34

Thermoregulation in pediatric anesthesia

Kelly A. Machovec and B. Craig Weldon

Maintenance of body temperature is a tightly regulated physiologic phenomenon involving integration of central and peripheral nervous systems. Thermoreceptors reside in the skin, with tenfold more cold receptors than warm receptors.[1] Cold information travels to the CNS via A delta nerve fibers, while heat information travels via unmyelinated C fibers.[1] Afferent signals from peripheral sites regarding body temperature travel to the central nervous system (CNS). Efferent responses are then generated and travel back to peripheral sites.

The hypothalamus is the primary CNS site for temperature control and signal integration. An efferent signal is generated once a particular hyperthermic or hypothermic threshold is reached. The *interthreshold range* defines the temperature range in which no efferent response to either hypothermia or hyperthermia is generated.[2] In unanesthetized humans, this range is only 0.5 °C[3] extending equally above and below a normal temperature of 37 °C. Under general anesthesia, the interthreshold range expands to 4 °C, from approximately 33 °C to 38 °C.[3] In this expanded range of temperature over which the body will not trigger a response, humans behave as poikilotherms, and will mimic the temperature of the environment. Note that the interthreshold range does not expand equally into hyperthermic and hypothermic zones; the threshold for hypothermia is lowered much more than the threshold for hyperthermia is raised, reflecting the more dangerous consequences of hyperthermia.[4–7] Despite the lowered threshold for response, once a thermoregulatory efferent response is generated, the magnitude of the response is not affected by general anesthesia.[4]

Efferent signals modulate responses to both hyperthermia and hypothermia. Such responses include behavioral changes, voluntary muscle activity, cutaneous vasodilation and vasoconstriction, shivering, and sweating. Behavioral changes and voluntary muscle activity are not relevant in anesthetized patients and will not be discussed further. Cutaneous vasoconstriction is the most effective method to reduce heat loss.[2] Vasoconstriction both decreases cutaneous blood flow and increases the insulation effect of body tissue. Sweating is an effective method to increase body heat loss; it is mediated by postganglionic cholinergic transmission.[2] Sweating accompanies cutaneous vasodilation, allowing heat to be lost through the skin and is a more effective response than shivering. Humans can expend up to five times the basal metabolic rate by sweating but can only double heat production by shivering.[3,8]

Importance of thermoregulation in neonates and infants

Newborns, both preterm and full term, have intact vasoconstrictor and vasodilator responses to temperature changes.[9] However, this population is prone to heat loss due to thin skin and a large body surface area to mass ratio. Heat is very easily lost through the infant's head due to thin skull bones, little hair, and a relatively large head with a highly perfused brain.[10] Covering the baby's head can limit heat loss and decrease oxygen consumption.[11] In fact, there is a direct relationship between oxygen consumption and the temperature gradient between the infant's skin and their environment. Gradients as low as 2–4 °C will minimize the increase in oxygen consumption.[12]

Heat loss mechanisms

In order of decreasing magnitude, body heat under anesthesia is lost by radiation, convection, evaporation, and conduction. *Radiation* is the transfer of

Essentials of Pediatric Anesthesiology, ed. Alan David Kaye, Charles James Fox and James H. Diaz. Published by Cambridge University Press. © Cambridge University Press 2015.

heat between two surfaces that are not in direct contact. It is the primary modality of heat loss under general anesthesia. Radiant heat loss is particularly problematic in infants and children, who have a large surface area to body weight ratio. Warming the operating room, and thus decreasing the temperature difference between the patient and the environment, minimizes radiant heat loss.

Convection describes the loss of body heat due to disruption of the layer of air immediately surrounding the body that normally acts as insulation; loss of this insulating air layer is due to operating room airflow, and exposes the patient to environmental air currents. Conceptually, convective heat loss is similar to the "wind chill."

Conduction is the transfer of heat between two surfaces that are in direct contact. Avoiding direct skin contact with metal objects, warming fluids and blood, and warming intracavity irrigation solutions may minimize conductive heat loss.

Evaporative heat is lost to the environment through the integumentary and respiratory systems. Thus, wet skin preparation solutions, wet drapes, increased minute ventilation, and large open surgical wounds increase evaporative losses.[13] Humidification of fresh gas combats respiratory heat losses.[14] Active humidification of fresh gases up to 90% humidity can increase core body temperature up to 0.25 °C, while lack of humidification may decrease core body temperature by 0.75 °C.[15]

Heat generation mechanisms

Mechanisms of heat generation include voluntary muscle activity, nonshivering thermogenesis, and shivering thermogenesis. As voluntary muscle activity is not relevant to the general anesthesia setting, this discussion is limited to the latter two entities.

Nonshivering thermogenesis involves metabolic heat production from specialized adipose tissue, or brown fat. Brown fat is present in the neonate at 20–30 weeks gestation,[16] and is primarily located in the interscapular region, neck, axilla, mediastinum, and perirenal/periadrenal regions.[17] Brown fat is brown in color due to the presence of large numbers of mitochondria; heat production results from the uncoupling of mitochondrial oxidative phosphorylation, which would normally produce adenosine triphosphate.[18] Hypothermia causes release of norepinephrine, which binds to β_3-adrenergic receptors in brown adipose tissue, causing release of free fatty acids which are metabolized to produce heat.[19] Glucocorticoids[20] and thyroid hormone[21] are also involved in activation of brown adipose. Nonshivering thermogenesis is a primary source of heat production in infants but is not sustainable for long periods of time. This mechanism, however, is not clinically significant in older children or adults.[2] General anesthetic agents inhibit heat generation by brown fat metabolism, including inhalational agents[22] and propofol.[23]

Shivering thermogenesis is triggered after behavioral modification (e.g., seeking warm shelter) and cutaneous vasoconstriction have failed to remedy hypothermia. Shivering is defined as rapid, disorganized skeletal muscle activity with the goal of heat production[24] and is involuntary in nature. Shivering is more pronounced in the trunk than the peripheral muscles[25] and can double metabolic heat production[2] but this may not be sustainable. Shivering does not occur in newborns[2] and may occur for nonthermoregulatory reasons, such as pain.[26,27]

Effects of hypothermia and hyperthermia

Hypothermia has many undesirable physiologic effects. Hypothermia results in shivering, impaired drug metabolism,[28–31] increased blood loss,[32,33] impaired wound healing, and increased postoperative infections.[34,35] Shivering results in increased oxygen consumption and increased levels of norepinephrine that, if severe, lead to vasoconstriction, decreased tissue perfusion, hypoxia, and acidosis. Importantly, hypothermia decreases minimal alveolar concentration for inhalational anesthetics and increases tissue solubility of the agents,[36,37] making anesthetic overdose possible in a hypothermic patient. Mild hypothermia (34–36 °C) does not delay awakening or postanesthetic recovery in infants or children.[38]

General anesthesia does not disrupt the effector mechanisms for hyperthermia,[39] including cutaneous vasodilation[40] and sweating.[3] Vasodilation increases heat dissipation via the cholinergic autonomic nervous system.[41,42]

Anesthesia and thermoregulation

Mild hypothermia (34–36 °C) is common under general anesthesia because of increased environmental exposure, decreased metabolic rate (and therefore

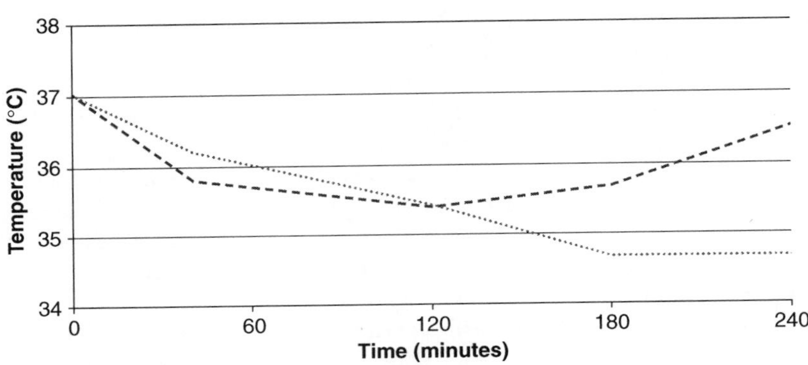

Figure 34.1 Three stages of heat loss in infants (dashed line) and adults (dotted line) under anesthesia. Phase 1 represents redistribution from core to peripheral tissues and lasts approximately 1 hour. Phase 2 is a period of heat loss to the environment. Phase 3 in adults represents steady state and in children is a period of rewarming. Adapted from Bissonnette B. Thermoregulation and paediatric anaesthesia. *Current Opinion in Anesthesiology* 1993; **6**: 537–42.

metabolic heat production),[43] central inhibition of thermoregulatory effector mechanisms,[3] and redistribution of body heat.[44]

Thermoregulation under general anesthesia can be divided into three phases[45,46] (Figure 34.1). The first phase is redistribution, where heat moves from the body's core, which contains the vessel-rich group and receives 75% of cardiac output, to the periphery. Core temperature decreases 0.5–1.5 °C during the first hour of anesthesia.[40] However, this does not represent true heat loss but rather a redistribution to the peripheral tissues. This redistribution is due to vasodilation induced by anesthetic agents.[47] Peripheral tissues act as a buffer, triggering vasoconstriction or vasodilation in response to signals from the central nervous system.

The second phase is the period of increased heat loss to the environment and decreased heat production.[4] Radiation and convection are the most important causes of heat loss during this phase. This phase may last 2–3 hours and is accompanied by increasing heat loss, with a total body heat deficit.

The third phase of thermoregulation differs in infants versus older children and adults. In older children and adults, this phase represents a steady state between heat production and heat loss, where core temperature remains stable. However, in infants and small children, this third phase is a time of rewarming. Infants are actually able to increase their core temperature under general anesthesia, likely due to nonshivering thermogenesis.[47]

As aforementioned, inhalational anesthetics expand the interthreshold range, reducing the threshold response for hypothermia more than increasing the threshold response for hyperthermia. However, the magnitude of the response is maintained once triggered, with all inhalational agents except desflurane, which may decrease the effector response.[48] Nitrous oxide decreases shivering thermogenesis.[49]

For intravenous anesthetics, opioids including alfentanil[50] and meperidine[51] decrease the threshold for vasoconstriction. Meperidine also decreases the threshold response for shivering, making it a clinically useful agent for this purpose. Midazolam minimally decreases the threshold for vasoconstriction,[52] while propofol decreases this threshold after a single bolus dose.[53] Dexmedetomidine decreases the threshold for vasoconstriction[54] and is also a useful treatment for shivering.[55] Atropine blocks sympathetic cholinergic transmission, thus increasing the threshold temperature for sweating.[56]

Regional anesthesia and thermoregulation

Core temperature decreases during the first hour of a regional anesthetic due to redistribution of heat from the core to the peripheral tissues,[57] similar to the first hour of a general anesthetic. However, unlike general anesthesia, central thermoregulation is not disrupted with regional anesthesia, and metabolic heat generation capabilities are intact.[44] Regional anesthetics disrupt afferent and efferent signaling between the central nervous system and the periphery. Therefore the magnitude of heat loss depends on the extent of the area blocked. Extensive blockade (e.g., thoracic epidural) and impaired vasoconstriction may prevent the steady state between heat loss and heat generation, potentially allowing extensive heat loss.[58–60] A study of combined inhalational anesthetic with caudal bupivacaine showed that the addition of the caudal did not change the vasoconstriction threshold from that induced by general anesthesia.[61]

Temperature monitoring

The American Society of Anesthesiologists recommends that body temperature be monitored when significant changes during the course of the anesthetic are expected (see American Society of Anesthesiologists Standards for basic anesthesia monitoring, available at www.asahq.org/publicationsAndServices/standards/02.pdf.). Core temperature monitoring at the nasopharynx, esophagus, bladder, and rectum offer the best combination of accuracy and precision.[62] Axillary temperature reflects core temperature when the temperature probe is correctly placed over the axillary artery.[14] The surgical procedure should be considered when choosing a core temperature monitoring site. For example, a laparotomy with peritoneal cavity irrigation may affect rectal temperature readings, while cardiac procedures may affect esophageal temperature readings.

References

1. Poulos DA. Central processing of cutaneous temperature information. *Federation Proceedings*. Dec 1981; **40**(14): 2825–9.
2. Sessler DI. Temperature monitoring and perioperative thermoregulation. *Anesthesiology*. Aug 2008; **109**(2): 318–38.
3. Sessler DI. Sweating threshold during isoflurane anesthesia in humans. *Anesthesia and Analgesia*. Sep 1991; **73**(3): 300–3.
4. Stoen R, Sessler DI. The thermoregulatory threshold is inversely proportional to isoflurane concentration. *Anesthesiology*. May 1990; **72**(5): 822–7.
5. Matsukawa T, Kurz A, Sessler DI, *et al.* Propofol linearly reduces the vasoconstriction and shivering thresholds. *Anesthesiology*. May 1995; **82**(5): 1169–80.
6. Xiong J, Kurz A, Sessler DI, *et al.* Isoflurane produces marked and nonlinear decreases in the vasoconstriction and shivering thresholds. *Anesthesiology*. Aug 1996; **85**(2): 240–5.
7. Annadata R, Sessler DI, Tayefeh F, Kurz A, Dechert M. Desflurane slightly increases the sweating threshold but produces marked, nonlinear decreases in the vasoconstriction and shivering thresholds. *Anesthesiology*. Dec 1995; **83**(6): 1205–11.
8. Horvath SM, Spurr GB, Hutt BK, Hamilton LH. Metabolic cost of shivering. *Journal of Applied Physiology*. May 1956; **8**(6): 595–602.
9. Lyons B, Taylor A, Power C, Casey W. Postanaesthetic shivering in children. *Anaesthesia*. May 1996; **51**(5): 442–5.
10. Fleming PJ, Azaz Y, Wigfield R. Development of thermoregulation in infancy: possible implications for SIDS. *Journal of Clinical Pathology*. Nov 1992; **45**(11 Suppl): 17–19.
11. Sinclair JC. Thermal control in premature infants. *Annual Review of Medicine*. 1972; **23**: 129–48.
12. Adamson SK, Jr., Gandy GM, James LS. The Influence of thermal factors upon oxygen consumption of the newborn human infant. *Journal of Pediatrics*. Mar 1965; **66**: 495–508.
13. Roe CF. Effect of bowel exposure on body temperature during surgical operations. *American Journal of Surgery*. Jul 1971; **122**(1): 13–15.
14. Bissonnette B, Sessler DI, LaFlamme P. Intraoperative temperature monitoring sites in infants and children and the effect of inspired gas warming on esophageal temperature. *Anesthesia and Analgesia*. Aug 1989; **69**(2): 192–6.
15. Bissonnette B, Sessler DI, LaFlamme P. Passive and active inspired gas humidification in infants and children. *Anesthesiology*. Sep 1989; **71**(3): 350–4.
16. Lean ME, James WP, Jennings G, Trayhurn P. Brown adipose tissue uncoupling protein content in human infants, children and adults. *Clinical Science*. Sep 1986; **71**(3): 291–7.
17. Aherne W, Hull D. The site of heat production in the newborn infant. *Proceedings of the Royal Society of Medicine*. Dec 1964; **57**: 1172–3.
18. Himms-Hagen J. Cellular thermogenesis. *Annual Review of Physiology*. 1976; **38**: 315–51.
19. Schiff D, Stern L, Leduc J. Chemical thermogenesis in newborn infants: catecholamine excretion and the plasma non-esterified fatty acid response to cold exposure. *Pediatrics*. Apr 1966; **37**(4): 577–82.
20. Jessen K. The cortisol fluctuations in plasma in relation to human regulatory nonshivering thermogenesis. *Acta Anaesthesiologica Scandinavica*. Apr 1980; **24**(2): 151–4.
21. Jessen K. The relation between thyroid function and human regulatory nonshivering thermogenesis. *Acta Anaesthesiologica Scandinavica*. Apr 1980; **24**(2): 144–50.
22. Ohlson KB, Mohell N, Cannon B, Lindahl SG, Nedergaard J. Thermogenesis in brown adipocytes is inhibited by volatile anesthetic agents. A factor contributing to hypothermia in infants? *Anesthesiology*. Jul 1994; **81**(1): 176–83.
23. Plattner O, Semsroth M, Sessler DI, *et al.* Lack of nonshivering

thermogenesis in infants anesthetized with fentanyl and propofol. *Anesthesiology*. Apr 1997; **86**(4): 772–7.

24. Hemingway A, Price WM. The autonomic nervous system and regulation of body temperature. *Anesthesiology*. Jul–Aug 1968; **29**(4): 693–701.
25. Bell DG, Tikuisis P, Jacobs I. Relative intensity of muscular contraction during shivering. *Journal of Applied Physiology (1985)*. Jun 1992; **72**(6): 2336–42.
26. Horn EP, Sessler DI, Standl T, *et al.* Non-thermoregulatory shivering in patients recovering from isoflurane or desflurane anesthesia. *Anesthesiology*. Oct 1998; **89**(4): 878–86.
27. Horn EP, Schroeder F, Wilhelm S, *et al.* Postoperative pain facilitates nonthermoregulatory tremor. *Anesthesiology*. Oct 1999; **91**(4): 979–84.
28. Fritz HG, Holzmayr M, Walter B, *et al.* The effect of mild hypothermia on plasma fentanyl concentration and biotransformation in juvenile pigs. *Anesthesia and Analgesia*. Apr 2005; **100**(4): 996–1002.
29. Caldwell JE, Heier T, Wright PM, *et al.* Temperature-dependent pharmacokinetics and pharmacodynamics of vecuronium. *Anesthesiology*. Jan 2000; **92**(1): 84–93.
30. Heier T, Clough D, Wright PM, *et al.* The influence of mild hypothermia on the pharmacokinetics and time course of action of neostigmine in anesthetized volunteers. *Anesthesiology*. Jul 2002; **97**(1): 90–5.
31. Smeulers NJ, Wierda JM, van den Broek L, Gallandat Huet RC, Hennis PJ. Effects of hypothermic cardiopulmonary bypass on the pharmacodynamics and pharmacokinetics of rocuronium. *Journal of Cardiothoracic and Vascular Anesthesia*. Dec 1995; **9**(6): 700–5.
32. Schmied H, Kurz A, Sessler DI, Kozek S, Reiter A. Mild hypothermia increases blood loss and transfusion requirements during total hip arthroplasty. *Lancet*. Feb 3 1996; **347**(8997): 289–92.
33. Rajagopalan S, Mascha E, Na J, Sessler DI. The effects of mild perioperative hypothermia on blood loss and transfusion requirement. *Anesthesiology*. Jan 2008; **108**(1): 71–7.
34. Greif R, Akca O, Horn EP, *et al.* Supplemental perioperative oxygen to reduce the incidence of surgical-wound infection. *New England Journal of Medicine*. Jan 20 2000; **342**(3): 161–7.
35. Kurz A, Sessler DI, Lenhardt R. Perioperative normothermia to reduce the incidence of surgical-wound infection and shorten hospitalization. Study of Wound Infection and Temperature Group. *New England Journal of Medicine*. May 9 1996; **334**(19): 1209–15.
36. Liu M, Hu X, Liu J. The effect of hypothermia on isoflurane MAC in children. *Anesthesiology*. Mar 2001; **94**(3): 429–32.
37. Antognini JF, Lewis BK, Reitan JA. Hypothermia minimally decreases nitrous oxide anesthetic requirements. *Anesthesia and Analgesia*. Nov 1994; **79**(5): 980–2.
38. Bissonnette B, Sessler DI. Mild hypothermia does not impair postanesthetic recovery in infants and children. *Anesthesia and Analgesia*. Jan 1993; **76**(1): 168–72.
39. Lopez M, Ozaki M, Sessler DI, Valdes M. Physiologic responses to hyperthermia during epidural anesthesia and combined epidural/enflurane anesthesia in women. *Anesthesiology*. Jun 1993; **78**(6): 1046–54.
40. Matsukawa T, Sessler DI, Sessler AM, *et al.* Heat flow and distribution during induction of general anesthesia. *Anesthesiology*. Mar 1995; **82**(3): 662–73.
41. Bennett LA, Johnson JM, Stephens DP, Saad AR, Kellogg DL, Jr. Evidence for a role for vasoactive intestinal peptide in active vasodilatation in the cutaneous vasculature of humans. *The Journal of Physiology*. Oct 1 2003; **552**(Pt 1): 223–32.
42. Wilkins BW, Chung LH, Tublitz NJ, Wong BJ, Minson CT. Mechanisms of vasoactive intestinal peptide-mediated vasodilation in human skin. *Journal of Applied Physiology (1985)*. Oct 2004; **97**(4): 1291–8.
43. Viale JP, Annat G, Bertrand O, *et al.* Continuous measurement of pulmonary gas exchange during general anaesthesia in man. *Acta Anaesthesiologica Scandinavica*. Nov 1988; **32**(8): 691–7.
44. Hynson JM, Sessler DI, Glosten B, McGuire J. Thermal balance and tremor patterns during epidural anesthesia. *Anesthesiology*. Apr 1991; **74**(4): 680–90.
45. Kurz A. Physiology of thermoregulation. Best practice and research. *Clinical Anaesthesiology*. Dec 2008; **22**(4): 627–44.
46. Sessler DI. Perioperative heat balance. *Anesthesiology*. Feb 2000; **92**(2): 578–96.
47. Bissonnette B. Thermoregulation and paediatric anaesthesia. *Current Opinion in Anaesthesiology*. 1993; **6**: 537–42.
48. Kurz A, Xiong J, Sessler DI, *et al.* Desflurane reduces the gain of thermoregulatory arteriovenous shunt vasoconstriction in humans. *Anesthesiology*. Dec 1995; **83**(6): 1212–19.
49. Cheung SS, Mekjavic IB. Human temperature regulation during subanesthetic levels of nitrous

oxide-induced narcosis. *Journal of Applied Physiology (1985)*. Jun 1995; **78**(6): 2301–8.

50. Kurz A, Go JC, Sessler DI, *et al.* Alfentanil slightly increases the sweating threshold and markedly reduces the vasoconstriction and shivering thresholds. *Anesthesiology*. Aug 1995; **83**(2): 293–9.
51. Ikeda T, Kurz A, Sessler DI, *et al.* The effect of opioids on thermoregulatory responses in humans and the special antishivering action of meperidine. *Annals of the New York Academy of Sciences*. Mar 15 1997; **813**: 792–8.
52. Kurz A, Sessler DI, Annadata R, *et al.* Midazolam minimally impairs thermoregulatory control. *Anesthesia and Analgesia*. Aug 1995; **81**(2): 393–8.
53. Leslie K, Sessler DI, Bjorksten AR, *et al.* Propofol causes a dose-dependent decrease in the thermoregulatory threshold for vasoconstriction but has little effect on sweating. *Anesthesiology*. Aug 1994; **81**(2): 353–60.
54. Talke P, Tayefeh F, Sessler DI, *et al.* Dexmedetomidine does not alter the sweating threshold, but comparably and linearly decreases the vasoconstriction and shivering thresholds. *Anesthesiology*. Oct 1997; **87**(4): 835–41.
55. Easley RB, Tobias JD. Pro: dexmedetomidine should be used for infants and children undergoing cardiac surgery. *Journal of Cardiothoracic and Vascular Anesthesia*. Feb 2008; **22**(1): 147–51.
56. Fraser JG. Iatrogenic benign hyperthermia in children. *Anesthesiology*. May 1978; **48**(5): 375.
57. Matsukawa T, Sessler DI, Christensen R, Ozaki M, Schroeder M. Heat flow and distribution during epidural anesthesia. *Anesthesiology*. Nov 1995; **83**(5): 961–7.
58. Ozaki M, Kurz A, Sessler DI, *et al.* Thermoregulatory thresholds during epidural and spinal anesthesia. *Anesthesiology*. Aug 1994; **81**(2): 282–8.
59. Leslie K, Sessler DI. Reduction in the shivering threshold is proportional to spinal block height. *Anesthesiology*. Jun 1996; **84**(6): 1327–31.
60. Frank SM, El-Rahmany HK, Cattaneo CG, Barnes RA. Predictors of hypothermia during spinal anesthesia. *Anesthesiology*. May 2000; **92**(5): 1330–4.
61. Bissonnette B, Sessler DI. Thermoregulatory thresholds for vasoconstriction in pediatric patients anesthetized with halothane or halothane and caudal bupivacaine. *Anesthesiology*. Mar 1992; **76**(3): 387–92.
62. Cork RC, Vaughan RW, Humphrey LS. Precision and accuracy of intraoperative temperature monitoring. *Anesthesia and Analgesia*. Feb 1983; **62**(2): 211–14.

Index